ADOLESCENT HEALTH

Understanding and Preventing Risk Behaviors

RALPH J. DICLEMENTE
JOHN S. SANTELLI
RICHARD A. CROSBY
EDITORS

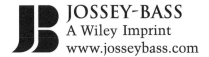

JOSSEY-BASS
A Wiley Imprint
www.josseybass.com

Published by Jossey-Bass
A Wiley Imprint
989 Market Street, San Francisco, CA 94103-1741—www.josseybass.com

Jossey-Bass books and products are available through most bookstores. To contact Jossey-Bass directly call our Customer Care Department within the U.S. at 800-956-7739, outside the U.S. at 317-572-3986, or fax 317-572-4002.

Jossey-Bass also publishes its books in a variety of electronic formats. Some content that appears in print may not be available in electronic books.

Library of Congress Cataloging-in-publication data has been applied for.

ISBN 13: 978-0-4701-7676-4
ISBN 10: 0-4701-7676-8

Printed in the United States of America
FIRST EDITION

PB Printing　　　10 9 8 7 6 5 4 3 2 1

CONTENTS

PART ONE: FOUNDATIONS AND THEORY IN ADOLESCENT HEALTH RISK BEHAVIOR

PART TWO: PREVENTING KEY HEALTH RISK BEHAVIORS

PART THREE: POPULATIONS, POLICY, AND PREVENTION STRATEGIES

FIGURES, TABLES, AND EXHIBITS

FIGURES

TABLES

EXHIBIT

RJD

To Sahara Rae—the brightest light in my universe, the axis on which my world revolves, and the center of my heart—with all my love. To my lovely, talented, and supportive wife—a partner in so many ways. To my wonderful family for being understanding and accepting.

JSS

To Jennifer, Isaac, and Jacob, who make life worthwhile, who keep me honest, and who tolerate my solitary scholarly propensities.

RAC

To my family and my colleagues—all of whom make life exciting, rewarding, and bring simple pleasures to life as a scholar.

FOREWORD

Practitioners and researchers interested in youth development and health promotion will find *Adolescent Health: Understanding and Preventing Risk Behaviors* an excellent source for informing their work. This volume serves as a textbook for graduate students in public health, medicine, social work, nursing, and other behavioral sciences. Knowledge about adolescent health issues should also be incorporated into schools of education so that future educators are informed about the need for collaborative interventions.

I wish that I could invite all the contributors to *Adolescent Health* to sit around in my living room, where we could chat informally about teenagers. The gathering would include most of the "gurus" of youth development who have labored for years to track the prevalence of problems and the outcomes of interventions. I think there would be a strong consensus that we have accumulated a large body of evidence that many young people growing up in this country face enormous barriers to maturing into successful adults. We would agree that other young people have the necessary equipment (support systems, fortitude, and resilience) to make it, as long as their institutions (family, school, community, and the media) don't fail them.

We would concur that this volume contains most of what practitioners need to know in order to help adolescents overcome developmental barriers and achieve healthy lifestyles. Risk areas (such as substance abuse, violence, pregnancy, and depression) are explored in depth and the interrelationships between them clarified. Areas of resiliency (youth assets and connectedness) are investigated and illuminated. From this rich source of research findings, we would conclude that young people must be attached to strong adults—if not their parents, then some other person. We would focus on the fact that children must receive attention early enough in their lives to prevent later problems and that they must have access to the requisite social skills to relate to their peers.

In addition to interventions focused on individuals, we would pay attention to the development of comprehensive community-level programs that link together what goes on in the schools with other interventions. Some of the participants in this discussion would be making the case for more refined "theories of change," while others would argue in favor of more research and evaluation. A strong rationale would be given for changing social policies—gun control, driving regulations, condom distribution, racial desegregation, and school reform. These subjects would generate plenty of steam.

I would not be surprised if the conversation in my living room eventually turned from research and policy to personal experiences with raising children. It is quite a shock when your own children start "acting out," experimenting with drugs and sex, skipping school, or downloading forbidden material from the Internet. I am currently dealing with my grandchildren's developmental issues—they are two beautiful young women, aged thirteen and fifteen. When their parents turned to me for advice, assuming that I was an authority on adolescent behavior, I replied (sheepishly), "I think you have to be stricter or more lenient." I am certain that the gurus gathered here would confirm that it is more difficult to solve one's personal problems with raising children and preventing risky behavior than to prescribe broad social measures.

I have observed, however, that my grandchildren receive almost unlimited attention from their parents: listening, shopping, driving, cajoling, monitoring, cooking special dishes, helping with math homework, and, most important, hugging. If the essence of this attention could be bottled and sold, many of the problem behaviors so clearly documented in this book might be averted.

Practitioners, researchers, students, and parents should find the material in *Adolescent Health* indispensable for gaining an understanding of the complex lives of teenagers today. Most of these authorities claim that more research is needed to complete the picture, particularly on intervention outcomes. However, as readers will observe, enough is known to focus on intervention. Our society owes each new generation the opportunity to grow into effective and healthy adults. The need today is urgent.

Joy G. Dryfoos

ACKNOWLEDGMENTS

We wish to acknowledge all our wonderful and talented contributors for their time, effort, and dedication. Their research, practice, and advocacy make life better for all adolescents. We thank Andrew Pasternack, our editor, for his encouragement, steadfast support, and valuable feedback; Seth Schwartz, whose acumen and assistance have been instrumental to creating this volume; and Seth Miller, for his diligence in producing it.

PREFACE

The primary aim of this volume is to inform health care professionals about adolescent risk-taking behavior; its epidemiology, consequences, prevention and treatment. Our book is intended as both a professional reference and classroom text. It takes a multi-faceted approach that includes an epidemiologic assessment of the impact of health risk behaviors, a synthesis of the empirical literature describing factors associated with the onset and maintenance of health risk behaviors, a description of relevant intervention strategies and programs designed to prevent or reduce health risk behaviors, and an examination of social and health policy issues relevant to each health risk behavior. Acknowledging that behavior does not occur in a political or social vacuum, the policy perspective is designed to provide a frame of reference for understanding the scope of the problem posed by specific health risk behaviors and the parameters and options available to effectively confront these adolescent health threats. Authors describe trends and changes in risk behaviors, morbidity and mortality over time; illustrate theoretical models useful for understanding adolescent risk-taking behavior and developing preventive interventions; review the state-of-the-science with respect to prevention strategies for each risk behavior; and identify effective treatment modalities. Special populations at risk and emergent crosscutting issues in risk and prevention research are also presented. Finally, each chapter provides an opportunity for the authors to offer directions for future research relevant to specific health risk behaviors. In each case, we have sought out the leading experts to contribute these chapters. We are humbled and grateful to benefit from their scientific acumen, their wealth of experience, and wise insights.

THE CONTRIBUTORS

Richard A. Crosby, PhD, DDI Endowed Professor and chair, Department of Health Behavior, College of Public Health at the University of Kentucky

Ralph J. DiClemente, PhD, Charles Howard Candler Professor, Rollins School of Public Health; professor, School of Medicine, Department of Pediatrics, Division of Infectious Diseases, Epidemiology, and Immunology, Emory University; associate director, Center for AIDS Research

John S. Santelli, MD, MPH, Harriet and Robert H. Heilbrunn Professor of clinical pediatrics and clinical population and family health; chairman, Heilbrunn Department of Population and Family Health, Mailman School of Public Health, Columbia University

Mona Abo-Zena, EdM, doctoral research assistant, Institute for Applied Research in Youth Development, Tufts University

David G. Altman, PhD, executive vice president, Research, Innovation, and Product Development, Center for Creative Leadership, Greensboro, North Carolina

Michael F. Ballesteros, PhD, deputy associate director of science, Division of Unintentional Injury Prevention, National Center for Injury Prevention and Control, Centers for Disease Control and Prevention

Neda Bebiroglu, MA, doctoral research assistant, Institute for Applied Research in Youth Development, Tufts University

Debra H. Bernat, PhD, clinical associate professor, School of Nursing, University of Minnesota

Lynne Michael Blum, MS, PhD, scientist, Johns Hopkins Bloomberg School of Public Health; president, Connected Kids, Baltimore, Maryland

Robert Wm. Blum, MD, MPH, PhD, William H. Gates Sr. Professor and chair, Department of Population, Family and Reproductive Health; director, Johns Hopkins Urban Health Institute, Johns Hopkins Bloomberg School of Public Health

Debra Braun-Courville, MD, assistant professor, Department of Pediatrics, Mount Sinai School of Medicine, Mount Sinai Adolescent Health Center

Aerika Brittian, MA, doctoral research assistant, Institute for Applied Research in Youth Development, Tufts University

Crystal A. Caudill, MPH, public health director, Wedco District Health Department

Heather Champion, PhD, enterprise associate, Center for Creative Leadership, Greensboro, North Carolina

Richard R. Clayton, PhD, professor and Good Samaritan Foundation Chair in Health Behavior; associate dean for research, College of Public Health, University of Kentucky

Susan L. Davies, PhD, associate professor, Department of Health Behavior, University of Alabama at Birmingham School of Public Health

Angela Diaz, MD, MPH, professor, Department of Pediatrics and Community and Preventive Medicine, Mount Sinai School of Medicine; director, Mount Sinai Adolescent Health Center

Geri R. Donenberg, PhD, professor and director, Healthy Youths Program, Institute for Juvenile Research, University of Illinois at Chicago

Julie S. Downs, PhD, assistant research professor, Department of Social and Decision Science, Carnegie Mellon University

Abigail English, JD, director, Center for Adolescent Health & the Law

Baruch Fischhoff, PhD, Howard Heinz University Professor, Department of Social and Decision Science and Department of Engineering and Public Policy, Carnegie Mellon University

Nicholas Freudenberg, DrPH, distinguished professor of public health, Hunter College, and Graduate Center, City University of New York

Quetzalcoatl Hernandez-Cervantes, PhD, assistant professor, School of Public Health, Michoacan, Mexico

Marjorie J. Hogan, MD, associate professor, Department of Pediatrics, University of Minnesota School of Medicine, Hennepin County Medical Center

Darrell Hudson, MPH, graduate research assistant, Department of Health Behavior and Health Education, University of Michigan School of Public Health

Charles E. Irwin Jr., MD, professor and vice chairman of pediatrics; director, Division of Adolescent Medicine, Department of Pediatrics, University of California, San Francisco

Sonia Isaac, MA, doctoral research assistant, Institute for Applied Research in Youth Development, Tufts University

Natalie C. Kaiser, MA, research associate, Department of Psychology, Loma Linda University

Chisina Kapungu, PhD, Prevention Research Postdoctoral Fellow, Institute for Health Research and Policy, University of Illinois at Chicago

Douglas Kirby, PhD, senior research scientist, ETR Associates, Inc., Scotts Valley, California

Sarah E. Kretman, MPH, MEd, Community health specialist, Regional Center For Healthy Communities–Metrowest, Cambridge, MA.

Richard M. Lerner, PhD, director, Institute for Applied Research in Youth Development, Tufts University

Stefanie Limberger, MEd, LPC, Institute for Juvenile Research, University of Illinois at Chicago

Alicia Doyle Lynch, MA, doctoral research assistant, Institute for Applied Research in Youth Development, Tufts University

Susan Morrel-Samuels, MA, MPH, managing director, Prevention Research Center of Michigan, Department of Health Behavior and Health Education, University of Michigan School of Public Health

Anne Nucci-Sack, MD, assistant professor, Department of Pediatrics, Mount Sinai School of Medicine; medical director, Mount Sinai Adolescent Health Center

Jason E. Owen, PhD, MPH, assistant professor, Department of Psychology, Loma Linda University

M. Jane Park, MPH, policy research director, Division of Adolescent Medicine, Department of Pediatrics, University of California, San Francisco

Mary Ann Pentz, PhD, director, Institute for Prevention Research; professor, Department of Preventive Medicine, Keck School of Medicine, University of Southern California

Michael D. Resnick, PhD, professor and Gisela and E. Paul Konopka Chair in Adolescent Health and Development; director, Healthy Youth Development—Prevention Research Center, Division of Adolescent Health and Medicine, Department of Pediatrics, University of Minnesota

Frederick P. Rivara, MD, MPH, Seattle Children's Hospital Guild Endowed Chair in Pediatrics, vice chair and professor, Department of Pediatrics, University of Washington

Audrey Smith Rogers, PhD, former staff epidemiologist, National Institute of Child Health and Development, National Institutes of Health

Mary Rojas, PhD, associate professor, Department of Pediatrics and Health Policy, Mount Sinai School of Medicine; director of research, Mount Sinai Adolescent Health Center

Laura F. Salazar, PhD, assistant professor, Rollins School of Public Health, Emory University

Jessica M. Sales, PhD, assistant professor, Rollins School of Public Health, Emory University

Melissa J. H. Segress, MS, managing director, Training Resource Center, College of Social Work, University of Kentucky

Elizabeth A. Shirtcliff, PhD, assistant professor, Department of Psychology, University of New Orleans.

Lydia A. Shrier, MD, MPH, director of clinic-based research, Division of Adolescent/ Young Adult Medicine, Children's Hospital Boston; assistant professor of pediatrics, Harvard Medical School

Renee E. Sieving, PhD, RN, associate professor, School of Nursing and Department of Pediatrics; Deputy Director, Healthy Youth Development—Prevention Research Center, University of Minnesota

David A. Sleet, PhD, FAAHB, associate director for science, Division of Unintentional Injury Prevention, National Center for Injury Prevention and Control, Centers for Disease Control and Prevention

Anthony Spirito, PhD, professor of psychiatry and human behavior, Center for Alcohol and Addiction Studies, Alpert Medical School of Brown University

Victor C. Strasburger, MD, professor of pediatrics and family and community medicine; chief, Division of Adolescent Medicine, Department of Pediatrics, University of New Mexico School of Medicine

Erin L. Sutfin, PhD, research assistant professor, Department of Social Sciences and Health Policy, Wake Forest University School of Medicine

Charu Thakral, PhD, instructor, University of Illinois at Chicago

Michael Windle, PhD, Rollins professor and chair, Department of Behavioral Sciences and Health Education, Rollins School of Public Health, Emory University

Rebecca C. Windle, MSW, senior associate, Department of Behavioral Sciences and Health Education, Rollins School of Public Health, Emory University

Andrew J. Winzelberg, PhD, research scientist, Department of Psychiatry and Behavioral Sciences, Stanford University

Marc A. Zimmerman, PhD, professor and chair, Department of Health Behavior and Health Education, University of Michigan School of Public Health

ADOLESCENT HEALTH

PART

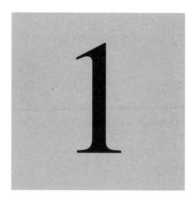

FOUNDATIONS AND THEORY IN ADOLESCENT HEALTH RISK BEHAVIOR

CHAPTER

1

ADOLESCENTS AT RISK: A GENERATION IN JEOPARDY

RICHARD A. CROSBY ▪ JOHN S. SANTELLI ▪ RALPH J. DICLEMENTE

LEARNING OBJECTIVES

After studying this chapter, you will be able to

- Identify key features of the adolescent period.
- Describe underlying factors that may influence adolescent risk taking behavior.

Adolescence is a period of rapid and transformative physical, psychological, sociocultural, and cognitive development. The physical changes of puberty—including growth and maturation of multiple organ systems such as the reproductive organs and brain—lay a biological foundation for the other developmental changes. The adolescent brain is rewired, with resulting maturation of cognitive abilities in early adolescence. When these new cognitive abilities are combined with life experiences, we often observe development of social judgment, including judgment about risk and safety. Adolescence is also marked by critical transformation in the relationship of a young person to the world, as the social circles of peers and the adult worlds of work, pleasure, and social responsibility become more central and the family circle becomes somewhat less prominent—at least temporarily. Adolescents must learn to deal with an expanding social universe and must develop the social skills to find friendship, romance, employment, and social standing within multiple social spheres. Finally, a critical task of adolescence is the establishment of a stable sense of identity and the development of autonomy or agency. This development of identity often occurs only after a period of exploration, of trial and error in social roles and social behaviors. Although most adolescents navigate the often turbulent course from childhood to adulthood to become healthy adults and productive citizens, many fail to do so. Too many fall prey to social and behavior morbidities and mortality, and many fail to achieve their full potential as workers, parents, and individuals. Many suffer substantial short-term impairment and disability, and for many this impairment extends into adulthood. Many of these failures of adolescent development are the result of preventable health risk behaviors.

Adolescence is marked by increasing involvement in health risk behaviors. Between the ages of twelve and twenty-five, we observe the initiation of myriad health risk behaviors, including alcohol and drug use, smoking, sexual behaviors, delinquency, and behaviors leading to intentional and unintentional injuries—all of which can adversely influence health in the short and long term. For example, alcohol and drug use are the proximate causes of unintentional injuries during adolescence; they also can lead to adult addiction and social and health impairment. Sexual behaviors often result in unplanned pregnancy and sexually transmitted diseases, including HIV infection. These adolescent risk behaviors may profoundly influence health in adulthood.

Paradoxically, the rise in health behavior–related morbidities is the result of public health success in controlling and eliminating infectious diseases. As the result of advances in medical and public health understanding and technologies such as clean water, sanitation, and vaccines, enormous progress was made throughout the nineteenth and twentieth centuries in controlling these traditional causes of morbidity and mortality. Today adolescents in the developed world are primarily at risk from diseases that originate from behavioral and social circumstances. For example, a teen in the United States is much more likely to die from handgun violence or a motor vehicle injury than polio or whooping cough.

How can we explain this explosion of risk taking within each new cohort of adolescents? Multiple explanations have been suggested, most of which are explored in this volume. From an evolutionary viewpoint, risk taking may have had important survival value, with inquisitive young humans exploring new lands and willing to develop new ways of surviving in hostile environments. As such, developmental psychology often discusses risk taking as normal adolescent exploration that is an important part of the learning process of a young person.

Social and cultural factors including family instability, poverty, and racism also seem to drive adolescent risk-taking behaviors. While these responses may seem maladaptive from a societal viewpoint, they can also be seen as adaptive responses to unsupportive circumstances. Risk taking may also exist simply as part of the adolescent's new identification with peers and the desire to attain adult status. Recent attempts to understand adolescent resiliency and the positive health impact of school and community connectedness can be seen as reciprocal processes: adolescents with greater social capital or with greater identification with society's benefits and values may be more likely to eschew risk behaviors. Finally, these processes of risk taking can be understood at the level of brain chemistry, at the level of individual autonomic responses, and even as social processes that support risk taking.

Today preserving health is a function of understanding and altering the risk behavior of entire populations. This realization is vital because it suggests that population-based strategies to improve public health must begin early, before risk behaviors become ingrained habits. The implication, then, is that adolescents should be the primary foci of health promotion efforts. To understand the rich potential to affect public health through intervention with adolescents, consider just a few examples.

The current epidemics of obesity and diabetes in the United States are an outgrowth of sedentary behaviors combined with the overconsumption of high-calorie or empty-calorie food products (such as soda, chips, burgers, and fries). Similarly, the epidemic of hypertension in the United States is being addressed by changing the dietary and exercise behaviors of adolescents before they develop essential hypertension. Clearly, the public health battle to prevent cancer involves the prevention of tobacco use above and beyond any other single risk factor. Given the strong addictive properties of nicotine, it becomes clear that prevention efforts aimed at nonsmokers or new smokers are highly likely to serve public health; thus, once again adolescents become the critical population.

DISCUSSION QUESTIONS

1. What biological and physiological changes occur during adolescence? How does the sociocultural environment interact with these changes to affect the development of individual identity and later risk-taking behavior?

2. Discuss reasons why preventive interventions should focus on adolescents as a means to preserve health and alter risk.

CHAPTER

2

TRENDS IN ADOLESCENT AND YOUNG ADULT MORBIDITY AND MORTALITY

FREDERICK P. RIVARA ▪ M. JANE PARK ▪ CHARLES E. IRWIN JR.

LEARNING OBJECTIVES

After studying this chapter, you will be able to

- Explain the trends in morbidity and mortality among adolescents and young adults over the last twenty-five years.

- Discuss how high-risk adolescent behavior can affect health outcomes in adulthood.

- Recognize that adolescents and young adults are not a homogeneous group; rather, they are part of larger subgroups with diverse risk profiles.

It is important to consider both early adolescents and young adults along with the middle adolescent ages of fourteen through eighteen when discussing the health of this population.

Adolescence is an age of transition between childhood and adulthood. During this critical time, health habits and behaviors are established that affect health not only during adolescence but throughout the lifespan. Viewed in this context, the health and health care of adolescents take on even greater importance and much greater urgency.

In this chapter, we have chosen to define *adolescence and young adulthood* as encompassing the ages of ten through twenty-four years. This range includes early adolescents, ages ten through thirteen, who are making the transition from childhood into adolescence, as well as individuals ages nineteen through twenty-four, who are making the transition into adulthood. Given the economic, social, educational, and cultural changes in the United States over the last few decades, it is important to consider both early adolescents and young adults along with the middle adolescent ages of fourteen through eighteen when discussing the health of this population.

POPULATION CHARACTERISTICS

The 63 million adolescents and young adults ages ten through twenty-four in the United States accounted for about 21 percent of the population in the country in 2006 (Centers for Disease Control and Prevention [CDC], 2007a). Approximately 60 percent of this population is non-Hispanic white, 15 percent non-Hispanic African American, 4 percent Asian or Pacific Islander, and 1 percent American Indian or Alaskan Native. Eleven million adolescents and young adults, or 17 percent, reported their ethnicity as Hispanic or Latino.

Since 1990, the Hispanic population of adolescents and young adults has increased by 92 percent, while the African American population in this age group has increased by 25 percent and the non-Hispanic white population has increased by only 2.7 percent (see Figure 2.1). Hispanics are thus the largest minority group of adolescents and young adults in the United States.

The United States continues to be a country of immigrants. In 1990, 19 percent of adolescents less than twenty years of age lived in immigrant families. This increased to 22 percent by 2004 (U.S. Census Bureau, 2004). In 2006, there were 10.2 million adolescents and young adults (16.4 percent) who were living in poverty, accounting for 27.7 percent of all people in poverty in the United States (U.S. Census Bureau, 2007). There were an additional 12.5 million who were living at incomes between 100 and 200 percent of the poverty level. Over 12.5 million adolescents and young adults— or one in five—were uninsured in 2007, accounting for 26.6 percent of the 47 million uninsured people in this country.

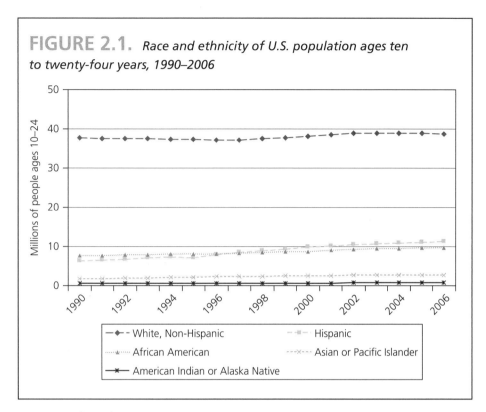

FIGURE 2.1. *Race and ethnicity of U.S. population ages ten to twenty-four years, 1990–2006*

Source: CDC (2007a).

MORTALITY

Overall mortality among individuals 10 through 24 years has decreased over the last twenty-five years (1980 to 2004), as shown in Figure 2.2. Mortality has fallen from 30.8 per 100,000 to 18.7 among 10- to 14-year-olds, from 97.9 to 66.1 among 15- to 19-year-olds, and 132.7 to 94.0 among 20- to 24-year-olds (CDC, 2007b). However, during this twenty-five-year period, the decline has not been constant for all age groups. Death rates among 15- to 19-year-olds increased by 10 percent between 1985 and 1991, and by 4.7 percent among 20- to 24-year-olds between 1985 and 1988, and again by 6.2 percent between 1999 and 2003. This trend is remarkable because these are the only age groups in the United States for whom mortality rates actually increased during this period. To better understand these trends in mortality, it is necessary to disaggregate the data and examine etiologic groups.

Mortality from Natural Causes

Mortality from cancer has decreased steadily among all three adolescent age groups over the last twenty-five years (see Figure 2.3). Cancer deaths dropped by 40.5 percent

Death rates among 15- to 19-year-olds increased by 10 percent between 1985 and 1991, and by 4.7 percent among 20- to 24-year-olds between 1985 and 1988, and again by 6.2 percent between 1999 and 2003.

among 10- to 14-year-olds, 33.3 percent among 15- to 19-year-olds, and 34.7 percent among 20- to 24-year-olds. Deaths from cardiac disease showed similar large declines, of 28.6 percent, 31.3 percent, and 18.9 percent in the three age groups, respectively. Respiratory disease–related death showed little progress among the 10- to 14-year-olds, but declined by approximately 25 percent in the two older age groups. Deaths from infectious causes were stable among the two younger cohorts, but actually increased by 60 percent (from 1.0 to 1.6) among 20- to 24-year-olds. This increase is due to deaths related to HIV infection, which accounted for 30,243 deaths among 20- to 24-year-olds from the beginning of the epidemic to 2002.

Mortality from Injuries

Injury—specifically unintentional injury, homicide, and suicide—accounts for almost three-quarters of all mortality in this age group. Overall injury mortality has declined substantially among people this age over the twenty-five-year period, although the aggregate data hide some important subgroup differences described below. Injury deaths decreased by 44.7 percent, 34.4 percent, and 32.3 percent among 10- to 14-,

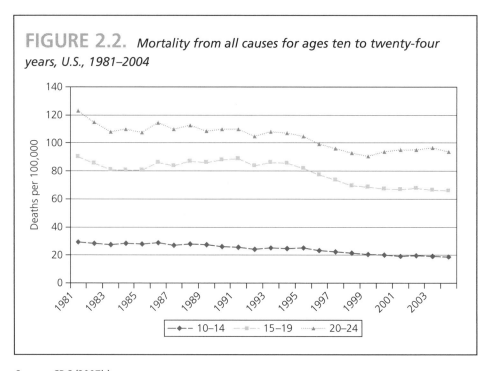

FIGURE 2.2. *Mortality from all causes for ages ten to twenty-four years, U.S., 1981–2004*

Source: CDC (2007b).

15- to 19-, and 20- to 24-year-olds, respectively. Aggregate data also hide the considerable gender differences in mortality. Males have higher mortality rates than females, across these three age groups and for all three causes of injury mortality. For ages 10 through 24, the gap is highest for homicide, with males at a rate more than five times that of females. For unintentional injury mortality, males have just under five times the rate of females; for suicide, this ratio is 2.5.

Unintentional Injuries Mortality due to unintentional injuries declined steadily over the last twenty-five years in all three age groups: 53.0 percent among 10- to 14-year-olds, 44.4 percent among 15- to 19-year-olds, and 39.6 percent among 20- to 24-year-olds (see Figure 2.4). The largest single cause of adolescent and young adult mortality is motor vehicle crashes. There have been substantial and similar decreases in death rates from motor vehicle crashes across all three age groups: 40.9 percent decrease among 10- to 14-year-olds, 41.2 percent among 15- to 19-year-olds, and 40.7 percent among 20- to 24-year-olds. Motor vehicle crash rates peak for ages 20 through 24 and then decrease throughout the life span until age 70, when they peak again.

Deaths related to HIV infection, which accounted for 30,243 deaths among 20- to 24-year-olds from the beginning of the epidemic to 2002.

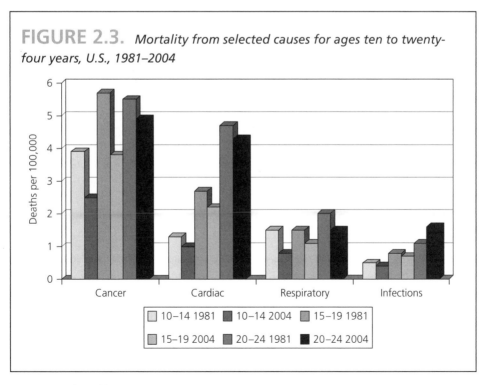

FIGURE 2.3. *Mortality from selected causes for ages ten to twenty-four years, U.S., 1981–2004*

Source: CDC (2007b).

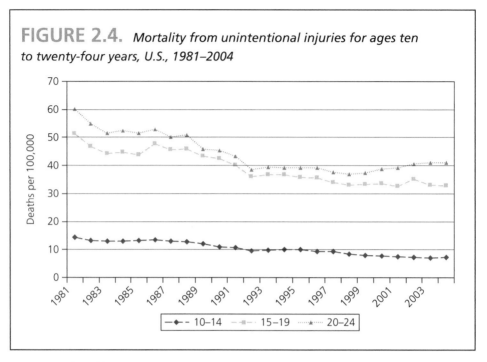

FIGURE 2.4. *Mortality from unintentional injuries for ages ten to twenty-four years, U.S., 1981–2004*

Source: CDC (2007b).

Homicide Homicide rates demonstrated the largest fluctuation among all causes of deaths for adolescents over the last twenty-five years (see Figure 2.5). In all three age groups, homicide death rates were lower at the end of the period than at the beginning. All three age groups, however, had increases in the homicide rates during the late 1980s and early 1990s, peaking in 1993 and then declining to levels last seen in the 1960s through 1970s. Nearly all of this increase was due to homicides involving guns. Although the causes of this increase (and subsequent decrease) are complex, the sudden appearance of crack cocaine on the East and West Coasts and then spreading inland played a large role (Blumstein, Rivara, & Rosenfeld, 2000).

Suicide Trends in suicide deaths among adolescents and young adults are complex (Figure 2.6). Suicide increased among 10- to 14-year-olds from 0.8 deaths per 100,000 in 1980 to 1.34 in 2004. However, during that twenty-five-year period suicides increased in this group of young adolescents to a peak of 1.72 per 100,000 in 1995 before slowly dropping to their current levels. This represents a 115 percent increase from the rate in 1980. Suicide rates among 15- to 19-year-olds were lower in 2004 than in 1980. Again, however, this masks a 34 percent increase during the 1980s. Only among 20- to 24-year-olds was there a slow, steady decline in suicide deaths by an average of 1 percent per year over this twenty-five-year period.

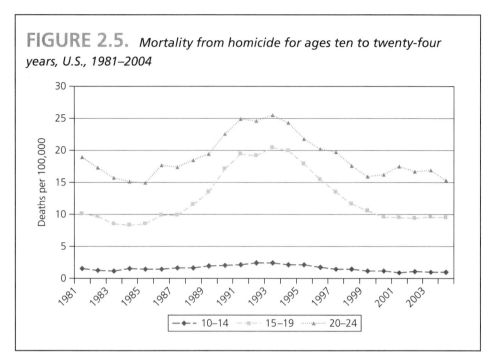

FIGURE 2.5. *Mortality from homicide for ages ten to twenty-four years, U.S., 1981–2004*

Source: CDC (2007b).

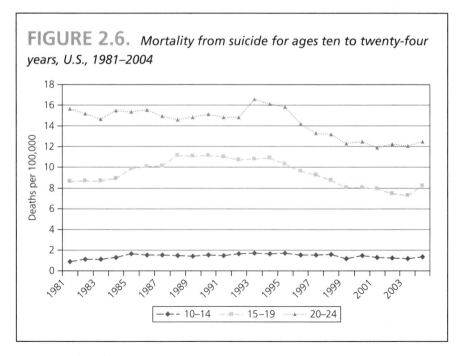

FIGURE 2.6. *Mortality from suicide for ages ten to twenty-four years, U.S., 1981–2004*

Source: CDC (2007b).

Unfortunately, suicide rates among 10- to 24-year-olds have risen recently by 8 percent in 2003–2004 (CDC, 2007c). This overall increase was due to a rise in suicide among 10- to 19-year-old females and 15- to 19-year-old males. Although firearms remain the most common method of suicide for ages 10 through 24, hanging and suffocation have become more common among all suicides in this age group and now represent the most common method for completed suicides among females.

HIGH-RISK BEHAVIORS AS UNDERLYING CAUSES OF DEATH

By traditional markers such as rates of mortality, chronic disease, and hospitalization, adolescents and young adults are healthy. Most health problems in this age group stem from high-risk behaviors that jeopardize health. Moreover, these behaviors also have implications for health outcomes in the long term, including premature death. In 1993, McGinnis and Foege published a seminal paper on the actual causes of death in the United States. This was updated in 2004 by Mokdad et al., who described actual causes of death in 2000 (Mokdad, Marks, Stroup, & Gerberding, 2004). Half of all deaths are due to potentially modifiable factors: tobacco, poor diet and physical inactivity, alcohol consumption, microbial agents, toxic agents, motor vehicle crashes, guns, sexual behavior, and illicit drugs. Most important for both this chapter and the rest of this book is that all these modifiable behaviors also occur in adolescents and young adults, and for some behaviors (such as smoking) the majority begin during adolescence. Some behaviors and negative outcomes—including use of tobacco, alcohol, and illicit drugs and the rate of sexually transmitted infections—peak in the late teens and early twenties.

Half of all deaths are due to potentially modifiable factors: tobacco, poor diet and physical inactivity, alcohol consumption, microbial agents, toxic agents, motor vehicle crashes, guns, sexual behavior, and illicit drugs.

Tobacco Use

An estimated 440,000 people die from smoking-related causes each year in the United States (Mokdad et al., 2004). Nearly all smoking-related deaths occur after the age of 35, but the majority of adults who smoke began during adolescence. Eighty-two percent of adults who smoke started smoking before age 18, and virtually no adult smokers start after the age of 25. Young adults ages 18 to 25 have the highest prevalence of recent smoking—60 percent higher than that of adults over the age of 25 (Substance Abuse and Mental Health Services Administration, 2007).

The trends in any daily use of tobacco in the prior thirty days show a steady decline of use by twelfth graders between 1980 (20.3 percent) and 1992, when daily smoking reached a nadir of 17.2 percent in this age group (see Figure 2.7; Substance Abuse and Mental Health Services Administration, 2007). However, rates subsequently increased to a peak of 24.6 percent in 1997 and have since declined to a low of 12.2 percent

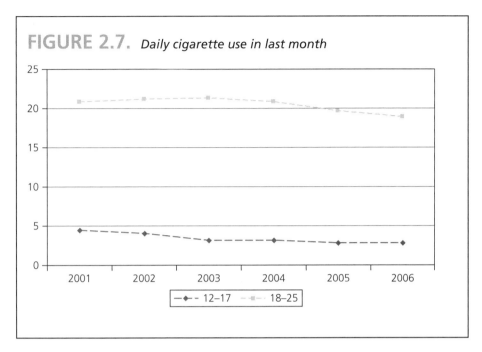

FIGURE 2.7. *Daily cigarette use in last month*

Source: Substance Abuse and Mental Health Services Administration (2007).

in 2006. Among young adults ages 19 through 28, the prevalence of daily smoking in the prior nineteen days decreased between 1986 and 1994, stabilized for a decade, and then decreased again in the last two years to 18.6 percent in 2006. Recent studies suggest that nicotine addiction and symptoms of dependence can begin very soon after the onset of smoking, and they emphasize the dangers of early smoking exposure among youth (Kandel & Chen, 2000; DiFranza, Savageau, Fletcher, O'Loughlin, et al., 2007; DiFranza, Savageau, Fletcher, Pbert, et al., 2007; Rubinstein, Thompson, Benowitz, Shiffman, & Moscicki, 2007).

Prevention of smoking-related deaths is likely to be more successful if undertaken on a population basis to prevent regular smoking initiation than on an individual basis to promote cessation, especially among adolescents. The available evidence indicates that smoking cessation programs for adolescents have some effectiveness, but the effect size is small (about a 3 percent absolute difference in cessation; Sussman, Sun, & Dent, 2006). School-based smoking prevention programs have been popular, but there is little evidence that these programs have long-term effects on prevention of smoking (Wiehe, Garrison, Christakis, Ebel, & Rivara, 2005). In contrast, programs to increase the tax on cigarettes and implement smoking counteradvertising can potentially reduce adolescent smoking by as much as 26 percent (Rivara, Ebel, et al., 2004) and can result in large cost *savings* of between $590,000 and $1.4 million per life saved (Fishman et al., 2005).

Poor Diet and Physical Inactivity

Between the publication of the paper by McGinnis and Foege (1993) and its update by Mokdad and colleagues (2000), overweight and obesity became a dramatically worse problem (Ogden et al., 2006). The changes in weight among adolescents and young adults in the United States as documented in the National Health and Interview Surveys over the last forty years clearly demonstrate this change. In 1966–1970, the mean weight of 12-year-old males was 42.9 kg and 46.6 kg for females this age. In 1999–2002, this had increased by 16.6 percent to 50.4 kg for males and by 11.6 percent to 52.0 kg for females (Ogden, Fryar, Carroll, & Flegal, 2004). Among 19-year-olds, mean weight increased by 7.7 percent among males and 14.1 percent among females between the 1971–1974 survey and the 1999–2002 survey. There were substantial changes in the weights of 20- to 29-year-olds as well; mean weight in males increased by 12.0 percent and among females by 18.4 percent between 1960–1962 and 1999–2002.

The CDC has defined *overweight* as a body mass index (BMI) of 95 percent or higher for age and gender. The proportion of adolescents ages 12 through 19 who were overweight has nearly tripled, from 6.1 percent in 1971–1974 to 17.4 percent in 2002–2004 (see Figure 2.8). This trend in overweight has not been uniform across ethnic and

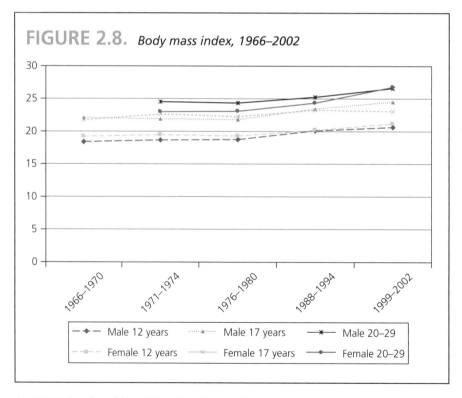

FIGURE 2.8. *Body mass index, 1966–2002*

Legend: — ◆ — Male 12 years   · · · ▲ · · · Male 17 years   — ✳ — Male 20–29
— ■ — Female 12 years   — ✕ — Female 17 years   — ● — Female 20–29

Source: National Health and Nutrition Examination Survey.

racial groups. In 2003–2004, non-Hispanic black girls ages 12 through 19 had the highest prevalence of overweight in this age group—25.4 percent. The prevalence of overweight also increased the most in this age group, nearly doubling between 1988–1994 and 2003–2004.

Overweight represents a mismatch between energy intake and energy expenditure, and is due to both poor diet and physical inactivity. The average number of calories consumed today is substantially higher than in the past. Moreover, the content of the diet has changed dramatically. One-third of children and adolescents consume fast food on a typical day (Bowman, Gortmaker, Ebbeling, Pereira, & Ludwig, 2004). Those who ate fast food consumed an average of 187 kcal more per day, including 9 grams more fat and 24 grams more carbohydrates. Overconsumption of fast food occurs in adolescence regardless of body weight, but overweight adolescents are less likely to compensate with increased energy intake at other times of the day, compared to nonoverweight adolescents (Ebbeling et al., 2004). Another significant source of "empty calories" among adolescents is soft drink consumption (Berkey, Rockett, Field, Gillman, & Colditz, 2004; AAP Committee on School Health, 2004). In one study, each additional sugar-sweetened drink consumed by children was associated with a 0.24 kg/m^2 increase in BMI (Ludwig, Peterson, & Gortmaker, 2001).

Unfortunately, a minority of adolescents engage in adequate physical activity. In 2005, only 36 percent of high school–aged adolescents had levels of physical activity that met recommended levels (CDC, 2006b). Males were more likely to meet the recommended levels than were females; non-Hispanic black girls ages 12 through 19 had the lowest proportion meeting recommended activity levels. Less than two-thirds of adolescents (64.1 percent) reported a more *moderate level of activity*, exercising for twenty minutes to promote cardiovascular fitness three or more times a week. This figure has changed little since it was first measured in 1993.

The health consequences of this poor diet and physical inactivity among adolescents are many, and they are both immediate and long term. The immediate consequences have included a marked increase in the number of adolescents with type II diabetes mellitus. In the 1999–2002 National Health and Nutrition Examination Survey, 0.5 percent of adolescents ages 12 through 19 years reported having diabetes, among whom 29 percent reported type II diabetes (Duncan, 2006). However, in a subsample of adolescents who did not report diabetes, 11 percent had impaired fasting glucose levels. This is equivalent to 39,000 adolescents ages 12 through 19 years with diabetes and 2.7 million with impaired glucose tolerance.

The longer-term consequences relate to the continuity in overweight over time. Although few adolescents will suffer the consequences of their obesity and lack of physical activity during their youth, nearly all overweight adolescents will be overweight as adults (Deshmukh-Taskar et al., 2006; Whitaker, Wright, Pepe, Seidel, & Dietz, 1997). In the Bogalusa

Overweight represents a mismatch between energy intake and energy expenditure, and is due to both poor diet and physical inactivity.

Although few adolescents will suffer the consequences of their obesity and lack of physical activity during their youth, nearly all overweight adolescents will be overweight as adults.

Heart Study, for example, nearly 90 percent of overweight adolescents became overweight adults (Freedman et al., 2005a; Freedman et al., 2005b).

Alcohol Use

Approximately 60,000 people of all ages die in the United States annually from alcohol-related causes (Rivara, Garrison, Ebel, McCarty, & Christakis, 2004). About half of these deaths are due to heavy episodic drinking and half are due to chronic medium and high levels of regular drinking. Deaths from chronic drinking are uncommon during adolescence and young adulthood, whereas episodic drinking is a significant cause of death in people this age, primarily because of alcohol-related motor vehicle crashes.

Alcohol use is common during adolescence and peaks during young adulthood, with 28 percent of 12- to 20-year-olds in 2005 reporting that they consumed alcohol in the prior month. Among ninth through twelfth graders, 43 percent had at least one drink of alcohol in the prior month, and one-quarter report binge drinking in the prior month (Substance Abuse and Mental Health Services Administration, 2007). As shown in data from the Youth Risk Behavior Surveillance System, there have been decreases in drinking among high school youth in the first part of this decade, but no changes in the last few years (CDC, 2006b).

Data from the National Survey on Drug Use and Health may be more accurate because they include youth who are not in school. The data are less encouraging in that no group of adolescents shows a sustained decrease in binge drinking from 2002 through 2008, and binge drinking in young adults age 21 to 25 has actually increased substantially (see Figure 2.9). This type of drinking represents the most hazardous drinking for youth, because it markedly increases the risk of adverse consequences such as motor vehicle crashes, violence, unwanted sexual activity, and risky sexual behavior (Davis, Hendershot, George, Norris, & Heiman, 2007; Goldstein, Barnett, Pedlow, & Murphy, 2007). These data also show that the prevalence of binge drinking among people of all ages peaks at age 21.

The other consequence of early initiation of alcohol consumption, especially heavy consumption, is the increased risk for later alcohol dependence and adverse effects from chronic heavy drinking. The median age of onset of alcohol-use disorders is ages 19 through 20. A number of studies have shown that the earlier drinking begins, the greater the risk of alcohol use disorders (Grant & Dawson, 1997; Hingson, Heeren, Levenson, Jamanka, & Voas, 2002; Hingson, Heeren, Winter, & Wechsler, 2003; Hingson, Heeren, & Zakocs, 2001; Hingson, Heeren, Zakocs, Winter, & Wechsler, 2003). More than 40 percent of those who begin drinking at age 14 or younger develop alcohol dependence, compared with 10 percent of those who begin drinking at age 20 or older (Hingson, Heeren, & Winter, 2006). Data from the National Longitudinal Survey of Youth indicate that 14 percent of males ages 17 through 20 who engage in hazardous drinking continue to do so at ages 30 through 31, compared with only 4 percent of adolescents who were not harmful drinkers (McCarty et al., 2004).

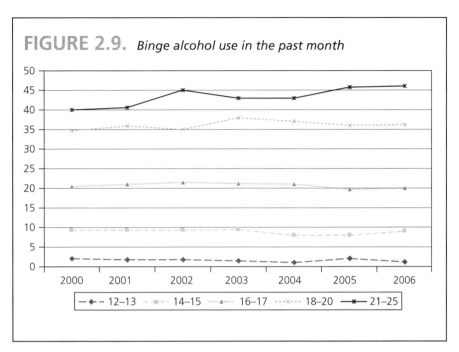

FIGURE 2.9. *Binge alcohol use in the past month*

Legend: 12–13, 14–15, 16–17, 18–20, 21–25

Source: Substance Abuse and Mental Health Services Administration (2007).

As with smoking, the most successful interventions to prevent hazardous drinking among adolescents and young adults and decrease the risk of harm from it are population-based measures. These include raising the legal drinking age to 21 years, lowering the legal blood alcohol limit for driving to 0.08 for those over 21 (and zero tolerance for those under 21), administrative revocation of licenses for drunk driving, and raising the alcohol tax. The federal tax on alcohol has not kept up with inflation, and raising it one dollar per six-pack of beer could reduce deaths from harmful drinking by 1,490 deaths annually, equivalent to 31,130 discounted years of potential life saved (Hollingworth et al., 2006).

Illicit Drugs

According to the National Survey on Drug Use and Health, the most common illicit drugs used by 12- to 17-year-olds in the prior month during 2006 were marijuana (6.7 percent of adolescents), psychotherapeutic agents (3.3 percent), inhalants (1.3 percent), and hallucinogens (0.7 percent; Substance Abuse and Mental Health Services Administration, 2007). Among 18- to 25-year-olds, the most common illicit drugs were marijuana (16.3 percent of adolescents), psychotherapeutic agents (6.4 percent), cocaine (2.2 percent), and hallucinogens (1.7 percent).

More than 40 percent of those who begin drinking at age 14 or younger develop alcohol dependence, compared with 10 percent of those who begin drinking at age 20 or older.

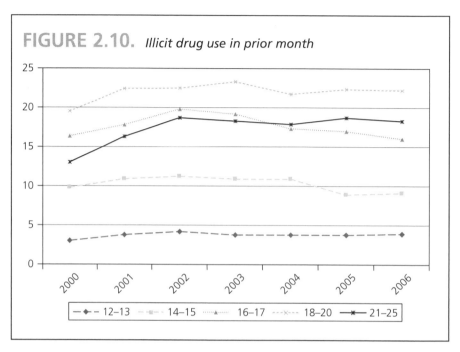

FIGURE 2.10. *Illicit drug use in prior month*

Source: Substance Abuse and Mental Health Services Administration (2007).

The peak age for illicit drug use among people of any age is 18 to 20 years. As shown in Figure 2.10, there has been some fluctuation over the decade, but no dramatic trends are evident in this graph. However, it is important to realize that in 2006 an estimated 2.8 million persons aged 12 or older used an illicit drug for the first time within the past twelve months; this averages to nearly 8,000 initiates per day. The average age of initiation among persons 12 through 49 years was 19; the average age for initiation of PCP use was 16.3 years.

There are also important geographic differences. Illicit use of prescription pain relievers (such as OxyContin) among 12- to 17-year-olds is highest (8.7 percent) in areas with populations of fewer than 250,000; in large metropolitan areas, 6.9 percent of youth of this age report past-month use (Substance Abuse and Mental Health Services Administration, 2007). Among 18- to 25-year-olds, the prevalence is 13.5 percent and 11.0 percent, respectively.

Sexual Behavior

Among high school students in grades nine through twelve, approximately one-third have been sexually active in the prior three months (see Figure 2.11). This proportion has decreased by 9.6 percent since 1991. By ages 18 through 19, the majority of both males and females have been sexually active in the prior twelve months with partners of the opposite sex (see Figure 2.12). This increases to approximately 85 percent for

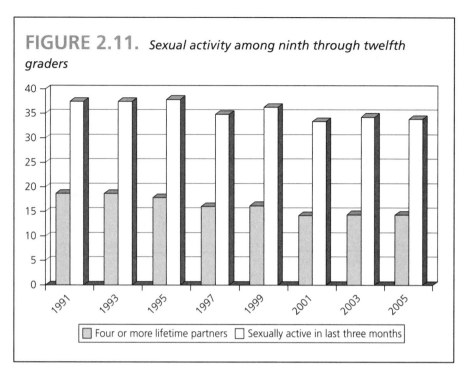

FIGURE 2.11. *Sexual activity among ninth through twelfth graders*

Source: CDC (2006b).

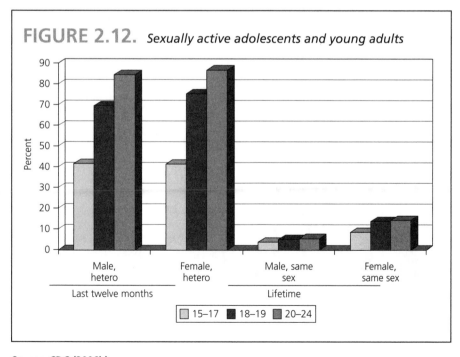

FIGURE 2.12. *Sexually active adolescents and young adults*

Source: CDC (2006b).

both sexes by ages 20 through 24. By ages 18 through 19, approximately 5 percent of males and 14 percent of females have had at least one same-sex partner.

Risky sexual behavior is relatively common among adolescents in the United States, although there has been some significant improvement in trends over the last decade (Mosher, Chandra, & Jones, 2005). According to the 2005 Youth Risk Behavior Surveillance, 3.7 percent of females and 8.8 percent of males had had first sex before age 13, compared to 5.1 and 15.1, respectively, in 1991 (CDC, 2006b). Among high school–aged youth, approximately 14 percent have had four or more sexual partners—a 23.6 percent reduction since 1991 (see Figure 2.11). Condom use among this group during last sexual intercourse has increased from 46.2 percent in 1991 to 62.8 percent in 2005 (see Figure 2.13). However, sexual activity after alcohol or drug use—a known risk factor for STD and unwanted pregnancy—continues at more than one in five sexual encounters in this age group.

Chlamydia rates in women ages 15 through 24 have increased over the last five years, whereas rates among 10- to 14-year-olds have decreased somewhat (Figure 2.14). This may not represent an actual increase in cases, but better case finding due to improved screening (CDC, 2006a). On the other hand, AIDS cases among adolescents, at a low around 1998–1999, have increased by 75.9 percent among 13- to 19-year-olds, and 46.5 percent among 20- to 24-year-olds, reflecting continued risk of STD among adolescents and young adults (Figure 2.15).

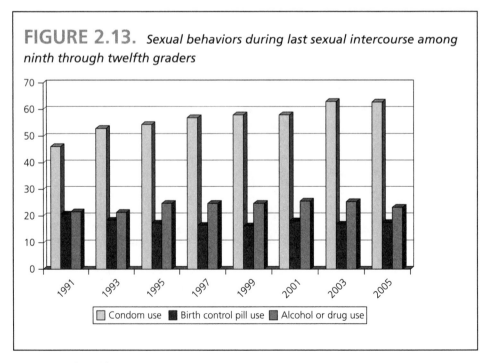

FIGURE 2.13. *Sexual behaviors during last sexual intercourse among ninth through twelfth graders*

Source: CDC (2006b).

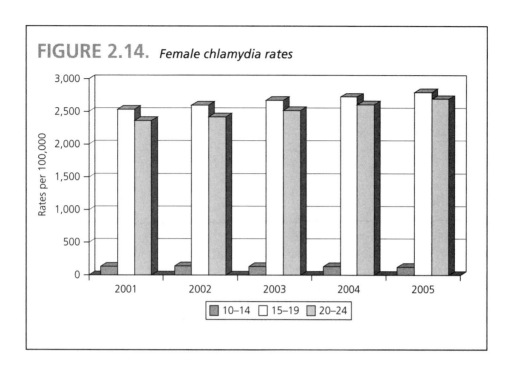

FIGURE 2.14. *Female chlamydia rates*

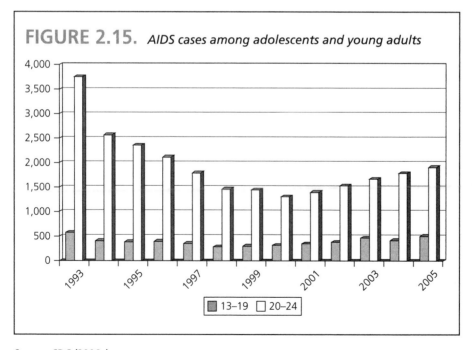

FIGURE 2.15. *AIDS cases among adolescents and young adults*

Source: CDC (2006a).

Births to teenagers continue to decline since the early 1990s, although there has been an upswing in 2006, the first reported increase since 1991 (Hamilton, Martin, & Ventura, 2007). The rate of births to women 15 through 19 years of age was 41.9 births per 1,000 women in 2006, compared to 40.5 in 2005. The 2005 rate was the lowest rate recorded in the last sixty-five years. The rate for teens ages 10 through 14 has remained low, at 0.6 births per 1,000 (Hamilton, Martin, & Ventura, 2007; Hamilton, Minino, et al., 2007). Equally encouraging is that the overall teenage pregnancy rates have also declined substantially, by 35 percent from the peak in 1990, at 115.8 per 1,000, to 76.4 per 1,000 in 2002 (Guttmacher Institute, 2006; Ventura, Abama, Mosher, & Henshaw, 2007).

Injury-Related Behavior

A variety of behaviors can dramatically affect an individual's risk of serious or fatal injury. Perhaps the most important is seat belt use. The proportion of high school students who report rarely or never wearing a seat belt has decreased by 61 percent since 1991, to 10.2 percent in 2005 (CDC, 2006b). Fewer adolescents report riding in the past month with a driver who had been drinking; in 2005 this figure was 28.0 percent, down from 39.9 percent in 1991 (a 30 percent decrease). Less than 10 percent of adolescents reported that they drove after drinking in 2005, compared to 16.1 percent in 1991. The proportion of respondents who reported carrying a weapon in the prior thirty days decreased from 26.1 percent to 18.5 percent in 2005.

MENTAL HEALTH

Mental health problems have a significant impact on functioning and well-being for people of all ages, including adolescents and young adults. This impact has been well documented using the "burden of disease" concept. This concept takes into account not only mortality and the age at death, but morbidity as well. This is especially relevant for considering the impact of chronic illness, in which most people do not die, but have lives marked by substantial disability. The unifying metric for this is the *disability-adjusted life year*, or *DALY* (McKenna, Michaud, Murray, & Marks, 2005), which takes into account the degree to which an individual with an illness is not able to function fully, the age of onset of the disability and its duration, as well as the number of deaths and the age at death. It is the sum of years of life lost due to death plus the years of healthy life lost due to disability from disease or injury.

According to the World Health Organization, in 2002 (the last year available) 12,781 DALYs per 100,000 population were lost from all causes in the United States. Noncommunicable diseases accounted for 10,367 DALYs, and neuropsychiatric disorders accounted for almost half of this, at 4,208 (World Health Organization, 2004). The single largest cause of DALYs lost in the United States was unipolar depression, accounting for 1,651 DALYs lost per 100,000 population in 2002.

As with risky behaviors, many mental health problems first emerge in adolescents and young adults. Recent data from the National Comorbidity Survey Replication demonstrate both the common prevalence of mental illness and the fact that most mental health problems first appear before adolescence ends (Kessler et al., 2007). In this population of adults ages 18 and older surveyed in 2001–2003, the most common mental health disorders during the lifetime were major depressive disorder (16.6 percent) and alcohol abuse (13.2 percent). As a class, anxiety disorders were most common (28.8 percent), followed by impulse control disorders (24.8 percent), mood disorders (20.8 percent), and substance abuse (14.6 percent; Kessler et al., 2007).

As shown in Table 2.1, the median age of onset for any mental health disorder was 14 years, with an interquartile range of 7 through 24 years. This means that 25 percent of people who develop a mental health disorder during their lifetimes will have onset by age 7, 50 percent by age 14, and 75 percent by age 24. Anxiety disorders had an even younger median age of onset. For impulse control disorders, 75 percent had their onset by age 15, and 95 percent by age 23. Mood disorders had the latest median age of onset; nevertheless, 25 percent first occurred by age 18. The prevalence of mood disorders then increases linearly through middle age. Substance use disorders generally do not appear until young adulthood, but then increase rapidly in prevalence so that by age 27, 75 percent of people with substance use disorders would have had their onset. The age of onset of the various mental health disorders appears to be very similar across countries where it has been studied (Kessler et al., 2007).

The National Comorbidity Survey Replication reported that approximately 1.5 percent of people had a lifetime prevalence of probable nonaffective psychoses

Twenty-five percent of people who develop a mental health disorder during their lifetimes will have onset by age 7, 50 percent by age 14, and 75 percent by age 24.

TABLE 2.1. Median age of onset of mental health disorders

	Median Age of Onset (years)	Interquartile Range (years)
Any disorder	14	7–24
Anxiety disorders	11	6–21
Any mood disorder	30	18–43
Any impulse control disorder	11	7–15
Any substance use disorder	20	18–27

Source: Kessler et al., 2007.

(Kessler et al., 2007). Treatment data from Australia indicate that the median age of presentation for the first episode of psychosis was 22 years, with an interquartile range of 19 through 25 years (Kessler et al., 2007). Thus, as with the disorders studied in the National Comorbidity Survey Replication, the majority of psychoses have their onset during adolescence and young adulthood (Kessler et al., 2007). Treatment of mental health disorders becomes more difficult and less successful with increasing duration of symptoms before therapy is begun. Among patients with DSM-IV disorders, only 41.1 percent had received treatment in the prior year (Wang et al., 2005).

SUMMARY

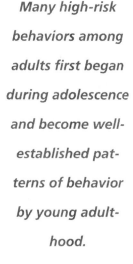

Many high-risk behaviors among adults first began during adolescence and become well-established patterns of behavior by young adulthood.

The period of adolescence and young adulthood is a complex time in the life course of an individual. Most of the morbidity and mortality that occurs during this period is related to individuals beginning to experiment with and assume a variety of adult roles. Many high-risk behaviors among adults first began during adolescence and become well-established patterns of behavior by young adulthood (Park, Mulye, Adams, Brindis, & Irwin, 2006).

The trends over the last twenty-five years in these markers of adolescent and young adult health have been mixed (Park et al., 2006). Deaths from natural causes have largely declined, except for the increase during the 1990s in deaths from HIV infection. Deaths from external causes of unintentional injuries have also dropped, in some cases fairly dramatically, though deaths from violence have not decreased. The recent increase in suicide deaths among middle adolescents is of major concern, and the underlying reasons for this change must be examined and addressed.

Many of the behavioral markers have also declined over the last two decades, indicating that most adolescents and young adults are healthy and leading lives that are likely to result in a healthy adulthood. However, this trend is not true for all behaviors or for all groups. For example, the recent increase in the rate of births to teens in middle adolescence is of major concern and may reflect changes in the economy, a relaxation of fear of HIV infection, and changes in social networking. The heterogeneity of the adolescent and young adult population and their profiles reflect the heterogeneity of American society. Though a cause for celebration, this heterogeneity also requires a thoughtful, nuanced approach to efforts to improve the health of the individual adolescent and young adult as well as that of the entire population.

KEY TERMS

Adolescence and young adulthood

Burden of disease concept

Disability-adjusted life year (DALY)

Moderate level of activity

Overweight

DISCUSSION QUESTIONS

1. How has adolescent risk behavior changed over the last twenty-five years in the early, middle, and late stages of adolescence?

2. Explain the relationship between adolescent-onset mental health problems and disability-adjusted life years (DALYs).

3. Which adolescent risk behavior outlined in this chapter is most amenable to change? Which would you target as a focus of intervention? Why?

REFERENCES

AAP Committee on School Health. (2004). Soft drinks in schools. *Pediatrics, 113*, 152–154.

Berkey, C. S., Rockett, H. R., Field, A. E., Gillman, M. W., & Colditz, G. A. (2004). Sugar-added beverages and adolescent weight change. *Obesity Research, 12*, 778–788.

Blumstein, A., Rivara, F. P., & Rosenfeld, R. (2000). The rise and decline of homicide—and why. *Annual Review of Public Health, 21*, 505–541.

Bowman, S. A., Gortmaker, S. L., Ebbeling, C. B., Pereira, M. A., & Ludwig, D. S. (2004). Effects of fast-food consumption on energy intake and diet quality among children in a national household survey. *Pediatrics, 113*, 112–118.

Centers for Disease Control and Prevention. (2006a). *Trends in reportable sexually transmitted diseases in the United States, 2005.* Vol. 2007.

Centers for Disease Control and Prevention. (2006b). Youth risk behavior surveillance: United States, 2005. *Morbidity and Mortality Weekly Report, 55*, 1–112.

Centers for Disease Control and Prevention. (2007a). Bridged-race population estimates, United States. Vol. 2007.

Centers for Disease Control and Prevention. (2007b). *Compressed mortality file.* Vol. 2007.

Centers for Disease Control and Prevention. (2007c). Suicide trends among youth and young adults aged 10–24 years: United States, 1990–2004. *Morbidity and Mortality Weekly Report, 56*, 905–908.

Davis, K. C., Hendershot, C. S., George, W. H., Norris, J., & Heiman, J. R. (2007). Alcohol's effects on sexual decision making: An integration of alcohol myopia and individual differences. *Journal of Studies on Alcohol and Drugs, 68*, 843–851.

Deshmukh-Taskar, P., Nicklas, T. A., Morales, M., Yang, S. J., Zakeri, I., & Berenson, G. S. (2006). Tracking of overweight status from childhood to young adulthood: The Bogalusa Heart Study. *European Journal of Clinical Nutrition, 60*, 48–57.

DiFranza, J. R., Savageau, J. A., Fletcher, K., O'Loughlin, J., Pbert, L., Ockene, J. K., et al. (2007). Symptoms of tobacco dependence after brief intermittent use: The Development and Assessment of Nicotine Dependence in Youth-2 study. *Archives of Pediatrics and Adolescent Medicine, 161*, 704–710.

DiFranza, J. R., Savageau, J. A., Fletcher, K., Pbert, L., O'Loughlin, J., McNeill, A. D., et al. (2007). Susceptibility to nicotine dependence: The Development and Assessment of Nicotine Dependence in Youth-2 study. *Pediatrics, 120*, e974–983.

Duncan, G. E. (2006). Prevalence of diabetes and impaired fasting glucose levels among US adolescents: National Health and Nutrition Examination Survey, 1999–2002. *Archives of Pediatrics and Adolescent Medicine, 160*, 523–528.

Ebbeling, C. B., Sinclair, K. B., Pereira, M. A., Garcia-Lago, E., Feldman, H. A., & Ludwig, D. S. (2004). Compensation for energy intake from fast food among overweight and lean adolescents. *Journal of the American Medical Association, 291*, 2828–2833.

Fishman, P. A., Ebel, B. E., Garrison, M. M., Christakis, D. A., Wiehe, S. E., & Rivara F. P. (2005).Cigarette tax increase and media campaign cost of reducing smoking-related deaths. *American Journal of Preventive Medicine, 29*, 19–26.

Freedman, D. S., Khan, L. K., Serdula, M. K., Dietz, W. H., Srinivasan, S. R., & Berenson, G. S. (2005a). The relation of childhood BMI to adult adiposity: The Bogalusa Heart Study. *Pediatrics, 115,* 22–27.

Freedman, D. S., Khan, L. K, Serdula, M. K., Dietz, W. H., Srinivasan, S. R., & Berenson, G. S. (2005b). Racial differences in the tracking of childhood BMI to adulthood. *Obesity Research, 13,* 928–935.

Goldstein, A. L., Barnett, N. P., Pedlow, C. T., & Murphy, J. G. (2007). Drinking in conjunction with sexual experiences among at-risk college student drinkers. *Journal of Studies on Alcohol and Drugs, 68,* 697–705.

Grant, B. F., & Dawson, D. A. (1997). Age at onset of alcohol use and its association with DSM-IV alcohol abuse and dependence: Results from the National Longitudinal Alcohol Epidemiologic Survey. *Journal of Substance Abuse, 9,* 103–110.

Guttmacher Institute. (2006). *U.S. teenage pregnancy statistics: National and state trends.* New York: Guttmacher Institute.

Hamilton, B. E., Martin, J. A., & Ventura, S. J. (2007). Births: Preliminary data for 2006. *National Vital Statistics Reports, 56,* 1–18.

Hamilton, B. E., Minino, A. M., Martin, J. A., Kochanek, K. D., Strobino, D. M., & Guyer, B. (2007). Annual summary of vital statistics: 2005. *Pediatrics, 119,* 345–360.

Hingson, R., Heeren, T., Levenson, S., Jamanka, A., & Voas, R. (2002). Age of drinking onset, driving after drinking, and involvement in alcohol related motor-vehicle crashes. *Accident Analysis and Prevention, 34,* 85–92.

Hingson, R. W., Heeren, T., & Winter, M. R. (2006). Age of alcohol-dependence onset: Associations with severity of dependence and seeking treatment. *Pediatrics, 118,* e755–763.

Hingston, R., Heeren, T., Winter, M. R., & Wechsler, H. (2003). Early age of first drunkenness as a factor in college students' unplanned and unprotected sex attributable to drinking. *Pediatrics, 111,* 34–41.

Hingson, R., Heeren, T., & Zakocs, R. (2001). Age of drinking onset and involvement in physical fights after drinking. *Pediatrics, 108,* 872–877.

Hingson, R., Heeren, T., Zakocs, R., Winter, M., &Wechsler, H. (2003). Age of first intoxication, heavy drinking, driving after drinking and risk of unintentional injury among U.S. college students. *Journal of Studies on Alcohol and Drugs, 64,* 23–31.

Hollingworth, W., Ebel, B. E., McCarty, C. A., Garrison, M. M., Christakis, D. A., & Rivara, F. P. (2006). Prevention of deaths from harmful drinking in the United States: The potential effects of tax increases and advertising bans on young drinkers. *Journal of Studies on Alcohol and Drugs, 67,* 300–308.

Kandel, D. B., & Chen, K. (2000). Extent of smoking and nicotine dependence in the United States: 1991–1993. *Nicotine and Tobacco Research, 2,* 263–274.

Kessler, R. C., Amminger, G. P., Aguilar-Gaxiola, S., Alonso, J., Lee, S., & Ustun, T. B. (2007). Age of onset of mental disorders: A review of recent literature. *Current Opinion in Psychiatry, 20,* 359–364.

Ludwig, D. S., Peterson, K. E., & Gortmaker, S. L. (2001). Relation between consumption of sugar-sweetened drinks and childhood obesity: A prospective, observational analysis. *Lancet, 357,* 505–508.

McCarty, C. A., Ebel, B. E., Garrison, M. M., DiGiuseppe, D. L., Christakis, D. A., & Rivara, F. P. (2004). Continuity of binge and harmful drinking from late adolescence to early adulthood. *Pediatrics, 114,* 714–719.

McGinnis, J. M., & Foege, W. H. (1993). Actual causes of death in the United States. *Journal of the American Medical Association, 270,* 2207–2212.

McKenna, M. T., Michaud, C. M., Murray, C. J., & Marks, J. S. (2005). Assessing the burden of disease in the United States using disability-adjusted life years. *American Journal of Preventive Medicine, 28,* 415–423.

Mokdad, A. H., Marks, J. S., Stroup, D. F., & Gerberding, J. L. (2004). Actual causes of death in the United States, 2000. *Journal of the American Medical Association, 291,* 1238–1245.

Mosher, W. D., Chandra, A., & Jones, J. (2005). Sexual behavior and selected health measures: Men and women 15–44 years of age, United States, 2002. *Advance Data, 362,* 1–56.

Ogden, C. L., Carroll, M. D., Curtin, L. R., McDowell, M. A., Tabak, C. J., & Flegal, K. M. (2006). Prevalence of overweight and obesity in the United States, 1999–2004. *Journal of the American Medical Association, 295,* 1549–1555.

Ogden, C. L., Fryar, C. D., Carroll, M. D., & Flegal, K. M. (2004). Mean body weight, height, and body mass index, United States, 1960–2002. *Advance Data, 347,* 1–17.

Park, M. J., Mulye, T. P., Adams, S. H., Brindis, C. D., & Irwin, C. E., Jr. (2006). The health status of young adults in the United States. *Journal of Adolescent Health, 39,* 305–317.

Rivara, F. P., Ebel, B. E., Garrison, M. M., Christakis, D. A., Wiehe, S. E., & Levy, D. (2004). Prevention of smoking-related deaths in the United States from interventions during childhood and adolescence. *American Journal of Preventive Medicine, 27,* 118–125.

Rivara, F. P., Garrison, M. M., Ebel, B., McCarty, C. A., & Christakis, D. A. (2004). Mortality attributable to harmful drinking in the United States, 2000. *Journal of Studies on Alcohol and Drugs, 65,* 530–536.

Rubinstein, M. L., Thompson, P. J., Benowitz, N. L., Shiffman, S., & Moscicki, A. B. (2007). Cotinine levels in relation to smoking behavior and addiction in young adolescent smokers. *Nicotine and Tobacco Research, 9,* 129–135.

Substance Abuse and Mental Health Services Administration. (2007). Results from the 2006 National Survey on Drug Use and Health. Rockville, MD: Department of Health and Human Services.

Sussman, S., Sun, P., & Dent, C. W. (2006). A meta-analysis of teen cigarette smoking cessation. *Health Psychology, 25,* 549–557.

U.S. Census Bureau. (2004). Foreign-born population of the United States: Characteristics of the population by generation. Vol. 2007.

U.S. Census Bureau. (2007). Current population survey: Annual social and economic supplement. Vol. 2007.

Ventura, S. J., Abama, J. C., Mosher, W. D., & Henshaw, S. K. (2007). *Recent trends in teenage pregnancy in the United States, 1990–2002.* Atlanta: National Center for Health Statistics.

Wang, P. S., Lane, M., Olfson, M., Pincus, H. A., Wells, K. B., & Kessler, R. C. (2005). Twelve-month use of mental health services in the United States: Results from the National Comorbidity Survey Replication. *Archives of General Psychiatry, 62,* 629–640.

Whitaker, R. C., Wright, J. A., Pepe, M. S., Seidel, K. D., & Dietz, W. H. (1997). Predicting obesity in young adulthood from childhood and parental obesity. *New England Journal of Medicine, 337,* 869–873.

Wiehe, S. E., Garrison, M. M., Christakis, D. A., Ebel, B. E., & Rivara, F. P. (2005). A systematic review of school-based smoking prevention trials with long-term follow-up. *Journal of Adolescent Health, 36,* 162–169.

World Health Organization. (2004). Revised global burden of disease estimates. Vol. 2007.

CHAPTER

3

THEORIES OF ADOLESCENT RISK TAKING: THE BIOPSYCHOSOCIAL MODEL

JESSICA M. SALES ▪ CHARLES E. IRWIN JR.

LEARNING OBJECTIVES

After studying this chapter, you will be able to

- Analyze a multidimensional framework in which socioenvironmental factors affect existing biological and psychological predispositions to influence risk-taking behavior.

- Summarize existing unidimensional theories of adolescent risk-taking behavior.

- Describe future directions for using the biopsychosocial model in understanding adolescent risk taking.

Adolescence is a stage of life characterized by marked physical, cognitive, social, and emotional change. Normative adolescent development consists of increased independence, a change in family relationships toward greater interdependence, prioritizing peer affiliations, identity formation, increased awareness of morals and values, and cognitive maturation, all of which are set against the backdrop of rapid physiological change. Along with the enormous "positive growth" seen during adolescence, this developmental stage also brings increased exploration and risk taking. *Risk* is defined as a chance of loss, and risk taking is often defined as engaging in risky behaviors that may have harmful consequences (Beyth-Marom & Fischoff, 1997).

Although risk-taking behaviors are considered to be a normative part of adolescence, these behaviors are nonetheless concerning to parents, teachers, clinicians, researchers, and society because they endanger adolescents' health and well-being. For instance, adolescents frequently engage in health-endangering and problematic behaviors including use of tobacco and alcohol, experimentation with drugs, unsafe sexual activities, poor eating habits, as well as delinquent actions (Sullivan & Terry, 1998; Grumbaum et al., 2004).

Unfortunately, the behaviors established during adolescence often become major contributors to the health problems of adults (Park, Mulye, Adams, Brindis, & Irwin, 2006). The potential long-term result of prevalent adolescent risk-taking behaviors include substance abuse, unwanted pregnancies, sexually transmitted infections (STIs) including HIV, obesity or other health problems caused by problem eating (eating disorders), and serious criminal activity. For instance, in 2006 the Monitoring the Future Study found that 45.3 percent of high school seniors had consumed alcohol and 18.3 percent had used marijuana in the past thirty days, and that the use of prescription-type drugs was high (Johnston, O'Malley, Bachman, & Schulenberg, 2006). Moreover, for the first time in fourteen years, the adolescent pregnancy rate rose in 2006 (Centers for Disease Control and Prevention [CDC], 2008), and recent reports indicate that one in four adolescent females have had an STI. Finally, juveniles accounted for 17 percent of all arrests and 16 percent of all violent crime arrests in 1999, including 14 percent of aggravated assault arrests, 17 percent of forcible rape arrests, and 24 percent of weapons arrests (Snyder, 2000). Adolescent death can be the ultimate consequence, with most cases of mortality (approximately 75 percent) in the United States during the adolescent period resulting from preventable causes like accidents, homicide, and suicide (Fingerhut & Anderson, 2008). Thus, understanding adolescent risk taking has become a public health priority.

A variety of factors, including biological, psychological, and environmental, have been found to be associated with adolescent risk-taking behaviors. However, many theories of risk-taking behavior are unidimensional and focus predominantly on one domain of factors—whether biological, psychological, or environmental—as they affect risk taking. To provide a more comprehensive framework for examining the range of factors thought to influence the likelihood of adolescents engaging in risk-taking behavior a theory or model must simultaneously take into account the roles of biology, psychosocial influences, and the environment. In line with this ideology, a recent report from the working group of the National Institutes of Health (NIH) Advisory Committee on research in the basic behavioral and social sciences has prioritized the need for a better understanding of the interaction among biology, environment, and behavior and emphasizes the utility of such an approach for advancing our understanding of behavior, particularly behaviors which place one at risk (Working Group of the NIH Advisory Committee, 2004). Consistent with the recommendations of the NIH Advisory Committee, the biopsychosocial model of risk taking (Irwin & Millstein, 1986) provides a framework in which social and environmental factors are brought to bear on existing biological and psychological predispositions to influence risk-taking behavior.

The remainder of this chapter reviews some of the unidimensional theories of risk taking—the biological, psychological, and environmental theories—and provides an overview of the multidimensional biopsychosocial model of risk taking. Empirical evidence supporting the biopsychosocial model is also presented. Future directions for the utility of the biopsychosocial model in advancing our understanding of adolescent risk taking are then discussed.

The National Institutes of Health Advisory Committee on research in the basic behavioral and social sciences has prioritized the need for a better understanding of the interaction among biology, environment, and behavior.

BIOLOGICALLY BASED THEORIES OF RISK TAKING

Biologically based theories suggest that risk-taking behaviors result from four sources: (1) genetic predispositions, (2) "direct" hormonal influences, (3) the influence of asynchronous pubertal timing (puberty that begins earlier or later than that of peers), and (4) brain and central nervous system development. Examples of each type of biological influence are presented here in turn.

Genetic Predispositions

The familial nature of health risk behaviors has led some to speculate about the role of genetic predispositions in risk-taking behaviors. Evidence from family studies demonstrates that risk-taking behaviors tend to cluster within families. For instance, certain families have a greater propensity for injury-related behavior. Schor (1987) found that a small number of families accounted for a disproportionately large number of injury-related health care visits, and individual members of these "high-injury" families had similar rates of unintentional injuries, with injury rates being stable over time. Moreover, genetic models have been employed to explain familial patterns of substance use. Many studies have demonstrated that children of alcoholics are more likely than children of nonalcoholics to abuse alcohol (Adger, 1991; Marlatt, Baer, Donovan, & Kivlahan, 1988). Twin-adoption studies have indicated that the association is more than the product of shared environment or learned behaviors, as children of alcoholic biological parents show a greater predisposition toward alcohol abuse even when raised by nonalcoholic adoptive parents (Cloninger, 1987).

Historically, the study of genetic influences on human behavior has been difficult and controversial, but with recent advances in gene mapping techniques, we now have the capability to further explore the role of genetic predispositions. For example, with regard to alcohol use, genetic studies support the Al allele of the D2 dopamine receptor gene (DRD2) as a risk marker for alcoholism and substance use disorders. Conner and colleagues (2005) found that male adolescents with the A1(+) allele tried and got intoxicated on alcohol more often than boys without this genetic marker, providing support for the DRD2 A1 allele as a marker identifying a subgroup of adolescent males at high risk for developing substance use problems. Identification of other genetic markers that predispose adolescents toward other risk-taking behaviors may be on the horizon.

Direct Hormonal Influences

Hormones have been postulated to play a role in the onset of adolescent risk-taking behavior, both directly and indirectly, through their role in pubertal development. For example, Udry, Billy, Morris, Groff, and Raj (1985) found that the rise in testosterone levels during adolescence was related to male coital debut. Female coital initiation was related to social controls and pubertal development (Udry, Talbert, & Morris, 1986).

Influence of Asynchronous Pubertal Maturation

The timing of pubertal maturation is related to both genetics and hormonal fluctuations. For example, the menarcheal ages of mothers and daughters are typically correlated, and physical development is preceded by elevations in respective sex steroid levels. Asynchronous pubertal maturation (maturation that is earlier or later than that of peers) is hypothesized to be a factor in risk taking (Irwin & Millstein, 1986). Adolescents who appear physically mature may be more apt to engage in "adult" behaviors such as smoking, drinking, and sexual intercourse (Brooks-Gunn, 1988). This potential early onset of risky behaviors could be the product of associating with an older peer group in which these behaviors may be more normative. Research indicates that early-maturing females are more likely to initiate sexual intercourse at younger ages (Phinney, Jensen, Olsen, & Cundick, 1990). Younger age at sexual debut is associated with less consistent contraception and increased numbers of lifetime sex partners, resulting in an increased risk for pregnancy and STDs (Kaestle, Halpern, Miller, & Ford, 2005; Ford et al., 2005; Manning, Longmore, & Giordano, 2000).

Brain and Central Nervous System Development

From a developmental neuroscience perspective, the slow maturation of the *cognitive-control system* in the brain, which regulates impulse control, makes adolescence a time of heightened vulnerability for risk-taking behavior (Steinberg, 2004). According to Steinberg (2007), adolescent risk taking is the product of both logical reasoning and psychosocial factors. Logical reasoning abilities are mostly fully developed by the age of fifteen, but psychosocial capacities (impulse control, emotion regulation, delay of gratification, and resistance to peer influence) that facilitate decision making and moderate risk taking are guided by the cognitive-control systems in the brain, which continues to mature well into young adulthood (Steinberg, 2004; 2007). The cognitive-control system, which consists mainly of outer regions of the brain such as the lateral prefrontal and parietal cortices and portions of the anterior cingulated cortex, is involved in executive function tasks like planning, thinking ahead, impulse control, and self-regulation (Giedd, 2008). Recent research from behavioral science is consistent with Steinberg's position. For instance, his laboratory-based research found that the presence of peers more than doubled the number of risks teenagers took in a video driving game and increased risk taking by 50 percent in college students, but had no effect among adults (Gardner & Steinberg, 2005).

Beyond Biology

Biological development during adolescence is accompanied by physiological changes in the ways in which adolescents perceive both themselves and the world around them. Cognitive development may occur in concert or asynchronously with physical development. When physical development precedes cognitive development (as is often the case with females experiencing early maturation), adolescents are at increased risk for behavioral morbidities. The social world may have unrealistic or unhealthy expectations of mature-appearing adolescents whose lack of experience and relative cognitive and social maturity (or immaturity) may increase their vulnerability. For example, when biological models are expanded to include environmental variables, the combined effects of biological (hormonal) and environmental (social) factors explain more of the variation in problem behaviors (smoking cigarettes or marijuana, drinking alcohol, or having sex) than either of these factors alone.

The combined effects of biological and environmental factors explain more of the variation in problem behaviors than either of these factors alone.

PSYCHOLOGICALLY BASED THEORIES OF RISK TAKING

Psychologically based theories of risk-taking behavior examine the roles of cognition, personality traits, and dispositional characteristics such as self-esteem in risk-taking behavior. Each of these roles is discussed in turn here.

The Role of Cognition

Cognitive theories of risk-taking behavior look at the ways in which individuals perceive risk and make decisions about risk taking. Adolescent risk perception theory has been influenced by the premise that adolescents are "optimistically biased" in their perception of risk or that they believe themselves invulnerable. The concept of invulnerability has been used to explain adolescent risk-taking behavior, although little evidence supports this assumption. In fact, people of all ages underestimate their likelihood of experiencing negative events. Adolescents do not appear to be more biased in that regard than adults.

A great deal of work has examined the role of decision making on risk taking. Fischoff (1992) identified five salient components of decision making: (1) identify alternative options, (2) identify possible consequences, (3) evaluate the desirability of the potential consequences, (4) assess the likelihood of those consequences, and (5) combine the information to make a decision. According to Keating (1990), by middle adolescence most individuals make decisions in a manner similar to adults. By fourteen or fifteen years of age, adolescents have the ability to generate and evaluate a range of alternative options. Although the decision-making process may be similar for adolescents and adults, the content of the aforementioned components may differ substantially based on, among other things, experience, biases, judgment, social pressure, and situations. In support of this position, Beyth-Marom, Austin, Fischoff, Palmgren, and Jacobs-Quadrel (1993) found that adolescent and adult patterns of response to potential risk were similar, with both producing more negative consequences than positive ones. However, overall adults reported more consequences than adolescents.

There is some evidence that adolescents give greater weight to proximal consequences than distal ones when making decisions.

There is some evidence that adolescents give greater weight to proximal (less severe) than distal (potentially more severe) possible consequences when making decisions. For example, Kegeles, Adler, and Irwin (1988) found that among a group of fourteen- to sixteen-year-olds, intentions to use condoms were not related to the adolescents' beliefs about the degree to which condoms prevent STDs or pregnancy. Rather, intentions to use condoms were correlated with the degree to which the adolescents perceived that condoms are easy to use, popular with peers, and would facilitate spontaneous sex. Adolescent smokers and nonsmokers have similar perceptions of their risk for long-term morbidities such as cancer (Greening & Dollinger, 1991). On the other hand, adolescent smoking prevention programs have successfully emphasized the immediate physiologic consequences of smoking (Flay, 1985).

With regard to perception of risk, adolescents are no worse than adults at perceiving risk or estimating vulnerability to risk (Reyna & Farley, 2006). For instance, Millstein and Halpern-Felsher (2002) demonstrated that increasing the salience of the risks associated with making a potentially dangerous decision had the same effect on adolescents and adults. Moreover, few age differences have been found in individuals' evaluations of the risks inherent in a variety of dangerous behaviors or in judgments about the seriousness of consequences resulting from risky behavior (Beyth-Marom, Austin, Fischoff, Palmgren, & Jacobs-Quadrel, 1993).

The Role of Personality

The relative influence of individual factors on adolescent decision making may reflect a general tendency toward unconventional behavior. Jessor's Problem Behavior Theory links "unconventionality" in personality (as well as perceived environment and behavioral systems) with an increased likelihood of engaging in problem behaviors such as risky sexual activity, substance use, and delinquency (Jessor & Jessor, 1977). Unconventionality in the personality system is represented by a greater value placed on independence than achievement, lower expectations for academic achievement, lesser religiosity, and greater tolerance for deviance. These factors have been correlated with problem drinking, marijuana use, and early sexual debut (Jessor, 1976; Jessor, Chase, & Donovan, 1980).

Sensation seeking as a personality trait has been used to explain risk-taking behavior. According to Zuckerman (1979), sensation seeking is a "trait defined by the need for varied, novel and complex sensations and experiences and willingness to take physical and social risks for the sake of such experiences." Zuckerman developed a Sensation-Seeking Scale to assess individual differences in optimal levels of arousal. There is a tendency for high-sensation seekers to perceive less risk in many activities than low-sensation seekers. But even when the evaluation of the risk involved is equal between the two groups, high-sensation seekers are likely to anticipate more positive potential outcomes than low-sensation seekers. Sensation seeking has been associated with risk-taking behaviors such as substance abuse, reckless motor vehicle use, delinquency, and risky sexual behavior (Andrucci, Archer, Pancoast, & Gordon, 1989; Newcomb & McGee, 1991; Tonkin, 1987; Zuckerman, 1991; Kalichman & Rompa, 1995). Interestingly, sensation seeking has been linked to a number of biological markers, including electrodermal and heart rate responses, cortical evoked potentials, and testosterone levels (Zuckerman, 1990).

The impulsivity seen among sensation-seekers may be seen in psychopathologic states that have been linked to an increased likelihood of risk-taking behaviors, primarily in male adolescents. Attention deficit hyperactivity disorder (ADHD) in males has been associated with an increased risk for delinquency. One study found that male youths with ADHD had arrest rates more than twice those of controls (Farrington, Loeber, & Van Kammen, 1990, as cited in U.S. Congress Office of Technology Assessment, 1991). Similarly, male youth with conduct disorders are at increased risk for alcohol and substance abuse (Kazdin, 1989). Finally, neuropsychological testing reveals a variety of cognitive differences between nonaggressive, matched control adolescents and aggressive, violent adolescents (Moffitt, 1990, as cited in Earls, Cairns & Mercy, 1993).

The Role of Dispositional Characteristics

Self-esteem, depression, and locus of control have often been cited as theoretical predictors of risk-taking behavior. Lower self-esteem has been associated with sexual debut in adolescent females (Orr, Wilbrandt, Brack, Rauch, & Ingersoll, 1989). Depressive mood and stress are related to initiation and intensity of adolescent tobacco use (Covey & Tam, 1990) and, more recently, to various risky sexual behaviors in both adolescent males and females (Crepaz & Marks, 2001). Depression and external locus of control have been implicated in substance use (Baumrind, 1987; Dielman, Campanelli, Shope, & Butchart, 1987). Additionally, Kohler (1996) examined the relationship between locus of control, sensation seeking, critical-thinking skills, and risk taking among adolescents. He found a significant correlation between risk taking and gender, critical thinking, and locus of control. Research has not supported a consistent role for any of these psychological factors, however (Dryfoos, 1990; McCord, 1990; Spitalnick, Younge, Sales, DiClemente, Crosby, & Salazar, under review).

Beyond the Psychological

In summary, cognitive factors such as risk perception and decision making contribute to adolescent risk taking. Adolescents' decision-making processes appear to differ little from their adult counterparts, although differences appear in the content of issues they bring to bear on their decisions. Adolescents lack adult experience interacting with the social and environmental world in general and engaging in decision making specifically. Their judgments cannot reflect the influence of these experiences. Secondly, the influence of peers peaks in early to middle adolescence, as reflected by the high levels of conformity at this age. As a result, decisions during this period may rely more heavily on peer input. Finally, adolescents appear to give greater weight to short-term potential consequences than long-term ones.

The relative strength of the influences on adolescent risk-related decision making may reflect young people's tendencies toward unconventionality and sensation seeking. Although the tendency toward sensation seeking is clearly related to increased rates of risk-taking behaviors, not all risk-taking behavior can be construed as sensation seeking. Psychological disequilibrium in the form of excessive aggression, impulsivity, and attention deficit and conduct disorders increase the likelihood of adolescents engaging in risk-taking behavior. And although depression has been linked to substance abuse and risky sexual behaviors, the role of depressive mood in other types of risk behavior has yet to be established. The evidence for a causal role for self-esteem and locus of control is unclear.

Biological and psychological factors are themselves important determinants of risk-taking behavior. They also are the personal filters through which social and environmental stimuli are interpreted and translated into action.

SOCIAL AND ENVIRONMENTAL THEORIES OF RISK TAKING

Social or environmental models of risk-taking behavior look at the roles of peers, parents, family structure and function, and institutions (school and church) in risk-taking behaviors. These theories examine how social and environmental contexts provide models, opportunities, and reinforcements for adolescent participation in risk-taking behaviors. The roles of family, peers, and society in risk-taking behaviors are presented in turn here.

The Role of Family

Adolescence is a time of emerging autonomy and individuation from the family. Recent evidence suggests that most adolescents maintain close relations with their parents despite the "minor perturbations" accompanying this transition (Steinberg, 1993). Moreover, the majority of adolescents cope successfully with the demands of physical, cognitive, and emotional development during this time period (Cicchetti & Rogosch, 2002). As a result, a model of transformation, realignment, and revision of roles and expectations has largely replaced traditional views of adolescent "storm and stress." Consistent with this view, parents continue to influence their children's behavior throughout adolescence.

Parents play an important role in determining adolescent involvement in risk behaviors. Adolescents may "learn" to engage in risk-taking behavior by observing their parents' behavior. Parental modeling of and permissive attitudes toward substance use have been implicated in the initiation of substance use in early adolescence (Hawkins & Fitzgibbon, 1993; Werner, 1991). Adolescents are less likely to abuse substances and to initiate sexual activity when parents provide emotional support and acceptance and have a close relationship with their children (Turner, Irwin, Tschann, & Millstein, 1993).

Family structure correlates fairly consistently with adolescent risk-taking behavior. Adolescents from single-parent families are more likely to use illicit substances (Flewelling & Bauman, 1990). Female adolescents from single-parent families are more likely to initiate intercourse and less likely to use contraception than their peers from intact families (Hayes, 1987; Mosher & McNalley, 1991). The nature of the relationship between family structure and adolescent risk-taking behavior is unclear. Newcomer and Udry (1987), for example, found that male adolescents' initiation of sexual intercourse was more closely related to disruption of a two-parent household than living in a single-parent household per se. The association of risk-taking behaviors with single-parent families may be related to lower levels of adolescent supervision. A recent study found a two-fold increase in substance use among eighth graders who took care of themselves after school as compared to their supervised peers (Richardson et al., 1989).

Parental monitoring has been widely studied as an important correlate of adolescent risk-taking behavior (Jaccard & Dittus, 1991). Monitoring and supervision incorporates both communication between parent and child, and supervision of the youth. Borawski, Ieveres-Landis, Lovegreen, and Trapl (2003) found that perceived parental monitoring combined with trust served as a significant protective factor against sexual activity for both genders, and against tobacco and marijuana use in females and alcohol use in male adolescents. Less parental monitoring has been associated with increased participation in antisocial activities, sexual risk taking, and increased substance use or abuse (Chilcoat, Breslau, & Anthony, 1996; Mulhall et al., 1996; Smith & Rosenthal, 1995; Steinberg, 1990).

Clearly the influence of family structure and monitoring on adolescent risk taking is related to characteristics of the parent-child relationship. In one study the effects of family structure on adolescent risk taking were no longer significant when sociodemographic variables and the emotional distance between parents and adolescent children were taken into account (Forman, Irwin, and Turner, 1990).

Parental influence on adolescent behavior appears to vary with the quality of the relationship between the adolescent and the parent. High levels of familial conflict are associated with increased rates of adolescent risk-taking behaviors. Bijur, Kurzon, Hamelsky, and Power (1991) noted that compared to youth from low-conflict families, British youth from families reporting a high degree of adolescent-parent conflict were almost three times as likely to report having injuries requiring hospitalization. Family cohesion, on the other hand, is associated with lower rates of sexual activity and substance use among early adolescents (Turner et al., 1993).

Parent-child relationships characterized by conflict, increased emotional distance, and nonresponsiveness increase the likelihood of adolescents engaging in risk behaviors.

Parental approaches to child rearing may influence adolescents' likelihood of engaging in risk-taking behaviors. Baumrind (1991) found an association between adolescent substance use and parenting styles. Adolescents whose parents were "authoritative" (demanding and responsive) were less likely to use substances than either those with "authoritarian" (demanding but unresponsive) or those with "permissive" (nondemanding but responsive) parents. Adolescent with "neglecting and rejecting" parents were the most likely to engage in substance abuse.

In summary, family approval and modeling of risk behavior has been linked to adolescent risk-taking behavior. Family structure is also related to adolescent risk-taking behavior; however, the relationship appears to be mediated by the nature of parent-child interactions. Parent-child relationships characterized by conflict, increased emotional distance, and nonresponsiveness increase the likelihood of adolescents engaging in risk behaviors.

The Role of Peers

One of the developmental tasks of adolescence involves individuation from the family and identification with a peer group. As a result, parental impact on risk-taking behavior may wane as peer influences increase throughout adolescence. According to Jessor and Jessor (1977), the relatively greater influence of peers compared to parents is associated with a greater tendency (or proneness) toward problem behaviors. Consistent with this theory, Jessor and colleagues found that the relative dominance of peer influence over parental influence predicted marijuana use, problem drinking, and precocious sexual debut (Jessor, Chase, & Donovan, 1980; Jessor, Costa, Jessor, & Donovan, 1983).

Peer influence has been cited as a factor in adolescent substance use (Kandel, 1985; Newcomb & Bentler, 1989; Heights & Jenkins, 1996), alcohol use (Urberg, Degirmencioglu, & Pilgram, 1997), delinquency (McCord, 1990), and sexual behaviors. Billy and Udry (1985) found, for example, that a white virgin adolescent female whose best male and female friends were sexually active was almost certain to become sexually active within two years. Also, adolescents are usually accompanied by one or more persons when committing crimes that range in seriousness from vandalism and drug use (Erickson & Jensen, 1977) to rape and homicide (Zimring, 1998).

One explanation of how peers exert influence on adolescent risk taking is put forth by Lashbrook (2000), who demonstrated that older adolescents may attempt to avoid negative emotions, such as feelings of isolation and inadequacy, by participating in risky behaviors with peers. Traditionally, "peer pressure" has been viewed as an etiologic factor in adolescent risk-taking behavior. However, it is still unclear whether risk behaviors are initiated in order to conform to an existing peer group or whether those inclined to engage in risk-taking behaviors are drawn to those who are similarly inclined.

The Role of Society

Societal influences such as mass media and community norms may also influence risk-taking behavior. Role models for such behavior are regularly presented by the media (including unprotected sexual behavior and alcohol use), though evidence for the influence of these models on actual behavior is lacking. Different communities and neighborhoods provide adolescents with opportunities and motivations to engage in risk-taking behavior. Local peer norms reflected in local rates of substance use and teen pregnancy create expectations of "typical" adolescent behavior (Crockett & Petersen, 1993). Local ordinances permitting cigarette vending machines or lower ages to purchase alcohol provide opportunities to engage in risk-taking behavior. Johnston, O'Malley, and Bachman (1993) have shown, however, that the perceived availability of marijuana in a community is not necessarily related to prevalence of use by adolescents. Declines in marijuana use by high school seniors have been accompanied by unchanged or even increased perceived availability in recent years.

Cultural expectations may influence the onset of risk-taking behavior. For example, despite similar ages of sexual debut, the United States has the highest rates of adolescent childbearing and abortion in the developed world (Martin et al., 2006). These rates are thought to be related to differing cultural attitudes toward adolescent sexuality and contraception (Geronimus, 2003). Even within the United States, contraception rates vary significantly by ethnicity and religious affiliation (Brewster, Cooksey, Guilkey, & Rindfuss, 1998; Santelli, Morrow, & Carter, 2004). Rates of adolescent substance use and early sexual debut also differ among different ethnic groups (Guerra, Romano, Samuels, & Kass, 2000; Cavanagh, 2004). (Ethnicity-associated differences may be confounded by factors related to socioeconomic status.)

Beyond Environment

The range of theories reflects the complexity of the interaction between adolescents and their social world. The biopsychosocial model provides a framework in which social environmental factors are brought to bear on existing biological and psychological predispositions to influence risk-taking behavior.

THE BIOPSYCHOSOCIAL MODEL OF RISK TAKING

The *biopsychosocial model* integrates two areas of research that have often been considered separately: (1) the relationship of biological development to psychosocial processing during adolescence, and (2) the relationship of risk-taking behaviors to psychosocial correlates of these behaviors. Specifically, according to this model, biological, psychological, and social or environmental factors influence adolescent risk-taking behaviors (Irwin & Millstein, 1986). The timing of biological maturation directly influences four areas of psychosocial functioning: cognition, perceptions of self, perceptions of the social environment, and personal values. According to this model, biological, psychological, and social or environmental variables—mediated by perceptions of risk and peer-group characteristics—then predict adolescent risk taking. Biological variables influencing adolescent risk-taking behavior include pubertal timing, hormonal effects, and genetic predispositions. Psychological variables associated with risk taking include self-esteem, sensation seeking, and cognitive and affective states. Social influences on adolescent risk taking include peers, parents, and school (see Figure 3.1).

Given the framework of the biopsychosocial perspective, Irwin and colleagues (Irwin, 1990; Irwin & Millstein, 1986; Irwin & Ryan, 1989) have elaborated on the theory to include conditions that may increase the probability that a given adolescent will engage in risk-taking behaviors (see Figure 3.2). Biological factors thought to

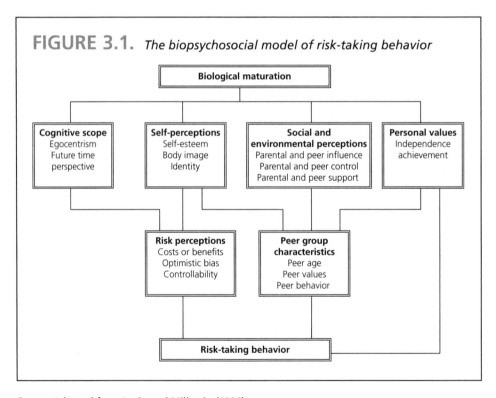

FIGURE 3.1. *The biopsychosocial model of risk-taking behavior*

Source: Adapted from Irwin and Millstein (1986).

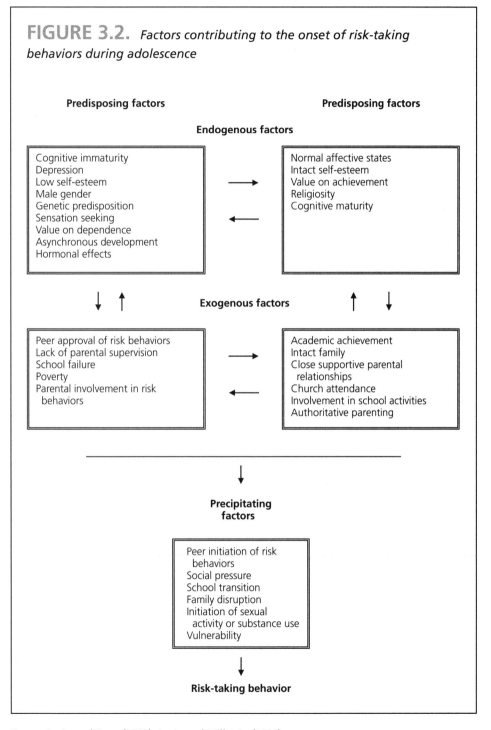

FIGURE 3.2. *Factors contributing to the onset of risk-taking behaviors during adolescence*

Predisposing factors   **Predisposing factors**

Endogenous factors

Cognitive immaturity
Depression
Low self-esteem
Male gender
Genetic predisposition
Sensation seeking
Value on dependence
Asynchronous development
Hormonal effects

Normal affective states
Intact self-esteem
Value on achievement
Religiosity
Cognitive maturity

Exogenous factors

Peer approval of risk behaviors
Lack of parental supervision
School failure
Poverty
Parental involvement in risk
  behaviors

Academic achievement
Intact family
Close supportive parental
  relationships
Church attendance
Involvement in school activities
Authoritative parenting

**Precipitating
factors**

Peer initiation of risk
  behaviors
Social pressure
School transition
Family disruption
Initiation of sexual
  activity or substance use
Vulnerability

Risk-taking behavior

Source: Irwin and Ryan (1989); Irwin and Millstein (1986).

predispose adolescents to risk-taking behaviors include male gender, genetic predispositions, and hormonal influences. Psychological predisposing factors include sensation seeking, risk perception, depression, and low self-esteem. Social and environmental predisposing factors include maladaptive parenting styles, parental modeling of risk behaviors, peer behaviors, and socioeconomic status. Finally, adolescent vulnerability to risk-taking behaviors may be increased situationally by family disruption, school transitions, substance use, and peer initiation of risk-taking behaviors.

Support for the Biopsychosocial Model

Support for the biopsychosocial model comes from a number of sources. Early maturational timing is associated with a more negative self-image and, among female adolescents, with earlier onset of sexual activity (Brooks-Gunn, 1988). Early maturation is a risk factor for the initiation of substance use in both male and female adolescents (Tschann et al., 1994). Studies by Jessor and Jessor (1977) support the role of perceived environment and personal values in the onset of adolescent risk-taking behavior—specifically, the predominance of peer over parental influence and the greater personal value placed on independence than achievement resulted in a greater likelihood of adolescents engaging in risk-taking behavior. Among Japanese students, results from a structural equation analysis showed that egocentrism contributes directly to health-endangering behaviors, whereas influences of self-esteem and perceived social norms are mediated by risk perception (Omori & Ingersoll, 2005). Moreover, Hughes and colleagues (1991) conducted a study with urban delinquent youth and concluded that alcohol and substance abuse during adolescence added to biological predispositions, educational difficulties, and coercive family environments, all of which contribute to delinquent behavior.

Several recent review articles also provide support for the utility of the biopsychosocial model in explaining disordered eating, conduct problems, and aggression and delinquency in adolescents. Disordered eating and the pursuit of muscularity in adolescent males are consistently associated with biological factors such as body mass index (BMI), psychological factors such as negative affect and self-esteem, and sociocultural factors such as perceived pressure to lose weight by parents and peers (Ricciardelli & McCabe, 2004). Dodge and Pettit (2003) conducted a review of the empirical findings pertaining to the development of chronic conduct problems in adolescence. They concluded that reciprocal influences among biological dispositions, contexts, and life experiences lead to recursive iterations over time that either worsen or diminish antisocial development. Additionally, adolescents' cognitive and emotional processes mediate the relationship between life experiences and conduct problems. Finally, a review by Celio, Karnik, and Steiner (2006) found that early maturation is a risk factor for aggression and delinquent behavior in adolescent girls. However, the way in which early physical maturation is perceived and treated by family, peers, and society often determines how adolescent girls respond. Thus, across various behavioral domains, research supports the utility of the biopsychosocial model for explaining adolescent risk taking.

SUMMARY

Because of the complexity of the biopsychosocial approach, it has been difficult to empirically examine all the factors making up the model in one study. However, with recent advances in technology and a concerted effort by researchers (and funding agencies) to engage in interdisciplinary collaborations to more thoroughly examine complex human behaviors, future research may be able to do so.

For instance, the recent mapping of the human genome allows for exploration of the biological underpinnings of behavior and cognition in ways not possible even a decade ago. Advances in gene mapping have led to findings implicating particular genes in alcoholism and substance use disorders (Conner et al., 2005). Also, genetic markers for impulsivity and depression are currently being explored, and the identification of other genetic markers that predispose adolescents toward various risk-taking behaviors may be on the horizon.

Advances in brain imaging science have allowed researchers to examine the brain across development stages and while engaging in problem solving. Neuroimaging studies have revealed that decision making in adult brains is composed of two networks: a highly interconnected cognitive-control network that biases decisions in favor of rational outcomes and a socioemotional network that biases decision making toward reward-based demands (Chein, 2008). The cognitive-control network can regulate the behavior of the socioemotional network, allowing for people to make rational, utilitarian decisions. However, neither of these systems is fully matured during adolescence, and each one develops along different timetables (Giedd, 2008). Therefore, these two underdeveloped networks and their differing rates of development pave the way for heightened risk taking during adolescence, which, as demonstrated by Gardner and Steinberg's (2005) work with teen drivers, may be further compounded by the influence of peers and other social and environmental factors. Although great scientific advances have been made through neuroimaging studies, our understanding of the relationship between neuroimaging findings and behavior is still in its infancy and a subject of great academic interest and active research. Demonstrating straightforward relationships between the size of, or neural activity in, a particular brain region and a specific behavior or ability has been rather elusive to date (Giedd, 2008).

Technological advances have also improved researchers' ability to assess adolescent risk taking, as well as psychological and environmental influences on risk taking. For example, it is now possible to detect through self-collected vaginal swab specimens (Yc PCR) the presence of semen in vaginal fluid. These can then be used as nondisease markers of unprotected intercourse (Zenilman, Yuenger, Galai, Turner, & Rogers, 2005). Novel techniques such as GeoCoding allow researchers to spatially place participants in their physical neighborhoods, which are then mapped onto census data to establish neighborhood profiles. These provide an objective measure of neighborhood-level social conditions including socioeconomic status, racial makeup, and population density.

Thus, in the coming years it will be possible to explore biological influence on behavior and the interaction between biology, psychology, environment, and adolescent risk-taking behavior in ways not possible before. The utility of complex models of adolescent risk taking like the biopsychosocial model will prove invaluable in guiding the next generation of adolescent risk-taking research.

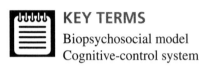

KEY TERMS

Biopsychosocial model   Risk
Cognitive-control system   Sensation seeking

DISCUSSION QUESTIONS

1. Compare and contrast biologically based theories of risk-taking behavior with psychologically based theories of risk-taking behavior. What are the main components of each?

2. Discuss the role of parents and peers using a social-environmental approach to understanding adolescent risk-taking behavior. How do relationships with parents and peers change during adolescence?

3. Of the future directions and novel approaches for using the biopsychosocial model described at the end of this chapter, which technological advance could prove most valuable in understanding adolescent risk taking? Explain your choice.

REFERENCES

Adger, H. (1991). Problems of alcohol and other drug abuse in adolescents. *Journal of Adolescent Health, 12,* 606–613.

Andrucci, G. L., Archer, R. P., Pancoast, D. L., & Gordon, R. A. (1989). The relationship of MMPI and sensation seeking scales to adolescent drug use. *Journal of Personality Assessment, 53,* 253–266.

Baumrind, D. (1987). A developmental perspective on adolescent risk taking in contemporary America. In C. E. Irwin (Ed.), *Adolescent social behavior and health. New Directions for Child Development,* No. 37 (pp. 93–125). San Francisco: Jossey Bass.

Baumrind, D. (1991). The influence of parenting style on adolescent competence and substance abuse. *Journal of Early Adolescence, 11,* 56–95.

Beyth-Marom, R., Austin, L., Fischoff, B., Palmgren, C., & Jacobs-Quadrel, M. (1993). Perceived consequences of risky behaviors: Adults and adolescents. *Developmental Psychology, 29,* 549–563.

Beyth-Marom, R., & Fischoff, B. (1997). Adolescents' decisions about risks: A cognitive perspective. In J. Schulenberg & J. L. Maggs (Eds.), *Health risks and developmental transitions during adolescence* (pp. 110–135). New York: Cambridge University Press.

Bijur, P. E., Kurzon, M., Hamelsky, V., & Power, C. (1991). Parent-adolescent conflict and adolescent injuries. *Journal of Developmental and Behavioral Pediatrics, 12,* 92–97.

Billy, J. O. G., & Udry, J. R. (1985). The influence of male and female best friends on adolescent sexual behavior. *Adolescence, 20,* 21–32.

Borawski, E., Ievers-Landis, C. E., Lovegreen, L. D., & Trapl, E. S. (2003). Parental monitoring, negotiated unsupervised time, and parental trust: The role of perceived parenting practices in adolescent health risk behaviors. *Journal of Adolescent Health, 33,* 60–70.

Brewster, K. L., Cooksey, E. C., Guilkey, D. K., and Rindfuss, R. R. (1998). The changing impact of religion on the sexual and contraceptive behavior of adolescent women in the United States. *Journal of Marriage and Family, 60,* 493–504.

Brooks-Gunn, J. (1988). Antecedents and consequences of variations in girls' maturational timing. *Journal of Adolescent Health Care, 9,* 1–9.

Cavanagh, S. E. (2004). The sexual debut of girls in early adolescence: The intersection of race, pubertal timing, and friendship group characteristics. *Journal of Research on Adolescence, 14,* 285.

Celio, M., Karnik, N. S., & Steiner, H. (2006). Early maturation as a risk factor for aggression and delinquency in adolescent girls: A review. *International Journal of Clinical Practice, 60,* 1254–1262.

Centers for Disease Control and Prevention. (2008). Births: Preliminary data for 2006. *National Vital Statistics Reports, 56,* 1–18.

Chein, J. (2008). Linking risk-taking behavior and peer influence in adolescents. *Neuropsychiatry Reviews, 9,* 1.

Chilcoat, H. D., Breslau, N., & Anthony, J. C. (1996). Potential barriers to parent monitoring: Social disadvantage, marital status, and maternal psychiatric disorder. *Journal of the American Academy of Child and Adolescent Psychiatry, 35*(12), 1673–1682.

Cicchetti, D., & Rogosch, F. A. (2002). A developmental psychopathology perspective on adolescence. *Journal of Consulting and Clinical Psychology, 70*(1), 6–20.

Cloninger, C. R. (1987). Neurogenetic adaptive mechanisms in alcoholism. *Science, 236,* 410–416.

Conner, B. T., Noble, E. P., Berman, S. M., Ozkaragoz, T., Ritchie, T., Antolin, T., & Sheen, C. (2005). DRD2 genotypes and substance use in adolescent children of alcoholics. *Drug and Alcohol Dependence, 79,* 379–387.

Covey, L. S., & Tam, D. (1990). Depressive mood, the single-parent home and adolescent cigarette smoking. *American Journal of Public Health, 80*(11), 1330–1333.

Crepaz, N., & Marks, G. (2001). Are negative affective states associated with HIV sexual risk behaviors? A meta-analytic review. *Health Psychology, 20*(4), 291–299.

Crockett, L. J., & Petersen, A. C. (1993). Adolescent development: Health risks and opportunities for health promotion. In S. G. Millstein, A. C. Petersen, & E. O. Nightingale (Eds.), *Promoting the health of adolescents: New directions for the twenty-first century* (pp. 13–37). New York: Oxford University Press.

Dielman, T. E., Campanelli, P. C., Shope, J. T., & Butchart, A. T. (1987). Susceptibility to peer pressure, self-esteem, and health locus of control as correlates of adolescent substance abuse. *Health Education Quarterly, 14,* 207–221.

Dodge, K. A., & Pettit, G. (2003). A biopsychosocial model of the development of chronic conduct problems in adolescence. *Developmental Psychology, 39,* 349–371.

Dryfoos, J. G. (1990). *Adolescents at risk.* Oxford, England: Oxford University Press.

Earls, F., Cairns, R. B., & Mercy, J. A. (1993). The control of violence and the promotion of nonviolence in adolescents. In S. G. Millstein, A. C. Petersen, & E. O. Nightingale (Eds.), *Promoting the health of adolescents: New directions for the twenty-first century* (pp. 285–304). New York: Oxford University Press.

Erickson, M., & Jensen, G. F. (1977). Delinquency is still a group behavior: Toward revitalizing the group premise of the sociology of deviance. *Journal of Criminal Law and Criminology, 68,* 262–273.

Fingerhut, L. A., & Anderson, R. N. (2008). The three leading causes of injury mortality in the United States, 1999–2005. Retrieved May 16, 2008, from www.cdc.gov/nchs/products/pubs/pubd/hestats/injury99-05/injury99-05.htm#other_ages AT.

Fischoff, B. (1992). Risk taking: A developmental perspective. In J. F. Yates (Ed.), *Risk-taking behavior* (pp. 132–162). New York: Wiley.

Flay, B. R. (1985). Psychosocial approaches to smoking prevention: A review of findings. *Health Psychology, 4*(5), 449–488.

Flewelling, R. L., & Bauman, K. E. (1990). Family structure as a predictor of initial substance use and sexual intercourse in early adolescence. *Journal of Marriage and Family, 52,* 171–181.

Ford, C. A., Pence, B. W., Miller, W. C., Resnick, M. D., Bearinger, L. H., Pettingell, S., & Cohen, M. (2005). Predicting adolescents' longitudinal risk for sexually transmitted infection: Results from the National Longitudinal Study of Adolescent Health. *Archives of Pediatric and Adolescent Medicine, 159*(7), 657–664.

Forman, S., Irwin, C. E. Jr., & Turner, R. (1990). Family structure, emotional distancing and risk-taking behavior in adolescence. *Pediatric Research, 27,* 5A.

Gardner, M., & Steinberg, L. (2005). Peer influence on risk-taking, risk preference, and risky decision making in adolescence and adulthood: An experimental study. *Developmental Psychology, 41,* 625–635.

Geronimus, A. T. (2003). Damned if you do: Culture, identity, privilege, and teenage childbearing in the United States. *Social Science & Medicine, 57,* 881–893.

Giedd, J. N. (2008). The teen brain: Insights from neuroimaging. *Journal of Adolescent Health, 42,* 335–343.

Greening, L., & Dollinger, S. J. (1991). Adolescent smoking and perceived vulnerability to smoking-related causes of death. *Journal of Pediatric Psychology, 16*(6), 687–699.

Grumbaum, J. A., Kann, L., Kinchen, S., Ross, J., Hawkins, J., Lowry, R., Harris, W. A., Mc Manus, T., Chyen, D., & Collins, J. (2004). Youth risk behavior surveillance: United States, 2003. *MMWR Surveillance Summaries, 53,* 1–96.

Guerra, L. M., Romano, P. S., Samuels, S. J., & Kass, P. H. (2000). Ethnic differences in adolescent substance initiation sequences. *Archives of Pediatric Adolescent Medicine, 154,* 1089–1095.

Hawkins, J. D., & Fitzgibbon, J. J. (1993). Risk factors and risk behaviors in prevention of adolescent substance abuse. *Adolescent Medicine: State of the Art Reviews, 4*(2), 249–262.

Hayes, C. (1987). *Risking the future: Adolescent sexuality, pregnancy, and childbearing* (Vol. 1). Washington, DC: National Academy Press.

Heights, R., & Jenkins, J. E. (1996). The influence of peer affiliation and student activities on adolescent drug involvement. *Adolescence, 122,* 297–309.

Hughes, J. R., Zagar, R., Sylvies, R. B., Arbit, J., Busch, K. G., & Bowers, N. D. (1991). Medical, family, and scholastic conditions in urban delinquents. *Journal of Clinical Psychology, 47,* 448–464.

Irwin, C. E., Jr. (1990). The theoretical concept of at-risk adolescents. *Adolescent Medicine: State of the Art Reviews, 1,* 1–14.

Irwin, C. E., Jr., & Millstein, S. G. (1986). Biopsychosocial correlates of risk-taking behaviors during adolescence. *Journal of Adolescent Health Care, 7,* 82S–96S.

Irwin, C. E., Jr., & Ryan, S. A. (1989). Problem behaviors of adolescence. *Pediatrics in Review, 10,* 235–246.

Jaccard, J., & Dittus, P. (1991). *Parent-teen communication: Toward the prevention of unintended pregnancies.* New York: Springer-Verlag.

Jessor, R. (1976). Predicting time of onset of marijuana use: A developmental study of high school youth. *Journal of Consulting and Clinical Psychology, 44,* 125–134.

Jessor, R., Chase, C. A., & Donovan, J. E. (1980). Psychosocial correlates of marijuana use and problem drinking in a national sample of adolescents. *American Journal of Public Health, 70,* 604–613.

Jessor, R., Costa, F., Jessor, L., & Donovan, J. E. (1983). Time of first intercourse: A prospective study. *Journal of Personality and Social Psychology, 44,* 608–626.

Jessor, R., & Jessor, S. L. (1977). *Problem behavior and psychological development: A longitudinal study of youth.* New York: Academic Press.

Johnston, L. D., O'Malley, P. M., & Bachman J. G. (1993). *National survey results on drug use from the Monitoring the Future Study, 1975–1992. Volume I: Secondary school students* (NIH publication no. 93-3597). Bethesda, MD: National Institute on Drug Abuse.

Johnston, L. D., O'Malley, P. M., Bachman, J. G., & Schulenberg, J. E. (2006). *Monitoring the Future: National results on adolescent drug use. Overview of key findings, 2005* (NIH publication no. 06-5882) Bethesda, MD: National Institute on Drug Abuse.

Kaestle, C. E., Halpern, C. T., Miller, W. C., & Ford, C. A. (2005). Young age at first sexual intercourse and sexually transmitted infections in adolescents and young adults. *American Journal of Epidemiology, 161*(8), 774–780.

Kalichman, S. C., & Rompa, D. (1995). Sexual sensation seeking and sexual compulsivity scales: Reliability, validity, and predicting HIV risk behaviors. *Journal of Personality Assessment, 65,* 586–602.

Kandel, D. B. (1985). On processes of peer influences in adolescent drug use: A developmental perspective, *Advances in Alcohol and Substance Abuse, 4*(3–4), 139–163.

Kazdin, A. E. (1989). Developmental psychopathology: Current research, issues and directions. *American Psychologist, 44,* 180–187.

Keating, D. P. (1990). Adolescent thinking. In S. S. Feldman & G. R. Elliot (Eds.), *At the threshold: The developing adolescent* (pp. 54–89). Cambridge, MA: Harvard University Press.

Kegeles, S. M., Adler, N. E., & Irwin, C. E., Jr. (1988). Sexually active adolescents and condoms: Changes over one year in knowledge, attitudes and use. *American Journal of Public Health, 78,* 460–461.

Kohler, M. P. (1996). Risk-taking behavior: A cognitive approach. *Psychological Reports, 78,* 489–490.

Lashbrook, J. T. (2000). Fitting in: Exploring the emotional dimension of adolescent peer pressure. *Adolescence, 35,* 277–294.

Manning, W. D., Longmore, M. A., & Giordano, P. C. (2000). The relationship context of contraceptive use at first intercourse. *Family Planning Perspectives, 32*(2), 104–110.

Marlatt, G. A., Baer, J. S., Donovan, D. M., & Kivlahan, D. R. (1988). Addictive behaviors: Etiology and treatment. *Annual Review of Psychology, 39,* 223–252.

Martin, J. A., Hamilton, B. E., Sutton, P. D., Ventura, S. J., Menacker F., & Kirmeyer, S. (2006). Births: Final data for 2004. *National Vital Statistics Reports, 55*(1), 1–101.

McCord, J. (1990). Problem behaviors. In S. S. Feldman & G. R. Elliot (Eds.), *At the threshold: The developing adolescent* (pp. 414–429). Cambridge, MA: Harvard University Press.

Millstein, S. G., & Halpern-Felsher, B. L. (2002). Perceptions of risk and vulnerability. *Journal of Adolescent Health, 31S,* 10–27.

Mosher, W. D., & McNalley, J. W. (1991). Contraceptive use at first premarital intercourse: United States, 1965–1988. *Family Planning Perspectives, 23,* 108–116.

Mulhall, P. F., Stone, D., & Stone, B. (1996). Home alone: Is it a risk factor for middle school youth and drug use? *Journal of Drug Education, 26*(1), 39–48.

Newcomb, M. D., & Bentler, P. M. (1989). Substance use and abuse among children and teenagers. *American Psychologist, 44,* 242–248.

Newcomb, M. D., & McGee, L. (1991). Influence of sensation seeking on general deviance and specific problem behaviors from adolescence to adulthood. *Journal of Personality and Social Psychology, 61,* 614–628.

Newcomer, S., & Udry, J. R. (1987). Parental marital status effects on adolescent sexual behavior. *Journal of Marriage and Family, 49,* 235–240.

Omori, M., & Ingersoll, G. M. (2005). Health-endangering behaviors among Japanese college students: Test of a psychological model of risk-taking behaviors. *Journal of Adolescence, 28,* 17–33.

Orr, D. P., Wilbrandt, M. L., Brack, C. J., Rauch, S. P., & Ingersoll, G. M. (1989). Reported sexual behaviors and self-esteem among young adolescents. *American Journal of Diseases of Children, 143,* 86–90.

Park, M. J., Mulye, T. P., Adams, S. H., Brindis, C., & Irwin, C. E., Jr. (2006). The health status of young adults in the U.S. *Journal of Adolescent Health, 29,* 305–317.

Phinney, V. G., Jensen, L. C., Olsen, J. A., & Cundick, B. (1990). The relationship between early development and psychosexual behaviors in adolescent females. *Adolescence, 98,* 321–332.

Reyna, V., & Farley, F. (2006). Risk and rationality in adolescent decision-making: Implications for theory, practice, and public policy. *Psychological Science in the Public Interest, 7,* 1–44.

Ricciardelli, L. A., & McCabe, M. P. (2004). A biopsychosocial model of disordered eating and the pursuit of muscularity in adolescent boys. *Psychological Bulletin, 30,* 179–205.

Richardson, J. L., Dwyer, K., McGuigan, K., Hansen, W. B., Dent, C., Johnson, C. A., Sussman, S. Y., Brannon, B., & Flay, B. (1989). Substance use among eighth-grade students who take care of themselves after school. *Pediatrics, 84,* 556–566.

Santelli, J. S., Morrow, B., & Carter, M. (2004). Trends in contraceptive use among US high school students in the 1990s. *Journal of Adolescent Health, 34,* 140.

Schor, E. L. (1987). Unintentional injuries: Patterns within families. *American Journal of Diseases of Children, 141,* 1280–1284.

Smith, A. M. A., & Rosenthal, D. A. (1995). Adolescents' perceptions of their risk environment. *Journal of Adolescence, 18,* 229–245.

Snyder, H. N. (2000). *Juvenile arrests, 1999*. Washington, DC: Office of Juvenile Justice and Delinquency Prevention.

Spitalnick, J. S., Younge, S., Sales, J. M., DiClemente, R. J., Crosby, R. A., & Salazar, L. F. (under review). Adolescent depression, HIV/STD-associated sexual risk taking, and outcomes of unprotected sex: A review of the empirical literature from the last 20 years. *Current Pediatric Reviews*.

Steinberg, L. (1990). Autonomy conflict and harmony in the family relationship. In S. S. Feldman & G. R. Elliot (Eds.) *At the threshold: The developing adolescent* (pp. 255–275). Cambridge, MA: Harvard University Press.

Steinberg, L. (2004). Risk-taking in adolescence: What changes, and why? *Annals of the New York Academy of Sciences, 1021,* 51–58.

Steinberg, L. (2007). Risk taking in adolescence: New perspectives from brain and behavioral science. *Current Directions in Psychological Science, 16,* 55–59.

Sullivan, M., & Terry, R. L. (1998). Perceived virulence of germs from a liked versus disliked source: Evidence of magical contagion. *Journal of Adolescent Health, 22,* 320–325.

Tonkin, R. S. (1987). Adolescent risk-taking behavior. *Journal of Adolescent Health Care, 8,* 213–220.

Tschann, J. M., Adler, N. E., Irwin, C. E., Jr., Millstein, S. G., Turner, R. A., & Kegeles, S. M. (1994). Initiation of substance use in early adolescence: The roles of pubertal timing and emotional distress. *Health Psychology, 13,* 326–333.

Turner, R. A., Irwin, C. E., Jr., Tschann, J. M., & Millstein, S. G. (1993). Autonomy, relatedness, and the initiation of health risk behaviors in early adolescence. *Health Psychology, 12*(3), 200–208.

Udry, J. R., Billy, J. O. G., Morris, N. M., Groff, T. R., & Raj, M. H. (1985). Serum androgenic hormones motivate sexual behavior in adolescent boys. *Fertility and Sterility, 43*(1), 90–94.

Udry, J. R., Talbert, L. M., & Morris, N. M. (1986). Biosocial foundations for adolescent female sexuality. *Demography, 23,* 217–227.

Urberg, K. A., Degirmencioglu, S. M., & Pilgram, C. (1997). Close friends and group influence on adolescent cigarette smoking and alcohol use. *Developmental Psychology, 33*(5), 834–844.

U.S. Congress Office of Technology Assessment. (1991). *Adolescent health. Volume II: Background and the effectiveness of selected prevention and treatment services* (Publication No. OTA-H-466). Washington, DC: U.S. Government Printing Office.

U.S. Preventive Services Task Force. (1989). *Guide to clinical preventive services*. Baltimore: Williams & Wilkins.

Werner, M. J. (1991). Adolescent substance abuse. *Maternal and Child Health Technical Information Bulletin*. Cincinnati, OH: National Center for Education in Maternal and Child Health.

Working Group of the NIH Advisory Committee. (2004). Report of the Working Group of the NIH Advisory Committee to the Director on Research Opportunities in the Basic Behavioral and Social Sciences. Retrieved May 16, 2008, from http://obssr.od.nih.gov/Documents/BSSRCC/Meetings/Minutes/Minutes_2005/Basic%20Beh%20Report_complete.pdf.

Zenilman, J. M., Yuenger, J., Galai, N., Turner, C. F., & Rogers, S. M. (2005). Polymerase chain reaction detection of Y chromosome sequences in vaginal fluid: Preliminary studies of a potential biomarker for sexual behavior. *Sexually Transmitted Diseases, 32*(2), 90–94.

Zimring, F. E. (1998). *American youth violence*. Oxford, England: Oxford University Press.

Zuckerman, M. (1979). *Sensation seeking: Beyond the optimal level of arousal*. Hillsdale, NJ: Erlbaum.

Zuckerman, M. (1990). The psychophysiology of sensation seeking. *Journal of Personality, 58,* 313–341.

Zuckerman, M. (1991). Sensation seeking: The balance between risk and reward. In L. P. Lipsett & L. L. Mitnick (Eds.), *Self-regulatory behavior and risk taking: Causes and consequences* (pp. 143–152). Norwood, NJ: Ablex Publishing.

CHAPTER

4

RESILIENCE IN ADOLESCENCE

LYNNE MICHAEL BLUM ▪ ROBERT WM. BLUM

LEARNING OBJECTIVES

After studying this chapter, you will be able to

▪ Define resilience and differentiate between risk and protective factors that affect adolescent health and development.

▪ Explain the relationship between stress and resilience.

▪ Compare the efficacy of health interventions that promote resilience with those that focus only on behavior change.

This chapter provides an overview of resilience and the risk and protective factors that lead to behaviors that will either promote or compromise adolescent health and development. As will be seen, there is substantial evidence that interventions that promote resilience have a higher likelihood of affecting health risk behaviors than interventions that focus exclusively on extinguishing the behavior.

Resilience research began in 1954, when Emmy Werner launched the Children of Kauai Study, which went on to follow a cohort of young people born on the island of Kauai, Hawaii, for nearly five decades. Werner wanted to understand why some children did well socially and emotionally in the face of adversity (Werner & Smith, 1982, 1992, 2001).

Since the early 1950s, there has been a plethora of research that has aimed at understanding Werner's original question, which Garmezy subsequently reframed as "What causes strength to overcome what causes harm?" (Garmezy, 1974). Centrally, resilience research has focused on why some who are reared in adversity "rebound," while others do not.

Garmezy (1991) defined *resilience* as "the capacity to recover and maintain adaptive behavior after insult." Those who are resilient are adaptive; they are not invincible (Werner & Smith, 1982) or invulnerable (Garmezy, 1985).

Early resilience research looked inside the young person for answers to Garmezy's question. Murphy and Moriarty (1976) found resilient young people to have *social charisma*—the capacity to relate well to others, the ability to experience a range of emotions, and the ability to regulate emotions (we will return to these points later in this chapter when we discuss adolescent neurodevelopment). Likewise, Rutter (1979) found resilient young people to have high creativity, effectiveness, and competence.

Not only does resilience appear to vary depending on life circumstances, research has shown that it can be enhanced by acquiring a set of skills.

As resilience research progressed, the lens broadened beyond the individual to the environments within which he or she lives. Research began to focus on three domains: attributes of young people themselves, family factors, and the social environments in which young people live (Luthar, 2003). Rutter (1993) came to understand resilience as interactive with risk and developmental in nature, stemming from biology and experiences earlier in life. He also concluded that protective factors may operate in different ways at different stages of development (for example, parental oversight and monitoring in infancy is highly protective, but in adolescence a comparable behavior may impede healthy development).

Likewise, over the past twenty years researchers have focused on processes and regulatory systems that account for resilience. Resilience is not viewed as a state or a personality characteristic but as a "developmental progression with new vulnerabilities and strengths emerging with changing life circumstances" (Luthar, 2006).

Not only does resilience appear to vary depending on life circumstances, research has shown that it can be enhanced by acquiring a set of skills. For example, Farber and Egeland (1987) reported enhancing resilience through developing skills with maltreated children. Furthermore, Luthar (1991) described how youth with depressed mothers assumed caretaking roles that over time were developmentally maladaptive (what she labeled as "false maturity").

After looking back over a half-century of research, the following conclusions can be drawn:

> Young people can be resilient but unhappy (maturing in an abusive environment does not preclude resilience in the face of unhappiness).

> Research has underscored the interrelationships of factors that are individual, environmental, and developmental in nature and how they interact to result in adaptive or maladaptive behaviors.

> Children do not consistently show resilience across all domains of their life, and we have come to understand specific components such as *educational resilience* (Wang & Gordon, 1994) and *emotional resilience* (Denny, Clark, Fleming, & Wall, 2004).

> Failure to address the emotional needs of resilient young people increases the risk of derailing their resilience in adulthood.

> Intervention strategies can enhance resilience.

The rest of this chapter will more specifically define the terms we use and present a conceptual model for both understanding resilience and developing interventions.

DEFINING THE TERMS

Luthar, Ciccetti, and Becker (2000) define *resilience* as "a dynamic process whereby resilient individuals display positive adaptation despite experiences of significant adversity or trauma." It is important to note that resilience in this definition is a *process,* not a trait. Furthermore, resilience exists only in the face of adversity.

Vulnerability refers to a state resulting from the presence of factors (neurodevelopmental, familial, or environmental) that increase the odds of maladaptive behaviors occurring. Conversely, *protection* occurs in the presence of factors that diminish negative outcomes and increase the odds of positive adaptation.

Cofer and Appley (1964) defined *stress* as "a state where well-being (or integrity) of an individual is endangered and he must devote all his energy to its protection."

What makes an event stressful is its capacity to change an individual's usual activity. Stress demands a response. The extent of the response, as well as the extent of the experience of stress, lies predominantly in the subjective meaning given the event, rather than in its objective reality. Antonovsky (1979) identified the following four stages in response to a problem:

1. *Problem confrontation*

2. *Tension:* the inner response to the problem that has been confronted

3. *Tension management:* the speed with which the problem is confronted and resolved

4. *Stress:* a state in which the energy expended to deal with the problem exceeds the energy needed for a resolution

As the stages of stress have become better understood, the factors that buffer or exacerbate stress have likewise become clearer, including *compensatory factors* (factors that counterbalance stressful events, such as ego strength); *protective factors* (factors that are interactive with stress, such as social skills); and *vulnerability processes* (traits that increase vulnerability to stress). It is clear that stress is a real phenomenon that is heavily influenced by the meanings the individual ascribes to an event. Some factors moderate and other factors exacerbate the impact of stress—physiologically, emotionally, and functionally.

Resilience is focused more on social functioning than mental health or other outcomes.

Stress can be viewed as the interaction between the individual's involuntary, biologically determined response set and the voluntary, environmentally and psychologically determined response set. Stress is not necessarily a risk itself. Arguably, moderate stress in supportive environments can act as a protective factor. When an individual faces a thief in the dark of night, stress can catapult the person into self-protective action (DiPietro, 2004). However, when stress overwhelms the individual's coping repertoire, it becomes a health risk leading to maladaptive responses. *Coping* refers to the process of adaptation to a stressor. As Compas (2004) notes, coping can be viewed as the behaviors and thoughts an individual mobilizes voluntarily or involuntarily when faced with a stress.

CONCEPTUAL FRAMEWORK

It is important to remember that resilience is the capacity to rebound in the face of adversity. An adverse life event triggers stress. Management of stress that leads to positive adaptations is considered resilience. The conceptual framework that drives our understanding of adaptive and maladaptive responses begins with stress. As shown in Figure 4.1, the concept of resilience is a functional notion that an individual is able to adapt to stressful situations in a positive, prosocial manner. Resilience is focused more on social functioning than mental health or other outcomes. Without stress, there is no test of resilience. Garmezy (1985) notes that the concept originated in metallurgy, referring to the capacity of a metal to return to its original shape after stress.

Large-scale factors such as war or natural disaster can certainly influence stress, but the most common macrolevel factors are poverty, discrimination, and inequality (Cicchetti & Dawson, 2002). A variety of proximal domains can also increase or moderate stress, ranging from neighborhood and community to family, school, and peers.

These factors together result in an individual's interpretation of an event as stressful or not. An individual's response is moderated by both biological (primarily neurodevelopmental) and individual (cognitive and temperamental) factors that result in both voluntary and involuntary responses to the stressor. These components taken together constitute the response that we call resilience (or lack of resilience).

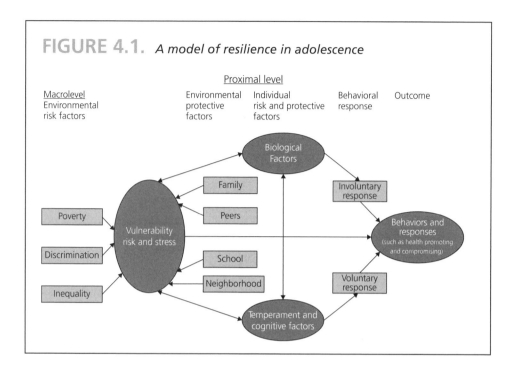

FIGURE 4.1. *A model of resilience in adolescence*

ECOLOGICAL FACTORS

In the pages that follow, we review the current literature on the various ecological factors associated with risk and resilience; our goal is not only to shed light on how these factors influence health behaviors but to show the interrelationships among them as well.

Neighborhood

As noted earlier in this chapter, poverty has a direct effect on stress, and it is a macro-level factor that affects stress response. But what is actually known about the effects that neighborhood has on risk and resilience? Much of the research has focused on the interrelationships between impoverished neighborhoods and risk (Furstenberg, 1993; Massey & Denton, 1993; Wilson, 1996). Living in economically disadvantaged neighborhoods is associated with lower grades (Dornbusch, Ritter, & Steinberg, 1991), lower educational attainment (Duncan, 1994), higher likelihood to drop out of school (Brooks-Gunn, Guo, & Furstenberg, 1993), more delinquency (Peppler & Loeber, 1994), and higher rates of precocious sexual activity and childbearing (Crane, 1991).

Exactly how neighborhoods exert their influence is less clear than their behavioral correlates. Wilson (1996) notes that there is a resource differential between high- and low-income neighborhoods that affects social as well as financial capital. Others have pointed to greater social disorganization in low-income communities as a major etiologic factor in the different outcomes. Conversely, Gephart (1997) has seen that a number of negative outcomes of economically disadvantaged communities can be moderated with high levels of monitoring, youth supervision, and consistent adult values across the community. Such consistent values are what Sampson, Raudenbush, and Earls (1997) refer to as *collective efficacy.*

Family

Family connectedness is the single most protective factor reducing negative outcomes for young people. In the United States, young people who feel connected to at least one parent are less likely to be involved with every risk behavior when compared with disconnected peers (Resnick et al., 1997). Parental connection has also been considered a more powerful explanation of the presence or absence of risk behaviors than race, income, and family structure combined (Blum et al., 2000).

The role that family plays in protecting young people from harm has been repeatedly seen across childhood and adolescence (Masten, 2001; Rutter, 2000; Werner, 2000). This consistency is especially salient in light of the myth (that prevailed until recently) that parental influence diminished after puberty. Early child research (for example, Sroufe, 2002) suggests that positive experiences with a nurturing parent early in life not only create a bond between child and caregiver but also give a young child the capacity to establish trust, which is a precondition for exploration of the world around them. As will be seen later in this chapter, early environmental factors directly and irreversibly affect neuromaturation as well.

> *Family connectedness is the single most protective factor reducing negative outcomes for young people.*

The protective role of family is not only seen in United States–based research but is also reflected globally. In a review of research from fifty-seven countries, the World Health Organization (2002) found parents to be consistently protective, especially with regard to three outcomes: early sexual intercourse, substance use, and depression.

When we look at the research on what constitutes effective parenting, a number of factors continue to emerge: behavioral monitoring (Galambos, Barker, & Almeida, 2003; Cavell, 2000; Schneider, Cavell, & Hughes, 2003); closeness and connectedness (Blum et al., 2000); emotional responsiveness (Wyman et al., 1999); knowing one's child and his or her friends, friends' parents, and teachers (Dishion & Kavanagh, 2003; Resnick et al., 1997); and setting clear and high behavioral and educational expectations.

In addition to these behavioral aspects of effective parenting, Baumrind has proposed a framework based on *parental styles* (Baumrind, 1965, 1966; Maccoby & Martin, 1983). The two central dimensions are warmth (what others have called connectedness) and behavioral monitoring or control. Baumrind posited that the authoritarian parent is high on control and low warmth, whereas the laissez-faire parent is high on warmth but low on control. The neglectful parental style is low on both dimensions. The most effective parenting style, Baumrind concluded, is high on both warmth and behavioral control.

In studying parenting styles empirically, Steinberg and his colleagues concluded that the authoritative parenting style—characterized by behavioral monitoring, clear boundaries, emotional responsiveness, closeness, negotiated rules, and consistent, nonviolent consequences—was the one most strongly associated with positive youth outcomes (Steinberg, Elmen, & Mounts, 1989). In fact, the authors conclude that it is important for at least one parent to use an authoritative approach because even if the other parent employs a different, less effective style, the authoritative approach will trump it.

There is consistent evidence among European American populations that shows positive associations between authoritative parenting and better academic performance (Steinberg, Mounts, Lamborn, & Dornbusch, 1991; Chen, Dornbusch, & Liu, 2007), social maturity and responsibility (Baumrind, 1971), and a variety of measures of competence, self-esteem, and mental health (Buri, 1989; Maccoby & Martin, 1983; Steinberg, Elmen, & Mounts 1989).

Among those who study parenting in different ethnic samples, Baumrind's paradigm has not been universally endorsed; in fact, some have argued that it is highly culture-bound. Chao (1994), for example, has found that the construct of authoritative parenting as the most effective style might not pertain to Asian Americans. Specifically, she suggests that Chinese heritage has more authoritarian elements, and high expectations have become the measure of effective parenting, rather than warmth. To Western eyes, this parental approach might appear more akin to the authoritarian than the authoritative approach.

Seeking a more universal paradigm for parenting, Barber and his colleagues explored the impact of the elements of effective parenting in twelve communities from nine countries (Barber, Maughan, & Olsen, 2005). In this framework the authors explored warmth and connectedness versus regulation and control (both behavioral and psychological) as separate dimensions. They concluded that psychological control (such as denying a young person affection, attention, or caring in order to achieve a goal of the adult) contributes cross-culturally to negative mental health and increases negative behaviors. Conversely, behavioral control (such as knowing where one's child is at all times) reduces negative behavior. Warmth and connectedness were likewise associated with both positive mental health and less risk behaviors.

In sum, there is emerging consensus among researchers with regard to Baumrind's (1991) and Maccoby and Martin's (1983) two essential components of parenting: *responsiveness* and *demandingness.* These constructs have been used in many studies of parenting. Although other investigators have used different terms—such as acceptance, warmth, support, or connectedness for responsiveness, and behavioral control or regulation for demandingness—the concepts behind responsiveness and demandingness appear to apply cross-culturally. The ways in which they manifest, however, seem to be heavily culturally determined (Blum & Mmari, 2006).

School

Outside of home, school is the primary social environment within which young people function (Osterman, 2000). There is ample evidence today that young people who feel connected to school not only do better academically but have better developmental outcomes as well (Catalano, Haggerty, Oesterle, Fleming, & Hawkins, 2004). Following are seven central elements that seem to influence positive school attachment (Klem & Connell, 2004):

- Having a sense of belonging and being part of a school
- Liking school

- Perceiving that teachers are supportive and caring

- Having good friends at school

- Being engaged in one's own current and future academic progress

- Believing that discipline is fair and effective

- Participating in extracurricular activities

When most or all of these elements are present, the evidence shows that young people are less likely to exhibit disruptive and violent behavior, carry or use a weapon, experiment with illegal substances, smoke cigarettes, drink to the point of getting drunk, appear emotionally distressed, consider or attempt suicide, or engage in early sexual intercourse (Blum & Libbey, 2004).

The central role of teachers in creating an environment of school connectedness cannot be overemphasized (Croninger & Lee, 2001). McNeely and Falci (2004) have shown that when young people who report high connectedness to a teacher are compared with those with low connectedness over a one-year interval, those with high connectedness are half as likely to initiate cigarette smoking (2.8 percent versus 5.3 percent), half as likely to report getting drunk on a regular basis (3.2 percent versus 6.2 percent), nearly half as likely to report regular marijuana use (2.6 percent versus 4.4 percent), and nearly half as likely to report a suicide attempt (1.3 percent versus 2.2 percent).

Another aspect of school connectedness is *engagement.* The National Research Council (2004; Lehr & Christenson, 2002) has identified the following four principles of engaging schools:

- *High academic standards.* Teachers hold students accountable for work completion and performance. All students are expected to excel; "tracking" is avoided.

- *Personalized learning.* Every student has a relationship with one caring adult. Schools are on a human scale (using, for example, schools within a school or career academics). Mentorship is available, and team teaching is often the educational approach.

- *Relevance.* The school uses exploratory strategies, service learning, the Internet, and neighborhood events for instruction.

- *Flexibility.* Instructional methods are varied, using cooperative learning, experiential learning, extended day and year, and educational remediation.

Peers

School and peers are closely intertwined; as Coleman (1961) showed, most teens' closest friends come from their school. Thus, peer groups are powerful socializing influences that may be positive or negative.

Positive peer relationships have been associated with decreased stress (Luthar, 2006), and even gang membership has been associated with positive self-esteem. Where young people associate with religious peers, they are less likely to initiate intercourse (Bearman & Brückner, 2001), less likely to smoke cigarettes (Nonnemaker, McNeely & Blum, 2003), less likely to be depressed (Seidman & Pedersen, 2003) and less likely to use substances (Miller, Davis, & Greenwald, 2000; Miller & Gur, 2002). Likewise, Steinberg, Dornbusch, and Brown (1992) found that among African American teens exposed to multiple risks, those who felt they could depend on peers for support did better academically than their unsupported peers.

On the other hand, the quality of one's peer group is strongly linked with a number of negative behaviors, including drug and alcohol use and gang membership (Case & Lawrence, 1991). Likewise, research has consistently shown that youth are more likely to conform to the views of their peers than their parents (Massey & Denton, 1993; Cauce, Stewart, Rodriguez, Cochran, & Ginzler, 2003; Leventhal & Brooks-Gunn, 2000). This tendency may prove to be especially difficult in low-income, high-deviance communities (Leventhal & Brooks-Gunn, 2000; Jarrett, 1999).

In school settings, peers often reinforce nonacademic norms of work avoidance (Bishop et al., 2004). Furthermore, Luthar (1995) found school popularity was associated with aggression and low academic effort.

Interpersonal aggression is a major issue among youth in schools. Bishop and colleagues (2004) point to one study reporting that 13.1 percent of boys and 6.7 percent of girls were teased, insulted, or made fun of nearly every day—and this percentage represents 2.3 million secondary school children! The more high-status the clique, the more its members will reject others. These groups set the norms for "coolness" in dress, attitudes, and behavior (Brown, 1990).

Brown (1990) draws the distinction between cliques and crowds. *Cliques* are small groups of friends who hang out together and are personally close. *Crowds* are reputation-based collectives (such as nerds, jocks, or burnouts). Clique norms develop from within the group; crowd norms are imposed externally depending on the stereotypic image. Cliques have powerful influence on academic achievement (Damico, 1975). Crowd membership reflects the behavioral roles one is most likely to play out. Traits most associated with popularity include—in rank order—cool clothes, attractiveness, sense of humor, sports ability, outgoingness, self-confidence, toughness, lack of attentiveness in class, working hard for grades, attentiveness in class, and intelligence.

ADOLESCENT NEURODEVELOPMENT, STRESS, AND RESILIENCE

Because stress is centrally mediated and stress response results from individual interpretation of events, it is important to gain a basic understanding of adolescent neuromaturation and the impact of stress on these processes. Remember that stress and resilience are closely intertwined, because resilience is only manifest in the presence

Adversity creates stress; thus, the factors that mediate, moderate, or exacerbate stress will determine the extent to which an individual is resilient.

of adversity. Adversity creates stress; thus, the factors that mediate, moderate, or exacerbate stress will determine the extent to which an individual is resilient.

A generation ago, the prevailing understanding of brain development was that brain growth ceased when the occipital sutures closed, at about age three. Today we have come to understand that neuromaturation is not complete until the midtwenties. In addition, we have come to understand that brain development progresses at different times for different regions of the brain. For example, the visual cortex matures early—generally in the first year of life—whereas the prefrontal lobe does not fully mature until more than two decades later.

The frontal and prefrontal cortex is the last region of the human brain to mature, and this stage occurs during adolescence. This region controls what is often referred to as executive functions: impulse control, planning, reasoning, regulation of emotions, weighing of risks, and learning from experience. It naturally follows that if the neuromaturation process is impaired, it could potentially affect a number of functions key to adult functioning and adaptability.

Stress and Neuromaturation

Brain development is not independent of environment; rather, it is *experience dependent.* For those who mature under conditions of chronic, severe stress—in what Garbarino has referred to as "toxic environments"—a cascade of neuroendocrinologic changes will then precipitate structural changes. This is not to say that all stress is harmful. In fact, a moderate amount of stress within a supportive environment is beneficial (DiPietro, 2005). But what occurs neurodevelopmentally under conditions of "toxic stress"?

First, stress has a direct effect on the pituitary gland, which stimulates the production of cortisol. Stress stimulation of the pituitary results in increased production of adrenocorticotropic hormone, which in turn stimulates adrenal overproduction of cortisol and also suppresses hypothalamic production of gonadotropin releasing factor. This decrease in turn suppresses estrogen and testosterone. Elevated levels of cortisol result in decreased synaptic and dendritic density (less production of dendrites early in life), which in turn will affect brain architecture and functioning throughout life. As the "fight-or-flight" response is neurohormonally mediated, key consequences of persistently elevated cortisol levels in adolescence include:

- A decrease in hormones associated with pubertal maturation

- A diversion of brain resources away from learning and development of cognitive skills for survival

- Interruption of normal neurotransmitter functions (such as serotonin)

Given that neurodevelopment is environment dependent, it is easy to see how persistent, severe stress may irreversibly alter neuromaturational pathways by affecting dendrite density, neurotransmitter receptors, serotonin, and structural changes in the hippocampus, corpus collosum, left hemisphere, and brain volume.

Such environments are, in fact, all too common. Persistent physical or sexual abuse is one example, as are persistently violent environments. Many youth reared in violent neighborhoods suffer from posttraumatic stress disorder, which is associated with the following issues:

- Diminished hippocampal volume

- Problems with executive functioning

- Diminished emotional control

- Problems with social relationships and academic achievement

Internal Traits

When the pioneers of resilience research asked why some children and youth could bounce back from adversity, they placed heavy emphasis on the competence-building traits of temperament and intelligence possessed by youth—as well as the traits of surrounding adults and others with the power to protect children. However, it is important to note that in subsequent research resilience as an individual characteristic did not explain more than a small proportion of variance in behavioral development. As Sameroff and Rosenblum (2006) note, "childhood resilience requires attention to the social risk factors that challenge individuals and their families." They go on to say, "In our analysis we have found that individual characteristics of mental health and higher intelligence contribute to competence. However, the effects of such individual resiliencies do not overcome the effects of high environmental risk. In our analyses we consistently found that groups of high resilience children in high risk environments had lower later mental health and cognitive competence than groups of low resilience children in low-risk environments" (Sameroff & Rosenblum, 2006). Furthermore, Luthar's (2006) review of the literature indicates that many attributes are shaped by the environment. For example, self-efficacy is shaped by parents giving permission for autonomy (Bandura, 1997). Self-esteem is affected by parental warmth (Sandler, Wolchick, Davis, Haine, & Ayers, 2003). Early onset of maltreatment has been shown to reduce internal locus of control (Capella & Weinstein, 2001). When teachers are perceived as cold and inconsistent, students feel less confident that they can succeed (Skinner, Zimmer-Gembeck, & Connell, 1998).

Temperament Traits *Temperament* refers to relatively stable, early appearing, biologically rooted individual differences in behavioral traits (Rothbart & Bates, 1998). Largely biologically determined, the traits are also affected by environment and experience. Therefore, children and youth with certain traits are predisposed to behave in ways that spur positive or negative responses, which in turn affect their temperament over time (Rothbart & Bates, 1998).

Temperament is one domain of individual characteristics that may promote resilience in children and youth (Compas, Connor-Smith, Saltzman, Thomsen, & Wadsworth,

2001). Wachs (2005) reviewed studies of children from infancy through adolescence and found that there is more evidence for the dimensions of temperament promoting or inhibiting resilience than for the pathways for individual differences in temperament translating into vulnerability or resilience. He notes that despite measurement differences in studies, the literature links the following traits to resilience: easy temperament, emotional reactivity, sociability, self-regulation, and attention or focus.

Wachs (2005) indicates children and youth with easy temperaments experience lower levels of behavioral problems, higher levels of social and emotional competence, lower rates of behavioral-emotional problems, and lower levels of substance abuse.

Wachs (2006) states that emotional reactivity to stress is critical. For those at risk, positive emotional reactivity is linked to resilience because of higher levels of social and emotional competence, lower rates of behavioral-emotional problems, and lower levels of substance abuse. Negative emotional reactivity is linked to reduced resilience, behavior problems, and lower rating of school competence for children under stress. Hauser and Allen's (2006) long-term study of teens hospitalized with psychiatric diagnoses reported that resilience was evidenced by self-reflection or awareness of their feelings and thoughts, self-efficacy or making choices about their lives, self-complexity in recognizing multiple facts to different situations; persistence and ambition in education and careers, and a positive self-view. Beardslee (2002) identified protective behaviors of teens with depressed parents as including awareness of what they were facing, recognition of their parent's illness, recognition that they were not responsible, capacity to articulate their feelings, and the ability to establish nurturing relationships with adults outside the family. Harter (2002) described resilient youth as having *personal authenticity,* which means taking responsibility for one's personal thoughts and emotions and acting on them. For example, those grieving the loss of a loved one showed better adjustment when they could recall positive experiences with the loved one.

Young people who experience stress and who also possess high social skills show lower levels of behavior problems and higher levels of cognitive performance and social-emotional competence (Wachs, 2006). Likewise, those with higher "approach" skills have lower levels of behavior problems compared to kids low in "approach" skills. Social competence and a quality relationship with a caregiver were strongly linked to latent resilience in a study of young teens ages eleven to fifteen who were referred to the child welfare system for maltreatment (Rajendran & Videka, 2006). In families with depressed parents, Beardslee (2002) found that resilient youth had a well-developed capacity to see things from others' viewpoints and to think about their needs. Bandura, Caprara, Barbaranelli, Gerbino, and Pastorelli (2003) have shown that high perceived empathic self-efficacy among teens was related to high prosocial behavior and less delinquency. Masten and Reed (2002) note that empathy and altruism are highlighted in the emerging *positive psychology movement.*

Masten (2001) expands on these characteristics of resilience, noting that the following traits have also been reported in the literature: intelligence, self-regulation, self-esteem, self-efficacy, and internal locus of control. Subsequently Masten (2004) created a "short list" of widely reported correlates and predictors of resilience in youth: problem-solving skills, effective emotional and behavior regulation, positive self-perceptions of efficacy and worth, belief that life has meaning, hopefulness, religious faith and affiliations, aptitudes and characteristics valued by society such as talent and attractiveness, prosocial friends, effective school bonding, and connections to competent, caring adults. These factors correlate repeatedly with fewer health risk behaviors.

Using her longitudinal study of the children of Kauai (Werner & Smith, 1992) and a review of related studies, Werner describes infants and toddlers who cope well in adverse conditions as having temperamental characteristics that elicit positive responses from caregivers. They are active, affectionate, cuddly, good natured, and easy to deal with. By preschool, they have developed a coping pattern that combines autonomy with an ability to ask for help when needed. Resilient adolescents are outgoing and autonomous, nurturing and emotionally sensitive. These traits also predict resilience in later years (Werner, 1995). We will elaborate separately on social and emotional attributes and cognitive and self-regulatory attributes.

Cognition and Self-Regulatory Attributes Recent findings in neuropsychology are relevant to the resilience literature. Intervention programs could be organized to increase executive functioning (organizing oneself to meet a goal), inhibitory control (inhibiting a reaction long enough to think through a response), planning, problem-solving, and attentional capacities (focusing and persisting on problem solving until a goal is reached).

Self-regulation refers to positive executive functioning: inhibition, future time orientation, consequential thinking, and the planning, initiation, and regulation of goal-directed behavior. The development of executive functioning is crucial to self-regulation, and deficiencies in executive functioning have been related to impulsivity and numerous poor outcomes. In one study young people who rated themselves and their parents as high in self-regulation skills showed lower levels of internalizing behavior problems (depression or anxiety) than peers low in these skills. Stressed youth high in impulsivity with poor self-regulation show higher externalizing behavior problems than those low in impulsivity. Buckner, Mezzacappa, and Beardslee (2003) found that good self-regulation contributed to resilience. Teens with strong self-regulation skills that came from low-income families experienced satisfactory mental health and emotional well-being, even after researchers considered self-esteem and nonverbal intelligence. Bandura et al. (2003) found that perceived self-efficacy to regulate positive and negative affect is related to teens' beliefs that they can manage academic, transgressive, and empathic aspects of their lives, and these forms of perceived self-efficacy related in turn to lower levels of depression, delinquency, and antisocial behaviors.

Masten (2004) describes the following factors as "regulating" a person's behavior and the outcomes from that behavior: executive functioning, emotion regulation, attachments to adults who monitor and support youth effectively, relationships with peers who regulate others effectively, bonding to prosocial socializing and community organizations, and opportunities for regulatory capacity building. She describes these regulatory skills as needing to develop in order to handle periods of rapid change and development and the impulses of teens when making decisions about driving, sexual intimacy, or using drugs to cope with stress.

Attention and Task Orientation Wachs (2005) notes that the hybrid trait of temperament and cognition allows children and youth to remain focused on meeting goals and expectations. Children and youth facing stressors (of divorce or family conflict) who are rated high in task orientation have fewer behavior problems or problems of substance abuse compared to peers low in these traits.

Dishion and Connel (2006) state that self-regulation is the index of youth resilience, and it is also the goal of intervention: children and youth who learn strategies to regulate themselves will improve their adjustment in problematic environments and stressful circumstances. The authors go on to describe the steps of self-regulation from the time the stress stimulus occurs in the environment to the time the person gives a response: the individual initially appraises the event and its emotional meaning; second, he or she regulates arousal (self-regulation) to take action to initiate problem solving, which in turn leads to a fuller cognitive-affective interpretation of the event, which then leads to the behavior response.

Werner (1995) observes that most studies of resilient children and youths report that intelligence and scholastic competence are positively associated with the ability to overcome great odds, because these youth have the skills to find strategies for coping with adversity either on their own or by actively asking for help. This finding has been replicated in studies of Asian American, Caucasian, and African American children (Clark, 1983). The findings indicate that intelligence is not itself the trait that predicts success, but rather the ability to use intellectual flexibility, think through and plan problem-solving strategies, and creatively apply strategies are markers for intellectual competence. According to a study by Gutmen, Sameroff, and Cole (2003), intelligent teens fared better in school than less intelligent teens when life stress levels were low; when stress was high, bright and less bright teens fared the same. In areas of poverty, teens with high IQ and creativity used their wits to survive, engaging strategies such as entrepreneurship rather than school success.

Yates and Masten (2004) note the following protective characteristics of youth who thrive in the face of adversity:

- Flexible coping strategies

- Internal locus of control, which allows them to attribute negative experiences to external factors, while retaining the capacity to value their own strengths and assets

- Intelligence and sense of humor are associated with flexible problem solving and with academic and social competence

- Social responsiveness with ability to elicit positive regard and warmth from caregivers

TABLE 4.1. Programs that build resilience

Programs	Social Competence	Problem Solving	School Connection	Academic Achievement	Leadership Skills*	Family Relations	Substance Use Abuse	Service	Ages	Evidence	Link	Setting
Across Ages	X	X	X	X	X	X	X	X	9–13	Mentoring on prosocial values, substance resistance, and school attendance	www.temple .edu/cil/Across ageshome.htm	All
Aggression Replacement Training (ART)	X	X							Adol	Increased prosocial skills; decreased impulsivity and felony recidivism	http://artgang0 .tripod.com/ prod01.htm	All
Community of Caring/Growing up Caring	X	X	X	X	X	X	X	X	K–12	Increased positive behavior, social competence, substance resistance, grade point average, and school attendance	www.communi tyofcaring.org	School
Keepin' It REAL	X	X			X		X	X	10–17	Increased behavioral and social outcomes, substance resistance, and antidrug values; decreased or cessation of substance use	http://keepinitreal .asu.edu	School

(Continued)

TABLE 4.1. *(Continued)*

Programs	Social Competence	Problem Solving	School Connection	Academic Achievement	Leadership Skills*	Family Relations	Substance Use Abuse	Service	Ages	Evidence	Link	Setting
Leadership and Resiliency Program (LRP)	x	x	x	x	x		x	x	14–17	Increased academic achievement, school attendance, school connectedness, and graduation rate	www.modelpro grams.samhsa. gov/pdfs/model/ leadership.pdf	All
Life Skills Train- ing	x	x					x		8–14	Decreased substance use	www.lifeskills training.com	School
Lions Quest	x	x	x	x	x	x	x	x	10–14	Increased problem- solving skills and academic achievement; increased positive behavior at one-year follow-up	www.lions-quest .org	School
Peace Works	x	x	x	x		x		x	pre-K– 12	Increased positive behavior, social skills, and achievement; decreased violence	www.peaceedu cation.com	School
Peace Builders	x	x	x	x		x			pre-K– 12	Increased violence prevention and health promotion	www.peacebuild ers.com	School

Program							Grade	Outcomes	Website	Setting
Peacemakers	x	x	x	x	x		K–9	Increased conflict resolution skills in and out of school	www.solution tree.com/Public/Media.aspx?	School
Positive Action	x	x	x	x	x	x	K–12	Increased positive behavior, school attendance, and achievement; decreased suspensions, crime, violence, and drug use	www.positive action.net	School
Project Venture	x	x		x	x	x	Adol	Increased school attendance; decreased substance use, depression, and aggression	http://niylp.org/programs/project_venture	All
Promoting Alternative Thinking Strategies (PATHS)	x	x	x	x	x	x	K–6	Increased self-control, conflict resolution, and social skills; decreased violence and aggression	www.prevention.psu.edu/projects/PATHS.html	School
Reconnecting Youth (RY)	x	x	x	x	x	x	14–18	Increased academic achievement, attendance, and graduation; decreased substance use and emotional distress	www.son.washington.edu/departments/pch/ry/curriculum.asp	School

(Continued)

TABLE 4.1. (Continued)

Programs	Social Competence	Problem Solving	School Connection	Academic Achievement	Leadership Skills*	Family Relations	Substance Use Abuse	Service	Ages	Evidence	Link	Setting
Resolving Conflict Creatively Program (RCCP)	x	x	x	x	x	x		x	K–HS	Increased academic achievement, attendance, and conflict resolution; decreased violence, suspension, and dropouts	www.esrnational.org	School
Responding in Peaceful and Positive Ways (RIPP)	x	x			x		x	x	MS–JH	Increased use of peer mediators, conflict resolution skills, and substance resistance; decreased violence	www.prevention opportunities.com	School
Second Step	x	x			x				4–14	Increased conflict resolution, problem-solving skills, social-emotional skills, empathy skills, and verbal mediation skills; decreased aggression and violence	www.cfchildren.org	School
SMART Team: Students Managing Anger and Resolution Together Team	x	x							11–15	Increased anger control, conflict resolution, and perspective taking skills; decreased belief in use of violence	www.krisbos worth.org	School

Program						Age	Outcomes	Website	
Strengthening Families Program (SFP)	x	x	x	x	x	pre-K–18	Increased family attachment, communication, and parenting skills, compliance with adults, problem solving, conflict resolution skills, and social competence; decreased conduct disorder	www.strengtheningfamiliesprogram.org	All
Teaching Students to be Peacemakers	x	x	x	x		5–14	Increased conflict resolution, social competency, and academic achievement	www.modelprograms.samhsa.gov/pdfs/model/TeachingStud.pdf	School
Teen Outreach Program	x	x	x	x	x	12–17	Decreased course failure, suspension rates, and pregnancy rates—but research design has been questioned	www.wymanteens.org	All
Voices: A Comprehensive Reading, Writing, and Character Education Program	x	x	x	x		K–6	Increased academic achievement	www.voicespublishing.com	School

With this review as background, we will now turn to what is known about interventions and explore the evidence that resilience can be fostered through deliberate interventions.

RESILIENCE AND EVIDENCE-BASED INTERVENTIONS

Little (1993), Dryfoos (1990), and Schorr (1988) have analyzed youth programs to identify the key elements for success. Looking across the three researchers, we find that resilience-based programs have the following characteristics:

- Built on communitywide, intersectoral collaborations that are not bounded by traditional agency roles or administrative constraints

- Focused on enhancing competence in young people at least as much as reducing a given risk behavior or undesirable outcome

- See youth as part of the solution, not just the focus of the problem

- Start early in the lives of young people, are continuous, and are developmentally appropriate

- Have staff who are collaborative, interdisciplinary, not overly "professionalized," willing to do what it takes to be successful, and value young people

These dimensions of resilience-based programming are echoed in Little's Four Cs (1993). These programs build the following qualities:

- *Competence* in areas that improve the quality of a child or youth's life, such as literacy, employability, interpersonal, vocational, and academic skills, and a sense of being able to contribute to his or her community

- *Connection* of youth to others through caring relationships manifest in mentoring, tutoring, leadership, and community service opportunities

- *Character* through values that give meaning and direction to the youth, such as individual responsibility, honesty, community service, responsible decision making, and integrity in relationships

- *Confidence*-building activities to give hope, self-esteem, and a sense of success in setting and meeting goals.

Table 4.1 lists programs that exemplify these dimensions and employ evidence-based best practices. The table also details which elements of resilience each program has been shown to build. Further information can be found at the program Web sites.

SUMMARY

Resilience is the capacity to rebound in the face of adversity. It is the ability to view a challenge not as an insurmountable barrier, but as a hurdle that with proper supports can be cleared. We have learned through a half century of research that those supports are not limited to individual traits. Rather, the factors that embrace resilience are the same factors that protect young people from harm. Some skills can be taught, and some must be learned from experience, but we now know that through deliberate strategies we can enhance resilience in young people, and in doing so we provide them the resources to make positive, adaptive, and health-promoting choices even in the face of adversity.

KEY TERMS

Cliques	Resilience
Collective efficacy	Self-regulation
Compensatory factors	Social charisma
Coping	Stress
Crowds	Temperament
Parental styles	Tension
Problem confrontation	Tension management
Protection	Vulnerability
Protective factors	Vulnerability processes

DISCUSSION QUESTIONS

1. Discuss how resilience is related to individual risk, particularly in adolescence, and how this concept varies depending on circumstantial life events.

2. How would you apply the conceptual framework outlined in this chapter to a particular adverse life event, such as teen pregnancy or an unexpected HIV diagnosis?

3. Describe various factors related to risk and resiliency that influence health behavior. Do you think culture plays a role in this relationship? How?

4. What are the pros and cons of developing an adolescent health behavior intervention that promotes resilience in the school setting?

5. Explain the following statement in terms of adolescent neurodevelopment: "Brain development is not independent of environment; rather, it is experience dependent." Provide examples to support your explanation.

REFERENCES

Antonovsky, A. (1979). *Health, stress and coping.* San Francisco: Jossey-Bass.

Bandura, A. (1997). *Self-efficacy: The exercise of control.* New York: Freeman.

Bandura, A., Caprara, G. V., Barbaranelli, C., Gerbino, M., & Pastorelli, C. (2003). Role of affective self-regulatory efficacy in diverse spheres of psychosocial functioning. *Child Development, 74*(3), 769–782.

Barber, B. K., Maughan, S. L., & Olsen, J. A. (2005). *Patterns of parenting across adolescence*. In J. G. Smetana (Ed.), *Changes in parental authority during adolescence. New Directions for Child and Adolescent Development*, No. 108. San Francisco: Jossey-Bass.

Baumrind, D. (1965). Parental control and parental love. *Children, 12*, 230–234.

Baumrind, D. (1966). The effects of authoritative parental control. *Child Development, 27*(4), 887–907.

Baumrind, D. (1971). Current patterns of parental authority. *Developmental Psychology Monograph: Part 2, 4*(1), 1–103.

Baumrind, D. (1991). Effective parenting during the early adolescent transition. In P. A. Cowen & M. Heatherington (Eds.), *Family Transitions* (pp. 111–163). Hillsdale, N.J.: Erlbaum.

Beardslee, W. R. (2002). *Out of the darkened room. When a parent is depressed: Protecting the children and strengthening the family*. New York: Little, Brown.

Bearman, P. S., & Brückner, H. (2001). Promising the future: Virginity pledges and the transition to first intercourse. *American Journal of Sociology, 106*(4), 859–862.

Bishop, J. H., Bishop, Ma., Bishop, Mi., Gelbwasser, L., Green, S., Peterson, E., Rubinsztaj, A., & Zuckerman, A. (2004). Why we harass nerds and freaks: A formal theory of student culture and norms. *Journal of School Health, 74*(7), 235–251.

Blum, R. W., Beuhring, T., Shew, M. L., Bearinger, L. H., Sieving, R. E., & Resnick, M. D. (2000). The effects of race/ethnicity, income and family structure on adolescent risk behaviors. *American Journal of Public Health, 90*(12), 1879–1884.

Blum, R. W., & Libbey, H. (2004). School connectedness: Strengthening health and education outcomes for teenagers. *Journal of School Health, 74*(7), 229–299.

Blum, R., & Mmari, K. (2004). Adolescent health in a global context. *Journal of Adolescent Health, 35*(5), 402–418.

Brooks-Gunn, J., Guo, G., & Furstenberg, F., Jr. (1993). Who drops out of and who continues beyond high school? A 20-year study of black youth. *Journal of Research in Adolescence, 3*, 271–294.

Brown, B. B. (1990). Peer groups and peer cultures. In S. S. Feldman & G. R. Elliot (Eds.), *At the threshold: The developing adolescent* (pp. 171–196). Cambridge, MA: Harvard University Press.

Buckner, J. C., Mezzacappa, E., & Beardslee, W. R. (2003). Characteristics of resilient youth living in poverty: The role of self-regulatory processes. *Development and Psychopathology, 15*, 139–162.

Buri, J. R. (1989). Self-esteem and appraisals of parental behavior. *Journal of Adolescent Research, 4*(1), 33–49.

Capella, E., & Weinstein, T. S. (2001). Turning around reading achievement: Predictors of high schools' academic resilience. *Journal of Educational Psychology, 93*, 758–771.

Case, A. C., & Lawrence, K. (1991). *The company you keep: The effects of family and neighborhood on disadvantaged youths*. Working paper no. 3705. Cambridge, MA: National Bureau of Economic Research.

Catalano, R. F., Haggerty, K. P., Oesterle, S., Fleming, C. B., & Hawkins, J. D. (2004). The importance of bonding to school for healthy development: Findings from the social development research group. *Journal of School Health, 74*(7), 252–261.

Cauce, A. M., Stewart, A., Rodriguez, M. D., Cochran, B., & Ginzler, J. (2003). Overcoming the odds? Adolescent development in the context of urban poverty. In S. S. Luthar (Ed), *Resilience and vulnerability: Adaptation in the context of childhood adversities* (pp. 343–363). New York: Cambridge University Press.

Cavell, T. A. (2000). *Working with parents of aggressive children: A practitioner's guide*. Washington, DC: American Psychological Association.

Chao, R. K. (1994). Beyond parental control and authoritarian parenting style for Chinese Americans and European Americans. *Child Development, 72*, 1832–1843.

Chen, Z. Y., Dornbusch, S., & Liu, Z. X. (2007). Direct and indirect pathways between parental constructive behavior and adolescent affiliation with achievement oriented peers. *Journal of Child and Family Studies, 16*(6), 837–858.

Cicchetti, D., & Dawson, G. (2002). Editorial: Multiple levels of analysis. *Development and Psychopathology, 14*, 417–420.

Clark, R. M. (1983). *Family, life, and school achievement: Why poor black children succeed or fail*. Chicago: University of Chicago Press.

Cofer, C., & Appley, M. (1964). *Motivation: Theory and research*. New York: Wiley.

Coleman, J. (1961). *The adolescent society*. New York: Free Press.

Compas, B. E. (2004). Processes of risk and resilience during adolescence: Linking contexts and individuals. In R. Lerner & L. Steinberg (Eds.), *Handbook of adolescent psychology* (2nd ed.). Hoboken, NJ: Wiley.

Compas, B. E., Connor-Smith, J. K., Saltzman, H., Thomsen, A. H., & Wadsworth, M. E. (2001). Coping with stress during childhood and adolescence: Progress, problems, and potential in theory and research. *Psychological Bulletin, 127,* 87–127.

Crane, J. (1991). The epidemic theory of ghettos and neighborhood effects on dropping out and teenage childbearing. *American Journal of Sociology, 96,* 1226–1259.

Croninger, R. G., & Lee, V. E. (2001). Social capital and dropping out of high schools: Benefits to at-risk students of teachers' support and guidance. *Teachers College Record, 103*(4), 548–581.

Damico, S. B. (1975). The effects of clique membership upon academic achievement. *Adolescence, 10*(37), 93–100.

Darling, N., & Steinberg, L. (1993). Parenting style as context: An integrative model. *Psychological Bulletin, 113*(3), 487–496.

Denny, S., Clark, T. C., Fleming, T., & Wall, M. (2004). Emotional resilience: Risk and protective factors for depression among alternative education students in New Zealand. *American Journal of Orthopsychiatry, 74,* 137–149.

DiPietro, J. (2004). The role of prenatal maternal stress in child development. *Current Directions in Psychological Science, 13,* 71–74.

Dishion, T. J., & Connel, A. (2006). Adolescents' resilience as a self-regulatory process: Promising themes for linking intervention with developmental science. *Annals of the New York Academy of Sciences, 1094,* 125–138.

Dishion, T. J., & Kavanagh, K. (2003). *Intervening in adolescent problem behavior: A family-centered approach.* New York: Guilford Press.

Dornbusch, S. M., Ritter, P. L., & Steinberg, L. (1991). Community influences on the relation of family statuses to adolescent school performance: Differences between African-Americans and non-Hispanic whites. *American Journal of Education, 38,* 543–567.

Dryfoos, J. (1990). *Adolescents at risk: Prevalence and prevention.* New York: Oxford University Press.

Duncan, G. J. (1994). Families and neighbors as sources of disadvantage in the schooling decisions of white and black adolescents. *American Journal of Education, 103,* 20–53.

Farber, A., & Egeland, B. (1987). Invulnerability among abused and neglected children. In E. J. Anthony & B. J. Cohler (Eds.), *The invulnerable child.* New York: Guilford Press.

Furstenberg, F. F., Jr. (1993). How families manage risk and opportunity in dangerous neighborhoods. In W. J. Wilson (Ed.), *Sociology and the public agenda* (pp. 231–258). Newbury Park, CA: Sage Publications.

Galambos, N. L., Barker, E. T., & Almeida, D. M. (2003). Parents do matter: Trajectories of change in externalizing and internalizing problems in early adolescence. *Child Development, 74,* 578–594.

Garmezy, N. (1974). The study of competence in children at risk for severe psychopathology. In E. J. Anthony & C. I. Koupernik (Eds.), *The child in his family. Vol. III: Children at psychiatric risk.* New York: Wiley.

Garmezy, N. (1985). Stress resistant children: The search for protective factors. In J. E. Stevenson (Ed.), *Recent Research in Developmental Psychopathology* (pp. 213–233). *Journal of Child Psychology and Psychiatry and Allied Disciplines,* Supp. no. 4. Oxford, England: Pergamon Press.

Garmezy, N. (1991). Resiliency and vulnerability to adverse developmental outcomes associated with poverty. *American Behavioral Science, 34,* 416–430.

Gephart, M. A. (1997). Neighborhood and communities as contexts for development. In J. Brooks-Gunn, G. J. Duncan, & J. L. Aber (Eds.), *Neighborhood poverty* (Vol. 1, pp. 1–43). New York: Russell Sage Foundation.

Gutmen, L. M., Sameroff, A. J., & Cole, R. (2003). Academic growth curve trajectories from 1st to 12th grade: Effects of multiple social risk factors and preschool child factors. *Developmental Psychology, 39,* 777–790.

Harter, S. (2002). Authenticity. In C. R. Snyder & S. J. Lopez (Eds.), *Handbook of positive psychology* (pp. 382–394). London: Oxford University Press.

Hauser, S. T., & Allen, J. P. (2006). Narrative in the study of resilience. *Psychoanalytic Study of the Child, 61,* 205–227.

Jarrett, R. L. (1999). Successful parenting in high-risk neighborhoods. *Future of Children, 9,* 45–50.

Klem, A. M., & Connell, J. P. (2004). Relationships matter: Linking teacher support to student engagement and achievement. *Journal of School Health, 74*(7), 262–273.

Lehr, C., & Christenson, S. (2002). Best practices in promoting a positive school climate. In A. Thomas & J. Grimes (Eds.), *Best practices in school psychology IV.* Bethesda, MD: National Association of School Psychologists.

Leventhal, T., & Brooks-Gunn, J. (2000). The neighborhoods they live in: The effects of neighborhood residence on child and adolescent outcomes. *Psychological Bulletin, 126,* 309–337.

Little, R. (1993). What's working for today's youth: The issues, the programs and the learnings. Paper presented at an Institute for Children, Youth, and Families Fellows' Colloquium, Michigan State University, E. Lansing.

Luthar, S. S. (1991). Vulnerability and resilience: The study of high-risk adolescents. *Child Development, 62,* 600–616.

Luthar, S. S. (1995). Social competence in the school setting: Prospective cross-domain associations among inner-city teens. *Child Development, 66,* 416–429.

Luthar, S. S. (2003). *Resilience and vulnerability: Adaptation in the context of childhood adversities.* New York: Cambridge University Press.

Luthar, S. S. (2006). Resilience in development: A synthesis of research across five decades. In D. Cicchetti & D. J. Cohen (Eds.), *Developmental psychopathology: Risk, disorder, and adaptation* (Vol. 3, 2nd ed.). New York: Wiley.

Luthar, S. S., Cicchetti, D., & Becker, B. (2000). The construct of resilience: A critical evaluation and guidelines for future work. *Child Development, 71,* 543–562.

Maccoby, E. E., & Martin, J. A. (1983). Socialization in the context of the family: Parent-child interaction. In P. H. Mussen (Ed.), *Handbook of child psychology* (Vol. 4, pp. 1–101). New York: Wiley.

Massey, D. S., & Denton, N. A. (1993). *American apartheid: Segregation and the making of the urban underclass.* Cambridge, MA: Harvard University Press.

Masten, A. S. (2001). Ordinary magic: Resilience processes in development. *American Psychologist, 56,* 227–238.

Masten, A. S. (2004). Regulatory processes, risk and resilience in adolescent development. *Annals of the New York Academy of Sciences,* 1021, 310–319.

Masten, A. S., & Reed, M. J. (2002). Resilience in development. In C. R. Snyder & S. J. Lopez (Eds.), *Handbook of positive psychology* (pp. 74–88). London: Oxford University Press.

McNeely, C., & Falci, C. (2004). School connectedness and the transition into and out of health risk behavior among adolescents: A comparison of social belonging and teacher support. *Journal of School Health, 74*(7), 284–292.

Miller, L., & Gur, M. (2002). Religiosity, depression and physical maturation in adolescent girls. *Journal of the American Academy of Child and Adolescent Psychiatry, 41,* 206–214.

Miller, L., Davies, M., & Greenwald, S. (2000). Religiosity and substance use and abuse among adolescents in the national co-morbidity survey. *Journal of the American Academy of Child and Adolescent Psychiatry, 39,* 1190–1197.

Murphy, L. B., & Moriarty, A. (1976). *Vulnerability, coping, and growth: From infancy to adolescence.* New Haven, CT: Yale University Press.

National Research Council and Institute of Medicine of the National Academy of Sciences; Board on Children, Youth and Families. (2004). *Engaging schools: Fostering high school students' motivation to learn.* Washington, DC: National Academies Press.

Nonnemaker, J. M., McNeely, C. A., & Blum, R. W. (2003). Public and private domains of religiosity and adolescent health risk behaviors: Evidence from the national longitudinal study of adolescent health. *Social Science and Medicine, 57,* 2049–2054.

Osterman, K. F. (2000). Students' need for belonging in the school community. *Review of Educational Research, 70*(3), 323–367.

Peppler, F., & Loeber, R. (1994). Do individual factors and neighborhood context explain ethnic differences in juvenile delinquency? *Journal of Quantitative Criminology, 10,* 141–158.

Rajendran, K., & Videka, L. (2006). Relational and academic components of resilience in maltreated adolescents. *Annals of the New York Academy of Sciences, 1094,* 310–319.

Resnick, M. D., Bearman, P. S., Blum, R. W., Bauman, K. E., Harris, K. M., Jones, J., Tabor, J., Beuhring, T., Sieving, R. E., Shew, M., Ireland, M., Bearinger, L. H., & Udry, J. R. (1997). Protecting adolescents from harm: Findings from the National Longitudinal Study on Adolescent Health. *Journal of the American Medical Association, 278,* 823–833.

Rothbart, M. K., & Bates, J. E. (1998). Temperament. In W. Damon (Series Ed.) & N. Eisenberg (Vol. Ed.), *Handbook of child psychology. Vol. 3: Social, emotional and personality development* (5th ed., pp. 105–176). New York: Wiley.

Rutter, M. (1979). Protective factors in children's responses to stress and disadvantage. In M. W. Kent & J. E. Rolf (Eds.), *Primary prevention in psychopathology. Vol. 8: Social competence in children* (pp. 49–74). Hanover, NH: University Press of New England.

Rutter, M. (1993). Resilience: Some conceptual considerations. *Journal of Adolescent Health, 14,* 626–631.

Rutter, M. (2000). Resilience reconsidered: Conceptual considerations, empirical findings, and policy implications. In J. P. Shonkoff & S. J. Meisels (Eds.), *Handbook of early childhood intervention* (2nd ed., pp. 651–682). New York: Cambridge University Press.

Sameroff, A. J., & Rosenblum, K. L. (2006). Psychosocial constraints on the development of resilience. *Annals of the New York Academy of Sciences, 1094,* 116–124.

Sampson, R. J., Raudenbush, S., & Earls, F. (1997). Neighborhoods and violent crime: A multilevel study of collective efficacy. *Science, 227,* 918–924.

Sandler, I., Wolchick, S., Davis, C., Haine, R., & Ayers, T. (2003). Correlational and experimental study of resilience for children of divorce and parentally bereaved children. In S. S. Luthar (Ed.), *Resilience and vulnerability: Adaptation in the context of childhood adversities* (pp. 213–240). New York: Cambridge University Press.

Schneider, W. J., Cavell, T. A., & Hughes, J. N. (2003). A sense of containment: Potential moderator of the relation between parenting practices and children's externalizing behaviors. *Development and Psychopathology, 15,* 95–117.

Schorr, L. (1988). *Within our reach: Breaking the cycle of disadvantage.* New York: Doubleday.

Seidman, E., & Pedersen, S. (2003). Holistic, contextual perspectives on risk, protection, and competence among low-income urban adolescents. In S. S. Luthar (Ed.), *Resilience and vulnerability: Adaptation in the context of childhood adversities* (pp. 318–342). New York: Cambridge University Press.

Skinner, E. A., Zimmer-Gembeck, M. J., & Connell, J. P. (1998). Individual differences and the development of perceived control. *Monographs of the Society for Research in Child Development, 63*(2–3), 1–220.

Sroufe, L.A. (2002). From infant attachment to promotion of adolescent autonomy: Prospective, longitudinal data on the role of parents in development. In J. G. Borkowski & S. L. Ramey (Eds.), *Parenting and the child's world: Influences on academic, intellectual, and social-emotional development. Monographs in Parenting* (pp. 187–202).

Steinberg, L., Elmen, J., & Mounts, N. (1989). Authoritative parenting, psychosocial maturity and academic success among adolescents. *Child Development, 60,* 1424–1436.

Steinberg, L. D., Dornbusch, S. M., & Brown, B. B. (1992). Ethnic differences in adolescent achievement: An ecological perspective. *American Psychologist, 47,* 723–729.

Steinberg, L. D., Mounts, N. S., Lamborn, S. D., & Dornbusch, S. M., (1991). Authoritative parenting and adolescent adjustment across varied ecological niches. *Journal of Research on Adolescence, 1,* 19–36.

Steward, S. M., & Bond, M. H. (2002). A critical look at parenting research from the mainstream: Problems uncovered while adapting Western research to non-Western cultures. *British Journal of Developmental Psychology, 20,* 379–392.

Wachs, T. (2005). Person-environment "fit" and individual development. In D. Teti (Ed.), *Handbook of research methods in developmental science* (pp. 443–466). Oxford, England: Blackwell.

Wachs, T. D. (2006). Contributions of temperament to buffering and sensitization processes in children's development. *Annals of the New York Academy of Sciences, 1094,* 40–51.

Wang, M. C., & Gordon, E. W. (1994). *Educational resilience in inner-city America: Challenges and prospects.* Hillsdale, NJ: Erlbaum.

Werner, E. E. (1995). Resilience in development. *Current Directions in Psychological Sciences, 4,* 81–84.

Werner, E. E. (2000). Protective factors and individual resilience. In J. P. Shonkoff & R. Meisels (Eds.), *Handbook of early childhood intervention* (pp. 115–132). New York: Cambridge University Press.

Werner, E. E., & Smith, R. S. (1982). *Vulnerable but invincible: A longitudinal study of resilient children and youth.* New York: McGraw-Hill.

Werner, E. E., & Smith, R. S. (1992). *Overcoming the odds: High-risk children from birth to adulthood.* Ithaca, NY: Cornell University Press.

Werner, E. E., & Smith, R. S. (2001). *Journeys from childhood to midlife: Risk, resilience, and recovery.* Ithaca, NY: Cornell University Press.

Wilson, W. J. (1996). *When work disappears: The world of the new urban poor.* New York: Knopf.

World Health Organization. (2002). Risk and resilience in adolescence: A global perspective. Geneva, Switzerland: Author.

Wyman, P. A., Cowen, E. L., Work, W. C., Hoyt-Meyers, L., Magnus, K. B., & Fagen, D. B. (1999). Caregiving and developmental factors differentiating young at-risk urban children showing resilient versus stress-affected outcomes: A replication and extension. *Child Development, 70,* 645–659.

Yates, T. M., & Masten, A. S. (2004). Fostering the future: resilience theory and the practice of positive psychology. In P. A. Linley & S. Joseph, (Eds.), *Positive psychology in practice.* Hoboken, NJ: Wiley.

CHAPTER

5

THEORIES AND MODELS OF ADOLESCENT DECISION MAKING

JULIE S. DOWNS ▪ BARUCH FISCHHOFF

LEARNING OBJECTIVES

After studying this chapter, you will be able to

- Explore research investigating the underlying decision-making processes adolescents use to make health decisions.

- Assess the decision-making skills and knowledge that adolescents bring to health decisions.

- Differentiate between normative analyses of decisions, descriptive accounts of how adolescents make decisions, and prescriptive interventions for improving decisions.

Adolescents' well-being depends critically on how well they make decisions, especially on matters with major physical and mental health consequences such as drinking, smoking, driving, education, sexuality, and violence. Adolescents' development depends critically on learning how to make such decisions, which inevitably entails some trial and error. Adolescents' ability to navigate the noisy process of development depends critically on an appropriate sense of self-efficacy, so that they take on decisions that they have a good chance of being able to handle, gradually increasing their range of autonomy.

Some observers dismiss adolescent decision making as an oxymoron. They see adolescents as irresponsible, thrill seeking, or liberated by a unique sense of invulnerability. These prejudices provide a ready audience for the fascinating results of early neuroimaging studies suggesting some distinctive features of the "adolescent brain," as revealed on tasks suited to that methodology. Like any sweeping generalization about a complex reality, this account can obscure as well as reveal important processes. For example, it belies the finding that adolescents tend to view themselves as *more* vulnerable, relative to their peers, than do adults (Quadrel, Fischhoff, & Davis, 1993). Adolescents greatly exaggerate their probability of dying prematurely, despite making other probability judgments with good construct and predictive validity (Bruine de Bruin, Parker, & Fischhoff, 2007a).

By the midteen years, teens typically have most of the same cognitive skills as adults (Reyna & Farley, 2006). Clearer differences between adolescents and adults arise in their familiarity with specific domains. In some domains adolescents may know more than adults as a result of how they spend their time (for example, on computers, cell phones, or in high school halls) or as a result of direct instruction (such as health education or drivers training). In other cases, they may know little or may even be misinformed (through advertising or rumors, for example). With new decisions, adolescents naturally lack the capabilities that come only with practice, such as quickly grasping the gist of familiar situations (Reyna & Farley, 2006) or having over-learned responses that they can exercise even under pressure.

With new decisions, adolescents naturally lack the capabilities that come only with practice, such as quickly grasping the gist of familiar situations.

Graduated drivers licensing illustrates one type of strategy for helping adolescents acquire the gist situational awareness and practiced psychomotor skills needed to make and execute sound choices in a very complex environment. Social skills training programs seek to do the same in settings where progress is essential if adolescents are to mature into adults (such as decisions about smoking, sex, or drinking), but where pitfalls can thwart development (such as addiction, unplanned pregnancy, or delinquency). As parents, educators, and policy makers, adults struggle to create the right balance of rights and responsibilities.

One measure of the difficulty faced by those providing guidance is seen in the observation by Justice Scalia in 2005 that the American Psychological Association had filed amicus briefs emphasizing both adolescents' capabilities (in a case supporting their reproductive rights) and their deficiencies (in a case opposing

The authors gratefully acknowledge support from National Science Foundation (Grant SES 0433152).

the adjudication of adolescents as adults). Both arguments could be valid. Decisions regarding health and violence differ in many ways, depending on the skills of the individual teens involved and the social and emotional pressures of the decisions that they face. However, such critical differences can get lost among sweeping generalizations about adolescents and their capabilities.

This chapter summarizes the research on the decision-making skills and knowledge that adolescents bring to health decisions. A different perspective would be to assess adolescents' competence to make various choices (Fischhoff, 2008). Health researchers and practitioners need to understand these limits, so that they expect neither too much nor too little from adolescents. They also need to understand the underlying processes, so that they can attempt to expand the range of health decisions that adolescents can make effectively.

Given the diversity and complexity of adolescents, decisions, and social environments, this research espouses no grand theories. Rather, it involves detailed assessments of decisions and the individuals making them. Overall theoretical accounts emerge from in a bottom up manner, from the integration of theories regarding the complex elements of people and tasks, rather than from a top-down general account of what people are like. The ingredients of these accounts are *normative analyses,* which identify the optimal choices for specific decisions and consider the values and capabilities of the individuals making them; *descriptive accounts* of how people interpret and integrate the elements of the choices they face; and *prescriptive interventions,* which seek to help people make better choices, bridging the gap between the normative ideal and the descriptive reality. These interventions enhance the normative and descriptive research by showing how well it has illuminated the problem.

A decision-making perspective provides a platform for integrating these diverse areas of research, extracting their practical importance for the choices that people make and how they make them.

Because it begins by characterizing decisions in analytical terms, this perspective looks at behavior through a cognitive lens. It accommodates noncognitive processes through their effects on how people approach their choices. Thus, for example, affective processes can cue specific task features, make judgments more or less optimistic, and affect task involvement. Impulsivity can arise from frustration over the inability to make choices or from drifting toward situations (such as sex or violence) where passions play a greater role. General feelings of self-efficacy (or internal locus of control) may predispose people to put more effort into getting decisions right, because they expect a return on their investment. Physiological or developmental factors can affect the outcomes that people seek to experience or avoid (such as fun, novelty, exploration, or social approval). Social and economic factors can affect the options among which individuals feel able to choose.

A decision-making perspective provides a platform for integrating these diverse areas of research, extracting their practical importance for the choices that people make and how they make them. Applied systematically, it can show general trends, such as adults' development of habitual responses that reduce their need for novel decision making and keep them from situations presenting impossible choices. Adults may also have more freedom from some coercive pressures (such as peers and parents) and less freedom from others (such as work and finance), affecting their ability to achieve desired ends.

KEY CONCEPTS AND RESEARCH FINDINGS

Decision science begins by creating a *normative* account of how a rational actor ought to make a decision. (The norms here are the axioms of utility theory, not the social norms familiar to psychologists.) *Rational actor models* assume that decision makers have a stable set of underlying preferences capable of evaluating any outcomes, and unlimited ability to perform the mental calculations needed to make such evaluations. If they are also well informed, rational actors will make *optimal* choices, in the sense of securing the best expected outcomes.

Rational actor models are implausible as a descriptive account of how most decisions are made. Indeed, violations of rationality were demonstrated (for example, Allais, 1952) almost as soon as its classic formulation (von Neumann & Morgenstern, 1944) was promulgated. Nonetheless, the conceptual clarity of rational actor models has aided the growth of more behaviorally realistic theories by making it easier to formulate hypotheses and aggregate results across studies. Comparison with a normative model also helps to focus and evaluate prescriptive attempts to facilitate better decision making by showing how much various imperfections matter.

An influential alternative approach describes behavior in terms of systematic deviations from rationality (Simon, 1956). It characterizes decision making in terms of psychologically plausible processes that seek to approximate optimal choices, but that don't require the cognitive skills, training, and capacity that rationality demands. One simplification strategy called *bounded rationality* uses a simplified (or "bounded") version of the actual decision, ignoring some options, uncertainties, or outcomes to get close enough to the optimal choice. A second simplification strategy called *satisficing* uses a heuristic (or rule of thumb) that can consider any aspect of a decision, but does not do so in rigorous detail. Rather, decision making proceeds until it identifies an option that passes critical thresholds (such as a vacation spot that is warm and inexpensive enough). Combinations are possible, such as using heuristics to simplify a choice set to the point where a boundedly rational analysis is possible.

Next, we consider separate elements of decision making: options, outcomes, and values. Here, we compare normative accounts of what a rational actor would do with descriptive accounts of what people actually do. We describe adolescent decision making in terms of differences from adult decision making (which it usually resembles in most respects), focusing on health-related tasks.

Considering Options

Decisions entail choices between options. Normatively, people should consider all possible options when making a choice. However, several constraints can truncate the set of options actually considered. One constraint is the limited time and energy available for identifying the potential options. When there are many possibilities, looking at them all can prevent understanding any of them (Long & Fischhoff, 2000). When reading long restaurant menus, for example, decision makers can feel that they have seen enough options and the time has come to start evaluating them. Truncating the search can improve decision making if it leads to examining promising options more thoroughly.

However, deeper examination of only a few options can undermine decision making if the option selection process is biased. Unlike restaurant selections, many decisions lack a list of options or an organizing principle outlining all categories of options. Instead, the available list may provide just appetizers with no hint as to what is missing. Familiar psychological processes can cause such biased selection by making some options disproportionately salient. For example, some options may be mentioned explicitly when a decision arises, whereas others are not. The status quo is typically an implicit option, and a favored one at that (Kahneman & Tversky, 1979). Inaction may not seem to be an option or may even be an admission of failure. Considering one option may highlight different possible outcomes than would emerge if that option's complement were considered instead (for example, skipping classes versus going to them).

When faced with explicit options, people might go no further, failing to ask if better options are "out there" or could be created from an ill-defined space of possibilities. Such restrictions on the option set could reflect a rational evaluation of the return on investment in additional searching. However, they could also reflect cognitive inertia, supported by not knowing how to structure the option creation process. Even when the explicit option space includes all viable alternatives, they may not be examined fully. People may instead unthinkingly rely on habitual behaviors that they have acquired by trial and error or instruction. When driving familiar routes, we think little about whether to make a particular turn unless something unusual captures our attention.

One likely difference between adolescents and adults is their repertoires of habits. In a rush, adolescents face many complex, uncertain decisions (about sex, drugs, schooling, careers, intimacy, and autonomy), with options that are barely delineated or are newly interpreted for their specific circumstances ("Exactly how do I say 'no' and still maintain my relationships?"). In contrast, adults have had more time to acquire effective habits (at least those adults who make it to adulthood with a modicum of success). As their tastes, interests, options, and beliefs change, they may also replace old habits with new ones. Happy hour may be less appealing (and less feasible) once a spouse or children enter the picture. As social circles and reputations solidify, less is riding on any given interaction. If their habits change gradually, it may be hard for them to reconstruct the process and realize how options that they have abandoned could still make sense for teens.

Other decisions don't evoke such habitual responses. The more important the decision, the greater the incentive to enumerate and examine options: which car to buy, which job to take, whether to have a child. Cognitively focused educational approaches are more likely to be effective for decisions like these, where people are predisposed to apply themselves analytically, as opposed to decisions where people wish to rely on simple heuristics or gut feelings, for which it may be better to teach solutions and their implementation.

Merely putting effort into decisions does not necessarily make them good ones, unless people have the needed cognitive skills. Parker, Bruine de Bruin, & Fischhoff

Merely putting effort into decisions does not necessarily make them good ones, unless people have the needed cognitive skills.

(2007) found that people who described themselves as attempting to maximize their outcomes reported poorer outcomes and performed more poorly on an individual-differences test of decision-making competence, compared to people who described themselves as attempting to satisfice (Bruine de Bruin, Parker, & Fischhoff, 2007b). Similarly, generating many options does not necessarily improve decision making. The value of this investment depends on one's ability to think of superior options and recognize them as such. Whether it is worth the effort depends on the importance of the decision and the efficiency of the process. Considering what to eat for lunch should not require systematic analysis, unless one is trying very hard to make a good impression. Even there, though, the critical advice may be simple, but perhaps not obvious to the inexperienced (for example, avoid spaghetti with tomato sauce on first dates and job interviews).

Utilities

Once the options are identified, their evaluation can begin. The first step is identifying the range of possible consequences that matters to the decision maker (for example, how much money could possibly be lost or gained or how long might a job take). The second step is determining the relative attractiveness (or aversiveness) of each possible consequence, known as its *utility* (or *disutility*). The utility could be a linear function of the outcomes if, say, a dollar is a dollar, however many one gets, or an hour is an hour, however long a job takes. Or it could take other forms. Decreasing marginal utility is common when the same incremental change matters less for higher values (going from $0 to $100, for example, versus from $1,000 to $1,100). But one can also anticipate getting increasingly frustrated as a task takes longer and longer.

The relative importance of one outcome compared to others depends on the range of possibilities for each. An outcome that is important in a general sense (such as money or life expectancy) might be unimportant in a particular decision if it does not vary across the options. For example, graduate students typically care a lot about money. However, within the set of apartments that they can conceivably afford, other concerns may dominate. Everyone values health, but needn't consider it when channel surfing. *Importance* is context dependent, and importance rating scales are thus meaningless unless interpreted in context.

Decision theory is agnostic about what people hold to be important. It cares only about people's ability to identify choices in their own, self-defined best interest. Elaborate procedures are used to discern what people value (Fischhoff & Manski, 1999). These follow two strategies. *Expressed preference procedures* ask people to describe those values. These procedures face the same threats as attitude measurement, such as overt misrepresentation, failure of introspection, stimulus and response range effects, and so on. *Revealed preference procedures* infer values from actual behavior. They face threats from the confounding effects of the other elements of the decision-making processes, such as how people assess the probabilities of achieving the outcomes, how people integrate different concerns in making their choices, and whether people act on those choices.

As imperfect as these procedures may be, they represent a commitment to looking at decisions from the decision makers' perspective. Indeed, although decision-making research is most clearly formulated in terms of completing the normative-descriptive-prescriptive arc, the normative analysis cannot begin without some descriptive understanding of decision makers' goals. This commitment means that even when researchers are focused on a particular goal shared by adolescents (such as avoiding sexually transmitted infections), they must consider other competing or conflicting objectives (such as social standing, experience, and fun), as well as the possibility that adolescents care less about shared objectives than adults might like (such as hoping to get much more out of life than just avoiding sexually transmitted infections).

Studying decision makers' values in a disciplined way is particularly important when researchers come from different backgrounds compared to decision makers. Thus, value elicitation might be essential when adults such as researchers or educators try to understand and help adolescents. As elsewhere, there is value in triangulating revealed and expressed preference methods. That is, it is good to observe what adolescents actually do—including the behaviors that they avoid—in sufficient detail to reveal reasonable hypotheses about the values that might underlie their choices. At the same time, it is also good to ask adolescents what is on their minds—in order to sort through potential motivating factors that are correlated—and identify those that had not occurred to adults.

An increasingly recognized threat to value assessment, and to effective decision making, is people not knowing what they want. That is, even when people hold strong general values, an inferential process is required to articulate their implications for specific choices. In such cases, seemingly subtle changes in problem representation can produce preference shifts. Such phenomena have long been the bread and butter of researchers studying context effects, such as the difference between people's willingness to "prohibit" an act and "not to allow" it. Such studies have typically emphasized the semantic content of evaluation tasks. Decision science's complementary contribution has been to offer more structural accounts of the vagaries in values.

One such account traced back to Coombs (1964), Thurstone (1924), and perhaps before, is that people have distributions of values from which they sample preferences whenever specific questions arise. In such cases, any two observations might seem inconsistent; however, a set of observations will reveal orderly variability. Over time, the distribution will tend to shift as people discover that they like some things more or less than they expected, and to tighten as people converge on that value. Shifting and uncertain preferences should be more likely with adolescents as they gradually learn what they like about new topics. When that is the case, it takes sustained observation to distinguish noisy preferences from chaotic ones.

These models typically assume stable preferences, which people learn to recognize. However, preferences can also change with experience. Of particular relevance to adolescence is the value that novelty per se can have, whether just as something new or as an opportunity to learn. Where novelty has value, experiences should have less value over time. Such habituation should be more common among adolescents than adults because more things are novel to them. In this light, adults' advice to "grow up" may in effect ask adolescents to reach a state that requires personal experience without allowing adolescents to live through those experiences.

A second decision science account involves situations in which people have conflicting values that they have not resolved. In such cases, people are particularly vulnerable to the perspectives made salient by the way questions are posed. Advertisers take advantage of this indeterminacy by trying to highlight values that favor their products. In principle, adolescents should be particularly vulnerable to such manipulation, insofar as they are still consolidating their self-identity and what things matter most to them.

A third account involves situations in which people choose to work through these uncertainties and contradictions. That is, of course, what happens in life. Sometimes we face easily weighed outcomes. At red lights, the utility of gaining a few seconds is clearly less than the expected disutility of possibly being hit by a bus. Sometimes, though, we are torn between competing values. A piece of cake may look delicious but conflict with dietary goals whose importance depends in turn on how we judge consequences like feeling good about ourselves, looking good at a reunion, and living to a ripe old age. Moreover, to some extent we realize that our values are time dependent, with current pleasures dominating later ones (and later pain). Temporal discounting—caring less about future outcomes—is one part of the puzzle and is often confounded with other concerns, like not being sure that we will live to enjoy future rewards or be able to collect on others' promises to deliver them (Frederick, Loewenstein, & O'Donoghue, 2002).

In order to avoid paralysis, we work through these conflicts, expressing preferences drawn from our basic values. An applied branch of decision science called *decision analysis* (Raiffa, 1968; von Winterfeldt & Edwards, 1986) tries to help people do so in an orderly way. Many of its tools seek to structure value elicitation in ways that avoid the kinds of bias described above. Similarly spirited prescriptive interventions can be found in various values-clarification procedures. Studies of such processes are relatively rare in descriptive research, as though the possibility of changing people, even for the better, leaves researchers nervous. Such studies would be particularly interesting with adolescents, given the possibilities for large, important changes.

Probabilities

The utilities assigned to possible outcomes capture their relative value. In many decisions, decision makers need to know the probability that choosing any given option will lead to each possible outcome. For example, when deciding whether to pull all-nighters, teens need to know how likely it is that the effort will improve their grade. Ideally, knowledge of such probabilities comes from long experience, allowing accurate estimation of relative frequencies. In lieu of experience, people are left with judgments. These expressions of belief about future events are called *subjective probabilities* when they have the internal consistency needed to satisfy the probability axioms (for example, the probability of an event and its complement should equal 100 percent).

Arguably, some subjectivity is inevitable. Even in deliberately standardized realms (such as casino gambles), people might wonder about the procedures (for example, are the slots rigged?). Even in statistics-rich domains, like baseball, judgment is needed to identify the relevant statistics. For example, is a batter's chance of hitting predicted best by his average for his career, the season, at home, or against left-handed pitchers? Conditioning on enough variables makes the event a unique one. Choosing the optimal reference class (or two or three) requires theoretical judgment. Recognizing the need for judgment, some scholars distinguish between *estimating* relative frequencies versus *assessing* probabilities. The former is akin to bounded rationality, following sophisticated procedures on a narrowly defined problem. The latter is akin to satisficing, taking a sophisticatedly broad view en route to admittedly flawed judgments.

The proper balance between seeing events as unique versus repeated is a central topic in decision science. Bayes's Theorem gives the normative answer. But descriptive research tells us that people don't often hit the right balance. On the one hand, people's existing beliefs can be very resistant to change, as they deliberately recruit supporting evidence and extract support from ambiguous evidence (*confirmation bias*). On the other hand, people can neglect the implications of statistical summaries of what usually happens in similar situations if they are confronted with salient evidence regarding a specific case (*base-rate fallacy*). Determining which conditions favor different patterns is a lively research area (Gilovich, Griffin, & Kahneman, 2002; Kahneman, Slovic, & Tversky, 1982). Once mastered, its conclusions should apply equally to adolescents and adults. There are no demonstrated developmental differences in how general and specific probabilities are combined. Like other higher cognitive skills, these appear to be consolidated by midadolescence, leaving teens with the capabilities and limitations of adults.

For example, fairly accurate predictions were made by a random national sample of fifteen- and sixteen-year olds (in the National Longitudinal Survey of Youth 1997) regarding the probabilities of major events in their lives, such as getting pregnant, being arrested, or working full-time (Bruine de Bruin et al., 2007a). The orderliness of their responses suggests that any biases in teens' probability judgments likely reflect problems with their beliefs, rather than difficulties with giving numerical probabilities. These predictions were later correlated with the experiences that the teens reported on subsequent waves of the survey. For most outcomes, there were large correlations between the probabilities that teens had initially given and whether they subsequently reported the event.

The group-level accuracy of some of these predictions follows general behavioral principles, plausibly applied to these tasks. For example, receiving a high school diploma and encounters with the law, both of which were predicted within a 3 percent margin of accuracy, are relatively public events for which teens might observe large, relatively unbiased samples such that relying on the availability heuristic would serve them well (Tversky & Kahneman, 1974). Females underestimated their risk of pregnancy and childbirth, possibly reflecting their not realizing how many pregnancies are hidden or how the chances will increase as they progress past puberty. It might also reflect misunderstanding of how unprotected sex happens, including the roles of passion and emerging social norms (Downs, Murray, et al., 2004). For those females who did not want to get pregnant, there may have been some element of wishful thinking, as there might have been with those who overestimated their chances of staying in school and working.

Each of these necessarily speculative accounts focuses on the information that teens have to process, while assuming that they have imperfect processing skills similar to those of adults. Whatever individuals' skills, they are at the mercy of the information available to them and their understanding of its limitations. Particular challenges arise with rare, important events that lack reliable, trustworthy reporting, requiring people to infer a lot from a little. Adolescents often find themselves in this kind of situation. They have not had time to observe many of life's most dire events, such as suicide, serious injury, addiction, or unplanned pregnancies. Conventional social practices often hide them. Summary information is often embedded in persuasive communications from well-meaning adults, which adolescents must learn to decode, much as they must learn to decode the communications of advertisers.

Whatever individuals' skills, they are at the mercy of the information available to them and their understanding of its limitations.

Thus, adolescents must make complex inferences about risks from imperfect information sources. For example, educational materials often depict unprotected sex as very risky (for example, "it only takes once" for sex to lead to pregnancy). When young women do not get pregnant after unprotected sex, some of them infer (logically, given their biased knowledge) that they are infertile. This inference leads to the conclusion that unprotected sex is safer than they thought, ultimately leading to higher-risk behaviors (Downs, Bruine de Bruin, Murray, & Fischhoff, 2004). Other possible inferential challenges arise after observing friends using drugs without overdosing, having sex without appearing to get pregnant or contract a disease, driving drunk without crashing, and so on. Risk analysts often use near misses to inform their understanding of rare events such as plane crashes. It would be a lot to ask teens to extract proper lessons intuitively from, say, observing the effects of binge drinking on controlling cars or sexual encounters if no severe consequences result. Adults would face similar difficulty in making inferences about poorly described unfamiliar events in their own lives (such as investments, career changes, or mortgages).

In contrast to the above relatively orderly and accurate predictions, adolescents greatly exaggerate the probability of premature death. Whereas 0.08 percent of U.S. teens die annually, survey respondents (0.10 percent of whom had died by the next wave of the survey) gave estimates that were two orders of magnitude higher: 18.6 percent chance of dying in the next year, 20.3 percent by age twenty. Moreover, most gave the same probability for dying in the next year and by age twenty, even though the first figure should normatively be much lower. Among those giving different judgments, only two-thirds gave a higher probability for the longer period. These judgments showed some elements of construct validity (such as positive correlations with reported neighborhood gang violence and personal gang membership), suggesting that they are not thoughtless responses. They include one known anomaly in probability judgments observed previously with adults (including technical experts): an apparent tendency to say fifty, in the sense of an uncertain "fifty-fifty," rather than a numerical probability when deeply uncertain about what to say but wanting to fulfill the researchers' demand for a number. Such epistemic uncertainty is seen here in a preponderance of responses at fifty within a distribution of probability judgments in which the median of other responses is 10 percent, still much too high. It represents another reflection of adolescents' heightened sense of vulnerability.

Integration

Options, values, and probabilities are the ingredients for a choice. Actually choosing requires applying a decision rule. For a rational actor, that entails assessing the *expected utility* of each option. The expected utility of each outcome equals its utility multiplied by its probability. Summing over the possible outcomes yields that option's overall expected utility. That is possible because all options have been translated into a common unit—utility. (A purely economic approach would translate everything into dollars.)

Summing expected utilities across outcomes treats them as *compensatory outcomes,* in the sense that being very good in one respect (such as most likely to be a lot of fun) compensates, at least somewhat, for being bad in another (such as some chance of pain). Other deliberate decision rules are possible and can be incorporated into normative analyses. For example, a *conjunctive decision rule* requires each expected outcome to pass a threshold (for example, at least some expected fun and not too costly). A *disjunctive decision rule* imposes a threshold on just one outcome (such as not risky at all). Such rules approach satisficing if the decision maker stops once the first acceptable option has been identified.

When outcomes are uncertain, the option with the highest expected utility may not turn out to be the one that provides the best outcomes. Experience may show some sound choices backfiring, with foolish ones occasionally lucking out. *Outcome bias* describes the tendency to judge choices by the outcomes that followed them, rather than by the thinking that went into them. It can be amplified by *hindsight bias,* as a result of which people can no longer recall (or reconstruct) the uncertainty surrounding the choices, and end up exaggerating how clear the experienced outcomes were.

Decision scientists have long known that in decisions of any complexity, complete expected utility calculations are infeasible. Researchers have adopted several strategies for dealing with that reality. One examines how people transform decision-making tasks into problem-solving ones, in which they can apply deterministic rules to identify the best options. Some of these rules have a formal structure. For example, elimination by aspects looks at all options in terms of the outcome that is most important in some general sense, eliminating those that are inferior in that respect. It then does the same for the second most important outcome and so on, until one option is left. Like any simplification strategy, this one can produce inferior choices when the features that it ignores matter. Tversky (1972) shows how elimination by aspects can

When outcomes are uncertain, the option with the highest expected utility may not turn out to be the one that provides the best outcomes.

produce intransitive preferences (preferring A to B, B to C, and C to A), violating a normative axiom. Other simplifying rules are domain-specific rules. Studying such rules helped the development of artificial intelligence (Newell & Simon, 1968).

A second approach to the descriptive implausibility of expected utility theory has been to create alternative computational rules, embodying principles that are more plausible psychologically. These alternative rules abandon the normative claims of expected utility theory (regarding how decisions should be made) for the sake of greater descriptive realism. The most prominent alternative is Kahneman and Tversky's (1979) *Prospect Theory*. It posits that people value options (called *prospects*) in terms of changes from a *reference point* (typically the status quo), rather than in terms of the resultant overall "wealth" (or *net asset position*). Although it might be normatively appropriate to look at everything (in effect, counting one's blessings), it is much more natural to look at changes from an adaptation level. Prospect theory also posits that the *value* assigned to a given change is greater if it is bad than if it is good (losses loom larger than equivalent gains). A third assumption is that people try to simplify the probabilities of these outcomes, showing insensitivity to differences in the midrange (for example, 30 percent versus 40 percent), while prizing outcomes that can be predicted with certainty.

Prospect theory has been elaborately examined and reformulated. Among its most renowned findings are *framing effects,* or reversals of preference achieved by manipulating the reference point. For example, comparing a salary increase to last year's salary may make it more acceptable than comparing it to the raise one expected or to some measure of inflation. Other researchers have proposed alternative reformulations of utility theory based on other psychologically intuitive principles, such as the desire to avoid regret (Loomes & Sugden, 1983).

A third integration strategy entails examining how sensitive the optimality of a choice is to the precision in decision makers' thinking. For example, von Winterfeldt & Edwards (1986) showed that for a broad class of decisions with continuous options (for example, drive X mph, spend Y hours on homework, or invest $Z), expected outcomes were relatively insensitive to errors. The downside of living in such a forgiving world is not receiving clear feedback on how good one's judgment was, leaving one vulnerable in situations where accuracy matters.

In a related result, Dawes and Corrigan (1974) found that predictive models with the computational form of utility theory (and prospect theory) are often forgiving of estimation errors in model inputs. Such *simple linear models,* including weighted sum models, consist of those where probabilities weight the utilities of outcomes. If the variables in a simple linear model are individually correlated with the criterion, the model will have some predictive success even if the weights are somewhat wrong, the bivariate relationships somewhat nonlinear, and there are some moderate interactions (not captured by simply adding individually weighted variables). With standardized variables (mean=0; standard deviation=1), regression weights perform no better than unit weights as long as they have the proper sign. The same would apply to other models as they approach standardization (for example, using the same rating scale for all variables).

The predictive power of simple linear models is good news for researchers with predictive intent. They can focus on identifying variables that correlate with the criterion and on measuring them well. The modeling will take care of itself. It is bad news for researchers with explanatory intent. Many different models, varying in their predictors, form, and weights, will have similar predictive success. Although each model implies a different explanatory account, essentially they are empirically indistinguishable. Researchers will naturally find ways to account for why one model fits better than another, in a single study or across studies. However, they might just be explaining random variation around the insight shared by the underlying constructs common to the various models.

Faced by these results, decision scientists have largely abandoned predicting individual choices, assured that this could always be done through collaboration with researchers who knew which concerns motivated individuals in particular domains. Instead they have focused on the processes governing the elements, such as how people assess probabilities and utilities, how they structure decisions, and how they evaluate their own competence. There is little research comparing adolescents and adults in terms of adherence to prospect theory or to any other integration rule. Nor is there any strong reason to expect the basic psychological processes (such as evaluating alternatives relative to a reference point) to be different at different ages.

DECISION SCIENCE AND SOCIAL COGNITION MODELS OF HEALTH BEHAVIOR

Many health researchers are familiar with the approach to decision making embodied in social cognitive models of behavior change, such as the health belief model (Becker & Rosenstock, 1987), the theory of reasoned action (Fishbein & Ajzen, 1975), and its extension in the theory of planned behavior (Ajzen, 1991). These models have had success in predicting behaviors in many domains and have informed interventions seeking changes in health behaviors.

These models share concepts with decision theory. They view people as making choices that reflect perceptions of the attractiveness of possible outcomes, weighted by their perceived likelihood (although each construct is measured somewhat differently). By focusing on specific domains, researchers bring subject-matter expertise regarding the outcomes that occupy decision-makers (such as conforming to social norms) and factors affecting likelihood judgments (such as perceived control or pluralistic ignorance). They may develop measures that can be reused across studies, decreasing costs and improving comparability, but necessarily sacrificing some precision in accounting for domain-specific factors. Thus, social cognitive models provide an efficient point of departure for practitioners, especially ones who care about theoretical understanding specifically to the extent that it facilitates achieving practical results. For them, the fact that social cognitive models are also simple linear models should matter little—that is, it should not matter if different models, and their underlying theories, cannot be distinguished empirically, as long as they include enough insight to predict or produce healthier behavior.

In contrast, *decision science* looks at each choice as a separate problem. It begins with a normative analysis that finds where a focal behavior fits into the big picture of individuals' goals, options, and constraints. As a result, the analysis can conclude that the behavior change desired by the researcher is not in the individuals' self-defined best interest. In other words, "misbehavior" may not be just a matter of misunderstanding the situation. Such cases raise the question of whether researchers are empowered to engage in persuasive attempts to change individuals' values or whether they would do better to change individuals' world so that the behavior that the researcher favors produces outcomes that the individuals also want.

As part of a broad review, Ogden (2003) criticizes applications of social cognitive models for failing to take their theoretical claims seriously. She notes that most studies find their criterion variable uncorrelated with at least one key predictor in their model. A typical response is to find reasons why the relationship might fail in their circumstances, rather than to challenge the model. This suggests that the models are valued more for their predictive power than for their theoretical content. As mentioned, that might satisfy the needs of practically oriented users, who may not appreciate or be concerned by the robustness (or shakiness) of the associated theory. As Ogden notes, a theory that cannot be tested is not a theory at all. (Invoking a theory might, however, effectively raise the status of social science research in settings dominated by natural scientists.)

In contrast, decision science offers no overarching theory of decision making. Expected utility theory provides aspirational predictions, showing what fully rational individuals would do. Providing a standard for evaluating actual performance helps to identify places where people could use help in making better choices, while prompting the search for processes that might undermine their performance. Those processes are typically studied in isolation, using primarily experimental procedures. This results in testable hypotheses (such as prospect theory, hindsight bias, and overconfidence) regarding elements of decision making. Normative analyses characterize the roles that these processes play in specific choices. Where social cognitive models have proven useful, they could provide points of departure for both the normative models and the descriptive work of decision science.

ADOLESCENTS AND ADULTS

Each of the preceding sections considered how adolescents might differ from adults, in light of either evidence making direct comparisons or general theoretical considerations. These comparisons consider differences in both psychology and circumstances. Generally speaking, there seems to be more variation in circumstances than in psychology. By the midteen years, cognitive performance on most decision-making skills appears to be similar for adults and adolescents. However, adolescents face different decisions in different and, arguably, more difficult informational environments. A full comparison of adult and adolescent decision making would also consider differences in social and emotional processes, looking for barriers to orderly decision making and interventions that might facilitate it.

Given the diversity of decisions that adults and adolescents face—not to mention the diversity of adults and adolescents—any sweeping generalization about differences between them may obscure as much as it clarifies. From a decision science perspective, any observed difference has practical importance to the extent that decisions are sensitive to it. Decision science assesses that relevance by asking how other processes affect each element of the normative-descriptive-prescriptive treatment of a decision. Consider the following three examples.

A full comparison of adult and adolescent decision making would also consider differences in social and emotional processes, looking for barriers to orderly decision making and interventions that might facilitate it.

1. Some evidence suggests that adolescents react more slowly to some risk-related stimuli. If decisions must be made so quickly that this time difference precludes recognizing a risk, then the decision that adolescents make could miss elements that adults recognize. Prescriptive interventions could train for the needed pattern recognition, as is done for drivers, pilots, and soldiers. Similar reasoning applies to older drivers who can no longer recognize or respond to familiar risks or whose driving environment has changed (although training for pattern recognition may be less feasible).

2. Adolescents are often held to be particularly prone to discount future outcomes, in part because they seem to be more willing to take risks that threaten their future well-being. *Pure temporal discounting* is the term for valuing outcomes less simply because they will be incurred later (next year versus today or two years from now versus next year). Decision science has studied how other concerns can mimic pure temporal discounting, while representing other underlying processes. For example, a future outcome may be valued less if one does not expect to live to enjoy it, if one does not expect it to be delivered, if one does not expect to enjoy it as much (as a result of changing tastes, for example), if one expects to derive greater benefit from savoring or learning from the experience by having it sooner, or if one expects to derive greater value from meeting an immediate need (such as money that provides a grubstake or recognition that launches a career). These expectations may be misinformed. However, even if they lead to poor choices, poor understanding is a different diagnosis from poor impulse control.

3. Adolescents are often held to be more impulsive than adults, and some observers point to neural and hormonal differences. However, looking at decisions from adolescents' perspective may reveal that their actions have benefits that adults do not appreciate. A youth culture may prize spontaneity, leading to deliberate choices that look superficially like impulsive ones. Inability to decide can leave people drifting toward situations in which social pressures change the decision calculus (such as a sexual encounter or violent confrontation). Not realizing just how difficult a decision can be may erode adolescents' (or adults') feelings of self-efficacy, leaving them less willing to try.

SUMMARY

Decision science employs a systematic strategy for all decisions. *Normative analysis* summarizes scientific knowledge regarding the decision, focused on the outcomes that matter to decision makers. *Descriptive research* characterizes the decision makers' perspectives in terms comparable to the normative analysis. *Prescriptive interventions* seek to close the critical gaps, a process that depends on the extent of descriptive understanding and the validity of the normative analysis. Decision science generates research regarding fundamental processes of decision making, such as probability assessment and value consistency. It accommodates research from other fields to the extent that their results involve effects large enough to affect choices.

Applied to adolescents, decision science has revealed a more positive picture, relative to the gloomy view that many people hold about adolescents' capabilities. That picture reflects (1) a gloomier view of adults, based on the well-documented litany of judgmental biases, (2) a conceptual framework that allows a clearer characterization of decision-making processes, and (3) a willingness to examine choices in terms of adolescents' many goals, not just those that adults wish them to have. Only decision-specific research can tell how competent adolescents are to make specific choices—or could be with properly focused help.

By the midteen years, adolescents seem to have most of the cognitive decision-making skills of adults. They know more about some things, less about others. They share some goals with adults, but not al. They may face harder decisions, with fewer automatic choices, under different social constraints, and with less emotional control. Future collaborations with decision scientists, especially in the development of prescriptive interventions, should be theoretically productive, while pushing other fields toward decision-relevant topics.

KEY TERMS

Base-rate fallacy
Bounded rationality
Confirmation bias
Conjunctive decision rule
Decision analysis
Decision science
Descriptive accounts
Disjunctive decision rule
Disutility
Expected utility
Expressed preference procedures
Framing effects
Hindsight bias
Normative analyses

Outcome bias
Prescriptive interventions
Prospect theory
Prospects
Pure temporal discounting
Rational actor models
Reference point
Revealed preference procedures
Satisficing
Self-efficiency
Simple linear models
Subjective probabilities
Utility

DISCUSSION QUESTIONS

1. How do decision makers use the information available to them in choosing between options? How might the quality of this information differ for adolescents and adults?

2. What are the key differences between social cognitive models of behavior change and decision science? What are the strengths and limitations to using each of these models as a framework for understanding how adolescents make decisions?

3. Given that adolescents and adults have similar cognitive skills, why are adolescents perceived to be worse decision makers? Explain and provide examples.

REFERENCES

Ajzen, I. (1991). The theory of planned behavior. *Organizational Behavior and Human Decision Processes, 50,* 179–211.

Allais, M. (1952). The foundations of a positive theory of choice involving risk and a criticism of the postulates and axioms of the American school. In M. Allais & O. Hagen (Eds.), *Expected utility hypotheses and the Allais Paradox* (pp. 27–147). Dordrecht, The Netherlands: D. Reidel.

Becker, M. H., & Rosenstock, J. M. (1987). Comparing social learning theory and the health belief model. In W. B. Ward (Ed.), *Advances in health education and promotion* (pp. 245–249). Greenwich, CT: JAI Press.

Bruine de Bruin, W., Parker, A. M., & Fischhoff, B. (2007a). Can teens predict significant life events? *Journal of Adolescent Health, 41,* 208–210.

Bruine de Bruin, W., Parker, A. M., & Fischhoff, B. (2007b). Individual differences in adult decision-making competence. *Journal of Personality and Social Psychology, 92,* 938–956.

Coombs, C. H. (1964). *A theory of data.* New York: Wiley.

Dawes, R. M., & Corrigan, B. (1974). Linear models in decision making. *Psychological Bulletin, 81,* 95–106.

Downs, J. S., Bruine de Bruin, W., Murray, P. J., & Fischhoff, B. (2004). When "it only takes once" fails: Perceived infertility after unsafe sex predicts condom use and STI acquisition. *Journal of Pediatric and Adolescent Gynecology, 17,* 224.

Downs, J. S., Murray, P. J., Bruine de Bruin, W., Penrose, J., Palmgren, C., & Fischhoff, B. (2004). Interactive video behavioral intervention to reduce adolescent females' STD risk: A randomized controlled trial. *Social Science and Medicine, 59,* 1561–1572.

Fischhoff, B. (2008). Assessing adolescent decision-making competence. *Developmental Review, 28,* 12–28.

Fischhoff, B., & Manski, C. F. (1999). (Eds.). Preference elicitation. Special (triple) issue of *Journal of Risk and Uncertainty, 19,* 1–3.

Fishbein, M., & Ajzen, I. (1975). *Belief, attitude, intention, and behavior: An introduction to theory and research.* Reading, MA: Addison-Wesley.

Frederick, S., Loewenstein, G., & O'Donoghue, T. (2002). Time discounting and time preference: A critical review. *Journal of Economic Literature, 40,* 351–401.

Gilovich, T., Griffin, D. W., & Kahneman, D. (2002). *Heuristics and biases: The psychology of intuitive judgment.* New York: Cambridge University Press.

Kahneman, D., Slovic, P., & Tversky, A. (1982). *Judgment under uncertainty: Heuristics and biases.* New York: Cambridge University Press.

Kahneman, D., & Tversky, A. (1979). Prospect theory: An analysis of decision under risk. *Econometrica, 47,* 263–291.

Long, J., & Fischhoff, B. (2000). Setting risk priorities: A formal model. *Risk Analysis, 20,* 339–351.

Loomes, G., & Sugden, R. (1983). Regret theory and measurable utility. *Economics Letters, 12,* 19–21.

Newell, A., & Simon, H. A. (1968). Simulation: Individual behavior. In D. L. Sills (Ed.), *International encyclopedia of the social sciences* (Vol. 14, pp. 262–268). New York: Macmillan and The Free Press.

Ogden, J. (2003). Some problems with social cognition models: A pragmatic and conceptual analysis. *Health Psychology, 22*, 424–428.

Parker, A. M., Bruine de Bruin, W., & Fischhoff, B. (2007). Maximizers versus satisficers: Decision-making styles, competence, and outcomes. *Judgment and Decision Making, 2*, 342–350.

Parker, A. M., & Fischhoff, B. (2005). Decision-making competence: External validation through an individual-differences approach. *Journal of Behavioral Decision Making, 18*, 1–27.

Quadrel, M. J., Fischhoff, B., & Davis, W. (1993). Adolescent (in)vulnerability. *American Psychologist, 48*, 102–116.

Raiffa, H. (1968). *Decision analysis.* Reading, MA: Addison-Wesley.

Reyna, V., & Farley, F. (2006). Risk and rationality in adolescent decision making: Implications for theory, practice, and public policy. *Psychology in the Public Interest, 7*(1), 1–44.

Simon, H. A. (1956). Rational choice and the structure of the environment. *Psychological Review, 63*, 129–138.

Thurstone, L. L. (1924). *The nature of intelligence.* New York: Harcourt Brace.

Tversky, A. (1972). Elimination by aspects: A theory of choice. *Psychological Review, 79*, 281–299.

Tversky, A., & Kahneman, D. (1974). Judgment under uncertainty: Heuristics and biases. *Science, 185*, 1124–1131.

Von Neumann, J., & Morganstern, O. (1944). *Theory of games and economic behavior.* Princeton, NJ: Princeton University Press.

Von Winterfeldt, D., & Edwards, W. (1986). *Decision analysis and behavioral research.* New York: Cambridge University Press.

CHAPTER

6

BIOLOGICAL UNDERPINNINGS OF ADOLESCENT DEVELOPMENT

ELIZABETH A. SHIRTCLIFF

LEARNING OBJECTIVES

After studying this chapter, you will be able to

- Recognize the influence of biological factors on behaviors during adolescence.
- List key biological changes that occur during the adolescent period.
- Explain how the organizational-activational hypothesis helps explain hormonal processes.

This chapter will explore the influence of biological factors on behaviors that change during adolescence. It will describe some of the biological changes that occur during adolescence, focusing on pubertal development, the hormonal changes that cause puberty to progress, and concomitant changes in the adolescent brain.

Understanding peripheral and central biological changes allows us to gain a better understanding about why social, emotional, and risky behavior changes during adolescence. This knowledge may in turn lead to a better understanding of how some biological changes in pubertal individuals can contribute to the emergence of problem behavior. A handful of behaviors that typically change during adolescence will be used as exemplars of this biosocial model.

It may seem out of place in a practical, outcome-based text to focus on biological underpinnings of adolescent development; therefore, a brief note about the policy implications of biological research is warranted. There are at least three possible policy-oriented reasons for exploring biological underpinnings of adolescent development, as follows:

1. Biologically informed methods may indicate a mechanism or provide a window into the *etiology* of a disorder or developmental phenomenon, particularly when we consider the interplay between biological and social forces.

2. Biological forces may indicate *who is the most vulnerable* to a particular disorder or, more interestingly, in what biological state or at what time an underlying vulnerability is most likely to be expressed.

3. Intervention research that indicates an initial biological vulnerability may be able to demonstrate *differential changes* in the outcomes in longitudinal investigations.

Thus, by incorporating biologically informed methods into our studies, we can gain insight into vulnerabilities and mechanisms and a deeper understanding of the developmental changes we are able to see or report. By understanding biological underpinnings, we may gain additional insights into the social contextual world of adolescents and how it interacts with their biology.

Hormones are emphasized here because they are remarkably responsive to the environment, constantly changing in response to our physical, social, and emotional world. Yet hormones are also the scaffolding for the genetic blueprint of the individual; over seconds, minutes, hours, and days, they activate genes nearly everywhere in the human body. Genes are unchanging, but hormones allow their expression to vary across time, social context, physical environments, and developmental stages (Gottlieb, 1996).

Hormones are also emphasized because they drive puberty—after critical events take place in the peripubertal brain. *Adolescence* has been defined as that awkward period between sexual maturation and the attainment of adult roles and responsibilities (Dahl, 2004). The first part of adolescence is marked by pubertal development and the activation of hormonal systems, and so understanding these biological changes will afford greater insight into the first changes in the early adolescent.

Although this review will emphasize hormones, I do not want to overplay their importance or perpetuate the long-standing myth of adolescents as victims of "raging hormones" (Buchanan, Eccles, & Becker, 1992). Many studies begin with such statements, then quickly dismiss the model after failing to support a simple hormone-behavior relationship. Raging hormones have become a straw man argument for adolescents before the nature of their biological changes has been sufficiently explored. Yet we know that a direct relationship between hormones and behavior is unlikely, because it takes so long for hormones to be released and longer still for them to turn genes on and off. Hormones rarely cause behavioral change. Rather, they are more likely to exaggerate one's propensity for that behavior. Acknowledging the complexities may help resolve the paradox of hormone-behavior relationships: hormones help us feel better, remember better, metabolize better, and interact better with others. Why, then, should adolescence be a risky time? The answer is not yet known, but a model more complex than a direct hormone-behavior relationship is necessary. Throughout I will emphasize when and where a hormonal effect is likely, and when a more complex model may be warranted.

THE ORGANIZATIONAL-ACTIVATIONAL HYPOTHESIS: HORMONAL CHANGES FROM FETAL THROUGH ADOLESCENT DEVELOPMENT

To understand the biological changes that occur in adolescence, one must begin by understanding hormonal activities in fetal and early postnatal development. Phoenix, Goy, and Young (1967) proposed the *organizational-activational hypothesis* to explain the observation that the same hormones that organize the body and the brain in fetal and early postnatal life will later activate the body and the brain after puberty (see Romeo, 2003, for a more recent review). During sexual differentiation in utero, the fetal testes release *androgens,* hormones that masculinize the brain and body (for example, testosterone). The male brain is also defeminized during fetal development, though *estrogens,* hormones which feminize the brain and body (for example, estradiol) are implicated. Testosterone crosses the blood-brain barrier more easily than estrogen, and then testosterone is converted to estrogen in the brain by the enzyme aromatase (Hutchison, 1997). The "default" sex is female, so no signal is necessary from the ovary to organize the female (Zahn-Waxler, Crick, Shirtcliff, & Woods, 2006). Most important, the hormonal cascade known as the *hypothalamic-pituitary-gonadal (HPG) axis,* which begins with the release of gonadotropin-releasing hormone (GnRH) from the hypothalamus and ends with the release of androgens and estrogens, is fully operational during pre- and early postnatal development. Newborn babies occasionally have acne, swollen testes, or enlarged nipples, all body changes that are advanced by hormones during puberty, providing observable evidence that this hormonal cascade is working early.

Organizational effects were first described regarding the development of structural differences between the male and female body, but were later extended to brain development and behavioral effects. Behaviors that implicate organizational effects include sexual, aggressive, and play behavior. Phoenix, Goy, and Young (1967) examined organizational effects in primates and showed that females who were administered testosterone prenatally showed more aggressive behavior, more "rough and tumble play" to near male-typical levels, and also male-like mounting behaviors (sexual behavior). These behaviors each involve an underlying neurocircuitry that is organized by hormones (Romeo, 2003). These organizational effects also translate to humans. Berenbaum and Resnick (1997) describe similar findings in girls with *congenital adrenal hyperplasia* (CAH), a condition in which the fetal adrenal gland secretes androgens instead of stress hormones, thereby exposing the developing female to near male-typical hormone levels. There is evidence for organizational effects in most behaviors that show consistent sex differences, particularly when there are behavioral differences between boys and girls in childhood (Cohen-Bendahan, van de Beek, & Berenbaum, 2005). Hormones aren't the complete story, though, because prenatal administration masculinizes females to an intermediate level between typical males and females. Nevertheless, these organizational effects are testaments to the powerful regulatory role that hormones exert during early critical periods.

What is the adaptive purpose of having hormones organize the bodies and brains of males and females? One model has received substantial empirical support, primarily in females. As outlined by Ellis (2004), *life history theory* postulates that early environmental forces shape children's developmental trajectories and influence the timing of puberty. When these environmental cues signify moderate amounts of stress or unstable family structures, the individual's developmental trajectory favors early maturation and the reproductive benefits of early sexual activity. Conversely, when these environmental cues signify a stable, supportive, resource-rich environment, the individual's developmental trajectory is more likely to delay sexual and pubertal maturation in favor of a prolonged period of social and cognitive maturation prior to the onset of sexual maturation and activity. Nutrition, birth- and early weight, family context, child-rearing practices, and stepfather presence have all been shown to influence the organization and development of the HPG axis. An active hormonal system in prenatal and postnatal life allows the individual to essentially "encode" this information about the quality of the early environment and translate those hormonal signals into shorter or longer latencies to sexual maturity in order to maximize reproductive potential years later. Organizational influences may not change hormone levels per se, but may change the timing at which hormonal signals begin to activate secondary sexual characteristics.

Life history theory postulates that early environmental forces shape children's developmental trajectories and influence the timing of puberty.

In late infancy, organizational effects diminish, the HPG axis is functionally turned off, and presumably the influence of these environmental forces on the hormonal system diminishes. In contrast to the popular view that puberty marks the advent of new abilities or functions, current models emphasize that the juvenile period is characterized by active inhibition of adultlike hormonal activity (Grumbach, 2002). The fact that the period of hormonal quiescence during childhood is actively facilitated by the brain is important because it suggests that the juvenile period is not just an extension of infancy and that the diminishing force of the HPG axis isn't due to the gonads being unable to support hormonal production. Rather, the active inhibition of hormones during childhood in essence *permits* childhood. This affords distinct advantages of delayed sexual maturity, including opportunities for additional neural, cognitive, and social development in line with the particular constraints of an individual's environment (Bjorklund, 1997). In stable, supportive early environments, the advantages of childhood outweigh the reproductive costs of delayed sexual maturity.

The active inhibition of hormones during childhood in essence permits *childhood.*

The active inhibition of the HPG axis during childhood takes place in the brain. Early in fetal development, the inhibitory neurotransmitter GABA is temporarily excitatory and is centrally involved in sexual dimorphisms of the developing brain during this window of excitation. As fetal development continues, GABA becomes inhibitory in interaction with gonadal hormones. In the juvenile state, GABA suppresses the hypothalamus from releasing GnRH, functionally "braking" the HPG axis before the hormonal cascade is initiated. During the same time in fetal development, the neurotransmitter glutamate interacts with gonadal hormones, but glutamate remains excitatory on GnRH neurons. Both GABA and glutamate neurons synapse with GnRH neurons, but GABA inhibits the ability of glutamate to stimulate GnRH release (Terasawa & Fernandez, 2001). Thus, GABA directly and indirectly inhibits the GnRH pulse generator in the juvenile state.

The active inhibition of the HPG axis during childhood takes place in the brain.

The onset of puberty is caused by a release of the brake on the *GnRH pulse generator* (Ojeda & Terasawa, 2002). The awakening of the GnRH pulse generator has become synonymous with the pubertal trigger. The GnRH pulse generator refers to the intermittent discharge of GnRH from the hypothalamus into the hypophysial portal circulation, marking the first stage of the HPG axis. Few neurons in the brain synthesize GnRH, whose primary role is to stimulate the synthesis and release of follicle-stimulating hormone (FSH) and luteinizing hormone (LH) from the anterior pituitary. The addition of the pulse generator term emphasizes that GnRH is released occasionally in juveniles, but bursts of GnRH must be frequent, of high amplitude, and regularly timed for puberty to proceed.

A decline in GABA activity in the hypothalamus causes the inhibition over the GnRH pulse generator to diminish; GABA's inhibition of glutamate release also diminishes, thereby permitting glutamate neurons to directly stimulate GnRH release. The third trigger of the GnRH pulse generator involves astroglial cells that regulate the secretion of GnRH neurons. Like neurons, astroglial cells generate and convey information within the brain, communicating primarily through local release of neurotransmitter precursors or growth factors. Glial-to-neuron communication is abundant in early puberty, but during later stages hormones primarily regulate the HPG axis. It is not known what causes the decline in GABA's control over the GnRH pulse generator, although several genes have been postulated, including a newly discovered gene called the KISS-peptin (Navarro, Castellano, Garcia-Galiano, & Tena-Sempere, 2007).

After puberty has been initiated in the brain, other permissive pubertal factors may accelerate maturation rate. *Permissive factors* contribute to the progression of puberty and may be necessary for puberty to continue, but are not sufficient stimulators to activate the GnRH pulse generator (Sisk & Foster, 2004). Neuropeptide Y, norepinephrine, dopamine, serotonin, endogenous opioids, leptin, and melatonin are all permissive factors. Most of the permissive pubertal factors have been implicated in mood disorders, especially those disorders that peak at adolescence.

Once puberty is initiated, positive and negative feedback mechanisms of gonadal hormones exert their effects at multiple levels of the HPG axis, with receptors on glutamate, GABA, and GnRH neurons.

Once puberty is initiated, positive and negative feedback mechanisms of gonadal hormones exert their effects at multiple levels of the HPG axis, with receptors on glutamate, GABA, and GnRH neurons (Terasawa & Fernandez, 2001). Many permissive factors, though hormone-independent in the prepubertal individual, were largely organized by gonadal hormones, interact heavily with other hormones and neurotransmitters, and are frequently dependent on concurrent gonadal hormones. They are also the likeliest candidates for environmental modulation of puberty. For example, leptin is a hormone related to satiety and appetite suppression. Prepubertal leptin levels are highly correlated with body mass index, serving as a marker for when sufficient weight and growth have been attained for sexual maturation to be permitted to continue. If there is a fall in circulating leptin below a critical level, delayed or interrupted sexual maturation results (Plant & Shahab, 2002).

What are the practical implications of this information about pubertal onset? If the dichotomy between hormone-dependent and -independent events is to be believed (a theme that will emerge again later in this chapter), then interventions or research aimed at understanding concurrent hormone interactions with behavior may best be applied after the maturation of the GnRH pulse generator. An intervention applied to an individual at pre- or mid- or postpubertal stages will not likely have the same effect on that individual's biology or behavior. As shown in Figure 6.1, the organization of the juvenile, pubertal, and postpubertal brain is enormously different.

First, the prepubertal individual will likely show few hormone-dependent behaviors outside of organizational effects, and the juvenile brain may primarily be influenced by central events. Second, in midpuberty, concurrent or activational hormone-dependent behaviors are being established and may be erratic, because feedback loops may still be immature and neural connections are still new; the maturation of the GnRH pulse generator in the early adolescent opens a wider window for opportunities for interactions with peripheral events including both hormones and environmental forces. Third, hormone-dependent behaviors in postpubertal individuals are more established and highly interactive with the social context. Our model for behavior, disease, and intervention

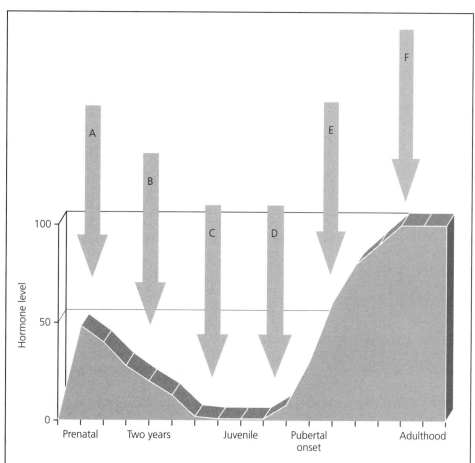

A. Prenatal testes release hormones. Organizational effects predominate.

B. Early on, the GnRH pulse generator is active. The effects of early experience are established, influencing the timing of puberty.

C. The GnRH pulse generator is actively inhibited during juvenile development. Few concurrent hormone-behavior associations are predicted.

D. The brake on the GnRH pulse generator is lifted. Permissive factors allow puberty to progress.

E. Gonadal hormones are elevated, permitting the development of secondary sexual characteristics. Because these circuits are activated after a long quiescence, the adolescent must acclimate to his or her new biological state.

F. Gonadal hormones are consistently or cyclically high in adulthood. Concurrent and stable activational hormone-behavior relationships are predicted.

FIGURE 6.1. *Gonadal hormones across childhood*

The idea that puberty is caused by hormone-dependent and hormone-independent events must be merged with the organizational-activational hypothesis and our knowledge that some developmental effects of gonadal hormones may be protracted.

cannot assume that the basic biology of individuals across different life stages is similar. The idea that puberty is caused by hormone-dependent and hormone-independent events must be merged with the organizational-activational hypothesis and our knowledge that some developmental effects of gonadal hormones may be protracted.

Downstream Effects of Activation of the Hypothalamic-Pituitary-Gonadal (HPG) Axis

The downstream effects of GnRH pulses are primarily responsible for sexual maturation (Styne & Grumbach, 2002). The hormonal cascade of the HPG axis begins with GnRH release. LH and FSH are then released in intermittent pulses into the peripheral bloodstream, primarily at night. It is only during late adolescence and adulthood that pulses can be detected during the day. LH and FSH, in turn, act on receptors in the gonads to stimulate the release of estrogens and androgens. In females, LH and FSH will be released cyclically from the anterior pituitary once negative and positive feedback of estrogen from the ovaries is established.

Gonadal hormones cause the maturation of secondary sexual characteristics such as pubic hair and breast and genital development. These are *activational effects,* when concurrent hormone levels activate the same structures that they originally organized in utero. Both sexes produce androgens and estrogens, though concentrations vary greatly.

Adrenarche, the maturation of the adrenal gland, occurs prior to the development of secondary sexual characteristics and the reawakening of the GnRH pulse generator, usually between six and eight years of age, and earlier in girls than boys (Tung, Lee, Tsai, & Hsiao, 2004). A steady release of dehydroepiandrosterone (DHEA), androstenedione, and DHEA-S from the adrenal gland marks the beginning of adrenarche. *Adrenal androgens* are hormones that are androgenic (like testosterone) but are released from the adrenal gland (like cortisol). Because the rise in adrenal androgens is gradual, effects are not apparent until years after adrenarche. Adrenal androgens cause the development of pubic hair, axillary hair, body odor, and acne (Auchus & Rainey, 2004).

Testosterone is an anabolic hormone that is directly and indirectly responsible for genital growth in males, including the growth of the penis and scrotum, muscular enlargement, and the maintenance of male-typical fat distributions (Styne & Grumbach, 2002). Testosterone is released primarily from the testes, though ovaries and adrenals also release testosterone. Once puberty is underway, testosterone influences GnRH, LH, and FSH release through negative feedback.

Estrogen, primarily estradiol, is released cyclically from the ovaries in females (Styne & Grumbach, 2002). Estrogen causes breast development and encourages female-typical body fat in concert with leptin. Together with progesterone, estrogen controls endometrial thickness and is responsible for stimulating the ovulatory surge by providing a positive feedback signal on the HPG axis. In both sexes, estrogen rises during late puberty to encourage long bone fusion. The effect of estrogen on bone growth is biphasic, with low estrogen stimulating and high estrogen inhibiting growth.

Adolescents also undergo a pubertal *growth spurt,* when they grow faster than at any other time of life, aside from fetal and early infant growth. Rising growth hormone is directly (and indirectly through estrogen and testosterone) responsible for the growth spurt. Another hormone involved in the pubertal growth spurt is insulin-like growth factor I (IGF-I), which rises very early. Unlike levels of growth hormone, initial rises in IGF-I levels are independent of gonadal hormones (Styne & Grumbach, 2002).

Brain Maturation Linked with Hormones

Gonadal hormones cause many changes in the body, and a growing literature likewise shows that the brain is also a target for gonadal hormones. Brain maturation in adolescence is both hormone-dependent and hormone-independent. This distinction is useful but imprecise, because hormone-dependent and -independent brain areas frequently interact. The *social information processing network (SIPN)* is an overarching model by Nelson, Leibenluft, McClure, and Pine (2005) to emphasize the synchrony between hormone-dependent and -independent maturational changes in the brain. Three neuronal circuits dedicated to the processing of social information mature at different times. The first circuitry, the detection node, is dedicated to categorizing social information and includes such areas as the inferior occipital cortex, the temporal cortex, and the fusiform face gyrus. The detection node is fully mature before adolescence.

The second circuitry, the affective node, matures during adolescence, specifically during puberty. The affective node involves brain areas related to reward and punishment, social and appetitive cues, and reproduction. Areas such as the amygdala, hypothalamus, ventral striatum, septum, and bed nucleus of the stria terminalis are regulated by gonadal hormones, particularly when social information is novel. In addition to global changes in the adolescent brain marked by competitive elimination, myelination, dendritic and axonal arborization (summarized in Giedd, 1997), amygdala volume increases, primarily in males, and hippocampal volume increases markedly in females. These regional changes are consistent with hormone-dependent maturational changes, as the amygdala is rich with testosterone receptors and the hippocampus is one of the main sites for estrogen-dependent synapse formation.

The affective node involves brain areas related to reward and punishment, social and appetitive cues, and reproduction.

Functional MRI (fMRI) studies have been used to probe the affective node and the processing of reward and punishment cues. Ernst and colleagues (2005) developed a wheel of fortune task to understand adolescents' propensity for risk taking and reward-seeking behavior. Their results revealed greater responses of the nucleus accumbens and amygdala when winning than losing. Whereas adults activated the amygdala, adolescents mostly activated the nucleus accumbens, suggestive of adolescents' heightened sensitivity to reward more than punishment. Another fMRI study has found that, compared to adults, adolescents showed greater activation in the anterior cingulate, orbitofrontal cortex, and right amygdala in response to viewing fearful faces (McClure et al., 2004). Similarly, when viewing subsequently remembered emotion-specific faces, adolescents had different levels of activity in the right temporal lobe, anterior cingulate, and hippocampus compared to adults (Nelson et al., 2003). These studies suggest that adults activate areas related to attentional demands when viewing emotion-laden faces, whereas adolescents spend more energy attending to the emotional content of the faces and consequently activate areas related to affective processing (McClure et al., 2004).

The third node of the SIPN is cognitive and regulatory. It involves structures related to theory of mind, such as the dorsomedial prefrontal cortex, as well as structures related to inhibitory and goal-oriented behavior, such as the dorsal and ventral prefrontal cortex. The cognitive node demonstrates slow development across childhood and does not fully mature until early adulthood. Its development is influenced by age and experience more than hormones, though hormones may have a secondary effect. Structures in the affective and cognitive nodes interact so extensively that the cognitive node will eventually regulate the affective node. In adolescents, the cognitive node may not be mature enough yet to dominate the affective node. Consequently, adolescents may be overwhelmed by socially relevant reward cues, failing to inhibit their behavior in emotion-laden situations (Dahl, 2004).

The SIPN model dovetails nicely with the developmental model for the organizational-activational hypothesis. Both of these models emphasize interactions across developmental epochs or across brain areas. Some changes in the adolescent brain (1) are relatively hormone-dependent or influenced by gonadal hormones, (2) follow a maturational trajectory with puberty, and (3) involve structural and functional changes in neurocircuitry related to emotion, appetitive responses, reward, and punishment. Maturation in other brain areas (1) is largely hormone-independent, (2) follows a maturational trajectory with age and experience that continues well past puberty, and (3) involves structures and functions related to inhibition and goal-oriented behavior. Hormones are more (for example, limbic structures) or less (for example, prefrontal areas) implicated in particular brain areas or with particular neural processes (for example, affective or reward stimuli versus inhibition or regulation). Similarly, the organizational-activational hypothesis emphasizes the disjunction in the timing of hormone-dependent and -independent events. Hormones are variably implicated in behaviors pre-, mid- or postpubertally. Understanding the adolescent brain rests on understanding the complex interaction of timing, location, and function. Yet even when a process is unlikely to directly implicate hormones, hormones may still be indirectly capable of influencing behavior, as when prenatal hormone exposure influences childhood play behavior or when pubertal maturation influences an adolescent's ability to cognitively inhibit a behavior or regulate emotion.

Behavioral Changes During Puberty

The interaction of timing, location, and function must be considered when we extend this model of adolescent brain development to behavior. As mentioned above, the organizational-activational hypothesis originally made this extension to behavior. Sexual, aggressive, and play behavior were all shown to be influenced by prenatal hormone exposure in nonhuman primates. The neural circuitry underlying these behaviors was also shown to be rich with hormone receptors (Romeo, 2003). If we extend this model to humans, we would predict that (1) behaviors that were organized by hormones (for example, behaviors that show consistent sex differences) would be affected during juvenile development, (2) the behaviors that were organized by hormones would further change when this neurocircuitry is activated (for example, at the onset of puberty), and (3) the behaviors that show activational effects would be influenced by hormones. The first prediction generally holds for organizational effects in humans (Berenbaum & Resnick, 1997), as sexual, aggressive, or risky behavior and play behavior are different in individuals prenatally exposed to high levels of androgens.

The second prediction requires evidence that these behaviors change during adolescence, and more specifically during puberty. The SIPN model further implies that we might predict changes only in behaviors implicated in the affective node (Nelson et al., 2005). Importantly, there is some correspondence between the behaviors that show organizational effects and the behaviors implicated in the maturation of the affective node. For example, it is easy to extend the organization of sexual behavior to the neurocircuitry involved in reproduction. Aggressive and risky behaviors likewise map onto the neurocircuitry involved in reward and punishment, although interactions with the cognitive and regulatory node are also likely, because risky behavior also involves inhibition.

The third prediction requires evidence that these behaviors—organized by hormones and implicated in the affective node after pubertal maturation—would likewise be related to gonadal hormones. The SIPN includes brain areas that are rich with hormone receptors, so there is some precedence to believe that hormones exert an effect on behaviors instantiated in these areas. The next section will briefly review some examples of behavioral changes in adolescence, emphasizing the hormonal underpinnings of these behaviors.

Example 1: Link with Aggression Is Not Simplistic Aggressive behavior does not appear exclusively at adolescence, but aggressive behavior peaks after puberty, with some behaviors directed pointedly toward adult males (Spear, 2000). Escalating symptoms of the aggressive child may also be exaggerated by permissive organizing hormonal factors (Zahn-Waxler et al., 2006). Much of the literature on testosterone has studied its effects on boys, because aggression is reliably higher in boys than girls.

Elevated testosterone is frequently present when aggression levels soar (Sapolsky, 1997). But testosterone doesn't cause aggression; rather, it exaggerates the aggressive impulses that were already present. Although the aggressive child may become a violent or delinquent adolescent when his testosterone levels rise at puberty, the aggressive tendencies were likely present before the rise in testosterone. For example, in a longitudinal study of fifteen- to seventeen-year-old boys, high testosterone led to an increased readiness to respond to provocation, but testosterone was unrelated to unprovoked aggression (Olweus, Mattsson, Schalling, & Low, 1980; Olweus, Mattsson, Schalling, & Low, 1988). A hormone replacement study in hypogonadal boys indicated that moderate doses of testosterone caused substantial increases in aggressive impulses, physical aggression against peers, and physical aggression against adults. These effects were not evident at low or high doses of testosterone, suggesting that testosterone may contribute to aggression only when it is rapidly rising; this phenomenon is called an *acclimation effect.*

Another causally limiting factor for testosterone-aggression associations is that testosterone may be indirectly linked with aggression, but directly linked with social dominance. Socially dominant individuals may respond aggressively if they are in a situation where their social status must be maintained. Boys who are socially dominant have higher testosterone, but not necessarily high physical aggression (Schaal, Tremblay, Soussignan, & Susman, 1996; Tremblay et al., 1998). Similarly, boys with high testosterone are perceived as popular and possessing leadership qualities only when they have nondeviant peers (Rowe, Maughan, Worthman, Costello, & Angold, 2004). Some effects of testosterone on aggression may also be mediated by the advanced muscular development that high testosterone permits.

Other hormones may be permissive for aggression in adolescence. High estrogen (Brooks-Gunn, Graber, & Paikoff, 1994) and androstenedione (Inoff-Germain et al., 1988) were associated with aggression in girls, particularly defiant and explosive aggression. Hypogonadal girls receiving estrogen showed increased aggressive impulses and physical aggression against peers and adults at low and medium doses. The fact that aggression did not continue to rise at a high dose suggests an acclimation effect (Finkelstein et al., 1997). Highly reactive boys had low DHEA levels (Inoff-Germain et al., 1988), and girls with low DHEA were more aggressive, particularly when they had experienced negative peer interactions (Brooks-Gunn & Warren, 1989).

Example 2: Adolescents Are Risk Takers Adolescents tend to be high novelty seekers and have low harm avoidance, especially during puberty. Spear (2000) aptly wrote that adolescents are risk takers: 80 percent of eleven-and-a-half- to fifteen-year-olds exhibited problem behaviors related to risk-taking and norm-violating behavior. Similarly, the leading causes of mortality in adolescence are directly and indirectly related to risk-taking behavior (Dahl, 2004). It is interesting that nonhuman primates also frequently take risks during adolescence. Occasionally risks can increase one's abilities and provide access to resources that might otherwise have been unavailable. For humans, risk-taking behavior can confer benefits in the form of popularity, friendships, social acceptance, and opposite-sex relationships. Adolescents who do not take risks are perceived as boring, although risk taking can present developmental snares.

Risk taking is associated with hormones. Warren and Brooks-Gunn (1989) found that impulse control decreased and then increased as estrogen levels rose. Susman and colleagues (1987) found higher androstenedione in boys expressing more acting-out behaviors. High testosterone was related to more risky behavior in both boys and girls for adolescents with poor-quality relationships with their parents (Booth, Johnson, Granger, Crouter, & McHale, 2003). These studies point to a role for hormones, even within the range of normative risky behavior.

Studies point to a role for hormones, even within the range of normative risky behavior.

Some adolescent novelty seeking and risk taking include drug use and experimentation. Over 25 percent of eighth graders report alcohol or drug use; over 50 percent of adolescents by their senior year have tried drugs, alcohol, and illegal substances (Spear, 2000). Initial drug abuse can be predicted by the interaction between puberty and socialization in family and peer networks. Families characterized by conflict and lack of parental warmth may inadvertently encourage youth to disengage from the family and engage with deviant peers who encourage persistent drug use (Dawes et al., 2000).

Adolescents may proceed from drug experimentation to abuse faster than adults because of a maturational dyssynchrony in the timing and sequencing of hormonal, physical, and social processes (Dawes et al., 2000). This dyssynchrony results in part because adolescents have altered activity in social and reward neurocircuitry. Reward dependence is a risk for development of substance abuse disorders. The brain is organized to find social stimuli rewarding, as a part of the neurocircuitry of the affective node of the SIPN. This same neurocircuitry is activated by drugs of abuse. Drugs may be co-opting the plasticity in the reward circuitry in part through activation by gonadal hormones (Keverne, 2004). It is interesting that this neurocircuitry is one of a few brain areas that show organizational influences by gonadal hormones during puberty. This adolescent vulnerability to drug addiction may become entrenched in the adult because drug use has permanently altered the social brain. Consequently, it may be particularly difficult to change this neurocircuitry after drug addiction is established during adolescence.

Relations between drug use and hormones are equivocal. Testosterone levels were higher in adolescents who had recently smoked cigarettes and who had an earlier age of pubertal onset (Martin et al., 2001), but subjects were age twenty-one at the time of testing. Another study found that adolescents at risk for substance abuse disorders had lower testosterone and dihydrotestosterone prior to a laboratory stressor (Dawes et al., 1999). Clearly, more research on the hormonal contribution to drug abuse is needed.

Example 3: The Biological Underpinnings of Same- and Opposite-Sex Relationships Are Different in Adolescent Boys and Girls Adolescents spend 33 percent of their waking hours with peers and only 8 percent with adults (Spear, 2000). The social behavior of adolescents differs qualitatively, as well as quantitatively, from children. Primate and human adolescents spend more time expressing affiliative and bonding behaviors with same- and opposite-sex peers (Spear, 2000). Adolescent friendships are marked by intimate and supportive communication with like-minded age mates (Steinberg & Morris, 2001). Adolescents—especially girls—are also highly influenced by negative events in peer relationships (Rudolph & Hammen, 1999), and this influence extends to biological alterations in stress reactivity in response to peer stressors (Stroud, Salavey, & Epel, 2002).

The *tend-and-befriend response* describes a recent theory on the female response to stress (Taylor et al., 2000). Females do not often respond to stress in the typical fight-or-flight manner, likely because they would often be compromised by pregnancy, lactation, or young children. Instead, they tend toward their offspring and bond socially with other females. These positive social behaviors reduce the stress response by stimulating the release of *oxytocin,* which induces feelings of relaxation (Carter & Keverne, 2002). Oxytocin is a peptide hormone released centrally into social and reward neurocircuitry (Insel, 2003).

Where do adolescents fit in this model? Oxytocin does not increase substantially at puberty, but estrogen facilitates the effects of oxytocin in the social neurocircuitry (one component of the affective node of the SIPN) and helps girls find social interactions rewarding. This model helps explain why adolescence marks the first stage when girls feel intense emotions about their peers, and friendships take on heightened importance (Carter & Keverne, 2002). Estrogen administration in hypogonadal females enhances feelings of close friendships (Schwab et al., 2001). Similarly, early breast development, under estrogenic control, encourages females to express interest in infants and feminine behavior (Brooks-Gunn & Warren, 1988).

Adolescent males present a different view. Oxytocin is not as important in males as *vasopressin,* a similar neuropeptide centrally released in the brain that likewise encourages social attachment and pair bonding (Insel, 2003). Testosterone suppresses oxytocin and vasopressin release, so the tend-and-befriend response is diminished in males compared to females (Geary & Flinn, 2002). This difference renders flexibility to the biological activity surrounding male social bonding and allows bonding to be more contextually dependent.

Adolescence also marks the first romantic relationships (Steinberg & Morris, 2001). Social neurocircuitry is also highly involved in initiating, maintaining, and strengthening romantic relationships and pair bonding. Oxytocin and vasopressin are released into the reward neurocircuitry when one interacts with one's romantic partner (Insel, 2003). Physical interactions are the most potent stimulators of these hormones, although they are not necessary. In animal models, sexual experiences are necessary to initiate changes in social and reward neurocircuitry (Insel, Winslow, Wang, & Young, 1998). That this neurocircuitry is being organized in new ways during adolescence by oxytocin and vasopressin, and is further enhanced by gonadal hormones, underscores the idea that the appetitive system (for example, the affective node) in adolescence is drastically different from that in any other developmental stage.

Much of the literature on social behavior and hormones, especially the animal literature, also involves the activation of circuitry devoted to sexual behavior (Romeo,

2003). This literature emphasizes that hormones are necessary to activate circuitry devoted to male and female sexuality, but once individuals gain sexual experience, hormones are no longer necessary. Occasionally, stronger findings are reported in females because small changes in testosterone can exert a powerful drive on female sexuality, whereas most males are well beyond the threshold permitting sexual behavior (Blaustein & Erskine, 2002). Although testosterone is intuitively related to sexual behavior, estrogen and DHEA likewise exert effects on sexual behavior (Finkelstein et al., 1998; McClintock & Herdt, 1996). Interestingly, sexual behavior during puberty is one of the few arenas in which organizational influences of hormones are generated after early postnatal life (Sisk & Foster, 2004). The hormonal rise at puberty and resultant sexual behaviors permanently alter the adolescent brain.

SUMMARY

With regard to adolescent behavior, there is good evidence that behaviors that were organized by hormones (such as risky behavior, aggression, and social and sexual behavior) change during adolescence, and further that these behaviors are related to individual differences in the gonadal hormones that were responsible for organizing their underlying neurocircuitry. A general theme is that a direct relationship between hormones and behaviors is relatively rare. Models that emphasize adolescents getting acclimated to their new biology or hormones being permissive or exaggerating an effect in certain contexts are more sophisticated. Though complex, these models provide more insight into the biological mechanisms underlying the complexities of adolescent development.

The organizational-activational hypothesis emphasizes that the timing of hormones' influence on the brain, body, and behavior of individuals is key to understanding hormone-behavior relationships. Even when a behavior is unlikely to directly implicate hormones, hormones may still be capable of indirectly influencing behavior. Before puberty, there will likely be few hormone-dependent behaviors outside of these early organizational effects. The adaptive purpose of organization effects that extend beyond early prenatal development and structural organization of the body is that being sensitive to early environmental signals helps to biologically embed this information about the early environment.

The onset of puberty, marked by the activation of the GnRH pulse generator, opens a wider window of opportunities for interactions with both hormonal and environmental events. The maturation of the GnRH pulse generator begins a hormonal cascade that results in the release of gonadal hormones. The SIPN emphasizes that the adolescent brain changes in both hormone-dependent and hormone-independent ways. Hormone-dependent changes are most likely to occur in concert with pubertal maturation in neurocircuitry related to reward and punishment,

Behaviors that were organized by hormones—such as risky behavior, aggression, and social and sexual behavior—are related to individual differences in the gonadal hormones that were responsible for organizing their underlying neurocircuitry.

social and appetitive cues, and reproduction. Near the onset of puberty, concurrent or activational hormone-dependent behaviors may be erratic as feedback loops are first becoming established and neural connections are still immature. Hormone-related behaviors are often more reliable once the entire HPG axis is mature and feedback loops are established. In the postpubertal individual, concurrent hormone effects on behavior may be stable.

Predictions for behavioral change or targets for behavioral interventions must specify what effect is anticipated, along with when and where. Hormone-behavior relationships are fundamentally different across childhood. An intervention applied to an individual will likely have different effects on that individual's biology or behavior, depending whether it is applied in pre-, mid-, or postpuberty. Rather than indicating who is the most vulnerable, this model emphasizes that a particular individual may be more or less at risk, depending on his or her biological state or developmental epoch. Just as this vulnerability or risk can change normatively across development, it may also be possible to design intervention research that considers biological mechanisms and vulnerabilities.

KEY TERMS

Acclimation effect
Activational effects
Adolescence
Adrenal androgens
Adrenarche
Androgens
Congenital adrenal hyperplasia (CAH)
Estrogens
GnRH pulse generator
Growth spurt

Hypothalamic-pituitary-gonadal (HPG) axis
Life history theory
Organizational-activational hypothesis
Oxytocin
Permissive factors
Social information processing network (SIPN)
Tend-and-befriend response
Testosterone
Vasopressin

DISCUSSION QUESTIONS

1. How do the biological changes that occur during puberty contribute to the emergence of problem behavior?

2. Describe the organizational purpose of hormones, from infancy to adolescence.

3. How might new understandings of permissive pubertal factors (such as leptin, dopamine, and serotonin) affect public health practice and intervention?

4. Is there an optimal time to administer a behavioral intervention (in pre-, mid-, or postpuberty)? Frame your discussion in the context of the hormone-behavior relationship.

REFERENCES

Auchus, R. J., & Rainey, W. E. (2004). Adrenarche: Physiology, biochemistry and human disease. *Clinical Endocrinology, 60*(3), 288–296.

Berenbaum, S. A., & Resnick, S. M. (1997). Early androgen effects on aggression in children and adults with congenital adrenal hyperplasia. *Psychoneuroendocrinology, 22*(7), 505–515.

Bjorklund, D. F. (1997). The role of immaturity in human development. *Psychological Bulletin, 122*(2), 153–169.

Blaustein, J. D., & Erskine, M. S. (2002). Feminine sexual behavior: Cellular integration of hormonal and afferent information in the rodent brain. In D. W. Pfaff, A. P. Arnold, A. M. Etgen, S. E. Fahrbach & R. T. Rubin (Eds.), *Hormones, brain, and behavior* (Vol. 1, pp. 139–214). San Diego, CA: Academic Press.

Booth, A., Johnson, D. R., Granger, D. A., Crouter, A. C., & McHale, S. (2003). Testosterone and child and adolescent adjustment: The moderating role of parent-child relationships. *Developmental Psychology, 39*(1), 85–98.

Brooks-Gunn, J., Graber, J. A., & Paikoff, R. L. (1994). Studying links between hormones and negative affect: Models and measures. *Journal of Research on Adolescence, 4*, 469–486.

Brooks-Gunn, J., & Warren, M. P. (1988). The psychological significance of secondary sexual characteristics in nine- to eleven-year-old girls. Child development (Vol. 59, pp. 1061–1069). Cambridge, MA: Blackwell.

Brooks-Gunn, J., & Warren, M. P. (1989). Biological and social contributions to negative affect in young adolescent girls. *Child development* (Vol. 60, pp. 40–55). Cambridge, MA: Blackwell.

Buchanan, C. M., Eccles, J. S., & Becker, J. B. (1992). Are adolescents the victims of raging hormones? Evidence for activational effects of hormones on moods and behavior at adolescence. *Psychological Bulletin, 111*(1), 62–107.

Carter, C. S., & Keverne, E. B. (2002). The neurobiology of social affiliation and pair bonding. In D. W. Pfaff, A. P. Arnold, A. M. Etgen, S. E. Fahrbach & R. T. Rubin (Eds.), *Hormones, brain, and behavior* (Vol. 4, pp. 589–660). San Diego, CA: Academic Press.

Cohen-Bendahan, C. C., van de Beek, C., & Berenbaum, S. A. (2005). Prenatal sex hormone effects on child and adult sex-typed behavior: Methods and findings. *Neuroscience and Biobehavioral Reviews, 29*(2), 353–384.

Dahl, R. E. (2004). Adolescent brain development: A period of vulnerabilities and opportunities. Keynote address. *Annals of the New York Academy of Sciences, 1021*, 1–22.

Dawes, M. A., Antelman, S. M., Vanyukov, M. M., Giancola, P., Tarter, R. E., Susman, E. J., Mezzich, A., & Clark, D. B. (2000). Developmental sources of variation in liability to adolescent substance use disorders. *Drug and Alcohol Dependence, 61*(1), 3–14.

Dawes, M. A., Dorn, L. D., Moss, H. B., Yao, J. K., Kirisci, L., Ammerman, R. T., & Tarter, R. E. (1999). Hormonal and behavioral homeostasis in boys at risk for substance abuse. *Drug and Alcohol Dependence, 55*(1), 165–176.

Ellis, B. J. (2004). Timing of pubertal maturation in girls: An integrated life history approach. *Psychological Bulletin, 130*(6), 920–958.

Ernst, M., Nelson, E. E., Jazbec, S., McClure, E. B., Monk, C. S., Leibenluft, E., Blair, J., & Pine, D. S. (2005). Amygdala and nucleus accumbens in responses to receipt and omission of gains in adults and adolescents. *Neuroimage, 25*(4), 1279–1291.

Finkelstein, J. W., Susman, E. J., Chinchilli, V. M., D'Arcangelo, M. R., Kunselman, S. J., Schwab, J., Demers, L. M., Liben, L. S., & Kulin, H. E. (1998). Effects of estrogen or testosterone on self-reported sexual responses and behaviors in hypogonadal adolescents. *Journal of Clinical Endocrinology and Metabolism, 83*(7), 2281–2285.

Finkelstein, J. W., Susman, E. J., Chinchilli, V. M., Kunselman, S. J., D'Arcangelo, M. R., Schwab, J., Demers, L. M., Liben, L. S., Lookingbill, G., and Kulin, H. E. (1997). Estrogen or testosterone increases self-reported aggressive behaviors in hypogonadal adolescents. *Journal of Clinical Endocrinology and Metabolism, 82*(8), 2433–2438.

Geary, D. C., & Flinn, M. V. (2002). Sex differences in behavioral and hormonal response to social threat: Commentary on Taylor et al. (2000). *Psychological Review, 109*(4), 745–753.

Giedd, J. (1997). Normal development. *Child and Adolescent Psychiatric Clinics of North America, 6*, 265–282.

Gottlieb, G. (1996). Developmental psychobiological theory. In R. B. Cairns, G. H. Elder, & A. Costello (Eds.), *Developmental science* (pp. 63–96). Cambridge, England: Cambridge University Press.

Grumbach, M. M. (2002). The neuroendocrinology of human puberty revisited. *Hormone Research, 57*(Suppl. 2), 2–14.

Hutchison, J. B. (1997). Gender-specific steroid metabolism in neural differentiation. *Cellular and Molecular Neurobiology, 17*(6), 603–626.

Inoff-Germain, G., Arnold, G. S., Nottelmann, E. D., Susman, E. J., Cutler, G. B., & Chrousos, G. P. (1988). Relations between hormone levels and observational measures of aggressive behavior of young adolescents in family interactions. *Developmental Psychology, 24*(1), 129–139.

Insel, T. R. (2003). Is social attachment an addictive disorder? *Physiology and Behavior, 79*(3), 351–357.

Insel, T. R., Winslow, J. T., Wang, Z., & Young, L. J. (1998). Oxytocin, vasopressin, and the neuroendocrine basis of pair bond formation. *Advances in Experimental Medicine and Biology, 449*, 215–224.

Keverne, E. B. (2004). Understanding well-being in the evolutionary context of brain development. *Philosophical Transactions of the Royal Society B: Biological Sciences, 359*(1449), 1349–1358.

Martin, C. A., Logan, T. K., Portis, C., Leukefled, C. G., Lynam, D., Staton, M., Brogli, B., Flory, K., & Clayton, R. R. (2001). The association of testosterone with nicotine use in young adult females. *Addictive Behaviors, 26*(2), 279–283.

McClintock, M., & Herdt, G. (1996). Rethinking puberty: The development of sexual attraction. *Current Directions in Psychological Science, 5*, 178–183.

McClure, E. B., Monk, C. S., Nelson, E. E., Zarahn, E., Leibenluft, E., Bilder, R. M., Charney, D. S., Ernst, M., & Pine, D. S. (2004). A developmental examination of gender differences in brain engagement during evaluation of threat. *Biological Psychiatry, 55*(11), 1047–1055.

Navarro, V. M., Castellano, J. M., Garcia-Galiano, D., & Tena-Sempere, M. (2007). Neuroendocrine factors in the initiation of puberty: The emergent role of KISS-peptin. *Reviews in Endocrine and Metabolic Disorders, 8*(1), 11–20.

Nelson, E. E., Leibenluft, E., McClure, E. B., & Pine, D. S. (2005). The social re-orientation of adolescence: A neuroscience perspective on the process and its relation to psychopathology. *Psychological Medicine, 35*(2), 163–174.

Nelson, E. E., McClure, E. B., Monk, C. S., Zarahn, E., Leibenluft, E., Pine, D. S., & Ernst, M. (2003). Developmental differences in neuronal engagement during implicit encoding of emotional faces: An event–related fMRI study. *Journal of Child Psychology and Psychiatry, 44*(7), 1015–1024.

Ojeda, S. R., & Terasawa, E. (2002). Neuroendocrine regulation of puberty. In D. Pfaff, A. Arnold, A. M. Etgen, S. Fahrbach, & R. T. Rubin (Eds.), *Hormones, brain and behavior* (Vol. 4, pp. 589–660). San Diego: Elsevier Science.

Olweus, D., Mattsson, A., Schalling, D., & Low, H. (1980). Testosterone, aggression, physical, and personality dimensions in normal adolescent males. *Psychosomatic Medicine, 42*, 253–269.

Olweus, D., Mattsson, A., Schalling, D., & Low, H. (1988). Circulating testosterone levels and aggression in adolescent males: A causal analysis. *Psychosomatic Medicine, 50*, 261–272.

Phoenix, C., Goy, R., & Young, W. (1967). *Sexual behavior: General aspects.* In L. Martini & W. Ganong (Eds.), *Neuroendocrinology* (Vol. 2). New York: Academic Press.

Plant, T. M., & Shahab, M. (2002). Neuroendocrine mechanisms that delay and initiate puberty in higher primates. *Physiology and Behavior, 77*(4–5), 717–722.

Romeo, R. D. (2003). Puberty: A period of both organizational and activational effects of steroid hormones on neurobehavioural development. *Journal of Neuroendocrinology, 15*(12), 1185–1192.

Rowe, R., Maughan, B., Worthman, C. M., Costello, E. J., & Angold, A. (2004). Testosterone, antisocial behavior, and social dominance in boys: Pubertal development and biosocial interaction. *Biological Psychiatry, 55*(5), 546–552.

Rudolph, K. D., & Hammen, C. (1999). Age and gender as determinants of stress exposure, generation, and reactions in youngsters: A transactional perspective. *Child Development, 70*(3), 660–677.

Sapolsky, R. M. (1997). *The trouble with testosterone: And other essays on the biology of the human predicament.* New York: Simon and Schuster.

Schaal, B., Tremblay, R. E., Soussignan, R., & Susman, E. J. (1996). Male testosterone linked to high social dominance but low physical aggression in early adolescence. *Journal of the American Academy of Child and Adolescent Psychiatry, 35*(10), 1322–1330.

Schwab, J., Kulin, H. E., Susman, E. J., Finkelstein, J. W., Chinchilli, V. M., Kunselman, S. J., Liben, L. S., D'Arcangelo, M. R., & Demers, L. M. (2001). The role of sex hormone replacement therapy on self-perceived competence in adolescents with delayed puberty. *Child Development, 72*(5), 1439–1450.

Sisk, C. L., & Foster, D. L. (2004). The neural basis of puberty and adolescence. *Nature Neuroscience, 7*(10), 1040–1047.

Spear, L. P. (2000). The adolescent brain and age-related behavioral manifestations. *Neuroscience and Biobehavioral Reviews, 24*(4), 417–463.

Steinberg, L., & Morris, A. S. (2001). Adolescent development. *Annual Reviews of Psychology, 52*, 83–110.

Stroud, L., Salavey, P., & Epel, E. (2002). Sex differences in stress responses: Social rejection versus achievement stress. *Biological Psychiatry, 52*(4), 318–328.

Styne, D. M., & Grumbach, M. M. (2002). Puberty in boys and girls. In D. Pfaff, A. Arnold, A. M. Etgen, S. Fahrbach, & R. T. Rubin (Eds.), *Hormones, brain and behavior* (Vol. 4, pp. 661–716). San Diego: Elsevier Science.

Susman, E. J., Inoff-Germain, G., Nottelmann, E. D., Loriaux, D. L., Cutler, G. B., Jr., & Chrousos, G. P. (1987). Hormones, emotional dispositions, and aggressive attributes in young adolescents. *Child Development, 58*(4), 1114–1134.

Taylor, S., Klein, L. C., Lewis, B. P., Gruenewald, T. L., Gurung, R. A. R., & Updegraff, J. A. (2000). Biobehavioral response to stress in females: Tend and befriend, not fight-or-flight. *Psychological Review, 107*, 411–429.

Terasawa, E., & Fernandez, D. L. (2001). Neurobiological mechanisms of the onset of puberty in primates. *Endocrine Reviews, 22*(1), 111–151.

Tremblay, R. E., Schaal, B., Boulerice, B., Arseneault, L., Soussignan, R., Paquette, D., & Laurent, D. (1998). Testosterone, physical aggression, dominance and physical development in early adolescence. *International Journal of Behavioral Development, 22*, 753–777.

Tung, Y. C., Lee, J. S., Tsai, W. Y., & Hsiao, P. H. (2004). Physiological changes of adrenal androgens in childhood. *Journal of the Formosan Medical Association, 103*(12), 921–924.

Warren, M. P., & Brooks-Gunn, J. (1989). Mood and behavior at adolescence: Evidence for hormonal factors. *Journal of Clinical Endocrinology and Metabolism, 69*(1), 77–83.

Zahn-Waxler, C., Crick, N. R., Shirtcliff, E. A., & Woods, K. (2006). The origins and development of psychopathology in females and males. In D. Cicchetti & D. Cohen (Eds.), *Handbook of developmental psychopathology* (2nd ed., pp. 76–139). New York: Wiley.

CHAPTER

7

POSITIVE YOUTH DEVELOPMENT

Contemporary Theoretical Perspectives

RICHARD M. LERNER ▪ MONA M. ABO-ZENA ▪ NEDA BEBIROGLU ▪ AERIKA BRITTIAN ▪ ALICIA DOYLE LYNCH ▪ SONIA S. ISSAC

LEARNING OBJECTIVES

After studying this chapter, you will be able to

- Recall the conceptual foundations of the positive youth development perspective and summarize key theoretical ideas.

- Demonstrate how the positive youth development perspective can be applied to human development.

- Define primary features of developmental systems theories.

This chapter presents the theoretical and empirical foundations of a conception of youth that emerged relatively recently. Termed the *positive youth development (PYD) perspective,* this orientation to young people has arisen because of interest among developmental scientists in using developmental systems, or dynamic models, of human behavior and development for understanding the plasticity of human development. This perspective recognizes the importance of relations between individuals and their real-world ecological settings as the bases of variation in the course of human development.

Accordingly, in this chapter we present the conceptual foundations of the PYD perspective and specify its key theoretical ideas. In turn, we will discuss the burgeoning empirical work that is framed by the PYD perspective. We will consider the implications of this research both for future scholarship and for policy and program applications of developmental science aimed at improving the life chances of diverse adolescents.

PRIOR THEORETICAL MODELS OF ADOLESCENT DEVELOPMENT

Since the founding of the scientific study of adolescent development (Hall, 1904) the predominant conceptual frame for the study of this age period has been one of "storm and stress," or of an ontogenetic time of normative developmental disturbance (Freud, 1969). Typically, these deficit models of adolescence were predicated on biologically reductionist theories of genetic or maturational determination (for example, Erikson, 1959) and resulted in descriptions of youth as "broken" or in danger of becoming broken (Benson, Scales, Hamilton, & Sesma, 2006), as both dangerous and endangered (Anthony, 1969), or as "problems to be managed" (Roth & Brooks-Gunn, 2003). In fact, if positive development was discussed in the adolescent development literature—at least prior to the 1990s—it was implicitly or explicitly regarded as the absence of negative or undesirable behaviors (Benson et al., 2006). A youth who was seen as manifesting behavior indicative of positive development was depicted as someone who was *not* taking drugs or using alcohol, *not* engaging in unsafe sex, *not* participating in crime or violence, and so forth.

For most of the twentieth century, the majority of literature and research about adolescence was based on this deficit conception of young people. However, several reports (for example, Bandura, 1964; Douvan & Adelson, 1966; Offer, 1969; also see Block, 1971) indicated that most young people do not have a stormy second decade of life. These reports also documented the diversity of adolescent development and the nature of the interrelations between individual and context involved in shaping the specific directions of change found across this period of life. Although such findings provided evidence for the potential presence of *plasticity* in human development

The preparation of this chapter was supported in part by a grant from the National 4-H Council.

(that is, for systematic variation in the course of ontogenetic change), the predominant lens for conceptualizing the nature of adolescence continued until the 1990s to use, implicitly or explicitly, a deficit model.

ORIGINS OF THE POSITIVE YOUTH DEVELOPMENT PERSPECTIVE

In the late 1990s and early 2000s, psychological science paid increasing attention to the concept of "positive psychology" (for example, Seligman, 2002). However, the emergence of a PYD perspective—a model that explicitly rejected the deficit conception of adolescence and replaced it with a strength-based conception—was not linked to this work.

Instead, the roots of the PYD perspective are found in the work of comparative psychologists (for example, Gottlieb, 1997; Schneirla, 1957) and biologists (for example, Novikoff, 1945a, 1945b; von Bertalanffy, 1933) who had been studying the plasticity of developmental processes that arose from the "fusion" (Tobach & Greenberg, 1984) of biological and contextual levels of organization. The use of these ideas about the import of levels of integration in shaping ontogenetic change began to affect the human developmental sciences in the 1970s (for reviews, see Cairns & Cairns, 2006; Gottlieb, Wahlsten, & Lickliter, 2006; Lerner, 2002, 2006; Overton, 2006). The theoretical papers by Overton (1973) and Lerner (1978) show how the nature-nurture controversy may be resolved by taking an integrative, relational perspective toward genetic and contextual influences on human development.

However, as research about adolescent development began to burgeon during the latter third of the twentieth century (Lerner & Steinberg, 2004)—and as this research continued to point to the potential plasticity of adolescent development, which arose because of the mutually influential relations among biological, individual, and contextual levels of organization within the ecology of youth development—developmental scientists interested in adolescence began to explore the use and implications of the ongoing developmental systems theory–predicated research in comparative psychology and biology (for example, Gottlieb et al., 2006; Suomi, 2004) for devising a new theoretical frame for the study of adolescence. This work converged with the efforts of developmental scientists interested in other portions of the life span (such as adulthood and aging), who were drawn to the study of adolescence because of its use as an ontogenetic laboratory for exploration of the use of developmental systems theory (for example, Lerner, Freund, De Stefanis, & Habermas, 2001). Accordingly, it is important to discuss the fundamental features of such theories and to explain how developmental systems models led to the elaboration of the PYD perspective.

DEFINING FEATURES OF DEVELOPMENTAL SYSTEMS THEORIES

The contemporary study of human development focused on concepts and models associated with developmental systems theories (Cairns & Cairns, 2006; Gottlieb et al.,

2006; Lerner, 2002, 2006; Overton, 2006). The roots of these theories may be linked to ideas in developmental science that were presented as early as the 1930s and 1940s at least (for example, Maier & Schneirla, 1935; Novikoff, 1945a, 1945b; von Bertalanffy, 1933), if not even significantly earlier, for example, in the concepts used by late nineteenth-century and early twentieth-century founders of the study of child development (see Cairns & Cairns, 2006). Following are several defining features of developmental systems theories.

1. *A relational metatheory.* Predicated on a postmodern philosophical perspective that transcends Cartesian dualism, developmental systems theories are framed by a *relational metatheory for human development.* These theories thus reject all splits between components of the ecology of human development (between nature- and nurture-based variables, for example) and between continuity and discontinuity and between stability and instability. Systemic syntheses or integrations replace dichotomizations or other reductionist partitions of the developmental system.

2. *The integration of levels of organization.* Relational thinking and the rejection of Cartesian splits are associated with the idea that all levels of organization within the ecology of human development are integrated or fused. These levels range from the biological and physiological through the cultural and historical.

3. *Developmental regulation across ontogeny involves mutually influential individual ↔ context relations.* As a consequence of the integration of levels, the regulation of development occurs through mutually influential connections among all levels of the developmental system, ranging from genes and cell physiology through individual mental and behavioral functioning to society, culture, the designed and natural ecology, and, ultimately, history. These mutually influential relations may be represented generically as Level 1 ↔ Level 2 (for example, family ↔ community) and, in the case of ontogeny, may be represented as individual ↔ context.

4. *Integrated actions and individual ↔ context relations as the basic unit of analysis within human development.* The *character of developmental regulation* means that the integration of actions—of the individual on the context and of the multiple levels of the context on the individual (individual ↔ context)—constitutes the fundamental unit of analysis in the study of the basic process of human development.

5. *Temporality and plasticity in human development.* As a consequence of the fusion of the historical level of analysis—and therefore of temporality—within the levels of the ecology of human development, the developmental system is characterized by the potential for systematic change—by plasticity. Observed trajectories of intraindividual change may vary across time and place as a consequence of such plasticity.

6. *Relative plasticity.* Developmental regulation may both facilitate and constrain opportunities for change. Thus, change in individual ↔ context relations is not limitless, and the *magnitude of plasticity* (the probability of change in a developmental

trajectory occurring in relation to variation in contextual conditions) may vary across the life span and history. Nevertheless, the potential for plasticity at both individual and contextual levels constitutes a fundamental strength of all humans' development.

7. *Intraindividual change, interindividual differences in intraindividual change, and the fundamental substantive significance of diversity.* The combinations of variables across the integrated levels of organization within the developmental system will vary at least in part across individuals and groups. This diversity is systematic and lawfully produced by idiographic, group differential and generic (nomothetic) phenomena. The range of interindividual differences in intraindividual change observed at any point in time is evidence of the plasticity of the developmental system and makes the study of diversity essential for the description, explanation, and optimization of human development.

8. *Optimism, the application of developmental science, and the promotion of positive human development.* The potential for and instantiations of plasticity legitimate an optimistic and proactive search for characteristics of individuals and ecologies that, together, can be arrayed to promote positive human development across life. Through the application of developmental science in planned attempts (interventions) to enhance (for example, through social policies or community-based programs) the character of humans' developmental trajectories, the promotion of positive human development may be achieved by aligning the strengths (operationalized as the potentials for positive change) of individuals and contexts.

9. *Multidisciplinarity and the need for change-sensitive methodologies.* The integrated levels of organization in the developmental system require collaborative analyses by scholars from multiple disciplines. Multidisciplinary knowledge and, ideally, interdisciplinary knowledge are sought. The temporal embeddedness and resulting plasticity of the developmental system require that research designs, methods of observation and measurement, and procedures for data analysis be change-sensitive and able to integrate trajectories of change at multiple levels of analysis.

In sum, the possibility of adaptive developmental relations between individuals and their contexts and the potential plasticity of human development—which is a defining feature of ontogenetic change within the dynamic, developmental system (Baltes, Lindenberger, & Staudinger, 2006; Gottlieb et al., 2006; Thelen & Smith, 2006)—stand as distinctive features of the developmental systems approach to human development. These features require methodological choices that differ in design, measurement, sampling, and data analytic techniques from those used typically by researchers using split or reductionist approaches to developmental science. Moreover, the emphasis on how the individual acts on the context to contribute to the relations with the context that regulate adaptive development (Brandtstädter, 2006) fosters an interest in person-centered (as compared to variable-centered) approaches to the study of human development (Magnusson & Stattin, 2006; Overton, 2006).

Furthermore, given that the array of individual and contextual variables involved in these relations constitute a virtually open set (for example, there are over 70 trillion potential human genotypes, and each of them may be coupled across life with an even larger number of life course trajectories of social experiences; Hirsch, 2004), the diversity of development becomes a prime substantive focus for developmental science (Lerner, 2004; Spencer, 2006). The diverse person—conceptualized from a strength-based perspective (in that the potential plasticity of ontogenetic change constitutes a fundamental strength of all humans; Spencer, 2006) and approached with the expectation that positive changes can be promoted across all instances of this diversity as a consequence of health-supportive alignments between people and settings (Benson et al., 2006)—becomes the necessary subject of developmental science inquiry.

It is in the linkage between the ideas of plasticity and diversity that a basis exists for the extension of developmental systems thinking to the field of adolescence and for the field of adolescence to serve as a "testing ground" for ideas associated with developmental systems theory. This synergy has had at least one key outcome: the forging of a new, strength-based vision of and vocabulary for the nature of adolescent development. In short, the plasticity-diversity linkage within developmental systems theory and method provided the basis for the formulation of the PYD perspective.

FEATURES OF THE PYD PERSPECTIVE

Beginning in the early 1990s, and burgeoning in the first half decade of the twenty-first century, a new vision and vocabulary for discussing young people has emerged. These innovations were framed by the developmental systems theories that were engaging the interest of developmental scientists. The focus on plasticity within such theories led in turn to an interest in assessing the potential for change at diverse points across ontogeny, from infancy through the tenth and eleventh decades of life (Baltes et al., 2006). Moreover, these innovations were propelled by the increasingly collaborative contributions of researchers focused on the second decade of life (for example, Damon, 2004; Lerner, 2004), practitioners in the field of youth development (for example, Floyd & McKenna, 2003), and policy makers concerned with improving the life chances of diverse youth and their families (for example, Cummings, 2003; Gore, 2003). These interests converged in the formulation of a set of ideas that enabled youth to be viewed as resources to be developed, not as problems to be managed (Roth & Brooks-Gunn, 2003). We will now discuss these ideas in connection with several key hypotheses.

PYD and Developmental Assets

Based on the idea that the potential for systematic intraindividual change across life (namely, for plasticity) represents a fundamental strength of human development, a key hypothesis is that when there is an alignment over time between the strengths of youth and the resources for healthy development present in the contexts of young people, PYD is promoted. A subsidiary hypothesis is that across the key settings of youth development (families, schools, and communities) there exist at least some supports for the promotion of PYD. Termed *developmental assets* (Benson et al., 2006), these resources constitute the social and ecological "nutrients" for the growth of healthy youth.

There is some controversy in the literature about the number of developmental assets that may exist in different social ecologies. For instance, are there forty developmental assets—half having their locus within the individual and the other half having their locus in the social ecology—as initially suggested by Search Institute (for example, Benson, Leffert, Scales, & Blyth, 1998)? Or are there only fourteen developmental assets—half associated with the individual and half associated with the social ecology—as recently reported by colleagues from the Institute for Applied Research in Youth Development (Theokas et al., 2005)? There are questions as well about whether developmental assets should be measured via youth reports, or perceptions, as is done in the survey research of Search Institute (for example, Leffert et al., 1998; Scales, Benson, Leffert, & Blyth, 2000) and/or through objective assessment of the actual ecology of youth development, as is done in the work of the Institute for Applied Research in Youth Development (Theokas & Lerner, 2006).

For instance, as part of the 4-H Study of PYD (Lerner et al., 2005; Jelicic, Bobek, Phelps, Lerner, & Lerner, 2007)—a longitudinal study of adolescent development supported by the National 4-H Council—Theokas and Lerner (2006) objectively assessed the following four ecological assets present in the homes, schools, and communities of youth:

1. *Other individuals:* for example, parents who spend high quantities of quality time with their children; high-quality, engaged teachers; and community mentors

2. *Institutions:* for example, structured, after-school programs, sport fields, libraries, and parks and hiking trails

3. *Collective activity:* for example, opportunities for youth and adults to work together on school committees, civic projects, or community organizations, such as the Chamber of Commerce or faith institutions

4. *Access:* for example, the availability of transportation to and from out-of-school-time activities or safe streets and neighborhoods

These actual assets were positively related to PYD and negatively related to indices of risk or problem behaviors (for example, internalizing problems such as depression or externalizing problems such as bullying) at levels generally higher than those associated with perceived assets. In addition, in all contexts—families, schools, and communities—the most important asset was always the people present in the lives of youth (Theokas & Lerner, 2006).

A question exists also about whether, from both theoretical and measurement standpoints, individual developmental assets can be differentiated from constructs related to indicators of PYD (Silbereisen & Lerner, 2007). In turn, if such differentiation is not feasible conceptually or empirically, then through what processes do youth contribute to the developmental regulations driving developmental changes? Consistent with research about the role of processes of self-regulation (and specifically the roles of selection, optimization, and compensation) and longevity and positive development among adults and other age groups (Baltes et al., 2006), results of other studies within the Institute using the 4-H data set indicate that adolescents who develop along a life path marked by pursuing positive, healthy goals, who possess the psychological, behavioral, and social capacities to effectively pursue these goals, and who manifest resilience in the face of failure or of blocked goals, show successful links with resources in their homes, schools, and communities that enable positive goals to be met and PYD to occur (for example, Gestsdottir & Lerner, 2007a, 2007b; Zimmerman, Phelps, & Lerner, 2007).

Finally, there remains a question about whether the mere accumulation of assets, whatever their source (family, school, or community) is the best predictor of PYD, or whether particular assets are of specific salience for youth living in specific communities. Although there is evidence for the idea that "more is better" (for example, Benson et al., 2006), recent theory and research have explored the more-is-better idea by focusing on a key domain of developmental assets—out-of-school time (OST) activities—for example, participation in sports, arts, service or volunteer organizations, hobby or interest clubs, or, in particular, youth development (YD) programs— those programs with a theory of change explicitly linked to the promotion of PYD (such as 4-H, Boys & Girls Clubs, Scouts, Big Brothers, Big Sisters, or YMCA).

Scales and colleagues (2000) found that youth reports of three or more hours a week of participation in sports, clubs, or organizations at school or in the community were the single developmental asset most frequently linked to several indicators of thriving (for example, school grades, leadership, physical health, and helping others) among the adolescents in the Search Institute sample. Lerner (2004) hypothesized that the link between YD programs and PYD emerges from what he calls the Big Three features of youth development programs: positive and sustained (for at least one year; Grossman & Rhodes, 2002) adult-youth relationships; skill-building activities; and opportunities to use these skills by participating in and leading valued community-based activities. Although reviews by Blum (2003), Eccles and Gootman (2002), and Roth and Brooks-Gunn (2003) differ in the number of attributes they propose as important for the conduct of youth programs effective in promoting PYD, all endorse the importance of the three attributes of after-school activities noted by Lerner (2004) as crucial for promoting exemplary positive development.

Indeed, Roth and Brooks-Gunn (2003) report that findings from evaluation research indicate that programs focusing on the development of *particular assets* are more likely than those focusing on enhancing the *quantity* of assets to be associated with the presence of key indicators of PYD. Speaking against the ubiquity of the more-is-better phenomenon and using data from the 4-H Study, Zarrett and colleagues have found that participation in particular *clusters of activities* seems more highly linked to greater levels of PYD and to lower levels of risk or problem behaviors than the *quantity* of OST activities (Zarrett, Fay, et al., in press; Zarrett, Lerner, et al., 2007; Zarrett, Phelps, et al., 2007). Moreover, the findings of Zarrett and colleagues suggest that there is a particular benefit of YD participation. For instance, high sports involvement is linked to low PYD and high levels of risk or problem behaviors. However, when high sports participation is combined with involvement in YD programs, then scores for PYD are at their highest (in comparison to other youth activity clusters) and scores for risk and problem behaviors are at their lowest—even lower than youth who are highly engaged in all categories of OST activities.

In short, developmental assets of youth and of their ecology are linked generally to the growth of PYD and the diminution of risk or problem behaviors. However, Phelps and colleagues (2007) discovered that this linkage is far from simple, and it is not an inverse relationship. There are multiple trajectories of PYD across the early adolescent years, and the directions of change for risk and problem behaviors are also quite varied. Inconsistent with the former mantra that the best way to prevent problem behaviors is to promote PYD (for example, Pittman, Irby, & Ferber, 2001)—thus implying that PYD and problems existed in a simple inverse relationship—Phelps and colleagues found that some youth show increases in both PYD and problem behaviors, some youth show decreases in both domains of functioning, and for most youth the combination of change trajectories is even more complex. Very few youth show a trajectory of linear increases of PYD coupled with linear decreases in risk and problem behaviors. Accordingly, policies and programs must be aimed at both the prevention of risks and problems and at the promotion of PYD. However, this conclusion requires that some specification be made of the substance and structure of PYD.

The Substance, Structure, and Import of PYD

Based on both the experiences of practitioners and on reviews of the adolescent development literature (Eccles & Gootman, 2002; Lerner, 2004; Roth & Brooks-Gunn, 2003), the *Five Cs* have been hypothesized as a way of conceptualizing PYD (and of integrating all the separate indicators of it, such as academic achievement and self-esteem). The Five Cs—competence, confidence, connection, character, and caring—have been linked to the positive outcomes of youth development programs reported by Roth and Brooks-Gunn (2003). In addition, the Five Cs are prominent terms used by practitioners, adolescents involved in youth development programs, and the parents of these adolescents in describing the characteristics of a "thriving youth" (King et al., 2005).

A hypothesis subsidiary to the postulation of the Five Cs as a means to operationalize PYD is that when a young person manifests the Cs across time (when the youth is thriving), he or she will be on a life trajectory heading toward an "idealized adulthood" (Rathunde & Csikszentmihalyi, 2006). Theoretically, an ideal adult life is marked by integrated and mutually reinforcing contributions to self (for example, maintaining one's health and one's consequent ability to remain an active agent in one's own development) and to family, community, and the institutions of civil society (Lerner, 2004). An adult engaging in such integrated contributions is a person manifesting adaptive developmental regulations (Brandtstädter, 2006).

Using data from the first wave of assessment (Grade 5) within the 4-H Study, Lerner and colleagues (2005) provided initial evidence for the empirical presence of the Five Cs (as first-order latent variables) and for the existence of PYD. The results of structural equation modeling analysis found evidence that the five first-order latent constructs accounted for variance in several theoretically meaningful "surface traits" (for example, measures of academic, social, and vocational abilities marked the construct of competence). In addition, these analyses found evidence for the convergence of the five first-order constructs on a second-order construct of PYD. Moreover, Lerner and colleagues (2005) found that PYD correlated positively within Grade 5 with the Sixth C of youth contribution and negatively with indices of risk and problem behaviors.

Jelicic and colleagues (2007) extended these within-grade findings in a subsequent longitudinal analysis. Results of random effects regression and structural equation modeling models indicated that, as expected, PYD in Grade 5 predicted higher youth contributions and lower risk behaviors and depression at Grade 6. There were significant sex differences for contribution (girls had higher scores) and for risk behaviors (boys had higher scores), but not for depression. Furthermore, the structural model fit was equivalent for boys and girls.

In sum, PYD may be indexed by the Five Cs; however, PYD is related to the development of youth contribution and to trajectories of youth risk and problem behaviors in complex and differentiated ways. Nevertheless, the current research findings derived from the 4-H Study of PYD indicate that through the alignment of youth strengths (as indexed by selection, optimization, and compensation scores, for example) with actual developmental assets in the ecology of youth (as indexed by individuals, institutions, collective action, and access, for example), the Five Cs and youth contribution may be promoted.

SUMMARY

Contemporary developmental science—predicated on a relational metatheory and focused on the use of developmental systems theories to frame research on dynamic relations between diverse individuals and contexts—constitutes an approach that may integrate the scholarship pertinent to these diverse levels of organization and, by so doing, may facilitate understanding of and promote positive human development. As we believe has been demonstrated here by reviewing the research associated with the PYD perspective, developmental systems approaches to developmental science offer a means to do good science—work informed by philosophically, conceptually, and methodologically useful information from the multiple disciplines having knowledge bases pertinent to the integrated, individual ↔ context relations comprising the ecology of human development. Such science is admittedly more difficult to enact than the ill-framed and methodologically flawed research that pursued split and reductionist paths taken during prior historical eras (Cairns & Cairns, 2006; Overton, 2006). Moreover, the current approach to developmental science underscores the diverse ways in which adolescents, in dynamic exchanges with their natural and designed ecologies, can create for themselves and others opportunities for health and positive development.

As Bronfenbrenner (2005) eloquently put it, it is these relations that make human beings human. Accordingly, the relational, dynamic, and diversity-sensitive scholarship that now defines excellence within developmental science may both document and extend the power inherent in each person to be an active agent in his or her own successful and positive development (Brandtstädter, 2006; Lerner, 2004; Magnusson & Stattin, 2006). A developmental systems perspective leads us to recognize that if we are to have an adequate and sufficient science of human development, we must integratively study individual and contextual levels of organization in a relational and temporal manner. Anything less will not constitute adequate science. And if we are to serve America's and the world's individuals, families, and communities through our science—if we are to help develop successful policies and programs through our scholarly efforts—then we must accept nothing less than the integrative temporal and relational model of diverse and active individuals that is embodied in the developmental systems perspective.

KEY TERMS

Character of developmental regulation
Contemporary developmental science
Developmental assets
Five Cs
Magnitude of plasticity

Plasticity
Positive youth development (PYD)
  perspective
Relational metatheory for human
  development

DISCUSSION QUESTIONS

1. How do the biological changes that occur during puberty contribute to the emergence of problem behavior?

2. Should the accumulation of assets be considered the best predictor of PYD? Why, or why not? Are some assets particularly salient for youth living in certain communities?

3. Discuss the concept of an "idealized adulthood" and how it relates to the Five Cs and PYD.

REFERENCES

Anthony, E. J. (1969). The reactions of adults to adolescents and their behavior. In G. Caplan & S. Lebovici (Eds.), *Adolescence: Psychosocial perspectives* (pp. 54–77). New York: Basic Books.

Baltes, P. B., Lindenberger, U., & Staudinger, U. M. (2006). Lifespan theory in developmental psychology. In R. M. Lerner (Vol. Ed.), *Handbook of child psychology: Vol. 1. Theoretical models of human development* (6th ed., pp. 569–664). Hoboken, NJ: Wiley.

Bandura, A. (1964). The stormy decade: Fact or fiction? *Psychology in the School, 1,* 224–231.

Benson, P., Leffert, N., Scales, P., & Blyth, D. (1998). Beyond the "village" rhetoric: Creating healthy communities for children and adolescents. *Applied Developmental Science, 2*(3), 138–159.

Benson, P. L., Scales, P. C., Hamilton, S. F., & Semsa, A., Jr. (2006). *Positive youth development: Theory, research, and applications.* In R. M. Lerner (Vol. Ed.), *Handbook of child psychology: Vol. 1. Theoretical models of human development* (6th ed., pp. 894–941). Hoboken, NJ: Wiley.

Block, J. (1971). *Lives through time.* Berkeley, CA: Bancroft Books.

Blum, R. W. (2003). Positive youth development: A strategy for improving adolescent health. In R. M. Lerner, F. Jacobs, & D. Wertlieb (Vol. Eds.), *Handbook of applied developmental science: Promoting positive child, adolescent, and family development through research, policies, and programs: Vol. 2. Enhancing the life chances of youth and families: Public service systems and public policy perspectives* (pp. 237–252). Thousand Oaks, CA: Sage Publications.

Brandtstädter, J. (2006). Action perspectives on human development. In R. M. Lerner (Vol. Ed.), *Handbook of child psychology: Vol. 1. Theoretical models of human development* (6th ed., pp. 516–568). Hoboken, NJ: Wiley.

Bronfenbrenner, U. (2005). *Making human beings human: Bioecological perspectives on human development.* Thousand Oaks, CA: Sage.

Cairns, R. B., & Cairns, B. D. (2006). The making of developmental psychology. In R. M. Lerner (Vol. Ed.), *Handbook of child psychology: Vol. 1. Theoretical models of human development* (6th ed., pp. 569–664). Hoboken, NJ: Wiley.

Cummings, E. (2003). Foreword. In D. Wertlieb, F. Jacobs, & R. M. Lerner (Vol. Eds.), *Handbook of applied developmental science: Promoting positive child, adolescent, and family development through research, policies, and programs: Vol. 3. Promoting positive youth and family development: Community systems, citizenship, and civil society* (pp. ix–xi). Thousand Oaks, CA: Sage.

Damon, W. (2004). What is positive youth development? *Annals of the American Academy of Political and Social Science, 591,* 13–24.

Douvan, J. D., & Adelson, J. (1966). *The adolescent experience.* New York: Wiley.

Eccles, J. S., & Gootman, J. A. (Eds.). (2002). *Community programs to promote youth development.* Washington, DC: National Academies Press.

Erikson, E. H. (1959). Identity and the life cycle. *Psychological Issues, 1,* 50–100.

Floyd, D. T., & McKenna, L. (2003). National youth serving organizations in the United States: Contributions to civil society. In R. M. Lerner, F. Jacobs, & D. Wertlieb (Vol. Eds.), *Handbook of applied developmental science: Promoting positive child, adolescent, and family development through research, policies, and programs: Vol. 3. Promoting positive youth and family development: Community systems, citizenship, and civil society* (pp. 11–26). Thousand Oaks, CA: Sage Publications.

Freud, S. (1969). Adolescence as a developmental disturbance. In G. Caplan & S. Lebovici (Eds.), *Adolescence* (pp. 5–10). New York: Basic Books.

Gestsdottir, S., & Lerner, R. M. (2007a). Intentional self-regulation and positive youth development in early adolescence: Findings from the 4-H Study of Positive Youth Development. *Developmental Psychology, 43*(2), 508–521.

Gestsdottir, S., & Lerner, R. M. (2007b). Hlutverk sjálfstjórnar fæskilegum þroska barna og unglinga. *Sálfræðiritið, 12,* 37–55.

Gore, A. (2003). Foreword. In R. M. Lerner & P. L. Benson (Eds.), *Developmental assets and asset-building communities: Implications for research, policy, and practice* (pp. xi–xii). Norwell, MA: Kluwer.

Gottlieb, G. (1997). *Synthesizing nature-nurture: Prenatal roots of instinctive behavior.* Mahwah, NJ: Erlbaum.

Gottlieb, G., Wahlsten, D., & Lickliter, R. (2006). The significance of biology for human development: A developmental psychobiological systems perspective. In R. M. Lerner (Vol. Ed.), *Handbook of child psychology: Vol. 1. Theoretical models of human development* (6th ed., pp. 210–257). Hoboken, NJ: Wiley.

Grossman, J. B., & Rhodes, J. E. (2002). The test of time: Predictors and effects of duration in youth mentoring programs. *American Journal of Community Psychology, 30,* 199–206.

Hall, G. S. (1904). *Adolescence: Its psychology and its relations to physiology. anthropology, sociology, sex, crime, religion, and education.* New York: Appleton.

Hirsch, J. (2004). Uniqueness, diversity, similarity, repeatability, and heritability. In C. Garcia Coll, E. Bearer, & R. M. Lerner (Eds.), *Nature and nurture: The complex interplay of genetic and environmental influences on human behavior and development* (pp. 127–138). Mahwah, NJ: Erlbaum.

Jelicic, H., Bobek, D., Phelps, E. D., Lerner, J. V., & Lerner, R. M. (2007). Using positive youth development to predict contribution and risk behaviors in early adolescence: Findings from the first two waves of the 4-H Study of Positive Youth Development. *International Journal of Behavioral Development, 31*(3), 263–273.

King, P. E., Dowling, E. M., Mueller, R. A., White, K., Schultz, W., Osborn, P., Dickerson, E., Bobek, D. L., Lerner, R. M., Benson, P. L., & Scales, P. C. (2005). Thriving in adolescence: The voices of youth-serving practitioners, parents, and early and late adolescents. *Journal of Early Adolescence, 25*(1), 94–112.

Leffert, N., Benson, P., Scales, P., Sharma, A., Drake, D., & Blyth, D. (1998). Developmental assets: Measurement and prediction of risk behaviors among adolescents. *Applied Developmental Science, 2*(4), 209–230.

Lerner, R. M. (1978). Nature, nurture, and dynamic interactionism. *Human Development, 21,* 1–20.

Lerner, R. M. (2002). *Concepts and theories of human development* (3rd ed.). Mahwah, NJ: Erlbaum.

Lerner, R. M. (2004). *Liberty: Thriving and civic engagement among American youth.* Thousand Oaks, CA: Sage.

Lerner, R. M. (2006). Developmental science, developmental systems, and contemporary theories of human development. In R. M. Lerner (Vol. Ed.), *Handbook of child psychology: Vol. 1. Theoretical models of human development* (6th ed., pp. 1–17). Hoboken, NJ: Wiley.

Lerner, R. M., Freund, A. M., De Stefanis, I., & Habermas, T. (2001). Understanding developmental regulation in adolescence: The use of the selection, optimization, and compensation model. *Human Development, 44,* 29–50.

Lerner, R. M., Lerner, J. V., Almerigi, J., Theokas, C., Phelps, E., Gestsdottir, S. Naudeau, S., Jelicic, H., Alberts, A. E., Ma, L., Smith, L. M., Bobek, D. L., Richman-Raphael, D., Simpson, I., Christiansen, E. D., & von Eye, A. (2005). Positive youth development, participation in community youth development programs, and community contributions of fifth-grade adolescents: Findings from the first wave of the 4-H Study of Positive Youth Development. *Journal of Early Adolescence, 25*(1), 17–71.

Lerner, R. M., & Steinberg, L. (Eds.). (2004). *Handbook of adolescent psychology* (2nd ed.). Hoboken, NJ: Wiley.

Magnusson, D., & Stattin, H. (2006). The person in the environment: Towards a general model for scientific inquiry. In R. M. Lerner (Vol. Ed.), *Handbook of child psychology: Vol. 1. Theoretical models of human development* (6th ed., pp. 400–464). Hoboken, NJ: Wiley.

Maier, N.R.F., & Schneirla, T. C. (1935). *Principles of animal behavior.* New York: McGraw-Hill.

Novikoff, A. B. (1945a). The concept of integrative levels and biology. *Science, 101,* 209–215.

Novikoff, A. B. (1945b). Continuity and discontinuity in evolution. *Science, 101,* 405–406.

Offer, D. (1969). *The psychological world of the teen-ager.* New York: Basic Books.

Overton, W. F. (1973). On the assumptive base of the nature-nurture controversy: Additive versus interactive conceptions. *Human Development, 16,* 74–89.

Overton, W. F. (2006). Developmental psychology: Philosophy, concepts, methodology. In R. M. Lerner (Vol. Ed.), *Handbook of child psychology: Vol. 1. Theoretical models of human development* (6th ed., pp. 18–88). Hoboken, NJ: Wiley.

Phelps, E., Balsano, A., Fay, K., Peltz, J., Zimmerman, S., Lerner, R., M., & Lerner, J. V. (2007). Nuances in early adolescent development trajectories of positive and of problematic/risk behaviors: Findings from the 4-H Study of Positive Youth Development. Child and Adolescent Clinics of North America, 16(2), 473–496.

Pittman, K., Irby, M., & Ferber, T. (2001). *Unfinished business: Further reflections on a decade of promoting youth development.* In P. L. Benson & K. J. Pittman (Eds.), *Trends in youth development: Visions, realities and challenges* (pp. 4–50). Norwell, MA: Kluwer.

Rathunde, K., & Csikszentmihalyi, M. (2006). The developing person: An experiential perspective. In R. M. Lerner (Vol. Ed.), *Handbook of child psychology: Vol. 1. Theoretical models of human development* (6th ed.; pp. 465–515). Hoboken, NJ: Wiley.

Roth, J. L., & Brooks-Gunn, J. (2003). What is a youth development program? Identification and defining principles. In. F. Jacobs, D. Wertlieb, & R. M. Lerner (Vol. Eds.), *Handbook of applied developmental science: Promoting positive child, adolescent, and family development through research, policies, and programs. Vol. 2. Enhancing the life chances of youth and families: Public service systems and public policy perspectives* (pp. 197–223). Thousand Oaks, CA: Sage.

Scales, P., Benson, P., Leffert, N., & Blyth, D. A. (2000). The contribution of developmental assets to the prediction of thriving among adolescents. *Applied Developmental Science, 4,* 27–46.

Schneirla, T. C. (1957). The concept of development in comparative psychology. In D. B. Harris (Ed.), *The concept of development* (pp. 78–108). Minneapolis: University of Minnesota.

Seligman, M.E.P. (2002). Positive psychology, positive prevention, and positive therapy. In C. R. Snyder & S. Lopez (Eds.), *Handbook of positive psychology.* New York: Oxford University Press.

Silbereisen, R. K., & Lerner, R. M. (2007). Approaches to positive youth development: A view of the issues. In R. K. Silbereisen & R. M. Lerner (Eds.), *Approaches to positive youth development* (pp. 3–30). London: Sage.

Spencer, M. B. (2006). Phenomenology and ecological systems theory: Development of diverse groups. In R. M. Lerner (Vol. Ed.), *Handbook of child psychology: Vol. 1. Theoretical models of human development* (6th ed., pp. 829–893). Hoboken, NJ: Wiley.

Suomi, S. J. (2004). How gene-environment interactions influence emotional development in rhesus monkeys. In C. Garcia Coll, E. Bearer, & R. M. Lerner (Eds.), *Nature and nurture: The complex interplay of genetic and environmental influences on human behavior and development* (pp. 35–51). Mahwah, NJ: Erlbaum.

Thelen, E., & Smith, L. B. (2006). Dynamic systems theories. In R. M. Lerner (Vol. Ed.), *Theoretical models of human development: Vol. 1. Handbook of child psychology* (6th ed., pp. 258–312). Hoboken, NJ: Wiley.

Theokas, C., Almerigi, J., Lerner, R. M., Dowling, E., Benson, P., Scales, P. C., & von Eye, A. (2005). Conceptualizing and modeling individual and ecological asset components of thriving in early adolescence. *Journal of Early Adolescence, 25*(1), 113–143.

Theokas, C., & Lerner, R. M. (2006). Observed ecological assets in families, schools, and neighborhoods: Conceptualization, measurement and relations with positive and negative developmental outcomes. *Applied Developmental Science, 10*(2), 61–74.

Tobach, E., & Greenberg, G. (1984). The significance of T. C. Schneirla's contribution to the concept of levels of integration. In G. Greenberg & E. Tobach (Eds.), *Behavioral evolution and integrative levels* (pp. 1–7). Hillsdale, NJ: Erlbaum.

von Bertalanffy, L. (1933). *Modern theories of development.* London: Oxford University Press.

Zarrett, N., Fay, K., Carrano, J., Li, Y., Phelps, E., & Lerner, R. M. (2007). *The multiple dimensions of participation: Variable- and pattern-centered approaches for examining effects of sports participation on youth development.* Medford, MA: Institute for Applied Research in Youth Development, Tufts University.

Zarrett, N., Lerner, R. M., Carrano, J., Fay, K., Peltz, J. S., & Li, Y. (2007). Variations in adolescent engagement in sports and its influence on positive youth development. In N. L. Holt (Ed.), *Positive youth development and sport.* Oxford, England: Routledge.

Zarrett, N., Fay, K., Carrano, J., Li, Y., Phelps, E., & Lerner, R. M. (In press). More than child's play: Variable- and pattern-centered approaches for examining effects of sports participation on youth development. *Developmental Psychology.*

Zimmerman, S., Phelps, E., & Lerner, R. M. (2007). *Intentional self-regulation in early adolescence: Assessing the structure of selection, optimization, and compensations processes.* Medford, MA: Institute for Applied Research in Youth Development, Tufts University.

2

PREVENTING KEY HEALTH RISK BEHAVIORS

CHAPTER

8

TOBACCO USE AND ADOLESCENT HEALTH

RICHARD R. CLAYTON ▪ CRYSTAL A. CAUDILL ▪ MELISSA J. H. SEGRESS

LEARNING OBJECTIVES

After studying this chapter, you will be able to

- Identify tobacco use as the largest preventable source of morbidity and mortality in the world.
- Determine when in the developmental period health effects from tobacco use occur.
- Articulate strategies for reducing the consequences of tobacco use during adolescence.

This chapter is about adolescents, tobacco use, and health outcomes. We need to be clear at the outset on two things. First, almost all of the health effects of tobacco use occur after years of chronic use; few of the health effects of tobacco use occur to adolescents or during adolescence. Second, because of this fact, there is very little rigorous research on the health effects of tobacco use among adolescents. Nevertheless, knowledge about the health effects of tobacco use that occur primarily among adults is critical because over eight out of ten adult smokers began their use of tobacco in their teens. Therefore, in this chapter we will review existing knowledge about the long-term effects of tobacco use that starts in adolescence and evidence concerning interventions designed to reduce tobacco use among adolescents. By way of introduction, there are several terms necessitating comment.

Adolescence. Up to this point in time, most academic disciplines and public commentators have treated adolescence as if it were one distinct stage of development. Dahl and Spear (2004) suggest that it is possible adolescence consists of a number of stages that may vary across individuals and settings. If there are multiple stages of adolescence, there is as yet no consensus on how many there are or what they might be named. Therefore, writings that claim to focus on adolescence may have a conceptual problem—the possibility of heterogeneity *within* the stage. For some, adolescence may consist of only a few stages characterized by large, signal events or changes that occur and clearly differentiate one stage from another. For others, adolescence may consist of many stages with some smooth and some jagged transitions in the trajectories from early to later stages of adolescence and then to young adulthood. Because the issue of stages in adolescence is unresolved and because there is limited scientific evidence on the number of stages in adolescence, we will refer to it as if it were one stage. However, we urge the reader of this chapter to think of adolescence as much more complex than the single-stage concept implies. Maughan (2005, p. 126) has aptly described the importance of this stage of development and its complexities: "Adolescence is marked by dramatic changes in a plethora of aspects of individual development—biological, cognitive, and emotional—that may have relevance for behavioral change; in addition, it heralds major changes in the nature of young people's relationships and in the contexts in which they spend their time."

Tobacco Use. There are obviously many forms and delivery devices for tobacco and nicotine: from cigarettes and pipes to small and large cigars, bidis, chew and moist snuff, kreteks, and "hookahs." However, a large majority of knowledge about and research on tobacco and adolescence concerns the use of cigarettes. Therefore, unless otherwise specified, in this chapter whenever we discuss tobacco use, we are referring to the use of cigarettes. Most importantly, cigarettes should be thought of as a *drug delivery device* designed specifically to deliver nicotine in the most efficient and effective manner.

Cigarettes should be thought of as a drug delivery device designed specifically to deliver nicotine in the most efficient and effective manner.

Health Outcomes. As mentioned earlier, almost all that is known about the health outcomes of tobacco use involves individuals who have smoked cigarettes for years, even though a large majority may have initiated their use when they were adolescents. Therefore, the knowledge base about *health outcomes attributable to tobacco use* overwhelmingly reflects chronic (long-term), not acute (short-term) exposure, and thus concerns adults more than adolescents.

SCOPE OF THE PROBLEM AND HEALTH OUTCOMES

Tobacco use is the largest preventable source of ill health and premature death in the world. By the year 2020, it is estimated that smoking will be the cause of 10 million deaths worldwide each year (Peto & Lopez, 2001). If you have trouble, as we do, with really big numbers, consider that the July 1, 2005, estimate of the population of New York City was 8,143,197. Therefore, by 2020, a population larger than the 2005 population of New York City will die each year because they smoked cigarettes.

Deaths Attributable to Tobacco Use

There are approximately 2.4 million total deaths in the United States each year. Of those, about 440,000 deaths are attributable to long-term, chronic tobacco use. To put this figure in perspective, it is equal to more than two fully loaded jumbo jets crashing each day for an entire year. For more perspective, consider that over the entire decade or more of the Vietnam War there were 58,000 American casualties, and close to 3,000 individuals lost their lives in the 9/11 disaster. To us, any untimely death is a reason for sorrow, so we mean no disrespect by citing the number of American casualties from the Vietnam War or 9/11. However, with regard to the magnitude of the effect, the mortality associated with smoking that has occurred year in and year out has no equal. In fact, smoking causes more deaths each year than the combined total of deaths attributable to alcohol, car accidents, suicide, AIDS, homicide, and illegal drugs.

To deal with this public health issue, the problem is not lack of knowledge. Virtually everyone knows and believes that smoking "causes" lung cancer. The first Surgeon General's Report on Smoking and Health appeared in 1964, and subsequent reports have made this scientific finding a well-known fact. More people die from lung cancer than any other type of cancer—these deaths represent 30 percent of all cancer deaths each year. If one were to consider the attention given to various types of cancer, one would think that breast cancer was the largest cause of cancer death among women. That is simply not the case. In fact, the number of lung cancer deaths among women passed the number of deaths from breast cancer in 1987, more than twenty years ago. Smoking is estimated to cause 87 percent of all lung cancer deaths. Smoking is also a major cause of the following other types of cancer: larynx, oral cavity, pharynx, esophagus, and bladder. Smoking is a contributing cause in the development of cancers of the pancreas, cervix, kidney, stomach, and some leukemias.

Cardiovascular disease is the leading cause of deaths in the United States, and smoking is a major risk factor for cardiovascular disease. Some 35 percent of all deaths attributable to smoking are from cardiovascular diseases.

Because over 80 percent of all smokers begin smoking when they are adolescents, these smoking-related deaths are a health outcome of a behavioral pattern that begins during adolescence.

Because over 80 percent of all smokers begin smoking when they are adolescents, these smoking-related deaths are a health outcome of a behavioral pattern that begins during adolescence. If we could significantly reduce the number of adolescents who smoke, or the number who begin smoking during adolescence, we could reduce these "adolescent" health outcomes.

Tobacco's Critical Role in Adolescent Health and Well-Being

It is clear that the huge number of deaths attributable to smoking is not occurring among adolescents. It usually takes a long time for the consequences of chronic tobacco use to become apparent. Why, then, are the health outcomes data reported earlier relevant to adolescent health? The answers are simple. First, over 80 percent of all continuing adult smokers began smoking in their teens. If we could reduce the incidence and the prevalence of smoking among adolescents, the morbidity and premature mortality attributable to smoking would decrease. Therefore, one approach to reducing the health outcomes caused by smoking is to encourage youth not to start using tobacco in the first place, thereby reducing the percentage of smokers in each birth cohort.

Second, the incidence and prevalence of tobacco use among adolescents are significantly affected by the fact that addiction to nicotine is exceptionally strong. In fact, the nicotine in cigarettes reaches the brain in approximately seven seconds after inhalation of smoke. A person who smokes twenty cigarettes a day and takes ten puffs from each cigarette is receiving two hundred hits of nicotine to the brain a day, each one taking only seven seconds to get there. Because chronic smokers often continue smoking even when they are sick, a twenty-a-day smoker consumes 7,300 cigarettes a year and gets 73,000 hits of nicotine to the brain. If that person smokes for twenty years, he or she will consume 1.46 million cigarettes. Furthermore, nicotine acts on the brain in smaller amounts than most other drugs. For example, a chronic smoker can completely satisfy his or her addiction to nicotine if the amount of nicotine in the brain is at or somewhat below 35 nanograms (35 billionths of a gram) per milliliter of blood; beyond that level he or she may get nauseous. By comparison, someone using cocaine hydrochloride (cocaine powder) might lay out five lines of cocaine and snort them. The expected blood cocaine level would be 100 nanograms per milliliter of blood.

The long-term outcomes of tobacco use are relevant to adolescent health because nicotine is a very addicting drug. Eight out of ten who start using tobacco begin during adolescence, and one out of two long-term smokers will die of a smoking-related illness. Further, the quality of life of chronic smokers is significantly lower than that of nonsmokers, particularly in terms of ease of breathing. It may take twenty to twenty-five years or so for a health outcome that is attributable to smoking to appear. Perhaps the best place to start reducing the untoward health outcomes from tobacco use is at the beginning, through various prevention efforts that occur during adolescence.

Lule and colleagues explain why tobacco is important in looking at the health outcomes for adolescents: "If we look only at disability-adjusted life years (DALYs) for the adolescent age group, adolescents appear to be relatively healthy. Nonetheless, more than 33 percent of the disease burden and almost 60 percent of premature deaths among adults can be associated with behaviors or conditions that began or occurred during adolescence—for example, tobacco and alcohol use, poor eating habits, sexual abuse, and risky sex" (Lule, Rosen, Singh, Knowles, & Behrman, 2006, p. 1106).

Epidemiology of Adolescents' Tobacco Use

Most of our knowledge about the epidemiology of tobacco use among adolescents comes from the following national data systems:

- The Monitoring the Future (MTF) annual surveys of twelfth graders (since 1975) and eighth and tenth graders (since 1991)

- The National Survey on Drug Use and Health (NSDUH) of youth twelve to seventeen years old, conducted in homes

- The Youth Risk Behavior Surveys, conducted in schools in many states by the Centers for Disease Control and Prevention

- The Youth Tobacco Survey, conducted by the American Legacy Foundation

We will now review incidence, prevalence, and trend data and also discuss some of the correlates of tobacco use among adolescents from these surveys.

Incidence of Tobacco Use Among Adolescents *Incidence* refers to new users—youth who have made the transition from never having smoked to having smoked cigarettes. The data shown below from the 2006 Monitoring the Future study of adolescents across the United States show two important things about adolescents and cigarette use (see Johnston, O'Malley, Bachman, & Schulenberg, 2007). First, the percentage of eighth graders in 2006 (14.7 percent) who had tried cigarettes by the end of the sixth grade (when most students are eleven years old) is higher than the percentage of tenth graders in 2006 (11 percent) or twelfth graders in 2006 (9.6 percent). This change suggests that there has been an increase in early use across these three birth cohorts. Second, the

Had Used Cigarettes by End of Sixth Grade		*Had Used Cigarettes by End of Eighth Grade*	
Eighth graders	14.7 percent	Eighth graders	24.6 percent
Tenth graders	11.0 percent	Tenth graders	24.5 percent
Twelfth graders	9.6 percent	Twelfth graders	22.4 percent

period between the end of the sixth grade and the end of the eighth grade is critical with regard to beginning to smoke. By the end of the eighth grade, almost the same percentage of youth in each cohort had smoked—about one in four or one in five.

The implications from a prevention and health promotion perspective are clear. If we are to reduce the incidence of smoking, our *primary prevention* interventions have to occur in early elementary school, before the sixth grade, to catch them *before* they start. From a *secondary prevention* perspective—catching them *soon after* they start—there should be concentrated interventions from the sixth through eighth grades to get those who have started to stop using cigarettes and discourage continuation toward chronic use of cigarettes.

The preceding data are from adolescents who completed questionnaires in their school as part of the Monitoring the Future study. The oldest of these students are in the twelfth grade and are probably eighteen years old. This study doesn't include school dropouts. Dropouts are more likely to smoke than those who stay in school. In addition, if one in four eighth, tenth, and twelfth graders in 2006 had already begun smoking, almost three-fourths of them are still at risk to start smoking. This illustrates what is called "right censoring." For us to determine the average age at onset of smoking, everyone in our sample needs to have gone through the periods when they are most at risk to start smoking. When nonright-censored data (from adults) for onset of smoking are examined in the National Survey on Drug Use and Health, it appears that the average or median age at onset of smoking has not changed much in the past twenty-five years. The median age (50 percent start at a later age and 50 percent start at a lower) at onset of smoking is sixteen.

Prevalence of Tobacco Use Among Adolescents *Current use of tobacco* is usually defined as any use in the previous thirty days. Trends refer to changes across years in the rate. The data listed after this paragraph indicate a substantial reduction in current use of cigarettes and smokeless tobacco from 1991 to 2006 among eighth, tenth, and twelfth graders. However, it is clear that between 1991 and the latter 1990s there was an increase in *prevalence* rates, followed by a decline. To date, there are no widely

Cigarette Use in Last 30 Days	*1991*	*2006*	*Highest Rate (Year)*	*Smokeless Tobacco Use in Last 30 Days*	*1991*	*2006*	*Highest Rate (Year)*
Eighth graders	14.3	8.7	21.0 (1996)	Eighth graders	6.9	3.7	7.7 (1994)
Tenth graders	20.8	14.5	30.4 (1996)	Tenth graders	10.0	5.7	10.5 (1994)
Twelfth graders	28.3	21.6	36.5 (1997)	Twelfth graders	—	6.1	12.2 (1995)

accepted hypotheses to explain why this bump in the rates occurred in the 1990s. Whatever happened, it is clear that it affected all three of these birth cohorts of adolescents and affected them at about the same time. This means that the relatively large shifts in the prevalence rate reflected in these trends probably exist at the macro or societal level, not at the intraindividual level. Johnston and his colleagues from the Monitoring the Future study suggest that the rates are influenced by changes in the perception of harm from cigarettes (and other drugs). As perceived harmfulness goes up, usage rates go down, and vice versa (Johnston, O'Malley, & Bachman, 2002).

STRATEGIES FOR REDUCING THE RISK OF TOBACCO USE AMONG ADOLESCENTS

In the United States, the problem of tobacco use among adolescents and its short- and long-term effects has been approached using a number of different strategies. Some of these strategies occur at the individual level, and others are population-based public health strategies utilizing laws, regulations, and policies designed to influence tobacco use among adolescents. In the sections that follow, several of these strategies will be described and discussed.

School-Based, Curriculum-Driven Prevention Programs

If the goal is to reduce the long-term health and other consequences of cigarette and other tobacco use among adolescents, then one approach is to catch kids where they spend a significant amount of their time (school), catch them before they start using cigarettes, and provide them with knowledge and skills that will persuade them to never start. This approach makes sense, at least on the surface. However, only a few school-based and curriculum-driven programs have had the desired effects.

One of the most comprehensive smoking prevention programs ever attempted is the Hutchinson Smoking Prevention Program (HSPP). The researchers identified forty school districts that had only one high school in the state of Washington (Peterson, Kealey, Mann, Marek, & Sarason, 2000). These forty districts were randomized into an experimental and a control condition, twenty districts in each group. Districts with only one high school were chosen to avoid having adolescents from treatment intervention middle schools and those from the control middle schools subsequently attending the same high school.

The intervention began in the experimental districts in the third grade, when most students were only eight years old. Every year from the third grade through the tenth grade, these students received a developmentally relevant "social influences" curriculum tailored to the modal age of the students each year. At the time this study began, the prevailing theories about why some adolescents smoked and others did not emphasized social influences such as peers and the media. Each year the curriculum contained all fifteen essential elements of school-based, curriculum-driven programs identified and endorsed by the National Cancer Institute and the Centers for Disease

Control and Prevention. The focus of this curriculum was exclusively on tobacco. The students in the control schools did not receive any formal curriculum, but did complete questionnaires each year.

Results on daily smoking when these students were in the twelfth grade were disappointing. Among males in the experimental districts, 26.32 percent were daily smokers, compared to 26.65 percent among males in the control districts; a difference of 0.33 percent. The results among females were equally depressing: 24.41 percent of those in experimental districts were daily smokers, compared to 24.66 percent in the control districts—a difference of 0.25 percent. And remember—these districts had only one high school, so those who did not receive the curriculum in elementary and middle school were not influenced by those who did receive it when they moved on to high school.

This study was theory- and evidence-based. In fact, the intervention was intensive—the most intensive and extensive ever attempted in terms of the number of hours for which the students in the experimental condition were exposed to the curriculum. The randomization of the school districts made this one of the most rigorous studies ever conducted. In fact, from the third grade through the twelfth grade and even two years beyond high school, the researchers were able to collect data on 93 percent of the original sample. This is an amazing figure. So what happened? The simple answer is theory failure: the social influences model on which the curriculum was built was not correct. At that point in time we obviously did not know with certainty the risk factors that spurred some young people to smoke and others not to smoke. However, one plausible alternative answer is that there are very large differences from school to school, but almost all the factors targeted in this study were at the individual level. For example, in the experimental schools, by the twelfth grade the percentage of daily smokers among males ranged from a low of 10 percent in one school to 42 percent in another school. Among females the range was equally large, from a low of 16 percent at one school to 34 percent at another school.

At that point in time we did not know with certainty the risk factors that spurred some young people to smoke and others not to smoke.

An entirely different story was found by Gilbert Botvin and his colleagues when they evaluated a school-based, curriculum-driven drug prevention program called Life Skills Training (Botvin, Baker, Dusenbury, Botvin, & Diaz, 1995). Unlike the Hutchinson study, the curriculum developed by Botvin focused on a number of drugs, including tobacco. The study by Botvin included fifty-six schools randomly assigned into two experimental conditions. (The teachers in experimental condition 1 were personally trained by Dr. Botvin and also received technical assistance from him and his team; the teachers in experimental condition 2 received their training from Dr. Botvin by videotape and received no further technical assistance.) The schools in the control group condition did not receive any drug prevention programming. The life skills training curriculum was delivered once a week for fifteen sessions in year 1 (the sixth grade), ten sessions in year 2 (the seventh grade), and five sessions in year 3 (the eighth grade). The two experimental conditions were further divided into a "high-fidelity" group (students who received 60 percent or more of the lessons) and a "low-fidelity" group (those who received less than 60 percent of the lessons). A total of almost one-third of the students in experimental condition 1 were classified as low fidelity, while one-fourth were so classified in experimental condition 2.

By the twelfth grade, Botvin and his colleagues found statistically significant differences between students in the two high-fidelity groups of the two experimental conditions and students in the control group. Surprisingly, there were no major differences between high-fidelity groups led by the teachers and those teachers who received training via videotape. Further, it is interesting that Botvin and his colleagues did not show data from the low-fidelity groups. There may be a reason for this oversight. Those in the low-fidelity groups in the two experimental conditions were virtually equal to the control group on all three measures of smoking. Stated differently, the students who received less than 60 percent of the lessons were no different in their smoking from students who received nothing at all. One could surmise that students in low-fidelity groups were at higher risk for virtually all problem behaviors including smoking, and they constituted between one-fourth and one-third of the students in the experimental conditions. Does this mean that the program worked for the "good kids" and had almost no effect on the high-risk kids, who are more likely to be absent or truant? The answer is probably yes. However, Botvin and colleagues (1995) reported a 75 percent reduction in smoking attributable to the Life Skills Training program.

Americans have an enormous amount of confidence that schools cannot only teach their children how to read, write, speak, and calculate, but also promote healthy behavioral patterns and discourage unhealthy ones. The two studies just described produced different results: the Hutchinson study (Peterson et al., 2000) found no influence on smoking, the Botvin et al. study (1995) reported a 75 percent reduction in smoking. Simply put, the power of school-based, curriculum-driven prevention programming in preventing adolescents' tobacco use is arguable.

Purchase, Use, and Possession Laws

One of the most widespread attempts to influence the use of cigarettes by adolescents is a prototypical public policy approach to a problem—get tough on the purchase, use, and possession (PUP) of cigarettes by making it tougher to buy them (see Clark, Natanblut, Schmitt, Wolters, & Iachan, 2000). By the first quarter of 2001, only six states and the District of Columbia did not have a PUP law. Some thirty-seven states had laws prohibiting the purchase of cigarettes by minors, thirty-two had laws prohibiting possession, and nineteen had laws prohibiting use. These laws were stimulated primarily by the so-called Synar Amendment. One provision of the Synar Amendment was to require random buy-bust attempts at retail tobacco outlets in every state. Marked improvements in the percentage of buy attempts that were successful were required. Failure to show improvement would lead to the federal government withholding dollars the states were to use for drug treatment programming.

All states have complied, but the PUP intervention has been largely unsuccessful. The reasons are fairly obvious: (1) there is a low likelihood of detection because of the low number of buy-bust attempts that can be implemented in states relative to the number of outlets for purchase of cigarettes, (2) there is often a relationship between the buyer and the clerk behind the counter in a so-called convenience store, and (3) citizens want law enforcement personnel to focus on more serious crimes. Further, the fines levied for violating the law are often small, and more often than not those fines are paid by the tobacco industry, not the owner of the store. The bottom line is that all states have shown that a relatively small percentage of buy-bust attempts result in a buy. However, if the number of successful buy attempts reported by the states is correct, one would expect a lower prevalence rate of cigarette use by adolescents. An alternative explanation is that there are many sources of cigarettes for adolescents. It is not necessary for an adolescent to personally buy his or her cigarettes.

In 1998 the Attorneys General for forty-six states signed an unprecedented Master Settlement Agreement with the major tobacco companies (four states had previously reached an agreement with the tobacco companies) that included payments to the states to compensate them for costs associated with treating illnesses of smokers and restrictions on the ways and places in which tobacco companies could promote their products. The tobacco industry used this development to their benefit. They significantly increased their point-of-purchase promotions. For example, in a study conducted over a four-month period in 1999, point-of-purchase promotions were observed in 3,031 retail outlets in 163 communities. In 92 percent of these stores, at least some form of point-of-purchase presence was observed (from internal or external advertising to self-service brand placement, multipack discounts, and tobacco-branded objects). In the outlets in these communities, 80 percent had interior advertising, 43 percent had low-height advertising at the eye level of children. Convenience stores account for the largest share of retail tobacco sales (McElrath et al., 2002). Seventy-five percent of teenagers shop at these types of stores at least once a week. Given the critical mass of promotion and advertising of tobacco products at the local level, it is not surprising that so many adolescents start smoking and then continue to smoke once they start.

The bottom line is that all states have shown that a relatively small percentage of buy-bust attempts result in a buy.

Mass Media Anti-Tobacco Campaigns

Very few explicit attempts have been made to influence point-of-purchase advertising and promotion in order to reduce adolescents' tobacco use. However, a number of mass media campaigns have been designed to influence tobacco use among adolescents. By far the most widely recognized and successful is the truth® campaign. It is national in scope and designed to attract teens by exposing the marketing and manufacturing practices used by the tobacco industry to recruit youth into smoking. In addition, the truth®

campaign uses innovative and relevant information to impress upon adolescents the toll of tobacco on individuals, families, and society at large. The ads themselves are purposefully edgy and sometimes "in your face" in style and format. They are boldly honest.

Evidence suggests that 22 percent of the overall decline in youth smoking rates between 2000 and 2002 is attributable directly to the truth® campaign (Farrelly, Davis, Haviland, Messeri, & Healton, 2005). This is a large effect. During this period it is estimated that there were approximately 300,000 fewer adolescent smokers because of the campaign. Furthermore, a *dose-response relationship* was found: the larger the number of ads viewed, the greater the likelihood the adolescent was a nonsmoker (Farrelly et al., 2005).

A number of mass media campaigns have been designed to influence tobacco use among adolescents.

Davis, Nonnemaker, and Farrelly (2007) used the data from the American Legacy Foundation's Media Tracking Surveys to compare the effects of the truth® campaign with the Think, Don't Smoke (TDS) campaign sponsored by Philip Morris tobacco company. Davis and his colleagues focused on perceived smoking prevalence among adolescents, a precursor to and predictor of smoking. We know that one's perception of the percentage of peers that are engaging in a behavior (perception of behavioral norms) influences one's own behavior. Davis and colleagues (2007) found that exposure to the truth® campaign was negatively and significantly associated with the perceived norms of smoking among adolescents. The Philip Morris TDS campaign was not associated with perceived smoking prevalence.

The bottom line here is that mass media campaigns have been very influential in their effects on adolescent smoking. This is a prototypical public health approach to health promotion and disease prevention. Effective campaigns grab the attention of the audience (in this case, adolescents), get them to encode, decode, and then apply the message into choices about their behavior. These results are pretty incredible, given the massive efforts by the tobacco industry to promote smoking.

The 1998 Master Settlement Agreement provided $206 billion to states, to be paid out between 2000 and 2025. Four states (Florida, Minnesota, Mississippi, and Texas) had previously reached a settlement that obligated the top five tobacco companies to pay more than $40 billion. The tobacco industry has increased its spending on marketing since the Master Tobacco Settlement was signed. From 1998 through 2005, the annual expenditures in billions were $6.9B, $8.4B, $9.8B, $11.5B, $12.7B, $13.4B, and $13.4B. The $13.4 billion spent in 2005 breaks down to $36 million a day—more than $45 for every person in the United States, and more than $290 for each U.S. adult smoker.

Roughly 75 percent of the 2005 tobacco industry marketing expenditures—close to $10 billion—were for price discounts paid to retailers and wholesalers to reduce the price of cigarettes. It is interesting that in 2005 cigarette companies spent $31 million on the sponsorship of sports teams or individual athletes. The five largest smokeless tobacco companies spent a little over $250 million on advertising and promotion, almost $16 million of which was on sports and sporting events in 2005.

Environmental Tobacco Smoke and Clean Indoor Air

The scientific evidence on health risks from exposure to *environmental tobacco smoke* (ETS—also known as secondhand smoke or passive smoke) is clear and persuasive. If a nonsmoker is in a room or an area where someone is smoking, that person is also smoking. Chronic exposure to environmental tobacco smoke is a known cause of lung cancer, heart disease, and chronic lung conditions such as bronchitis and asthma, particularly in children and low-birth-weight neonates. Exposure to ETS is estimated to result in at least 36,000 deaths annually in the United States and over one million illnesses in children, including the exacerbation of asthma in children (400,000 cases per year), acute lower respiratory illness (150,000 cases per year), otitis media (infection and inflammation of the inner ear and eardrum) in children (700,000 cases per year), 10,000 cases of low birth weight, and 2,000 cases of sudden infant death syndrome.

The scientific evidence on health risks from exposure to environmental tobacco smoke is clear and persuasive.

With all the evidence pointed in the negative direction, one of the most effective tobacco control measures involves restricting where individuals can smoke—so-called clean indoor air regulations, which have applied primarily to public places such as restaurants, bars, and workplaces. Of special relevance to adolescent health, substantial evidence indicates that exposure to ETS increases adolescents' chances of becoming smokers (see Wakefield et al., 2000). For example, Farkas, Gilpin, White, and Pierce (2000) found that adolescents who lived in smoke-free households were only 74 percent as likely to be smokers as those who lived in homes with no home smoking restrictions. Adolescents who worked in smoke-free workplaces were 68 percent as likely to be smokers, compared to those who worked in places with no restrictions on worksite smoking.

A growing body of evidence suggests that exposure to ETS during adolescence has an impact on academic achievement test scores. Collins, Wileyto, Murphy, and Munafo (2007) examined test scores at age sixteen and eighteen for a large cohort of adolescents who were born March 3 through 9, 1958, in the United Kingdom. These tests are classified as O-level (ordinary) and A-level (advanced), with O-level similar to an achievement test and A-level similar to the SAT in the United States. They found that adolescent exposure to ETS, not prenatal tobacco exposure, predicted failure on both the O-level and the A-level achievement tests. This occurred even after statistical controls for other factors known to affect achievement were considered. Because there is an inverse relationship between smoking and educational achievement (the lower the education, the higher the likelihood of smoking) and between socioeconomic status and a large number of indices of poor health, ETS exposure during adolescence is connected to ultimate health and smoking status. Therefore, from a health perspective the best conditions for adolescents with regard to tobacco use are to live in homes with explicit no-smoking policies, work in places with explicit no-smoking policies, and live in communities with comprehensive bans on smoking in public places (see Levy & Friend, 2003).

Increases in State-Level Tobacco Excise Taxes

The conclusion of the 1998 Institute of Medicine report "Taking Action to Reduce Tobacco Use" states, "the single most direct and reliable method for reducing consumption is to increase the price of tobacco products, thus encouraging the cessation and reducing the level of initiation of tobacco." Raising the price is a population-based public health approach to tobacco control and prevention.

As of January 1, 2007, the state excise tax on cigarettes varied widely, from a low of 7 cents per pack in South Carolina to 257.5 cents per pack in New Jersey. The median state excise tax per pack in 2007 across all states is 104.6 cents per pack.

The rationale for increasing state excise taxes on cigarettes was relatively simple. First, research shows that a 10 percent increase in the state excise tax produces a 7 percent decrease in the prevalence of adolescent smoking and a decrease of 3 to 5 percent in adult smoking. Such decreases suggest that one of the most effective approaches to reducing cigarette consumption among adolescents is to increase the state excise tax. Remember, these percentages refer to percent, not percentage points. Second, increased state excise taxes on cigarettes reduce consumption and consequently reduce health care costs. Third, higher taxes increase state revenue, despite the reductions in smoking and tobacco sales.

If the federal excise tax on a pack of cigarettes had been keyed to the Consumer Price Index, it would now stand at $1.51 per pack, not 39 cents per pack.

In 1960 the federal excise tax on cigarettes was 8 cents, about one-third of the 26 cents charged for a pack of cigarettes at the time. In 2007, the average cost of a pack of cigarettes is $4.00. This means that the current 39 cent federal excise tax is less than 10 percent of the mean retail price of a pack of cigarettes. If the federal excise tax on a pack of cigarettes had been keyed to the Consumer Price Index, it would now stand at $1.51 per pack, not 39 cents per pack. This would require an additional $1.12 per pack. In spite of the fact that increases in the price of cigarettes have a major influence on reducing tobacco use among both adults and adolescents, there is significant resistance in Congress to increasing the federal excise tax on cigarettes.

SUMMARY

We can draw a number of important conclusions about tobacco, adolescents, and health outcomes from tobacco use. Following are a few of the most salient points:

- Smoking is a complex behavior. Over 80 percent of adult smokers begin using tobacco when they are adolescents.

- Cigarettes are an extremely efficient and effective drug delivery device. Nicotine is an addictive drug.

- The long-term health consequences of chronic tobacco use are clear. Although not all smokers get cancer or cardiovascular disease, the chances that a smoker will suffer and eventually die from cancer or cardiovascular disease are significantly higher than the chances for a nonsmoker.

- A number of strategies have been developed and implemented to reduce the consequences of tobacco use, which usually begins during adolescence.

- Strategies that appear logical and promising on the surface have not always proven so. These include school-based, curriculum-driven prevention programming and purchase, use, and possession (PUP) laws. Their effect on reducing the number of new users of tobacco and the prevalence of smoking has been minimal.

- Population-based public health approaches have proven to be effective. These include mass media campaigns, bans on smoking in public places, and increases in state excise taxes.

- If our society is to reduce the health consequences associated with tobacco use, we have to intervene early to reduce the number of new users (incidence) and the percentage of youth making the transition from no use to continuation to progression to dependence on nicotine.

Adolescent health and tobacco use are integrally connected. This is true because dependence on nicotine that starts during adolescence is one of the first steps in a life-long behavior pattern (smoking) that significantly increases risk of morbidity and mortality. Therefore, a strategy for decreasing the health consequences of tobacco use that often begins during adolescence is to change the addictive potential of nicotine. This can be accomplished by reengineering how cigarettes are produced. Tobacco manufacturers control the amount of nicotine that is delivered by engineering the size of the particles that carry nicotine to the lungs and then to the brain. Unfortunately, no federal agency currently regulates tobacco products. Because the Food and Drug Administration (FDA) requires companies that manufacture and market drugs to show that they are safe and efficacious (and predictably do what they are supposed to do), we would expect that agency to also regulate tobacco. When consumers use cigarettes the way they are supposed to be used, they are responsible for 440,000 deaths a year. Why is our society more concerned about drugs that have few, if any, consequences when another drug delivered by a very efficient and effective delivery device causes such significant ill health and premature death?

KEY TERMS

Adolescence	Incidence
Current use of tobacco	Prevalence
Dose-response relationship	Primary prevention
Environmental tobacco smoke (ETS)	Secondary prevention
Health outcomes attributable to tobacco use	Tobacco use

DISCUSSION QUESTIONS

1. Given the number of preventable deaths each year that are attributed to tobacco use, would you agree that tobacco use is the number one public health problem in this country? Why or why not?

2. Which is a better strategy for reducing negative health outcomes associated with smoking—primary or secondary prevention ? Why?

3. What are the strengths and weaknesses of the Botvin et al. study (1995) and the Hutchinson study (Peterson et al., 2000)?

4. Brainstorm an ideal public health intervention focusing on tobacco use among adolescents. How and where would you intervene? What intervention components would you include? What age group would you target?

REFERENCES

Botvin, G. J., Baker, E., Dusenbury, L., Botvin, E. M., & Diaz, T. (1995). Long-term follow-up results of a randomized drug abuse prevention trial in a white, middle-class population. *Journal of the American Medical Association, 273*(14), 1106–1112.

Clark, P. I., Natanblut, S. L., Schmitt, C. L., Wolters, C., & Iachan, R. (2000). Factors associated with tobacco sales to minors. *Journal of the American Medical Association, 284*(6), 729–734.

Collins, B. N., Wileyto, E. P., Murphy, M.F.G., & Munafo, M. R. (2007). Adolescent environmental tobacco smoke exposure predicts academic achievement test failure. *Journal of Adolescent Health, 41,* 363–370.

Dahl, R. E., & Spear, L. P. (2004). *Adolescent brain development: Vulnerabilities and opportunities.* New York: New York Academy of Sciences.

Davis, K. C., Nonnemaker, J. M., & Farrelly, M. C. (2007). Association between national smoking prevention campaigns and perceived smoking prevalence among youth in the United States. *Journal of Adolescent Health, 41,* 430–436.

Farkas, A. J., Gilpin, E. A., White, M. M., & Pierce, J. P. (2000). Association between household and workplace smoking restrictions and adolescent smoking. *Journal of the American Medical Association, 284*(6), 717–722.

Farrelly, M. C., Davis, K. C., Haviland, M. L., Messeri, P., & Healton, C. G. (2005). Evidence of a dose-response relationship between "truth" antismoking ads and youth smoking prevalence. *American Journal of Public Health, 95,* 425–431.

Institute of Medicine. (1998). Taking action to reduce tobacco use. Washington, DC: National Academies Press.

Johnston, L. D., O'Malley, P. M., & Bachman, J. G. (2002). *Monitoring the Future national results on adolescent drug use: Overview of key findings, 2001.* (NIH Publication No. 02-5105). Bethesda, MD: National Institute on Drug Abuse.

Johnston, L. D., O'Malley, P. M., Bachman, J. G., & Schulenberg, J. E. (2007). *Monitoring the Future national survey results on drug use, 1975–2006: Vol. I. Secondary school students.* (NIH Publication No. 07-6205). Bethesda, MD: National Institute on Drug Abuse.

Levy, D. T., & Friend, K. B. (2003). The effects of clean indoor air laws: What do we know and what do we need to know? *Health Education Research, 18,* 592–609.

Lule, E., Rosen, J. E., Singh, S., Knowles, J. C., & Behrman, J. R. (2006). Adolescent health programs. In D. T. Jamison, J. G. Breman, A. R. Meashan, G. Alleyne, M. Claeson, D. B. Evans, P. Jha, A. Mills, & P. Musgrove (Eds.), *Disease control priorities in developing countries* (2nd ed., pp. 1109–1125). Washington, DC: The World Bank Group.

Maughan, B. (2005). Developmental trajectory modeling: A view from developmental psychopathology. *Annals of the American Academy of Political and Social Science, 602,* 118–130.

McElrath, Y. T., Wakefield, M., Giovino, G., Hyland, A., Barker, D., Chaloupka, F., Slater, S., Clark, P., Schooley, M., Pederson, L., & Pechacek, T. (2002). Point of purchase tobacco environments and variation by store type: United States, 1999. *Morbidity and Mortality Weekly Report, 51*(9), 184–187.

Peterson, A. V., Kealey, K. A., Mann, S. L., Marek, P. M., & Sarason, I. G. (2000). Hutchinson Smoking Prevention Project: Long-term randomized trial in school-based prevention—Results on smoking, *Journal of the National Cancer Institute, 92*(24), 1979–1991.

Peto, R., & Lopez, A. D. (2001). The future worldwide health effects of current smoking patterns. In E. C. Koop, C. E. Pearson, & M. R. Schwartz (Eds.), *Critical issues in global health* (pp. 154–161). San Francisco: Jossey-Bass.

Wakefield, M. A., Chaloupka, F. J., Kaufman, N. J., Orleans, C. T, Barker, D. C., & Ruel, E. E. (2000). Effect of restrictions on smoking at home, at school, and in public places on teenage smoking: Cross-sectional study. *British Medical Journal, 321,* 333–337.

CHAPTER

9

UNDERSTANDING AND PREVENTING RISKS FOR ADOLESCENT OBESITY

MARY ANN PENTZ

LEARNING OBJECTIVES

After studying this chapter, you will be able to

- Assess adolescent obesity risk by comparing overweight and obesity rates among different age groups.

- Demonstrate an understanding of adolescent obesity risk from a developmental perspective.

- Evaluate obesity risk factors in adolescence by the intrapersonal, social situation, and environmental context.

Overweight and obesity have multiple adverse health, social, and economic consequences and have been associated with several types of disease, including heart disease, diabetes (in both adults and adolescents), and several types of cancer, including endometrial, prostate, gallbladder, kidney, and postmenopausal breast cancer (Allison, Fontaine, Manson, Stevens, & VanItallie, 1999; Mokdad et al., 2003; Schottenfeld & Beebe-Dimmer, 2005). Obesity continues to increase rapidly in all age groups in the United States, suggesting even greater health burdens in the future (Conway & Rene, 2004). To put this problem in context, up to 31 percent of adults are now considered overweight (Conway & Rene, 2004). Estimates of overweight have also increased significantly in children and early adolescents aged four through twelve, and the prevalence of overweight children and adolescents in the six- through nineteen-year-old age range is upward of 15 percent (Bolen, Rhodes, Powell-Griner, Bland, & Holtzman, 2000; Elizabeth & Baur, 2007). In adolescents, health risks may be compounded by psychosocial problems associated with obesity, including depression, stress, low self-efficacy and self-image, peer victimization (bullying), and externalizing problem behaviors such as delinquency and acting out (Anderson, Cohen, Naumova, Jacques, & Must, 2007; Jasuja, Chou, Riggs, & Pentz, 2008; Pentz, Mac-Kinnon, & Pentz, 1988; Shaw, Ramirez, Trost, Randall, & Stice, 2004; Nguyen-Michel, Unger, & Spruijt-Metz, 2007).

Coupled with these statistics are findings on obesogenic trajectories of children and adolescents showing that the largest increases for both male and female youth appear to occur between the ages of ten and fifteen (Bolen et al., 2000; Committee on Nutrition, 2003; Toschke, Ruckinger, Reinehr, & von Kries, 2007). Because the trend toward obesity in adolescents may be gradual or misinterpreted as temporary weight changes associated with the onset of puberty (Davison & Birch, 2001; Mei, Gummer-Strawn, Thompson, & Dietz, 2004), it may be more logical to understand and prevent risks for obesity from a developmental trajectory perspective that focuses on universal prevention, rather than from a more clinical perspective of obesity reduction. This chapter addresses adolescent obesity risk and prevention from the developmental perspective, with discussion of intervention aimed at universal prevention.

HEALTH PROMOTION AND RISK PREVENTION

Some types of adolescent health risk behaviors are predefined as risk behaviors by virtue of being illegal, such as drug use and delinquency. In contrast, obesity and its two most proximal risk factors—dysregulated or poor eating behavior and sedentary behavior—are legal and somewhat normative. This difference requires defining what is meant by obesity risk for a population that is characterized by increasing overweight. Currently, *overweight,* or immediate obesity risk, is defined by international standards as an age- and gender-adjusted body mass index (BMI) greater than the 85th percentile, and *obesity* is an adjusted BMI greater than the 95th percentile (Cole, Bellizzi, Flegal, & Dietz, 2000).

Understanding Obesity Risk

Overweight and obesity are primarily the result of an imbalance between energy intake and energy expended over time (Hill, Melanson, & Wyatt, 2000), or considered another way, between *eating behavior* and *physical activity behavior*. Thus, based on the concept of energy imbalance—aside from genetic, metabolic, and demographic factors—*obesogenic trajectories* vary according to dietary and eating habits (representing energy intake) and physical activity (energy expended; Sothern, 2004). Obesogenic trajectories are similar in concept to trajectories that can be identified for virtually any health or health risk behavior, usually through the analytic process of growth mixture modeling (Li, Goran, Kaur, Nollen, & Ahluwalia, 2007; Windle et al., 2004). In this case, an individual may develop her own trajectory of BMI, and subgroups of individuals may share the same trajectory. Trajectories of obesity risk can also be examined in terms of trajectories of eating behavior or physical activity that serve as predictors of BMI, although there appears to be no research yet on either of these obesity risk trajectories in adolescents. In contrast, linking trajectories of risk factors to outcomes is increasingly used in other fields, for example, linking trajectories of sensation seeking to adolescent drug use (Crawford, Pentz, Chou, Li, & Dwyer, 2003). Several examples of translation of research on adolescent drug use and problem behavior to obesity are discussed throughout this chapter.

Eating behavior contains multiple variables or constructs in the energy balance equation.

Eating behavior contains multiple variables or constructs that contribute to energy balance. High sugar intake, high fat and low fiber intake, overconsumption of large portions of food, dysregulated or impulsive eating, and number and timing of eating episodes per day have all been related to adolescent obesity risk (Hill, Melanson, & Wyatt, 2000). The relative impact and interaction effects of these eating variables on adolescent obesity risk are still not well understood and may be driven by other factors that do not appear to be directly associated with eating. For example, research on children and adolescents in foster care suggests that executive cognitive function and impulse control may be diminished compared to other youth as a result of lower levels of circulating cortisol during normally active daytime periods (Fisher, Gunnar, Dozier, Bruce, & Pears, 2006). These lower levels affected learning in school and conduct problems at home. Results of studies such as these raise the possibility that low cortisol levels may predispose an adolescent to low executive function (decision making) and low impulse control, which in turn mediate poor food choices and eating behaviors.

Like eating behavior, physical activity contains multiple constructs. As adolescents gain independence from parents and extend the range of activities that are available to them and under their control, physical activity that poses a risk for obesity becomes more complex to measure (Nelson, Gordon-Larsen, Adair, & Popkin, 2005). At the very least, strenuous physical activities such as sports may mitigate obesity risk, while sedentary behaviors such as increased television viewing and time on the computer may heighten risk. Time spent walking, which lowers obesity risk in all age groups, may be highly variable or decrease significantly in adolescence, as this activity is replaced with time spent in cars with friends (Saksvig et al., 2007).

Obesity Risk in Adolescence

Obesity risk starts early, first with adiposity rebound (the point in early childhood when minimal obesity ends), then in early adolescence (Cole et al., 2000; Committee on Nutrition, 2003). Of these two developmental periods, early adolescence may be associated with greater risk, since obesogenic trajectories have been shown to rise more dramatically starting at about age ten or eleven, which typically marks the end of childhood and entry into early adolescence (Crimmins et al., 2007; Toschke et al., 2007). The rise occurs across both males and females and across different ethnic groups, including white youth (Li et al., 2007; Shaw et al., 2004). There are a few differences among these groups, though the differences may be subject to interactions with other factors (Tschumper, Nägele, & Alsaker, 2006). For example, female adolescents may show steeper obesogenic trajectories than males, which appear to be associated with a greater decline in exercise among females compared to males (Tschumper et al., 2006). This trend has been linked to a lower perceived value of exercise among females when they reach adolescence—exercise is not considered "cool" or is considered masculine in their peer social networks (Spruijt-Metz & Saelens, 2006; Voorhees et al., 2005). However, for females on sports teams, this decline may not occur. Alternatively, BMI may appear to increase in males compared to females, but this change may represent development of greater muscle mass associated with pubertal changes rather than obesity risk. In terms of ethnic differences, Hispanic adolescents may have a somewhat higher risk for obesity than either African American adolescents or Caucasian adolescents (35.4 percent versus 28.7 percent versus 20.6 percent, respectively; Bolen et al., 2000). However, these differences may interact with acculturation and differences in perceived meaning of exercise, which in turn have been linked to lower physical activity, more sedentary television viewing, and higher rates of fast food consumption (Lowry, Wechsler, Galuska, Fulton, & Kann, 2002; Spruijt-Metz & Saelens, 2006; Unger et al., 2004).

Regardless of possible demographic differences in obesogenic trajectories, several factors contribute to increased obesity risk in early adolescence overall. Broadly speaking, these factors can be considered in terms of physiological factors related to puberty, developmental tasks expected of adolescents, and emerging social influences outside of the family.

Physiological factors related to puberty. The first set of factors relates to puberty. The early adolescent period is typically associated with reaching puberty. *Puberty* is characterized by neural plasticity, which affects executive cognitive function (Chambers, Taylor, & Potenza, 2003); hormonal change, which affects emotional arousal, impulse control, and circulating metabolites (Lee et al., 2007); and changes in physical characteristics, which shape self- and other-perceptions of attractiveness (Toschke et al., 2007). Emotional dysregulation, poor impulse control, metabolic changes, and negative body image, in turn, have been shown to have significant relationships to obesity risk in adolescents, particularly through eating behavior (Golub et al., 2008).

Developmental tasks of adolescence. The second general factor relates to developmental tasks that are expected of adolescents. Emerging from late childhood, youth are expected to have started developing social competence, cognitive skills related to decision making, and emotional regulation (affect) or self-management (Nigg, Quamma, Greenberg, & Kusche, 1999). However, mastery of these tasks is not expected until adolescence, the next stage of development. The most important social competence skills are those that involve forging relationships with peers, the intent of which is to help adolescents establish their own identity and autonomy from parents. The most important cognitive skills may be those that represent executive function—skills involved in organization, planning, deliberate intention, self-monitoring, self-control, and working memory to repeat trial behavior (Nigg et al., 1999). Affect influences executive cognitive function and behavior and may also have a reciprocal relationship with these factors over time (Riggs, Greenberg, Kusché, & Pentz, 2006). Parents help adolescents achieve these tasks by using positive parent-child communication, modeling healthy eating and exercise behavior, and setting clear rules for emotional control and behavior at home, at school, and in other environments. Whether directly or indirectly, failure to achieve these developmental tasks may heighten risk for obesity. For example, it has been suggested that lack of self-regulation and decision-making skills is a prominent factor in explaining repetitive sequences of overeating and eating nonhealthy foods (Davis, Levitan, Muglia, Bewell, & Kennedy, 2004) and choosing immediate sedentary activities (such as watching television) rather than alternatives (Fleming-Moran & Thiagarajah, 2005; Nelson et al., 2005). Lack of planning and cognitive decision making also maintains these unhealthy sequences (Baranowski, Cullen, Nicklas, Thompson, & Baranowski, 2003).

> *Failure to achieve these develop- mental tasks may heighten risk for obesity.*

Emerging social influences. This third factor primarily involves peers. As adolescents spend more time away from home, in school, extracurricular activities, and leisure time activities, the influence of peers increases. Peers constitute a modeling influence on eating and physical activity behaviors (Grosbras et al., 2007), as well as social support for these behaviors (Duncan, Duncan, & Strycker, 2005). Obesity risk increases to the extent that peers congregate at fast food places, eat energy-dense foods to the exclusion of other foods, and concentrate their leisure time on sedentary activities such as television viewing and video games (Boynton-Jarrett et al., 2003). At the same time, the family still exerts a social influence through the modeling of eating behavior and food selection and preparation (Campbell et al., 2007).

Risk Factors by Context

Whether one focuses on eating behavior, physical activity, or both to understand obesogenic trajectories in adolescence, and whether one concentrates on puberty, developmental tasks, or emerging social influences for their relationship to adolescent obesity risk, the immediate drivers of eating and activity involve a multitude of specific attitudes, behaviors, social-situational, and environmental *contexts*. These contexts are admittedly complex and have become the emerging focus of recent National Institutes of Health (NIH) efforts to understand and prevent obesity risk in children and adolescents (Huang & Horlick, 2007). For example, the simple physical activity of an adolescent walking rather than riding a bus to school may depend on proximity to the school, wait time for the bus, weather conditions, and safety of walking routes to that school (for example, Kipke et al., 2007; Molnar, Gortmaker, Bull, & Buka, 2004; Gyurcsik, Spink, Bray, Chad, & Kwan, 2006). The influence of different contexts on this one activity becomes even more complex when one considers the multiple contexts involving the school; for example, whether there is opportunity to engage in physical activity during the school day and whether school food policies support healthy food choices (Blanchard et al., 2005; Gordon-Larsen, McMurray & Popkin, 2000; Kubik, Lytle, & Story, 2005; Wardle, Brodersen, & Boniface, 2007). Thus, multiple epidemiological studies have already identified several of the individual factors that affect child and adolescent obesity risk. In a review of epidemiological studies, the Committee on Nutrition (2003) classified some of these into sets, such as the sets of influence that represent the family context for eating and exercise behavior. However, what has been missing is an organizing principle or theory to understand how these risk factors cluster and how they may interact to affect obesity risk.

The next section considers obesity risk factors by intrapersonal, social-situational, and environmental context and uses four theoretical models drawn from the fields of drug use and violence prevention to illustrate how these factors operate. Theories from these fields are particularly relevant to adolescent obesity prevention for at least two reasons. First, there may a be a neurobiological link between drug use risk and obesity risk through the endocannabinoid system, which drives sensation seeking, low impulse control, craving, and, ultimately, compulsive behaviors (Beaver et al., 2006; DiMarzo & Matia, 2005; Volkow & Wise, 2005; Wang, Volkow, Thanos, & Fowler, 2004) and which is sensitive to the hormonal changes associated with puberty (Chambers, Taylor, & Potenza, 2003). Second, many of the same contextual risk factors that have been recently identified for adolescent obesity were previously found for drug use and violence in adolescents (Pentz, 2004; Pentz, Jasuja, Rohrbach, Sussman, & Bardo, 2006).

Theoretical Approaches to Understanding Adolescent Obesity Risk by Context

The *Social Development Model* was originally developed to elucidate and inform epidemiological studies of drug use and delinquency. Hawkins, Catalano, and Miller (1992) posited that an individual could exhibit positive (protective) or negative (risk) behaviors, or both, depending on the social context for behavior (S), personal behavioral skills (P), and the environmental opportunity for reward and practice of prosocial (as opposed to antisocial) behavior (S or E). Several individual risk factors from their work are relevant to adolescent obesity risk. Among these are sensation seeking related to low impulse control (P), previous maladaptive or negative behaviors (P), exposure to poor or negative modeling influences by peers and by parents (S), lack of parental supervision (S), perceived or actual lack of a safe neighborhood (E), and perceived and actual norms for negative behavior (S and E). In the case of obesity risk, maladaptive or negative behaviors refer to poor eating habits and sedentary as opposed to physical activity. Other risk and protective factors from this model may not be applicable to obesity risk, or at least no clear links have been found thus far. These include achievement orientation at school, school bonding, prevalence of crime in a neighborhood, and opportunities for reinforcement of positive behaviors.

The second theoretical model is *Problem Behavior Theory* (Donovan, Jessor, & Costa, 1988). This theory hypothesizes that P- and E-level risk factors interact to affect multiple problem behaviors, particularly risky sexual behavior, drug use, and delinquency. The theory targets the adolescent years associated with school transitions, whether to middle or high school. Adolescents are transition-prone to the extent that they are influenced by the behaviors of older peers during these transitions. Risk taking for the purpose of sensation seeking (a P-level dispositional factor) attempts to emulate older peers (an S-level social modeling influence), and ill use of leisure time (represented by E-level factors such as discretionary spending money, job status, and access to cars) are major features of this theory. The theory was later applied to understanding health-promoting as well as problem behavior (Donovan, Jessor, & Costa, 1993). All the factors in this theory potentially apply to poor eating and physical activity choices and modeling influences.

The third model is Greenberg and colleagues' *Cognition-Affect-Behavior-Dynamic* (CABD) *Regulation Model,* which was developed to explain risk for conduct problems and aggression in children (Greenberg, 2006; Riggs, Elfenbaum, & Pentz, 2006). Prominent P-level risk factors from this model include poor executive cognitive function—specifically, poor personal decision-making skills and poor emotional regulation or affective control—both of which are hypothesized to have dynamic relationships to behaviors representing both impulse control and social competence. S or social factors focus primarily on parent-child and teacher-child interactions and to some extent peer-peer interactions in play and school situations. E-level factors are not a major feature of this model. The factors most relevant to adolescent obesity risk and prevention are executive cognitive function and emotional regulation, as they may relate to eating behavior.

The fourth theory is *Integrative Transactional Theory* (ITT; Pentz, 1999), which was designed to explain development and prevention of risk for drug use and violence in adolescence. This model clusters a total of seventeen risk factors under the three contexts of person (P), social situation (S), and environment (E). The risk factors are hypothesized to have synergistic and reciprocal effects across contexts. For example, a P-level factor of intentions to try a drug will lead to or generate an S-level factor of peer influence on drug use, since an adolescent intending to try a drug may seek out a peer who is already using or who has a drug available (E-level factor). This chain of events may in turn result in greater exposure of the adolescent to a social norm of drug use over time. P-level factors in ITT include prior behavior, intentions to use, prior decision-making skills, appraisal or meaning of drug use (including for sensation seeking), prior social support seeking (whether of drug users or nonusers), and physiological reactions to use. S-level factors include peer modeling influences, parent and family modeling influences (drug use as well as parenting), prior peer interactions, social support, social norms, and social transitions. E-level factors include media influences, availability of prevention resources (including community organizations for prevention and fiscal resources), availability of drugs, community norms, and school and community policies. Most of these are relevant to adolescent obesity risk. Some, however, require adaptation in order to logically translate to obesity risk. For example, the P level of intentions to use drugs could be reframed as intentions to select a certain type of food or physical activity, and the P-level physiological reactions to use could be reframed as individual differences in reward drive associated with food (Beaver et al., 2006). Support seeking could be reframed as eating or exercising as a means of coping. The ITT model adapted to adolescent obesity risk is shown in Figure 9.1. Variables that are reframed for obesity risk are shown in italics.

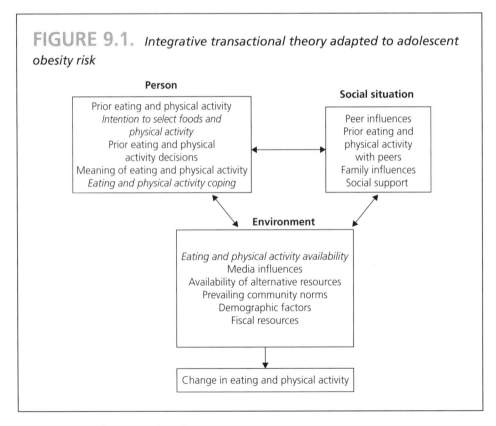

FIGURE 9.1. *Integrative transactional theory adapted to adolescent obesity risk*

Source: Adapted from Pentz (1999).

Overall, P- and S-level risk factors have figured more prominently than E-level factors in research on adolescent drug use (Pentz, 1999, 2003). This differential emphasis may reflect either the greater difficulty in conducting rigorous research on E-level factors or the greater concentration on behavioral demand reduction versus supply reduction that has characterized most epidemiological studies of adolescent drug use. For understanding adolescent obesity risk, however, E-level factors may be just as important, if not more so, than P and S factors. Because eating and physical activity, unlike drug use, are legal and necessary for survival, the E-level influences of marketing, product availability, access, and financial resources are expected to be much greater than those for drug use (Gyurcsik et al., 2006).

The influences of marketing, product availability, access, and financial resources are expected to be much greater for obesity risk than for drug use.

Prevention of Adolescent Obesity Risk

Excluding clinic-based intervention studies, obesity prevention interventions can be roughly categorized into programmatic (primarily school) or environmental interventions (such as cafeteria or food vending policies; Committee on Nutrition, 2003; French & Story, 2006; Institute of Medicine, 2004). Most of these have been implemented in schools, with either children or adolescents (Committee on Nutrition, 2003; Connelly, Duaso, & Butler, 2007). Although several have produced short-term changes in eating patterns and/or physical activity, relatively few have demonstrated changes in BMI, with most changes in obesity risk factors concentrated in girls (for example, Austin et al., 2007) or under intervention conditions requiring compulsory physical activity (Connelly et al., 2007; Dietz & Gortmaker, 2001). Participants at a recent NIH meeting on childhood obesity were in general agreement that few interventions could be considered evidence-based in terms of producing long-term changes in weight, including BMI (Pentz, 2004). Thus, at this point in time, there are no generally recognized evidence-based programs for adolescent obesity prevention, although recent Cochrane data-based reviews of prevention trials have identified several promising approaches, primarily those focusing on physical activity (Campbell, Waters, O'Meara, Kelly, & Summerbell, 2002). The relative lack of evidence-based obesity prevention programs for adolescents suggests a need for expediting the translation of findings from effective Type I studies of prevention in other health behavior areas such as drug abuse to obesity (Pentz, Jasuja, Rohrbach, Sussman, & Bardo, 2006; Reynolds & Spruijt-Metz, 2006).

There may be several possible reasons for the lack of efficacious programs for adolescent obesity prevention. Three of them are discussed in the following sections: insufficient theoretical basis, insufficient attention to context, and the need for comprehensive, multicomponent intervention.

Insufficient theory. The most prevalent theories upon which obesity prevention programs have been based are social learning theory, which attempts to modify modeling and practice behaviors; social cognitive theory, which addresses self-efficacy; and either reasoned action or planned behavior theories, which address attitudes toward health and personal expectations for nutrition and exercise (Baranowski et al., 2003; Committee on Nutrition, 2003). Although these theories account for between approximately 6 and 30 percent of attitudinal and intentional change, they account for relatively little intervention effect on actual obesity risk behavior (Baranowski et al., 2003), and unlike, for example, the CABD model developed for child conduct problems, they do not address emotion as it relates to impulse control or planning (Greenberg, 2006). Given that low impulse control and lack of decision making or planning are major risk factors for obesity risk in adolescence, it is possible that the inability of most obesity prevention programs to show either large or sustained effects may be related to a lack of attention to emotion, particularly poor impulse control. For example, Baranowski et al. (2003) posited that social cognitive theories can be applied to breaking down decisions in eating and physical activity events into discrete contextual steps (most of them in social contexts), with each step being a potential focus for prevention, such as the decision on where to eat a particular food. However, each of these steps depends on rational decision making and does not take into account rapid, impulsive behavior that may override rational decision making in adolescence.

Recently, Izard (2002) developed a theory that articulates emotion as a set of principles, much like Baranowski et al.'s (2003) steps in cognitive decision making: awareness and use of both positive and negative emotions, emotional regulation, recognition of emotional states, emotional activation for a purpose, communication of emotions to others, and connecting emotions with cognitive skills. Conceivably, these principles, combined with Baranowski's cognitive steps, could be incorporated into an adolescent obesity prevention program, along with one or more of the theories reviewed from the drug use field that would account for changes in cognitive, behavioral, and emotional mediators of obesity risk such as emotion-driven eating (Nguyen et al., 2007).

Insufficient attention to context. The theories from the field of drug use described earlier assume that risk behavior occurs in multiple contexts and that contexts interact to affect risk. One possible reason that effective obesity prevention programs are lacking is that they may not be designed to change all the contexts that affect eating and physical activity behavior on a daily basis, including in school, in the community, at home, and at different times during the day (Birch & Davison, 2001; Blanchard et al., 2005; Campbell et al., 2002; Davison & Birch, 2001).

Recent reviews of obesity prevention studies have noted that school-based programs, which make up the bulk of adolescent obesity prevention, tend to focus heavily on nutrition and health education, physical activity, and/or food and exercise availability at school (Committee on Nutrition, 2003; Franks et al., 2007; Peterson & Fox, 2007; Salmon, Phongsavan, Murphy, & Timperio, 2007; Sharma, 2007). A few of these also focus on parents' food selection and preparation, family exercise, and, to a lesser extent, family goal setting (Committee on Nutrition, 2003). The main risk factors addressed in these programs have included changing negative peer and parent modeling of eating and exercise, low parent monitoring, and availability of TV

Chou, C.-P., Montgomery, S. B., Pentz, M. A., Rohrbach, L. A., Johnson, C. A., Flay, B. R., & MacKinnon, D. (1998). Effects of a community-based prevention program on decreasing drug use in high-risk adolescents. *American Journal of Public Health, 88*(6), 944–948.

Cole, T. J., Bellizzi, M. C., Flegal, K. M., & Dietz, W. H. (2000). Establishing a standard definition for child overweight and obesity worldwide: International survey. *British Medical Journal, 320*(7244), 1240–1243. Retrieved September 14, 2008, from www.bmj.com/cgi/content/full/320/7244/1240.

Committee on Nutrition. (2003). Prevention of pediatric overweight and obesity. *Pediatrics, 112*(2), 424–430.

Connelly, J. B., Duaso, M. J., & Butler, G. (2007). A systematic review of controlled trials of interventions to prevent childhood obesity and overweight: A realistic synthesis of the evidence. *Public Health, 121*(7), 510–517.

Conway, B., & Rene, A. (2004). Obesity as a disease: No lightweight matter. *Obesity Review, 5*(3), 145–151.

Crawford, A., Pentz, M. A., Chou, C. P., Li, C., & Dwyer, J. (2003). Parallel developmental trajectories of sensation seeking and regular substance use in adolescents. *Psychology of Addictive Behaviors, 17*(3), 179–192.

Crimmins, N. A., Dolan, L. M., Martin, L. J., Bean, J. A., Daniels, S. R., Lawson, M. L., Goodman, E., & Woo, J. G. (2007). Stability of adolescent body mass index during three years of follow-up. *Journal of Pediatrics, 151*(4), 383–387.

Davis, D., Levitan, R. D., Muglia, P., Bewell, C., & Kennedy, J. L. (2004). Decision-making deficits and overeating: A risk model for obesity. *Obesity Research 12,* 929–935.

Davison, K. K., & Birch, L. L. (2001). Childhood overweight: A contextual model and recommendations for future research. *Obesity Review 2*(3), 159–171.

Dietz, W. H., & Gortmaker, S. L. (2001). Preventing obesity in children and adolescents. *Annual Review of Public Health, 22,* 337–353.

DiMarzo, V., & Matia, I. (2005). Endocannabinoid control of food intake and energy balance. *Nature Neuroscience, 8*(5), 585–589.

Donovan, J. E., Jessor, R., & Costa, F. M. (1988). Syndrome of problem behavior in adolescence: A replication. *Journal of Consulting and Clinical Psychology, 56*(5), 762–765.

Donovan, J. E., Jessor, R., & Costa, F. M. (1993). Structure of health-enhancing behavior in adolescence: A latent-variable approach. *Journal of Health and Social Behavior, 34*(4), 346–362.

Driskell, M. M., Dyment, S., Mauriello, L., Castle, P., & Sherman, K. (2008). Relationships among multiple behaviors for childhood and adolescent obesity prevention. *Preventive Medicine, 46*(3), 209–215.

Duncan, S. C., Duncan, T. E., & Strycker, L. A. (2005). Sources and types of social support in youth physical activity. *Health Psychology, 24*(1), 3–10.

Elizabeth, D. W., & Baur, L. A. (2007). Adolescent obesity: Making a difference to the epidemic. *International Journal of Adolescent Medicine and Health, 19*(3), 235–243.

Fisher, P. A., Gunnar, M. R., Dozier, M., Bruce, J., & Pears, K. C. (2006). Effects of therapeutic interventions for foster children on behavioral problems, caregiver attachment, and stress regulatory neural systems. *Annals of the New York Academy of Sciences, 1094,* 226–234.

Fleming-Moran, M., & Thiagarajah, K. (2005). Behavioral interventions and the role of television in the growing epidemic of adolescent obesity: Data from the 2001 Youth Risk Behavioral Survey. *Methods of Information in Medicine, 44*(2), 303–309.

Franks, A., Kelder, S. H., Dino, G. A., Horn, K. A., Gortmaker, S. L., Wiecha, J. L., & Simoes, E. J. (2007). School-based programs: Lessons learned from CATCH, Planet Health, and Not-on-Tobacco. *Preventing Chronic Disease, 4*(2), A33.

French, S., & Story, M. (2006). Obesity prevention in schools. In M. Goran & M. Sothern (Eds.), *Handbook of pediatric obesity* (pp. 291–310). Boca Raton, FL: Taylor & Francis.

Golub., M. S., Collman, G. W., Foster, P. M., Kimmel, C. A., Rajpert-De Meyts, E., Reiter, E. O., Sharpe, R. M., Skakkeback, N. E., & Toppari, J. (2008). Public health implications of altered puberty timing. *Pediatrics, 121*(Suppl. 3), S218–S230.

Gordon-Larsen, P., McMurray, R., & Popkin, B. M. (2000). Determinants of adolescent physical activity and inactivity patterns. *Pediatrics, 105*(6), 1–8.

Gordon-Larsen, P., & Reynolds, K. (2006). Influence of the built environment on physical activity and obesity in children and adolescents. In M. Goran & M. Sothern (Eds.), *Handbook of pediatric obesity* (pp. 251–270). Boca Raton, FL: Taylor & Francis.

Greenberg, M. T. (2006). Promoting resilience in children and youth: Preventive interventions and their interface with neuroscience. *Annals of the New York Academy of Sciences, 1094,* 138–150.

Grosbras, M.-H., Jansen, M., Leonard, G., McIntosh, A., Osswald, K., Poulsen, C., Steinberg, L., Toro, R., & Paus, T. (2007). Neural mechanisms of resistance to peer influence in early adolescence. *Journal of Neuroscience, 27*(30), 8040–8045.

Gyurcsik, N. C., Spink, K. S., Bray, S. R., Chad, K., & Kwan, M. (2006). An ecologically based examination of barriers to physical activity in students from grade seven through first-year university. *Journal of Adolescent Health, 38,* 704–711.

Hawkins, J. D., Catalano, R. F., & Miller, J. Y. (1992). Risk and protective factors for alcohol and other drug problems in adolescence and early adulthood: Implications for substance abuse prevention. *Psychological Bulletin, 112*(1), 64–105.

Hill, J., Melanson, E., & Wyatt, H. (2000). Dietary fat intake and regulation of energy balance: Implications for obesity. *Journal of Nutrition, 130*(Suppl. 2), 284S–288S.

Huang, T. T., & Horlick, M. N. (2007). Trends in childhood obesity research: A brief analysis of NIH-supported efforts. *Journal of Law, Medicine, and Ethics, 35*(1), 148–153.

Institute of Medicine. (2004). Overview of the IOM's Childhood Obesity Prevention Study. Retrieved April 14, 2008, from www.iom.edu/report.asp?id=22596.

Irwin Jr., C. E., Eyre, S., & Millstein, S. (1997). Risk-taking behavior in adolescents: The paradigm. *Annals of the New York Academy of Sciences, 817,* 1–35.

Izard, C. E. (2002). Translating emotion theory and research into preventive interventions. *Psychological Bulletin, 128*(5), 796–824.

Jasuja, G. K., Chou, C. P., Riggs, N. R., & Pentz, M. A. (2008). Early cigarette use and psychological distress as predictors of obesity risk in adulthood. *Nicotine and Tobacco Research, 10*(2), 325–335.

Kipke, M. D., Iverson, E., Moore, D., Booker, C., Ruelas, V., Peters, A. L., & Kaufman, F. (2007). Food and park environments: Neighborhood-level risks for childhood obesity in East Los Angeles. *Journal of Adolescent Health, 40*(4), 325–333.

Kubik, M. Y., Lytle, L. A., & Story, M. (2005). Schoolwide food practices are associated with body mass index in middle school students. *Archives of Pediatrics and Adolescent Medicine, 159*(12), 1111–1114.

Li, D., Goran, M. I., Kaur H., Nollen, N., & Ahluwalia, J. S. (2007). Developmental trajectories of overweight during childhood: Role of early life factors. *Obesity, 15*(3), 760–771.

Lowry, R., Wechsler, H., Galuska, D. A., Fulton, J. E., & Kann, L. (2002). Television viewing and its associations with overweight, sedentary lifestyle, and insufficient consumption of fruits and vegetables among U.S. high school students: Differences by race, ethnicity, and gender. *Journal of School Health, 72*(10), 413–421.

Mei, Z., Gummer-Strawn, L. M., Thompson, D., & Dietz, W. H. (2004). Shifts in percentiles of growth during early childhood: Analysis of longitudinal data from the California Child Health and Development Study. *Pediatrics, 113,* 617–627.

Mokdad, A. H., Ford, E. S., Bowman, B. A., Dietz, W. H., Vinicor, F., Bales, V. S., & Marks, J. S. (2003). Prevalence of obesity, diabetes, and obesity-related health risk factors. *Journal of the American Medical Association, 289,* 76–79.

Molnar, B. E., Gortmaker, S. L., Bull, F. C., & Buka, S. L. (2004). Unsafe to play? Neighborhood disorder and lack of safety predict reduced physical activity among urban children and adolescents. *American Journal of Health Promotion, 18*(5), 378–386.

Nelson, M. C., Gordon-Larsen, P., Adair, L. S., & Popkin, B. M. (2005). Adolescent physical activity and sedentary behavior: Patterning and long-term maintenance. *American Journal of Preventive Medicine, 28*(3), 259–266.

Nguyen-Michel, S. T., Unger, J. B., & Spruijt-Metz, D. (2007). Dietary correlates of emotional eating in adolescence. *Appetite, 49*(2), 494–499.

Nigg, J. T., Quamma, J. P., Greenberg, M. T., & Kusche, C. A. (1999). A two-year longitudinal study of neuropsychological and cognitive performance in relation to behavioral problems and competencies in elementary school children. *Journal of Abnormal Child Psychology, 27,* 51–63.

Pentz, M. A. (1999). Prevention aimed at individuals: An integrative transactional perspective. In B. S. McCrady & E. E. Epstein (Eds.), *Addictions: A comprehensive guidebook for practitioners* (pp. 555–572). New York: Oxford University Press.

Pentz, M. A. (2003). Evidence-based prevention: Characteristics, impact, and future direction. *Journal of Psychoactive Drugs, 35,* 143–152.

Pentz, M. A. (2004). Applying theory and methods of community-based drug abuse prevention to pediatric obesity prevention. Bethesda, MD: U.S. Department of Health and Human Services. Retrieved March 23, 2005, from www.niddk.nih.gov/fund/other/management_pediatric_obesity/SUMMARY_REPORT.pdf.

Pentz, M. A., Dwyer, J. H., MacKinnon, D. P., Flay, B. R., Hansen, W. B., Wang, E.Y.I., & Johnson, C. A. (1989). A multicommunity trial for primary prevention of adolescent drug abuse: Effects on drug use prevalence. *Journal of the American Medical Association, 261*(22), 3259–3266.

Pentz, M. A., Jasuja, G. K., Rohrbach, L. A., Sussman, S., & Bardo, M. (2006). Translation in tobacco and drug abuse prevention/cessation research. *Evaluation and the Health Professions, 29*(2), 246–271.

Pentz, M. A., Johnson, C. A., Dwyer, J. H., MacKinnon, D. P., Hansen, W. B., & Flay, B. R. (1989). A comprehensive community approach to adolescent drug abuse prevention: Effects on cardiovascular disease risk behaviors. *Annals of Medicine, 21*(3), 219–222.

Pentz, M. A., MacKinnon, D. P., & Pentz, C. (1988). Adolescent stress, drug use, and blood pressure. *American Journal of Epidemiology, 128,* 891–892.

Pentz, M. A., Mihalic, S.F., & Grotpeter, J. K. (1997). The Midwestern Prevention Project. In D. S. Elliot (Ed.), *Blueprints for violence prevention.* Boulder, CO: Center for the Study and Prevention of Violence, University of Colorado.

Peterson, K. E., & Fox, M. K. (2007). Addressing the epidemic of childhood obesity through school-based interventions: What has been done and where do we go from here? *Journal of Law, Medicine, & Ethics, 35*(1), 113–130.

Reynolds, K. D., & Spruijt-Metz, D. (2006). Translational research in childhood obesity prevention. *Evaluation and the Health Professions, 49*(2), 219–245.

Riggs, N. R., Elfenbaum, P., & Pentz, M. A. (2006). Parent program component analysis in a drug abuse prevention trial. *Journal of Adolescent Health, 39,* 66–72.

Riggs, N. R., Greenberg, M. T., Kusché, C. A., & Pentz, M. A. (2006). The mediational role of neurocognition in the behavioral outcomes of a social-emotional prevention program in elementary school students: Effects of the PATHS curriculum. *Prevention Science, 7,* 91–102.

Riggs, N. R., Kobayakawa-Sakuma, K. L., & Pentz, M. A. (2007). Preventing risk for obesity by promoting self-regulation and decision-making skills: Pilot results from the PATHWAYS to Health Program (PATHWAYS). *Evaluation Review, 31*(3), 287–310.

Saksvig, B. I., Catellier, D. J., Pfeiffer, K., Schmitz, K. H., Conway, T., Going, S., Ward, D., Strikmiller, P., & Treuth, M. S. (2007). Travel by walking before and after school and physical activity among adolescent girls. *Archives of Pediatrics and Adolescent Medicine, 161*(2), 153–158.

Salmon, J. B. M., Phongsavan, P., Murphy, N., & Timperio, A. (2007). Promoting physical activity participation among children and adolescents. *Epidemiologic Reviews 29,* 144–159.

Schottenfeld, D., & Beebe-Dimmer, J. L. (2005). Advances in cancer epidemiology: Understanding causal mechanisms and the evidence for implementing interventions. *Annual Review of Public Health, 26,* 37–60.

Sharma, M. (2007). International school-based interventions for preventing obesity in children. *Obesity Review, 8*(2), 155–167.

Shaw, H., Ramirez, L., Trost, A., Randall, P., & Stice, E. (2004). Body image and eating disturbances across ethnic groups: More similarities than differences. *Psychology of Addictive Behavior, 18*(1), 12–18.

Sothern, M. S. (2004). Obesity prevention in children: Physical activity and nutrition. *Nutrition, 20*(7–8), 704–708.

Spruijt-Metz, D., & Saelens, B. (2006). Behavioral aspects of physical activity in childhood and adolescence. In M. Goran & M. Sothern (Eds.), *Handbook of pediatric obesity: Etiology, pathophysiology, and prevention* (pp. 227–250). Boca Raton, FL: CRC Press.

Toschke, A. M., Ruckinger, S., Reinehr, T., & von Kries, R. (2007, August 22). Growth around puberty as predictor of adult obesity. *European Journal of Clinical Nutrition (e-pub).*

Tschumper, A., Nägele, C., & Alsaker, F. D. (2006). Gender, type of education, family background and overweight in adolescents. *International Journal of Pediatric Obesity, 1*(3), 153–160.

Unger, J. B., Reynolds, K., Shakib, S., Spruijt-Metz, D., Sun, P., & Johnson, C. A. (2004). Acculturation, physical activity, and fast-food consumption among Asian-American and Hispanic adolescents. *Journal of Community Health, 29*(6), 467–481.

Volkow, N. D., & Wise, R. A. (2005). How can drug addiction help us understand obesity? *Nature Neuroscience, 8*(5), 555–560.

Voorhees, C. C., Murray, D., Welk, G., Birnbaum, A., Ribisl, K. M., Johnson, C. C., Pfeiffer, K. A., Saksvig, B., & Jobe, J. B. (2005). The role of peer social network factors and physical activity in adolescent girls. *American Journal of Health Behavior, 29*(2), 183–190.

Wang, G.-J., Volkow, N. D., Thanos, P. K., & Fowler, J. S. (2004). Similarity between obesity and drug addiction as assessed by neurofunctional imaging: A concept review. *Journal of Addictive Diseases, 23*(3), 39–53.

Wardle, J., Brodersen, N. H., & Boniface, D. (2007). School-based physical activity and changes in adiposity. *International Journal of Obesity, 31*(9), 1464–1468.

Werch, C., Moore, M. J., DiClemente, C. C., Bledsoe, R., & Jobli, E. (2005). A multihealth behavior intervention integrating physical activity and substance abuse prevention for adolescents. *Prevention Science, 6*(3), 213–226.

Windle, M., Grunbaum, J. A., Elliott, M., Tortolero, S. R., Berry, S., Gilliland, J., Kanouse, D. E., Parcel, G. S., Wallander, J., Kelder, S., Collins, J., Kolbe, L., & Schuster, M. (2004). Healthy passages: A multilevel, multi-method longitudinal study of adolescent health. *American Journal of Preventive Medicine, 27*(2), 164–172.

CHAPTER

10

ADOLESCENT ALCOHOL USE

MICHAEL WINDLE ▪ REBECCA C. WINDLE

LEARNING OBJECTIVES

After studying this chapter, you will be able to

- Identify short-term and long-term adverse health outcomes for adolescents who consume alcohol.

- Interpret prevalence data for adolescent alcohol use across age, gender, and ethnicity.

- Examine strengths and limitations of existing health promotion and risk reduction programs for alcohol use.

Alcohol is the drug most commonly consumed by teenagers, exceeding both cigarettes and marijuana (Centers for Disease Control and Prevention [CDC], 2005; Johnston, O'Malley, Bachman, & Schulenberg, 2006). Referring to data collected in 2003, Miller, Naimi, Brewer, and Jones (2007) stated that 44.9 percent of ninth through twelfth graders reported *current alcohol consumption* (meaning they had consumed alcohol on at least one day in the past thirty days). Among those who reported current drinking, a majority (64.2 percent) also reported heavy episodic, or binge, drinking (five or more drinks of alcohol in a row) at least once during that same time period. Miller et al. further reported a dose-response relationship between current *binge drinking* and other proximal health risk behaviors, with more frequent binge drinking (versus drinking without binging) increasingly related to a higher prevalence of other health risk behaviors (such as drug use, suicidal behaviors, current sexual activity, and interpersonal violence).

Recently, the Committee on Developing a Strategy to Reduce and Prevent Underage Drinking from the National Research Council and Institute of Medicine stated: "The problem of underage drinking in the United States is endemic and, in the committee's judgment, is not likely to improve in the absence of significant new intervention" (National Academy of Sciences, 2004). The Acting Surgeon General of the United States, Kenneth Moritsugu, concluded that "too many Americans consider underage drinking a rite of passage to adulthood" (Health and Human Services Press Office, 2007).

"The problem of underage drinking in the United States is endemic and . . . is not likely to improve in the absence of significant new intervention."

Widespread teen alcohol use has adverse health, social, and economic consequences for youth and society. Miller, Levy, Spicer, and Taylor (2006) estimated the national economic costs attributable to underage drinking (alcohol consumption prior to the age of twenty-one). They calculated that in 2001 underage drinkers accounted for 16.2 percent of all U.S. alcohol sales. The economic costs of alcohol-attributable youth problems, such as drinking and driving, interpersonal violence, property crimes, and suicide, totaled $61.9 billion (in 2001 dollars). These costs included medical care costs, lost work and other monetary costs, and quality-of-life costs.

The three major causes of mortality among twelve- to twenty-year-olds in the United States are, in order, unintentional injuries (with motor vehicle traffic accidents accounting for the majority of deaths), homicides, and suicides (Subramanian, 2006). Teens' alcohol use, and especially heavy use, is strongly associated with each of these mortality causes (Miller et al., 2006; Windle, Miller-Tutzauer, & Domenico, 1992; Windle & Windle, 2005). For example, in 2003, motor vehicle traffic crashes were the leading cause of death among twelve- to twenty-year-olds (Subramanian, 2006). In that same year, a report by the National Highway

Preparation of this chapter was supported by National Institute on Alcoholism and Alcohol Abuse, grant number R01-AA07861, awarded to Michael Windle.

Traffic Safety Administration (Pickrell, 2006) indicated that, among drivers twenty years of age or younger who were involved in fatal traffic accidents, approximately 20 percent had consumed alcohol at the time of the crash. In addition, the median blood alcohol concentration (BAC) for this age group ranged from .12 to .14, well above the legal limit of intoxication (which is .08 or higher).

There may be both short- and long-term adverse health consequences for teens who consume alcohol. Short-term consequences include unintentional injury and death due to alcohol use (from motor vehicle crashes, drowning, or falls), alcohol-related violence such as assaults and homicides, suicide attempts and completions, and risky sexual behaviors. Longer-term consequences include sexually transmitted diseases (such as chlamydia) and HIV, which are contracted after the combination of alcohol use and unprotected intercourse, the development of alcohol disorders and other comorbid disorders (such as illicit substance disorders or major depressive disorder), and more recent research suggests that normal brain development occurring during adolescence may be compromised by teens' heavy alcohol use (Talpert & Schweinsburg, 2005). The impact of alcohol on brain development may have consequences for longer-term intellectual and cognitive functioning and for job performance and occupational attainment.

The impact of alcohol on brain development may have consequences for longer-term intellectual and cognitive functioning and for job performance and occupational attainment.

EPIDEMIOLOGY OF ALCOHOL USE AMONG TEENS

In the United States, alcohol consumption among adolescents is statistically normative. In 2005, three-quarters of seniors in high school reported having consumed alcohol during their lifetime. Nearly one-half (47 percent) consumed alcohol in the past thirty days, and three in ten reported being drunk in the past thirty days (Johnston et al., 2006). A number of large epidemiologic studies periodically assess adolescents' and young adults' alcohol (and other substance) use; the three that are cited in this chapter are the *Monitoring the Future Survey* (*MFS,* sponsored by the National Institute on Drug Abuse), the *National Survey of Drug Use and Health* (*NSDUH,* sponsored by the Substance Abuse and Mental Health Services Administration, SAMHSA), and the national *Youth Risk Behavior Surveillance Survey* (*YRBSS,* sponsored by the CDC). The MFS and the YRBSS provide data from nationally representative samples of teens attending public and private schools. The NSDUH is based on a representative household sample of the U.S. civilian and noninstitutionalized population twelve years of age and older.

Among epidemiologic studies measuring teens' alcohol consumption, different indexes have been used to measure alcohol use, problematic levels of alcohol consumption, alcohol-related consequences, and clinical levels of alcohol use. Common indicators of alcohol use are lifetime use, past year use, past *thirty-day use* (having used alcohol on at least one day in the past thirty days), and age of initiation. Indicators of more severe or problematic use include binge drinking at least one time in the past two weeks or the past thirty days, having been drunk in the past thirty days, and the daily use of alcohol, which is typically defined for adolescents as having consumed alcohol on twenty or more of the last thirty days. Another index to evaluate the impact of alcohol use on health-compromising outcomes is found in adverse physical consequences (such as hangovers and medical illnesses) and social consequences (missing classes or work and alcohol-related aggression) associated with alcohol use—also referred to as alcohol-related problems. Finally, indicators of clinical diagnostic levels of alcohol abuse and dependence provide insight into the tertiary healthcare needs of youth by the healthcare system.

In Table 10.1, we present prevalence data from the 2005 MFS. The data are disaggregated by grade, gender, ethnicity, and index of alcohol use. Several patterns of alcohol use are indicated by the data in this table. First, for all three alcohol indicators, use substantially increases as teens move from early to middle and late adolescence. Second, while younger males and females are similar in their use of alcohol, older male adolescents are more likely to currently drink alcohol and to use alcohol in heavier amounts relative to same-age female adolescents. Third, black adolescents across school grades reported lower levels of current and heavy alcohol use relative to white and Hispanic teens. At younger ages, Hispanic teens were slightly more likely to use alcohol than white teens, but white adolescents were more likely to consume alcohol by their senior year relative to Hispanic adolescents. In summary, although absolute prevalence rates may differ, data from the MFS, YRBSS, and NSDUH support the previously mentioned patterns of alcohol use in terms of age, gender, and race/ethnic group differences (CDC, 2005; Johnston et al., 2006; SAMHSA, 2006a).

Alcohol-related problems may adversely affect not only the alcohol user but also others in the user's environment (Wechsler, Dowdall, Maenner, Gledhill-Hoyt, & Lee, 1998). For example, drinking and driving has the potential to adversely affect the health and well-being of the driver who is drinking, any passengers in the vehicle, and others who are walking, riding a bike, or driving a car. The prevalence of alcohol-related problems is high among adolescents. Table 10.2 presents prevalence data on alcohol-related problems from a community-based longitudinal study currently being conducted by the authors of this chapter.

The study, currently in its twentieth year of funding and referred to as Lives Across Time: A Longitudinal Study of Adolescent and Adult Development has been funded by the National Institute on Alcohol Abuse and Alcoholism since its inception. The sample consists of predominantly white, middle-class participants. At each of four waves of data collection, participants were asked to report whether they had experienced fifteen different alcohol-related problems during the previous six months. Problems included getting into fights or heated arguments when drinking, having a drinking-and-driving accident, passing out from drinking, and missing work or school because of drinking. The data indicated that at each time of measurement (except at Time 4 for all participants and for female participants) more than half of adolescents

TABLE 10.1. Prevalence of alcohol consumption indicators by race/ethnicity, gender, and school grade, 2005 (in percent)

School Grade	Prevalence of Past-30-Day Alcohol Use			Prevalence of Having Been Drunk in Past 30 Days			Five or More Drinks in a Row in Past Two Weeks		
	8th	10th	12th	8th	10th	12th	8th	10th	12th
Race/ethnicity									
White	17.9	37.0	52.3	6.6	21.0	36.5	10.8	23.5	33.0
Black	14.9	23.0	29.0	3.8	8.0	15.4	8.2	11.0	11.6
Hispanic	20.6	38.2	43.3	7.0	17.3	22.2	14.8	26.0	24.7
Gender									
Male	16.2	32.8	50.7	5.9	18.2	33.6	10.2	22.0	33.4
Female	17.9	33.6	43.3	6.2	16.8	26.4	10.6	19.9	22.7
Total	17.1	33.2	47.0	6.0	17.6	30.2	10.5	21.0	28.1

Source: Monitoring the Future Surveys (Johnston et al., 2006).

TABLE 10.2. Percentage of participants in Lives Across Time longitudinal study reporting alcohol-related problems

Number of Alcohol-Related Problems	Time 1 (X Age = 15.83; SD = 0.68)			Time 2[a] (X Age = 17.31; SD = 0.68)			Time 3 (X Age = 24.12; SD = 1.27)			Time 4 (X Age = 29.39; SD = 1.14)		
	All	M	F	All	M	F	All	M	F	All	M	F
0 problems	38.0	40.3	35.9	40.3	40.4	40.3	38.7	29.5	46.0	51.8	42.7	58.9
1 to 3 problems	32.6	31.7	33.4	33.5	28.4	38.2	38.1	38.2	38.2	34.7	38.1	32.3
4 to 6 problems	20.5	20.0	20.9	17.8	20.5	15.3	14.2	19.1	10.3	8.9	13.7	5.1
7 or more problems	8.9	8.0	9.8	8.4	10.7	6.3	8.9	13.3	6.6	4.5	5.5	3.7

Note: Ns for participants: Time 1 = 973; Time 2 = 1047; Time 3 = 795; Time 4 = 760. Ns include those participants who reported drinking alcohol in the past six months.

[a]At Times 2 through 4, there were significant gender differences at the $p \leq .001$ level, with a higher percentage of males reporting more alcohol-related problems. At Time 1, there were no significant gender differences for alcohol-related problems.

and young adults reported experiencing at least one alcohol-related problem. At Time 1, when participants were middle adolescents, almost 30 percent reported four or more problems in the past six months. At Time 3, 70 percent of young adult males reported at least one problem, and 32 percent reported four or more problems. Significant gender differences were not evident at Time 1, but significant differences were seen at Times 2 through 4, with a higher percentage of males reporting more alcohol-related problems.

The prevalence of alcohol use among teens begins to increase in early adolescence, steadily increases throughout the high school years, reaches a peak in the early twenties, and begins to decline thereafter.

Survey data indicate that the years with the highest prevalence of alcohol disorders are late adolescence and early young adulthood (SAMHSA, 2006b). For example, data from the NSDUH indicate that for both males and females and for whites, blacks, and Hispanics, the highest rate of alcohol disorders is in the years eighteen through twenty-five. Other national surveys have likewise found that eighteen- to twenty-four-year-olds reported the highest rates of alcohol dependence, after which rates began to gradually decline (Grant, 1997). This decrease, or "maturing out," of alcohol disorders after the midtwenties has been attributed in part to young adults' movement toward assuming greater levels of responsibility and conventionality and adopting adult roles that are incongruent with pathological levels of alcohol use, such as completing one's education, entering the full-time work force, getting married, and having children (Labouvie, 1996; Miller-Tutzauer, Leonard, & Windle, 1991; Sher & Gotham, 1999).

In summary, the epidemiologic data indicate that the prevalence of alcohol use among teens begins to increase in early adolescence, steadily increases throughout the high school years, reaches a peak in the early twenties, and begins to decline thereafter. Higher levels of alcohol use are associated with a broad range of morbidities and with the three highest mortality indicators among teens—fatal crashes, homicide, and suicide. Heavy alcohol use among teens not only has adverse effects for teens, but may also adversely affect others via injuries and violence associated with alcohol use by teens (such as victims of adolescent alcohol-related crashes or enhanced aggressive tendencies).

PROMOTING HEALTH AND PREVENTING RISK OF ALCOHOL USE AMONG YOUTH

A broad range of alcohol prevention programs currently target different units or levels of analysis—from school to family to individual levels. For example, *extant programs* include family-focused interventions (see Kumpfer, Alvarado, & Whiteside, 2003, for a review), interventions with high-risk youth, social policy interventions (such as alcohol taxes, minimum legal drinking age, and zero-tolerance laws), and treatment programs for youth with alcohol disorders (see Windle, 1999, for a review). Owing to space constraints, we have focused on some prominent universal prevention programs, because the majority of alcohol and drug prevention programs with youth in the United States involve universal interventions.

Universal programs include all persons in a particular population (all students in a school, for example) without regard to level of risk. These programs generally include classroom curricula that are administered to students within school settings; they may also include schoolwide climate change programs, parent programs, mass media programs, and communitywide interventions (Stigler, Perry, Komro, Cudeck, & Williams, 2006). The majority of universal interventions are based on a *social-influence model,* which suggests that the primary influences affecting youths' substance use behaviors are social factors such as peer, family, and media influences (Bauman & Ennett, 1996; Norman & Turner, 1993). These programs are thus aimed both at helping adolescents acquire skills that will enable them to effectively resist social pressures—especially peer pressures—to use substances and at promoting prosocial attitudes and norms against substance use. Most alcohol and drug prevention curricula for youth are administered during the late elementary and junior high grades, because this is the age period when alcohol and other substance use is often initiated.

Tobler and colleagues (2000) conducted a meta-analysis of 207 universal, school-based drug prevention programs based on effect sizes reported in published studies. Key findings from this meta-analysis were that *interactive prevention programs* (such as programs that encouraged social interactions with peers and focused on interpersonal skills, refusal skills, and changes in normative beliefs) had substantially larger effect sizes than *noninteractive prevention programs* (such as didactic programs in which teachers provide information to students about the adverse effects of drug use). Furthermore, effective programs (1) were more likely to have a smaller number of participants (programs with three hundred participants were more effective than those with a thousand participants), (2) were of higher intensity (offered more delivery hours), and (3) were more comprehensive with regard to changes at multiple levels (such as individual, parent, school, and community levels).

Among some of the most highly visible universal adolescent alcohol and substance use prevention programs are Project ALERT (Ellickson, McCaffrey, Ghosh-Dastidar, & Longshore, 2003; Ghosh-Dastidar, Longshore, Ellickson, & McCaffrey, 2004), Life Skills Training (Botvin, Griffin, Diaz, & Ifill-Williams, 2001; Griffin, Botvin, Nichols, & Doyle, 2003), the Alcohol Misuse Prevention Study (Dielman, Shope, Leech, & Butchart, 1989; Shope, Dielman, Butchart, Campanelli, & Kloska, 1992; Wynn, Schulenberg, Maggs, & Zucker, 2000), the communitywide Midwestern Prevention Project (Pentz et al., 1989; Johnson et al., 1990; Chou et al., 1998), and the communitywide Project Northland (Perry et al., 2000; Perry et al., 2002; Stigler et al., 2006). The family-focused Iowa Strengthening Families Program (Spoth, Redmond, & Shin, 2001; Spoth, Shin, Guyll, Redmond, & Azevedo, 2006) is not a "traditional" universal, school-based program but it is included in this list because it is methodologically rigorous and evaluations of the program have been extensively published in the research literature.

Although outcome variables for these programs have differed—from preventing or delaying drinking onset to reductions in current alcohol use, slowing the rate of increase in alcohol use, reductions in binge drinking, reductions in expectations for future alcohol use, perceptions of peer alcohol use, and refusal skills to withstand peer pressures to drink—each program has reported successes in short- and medium-term posttest evaluations, and some in longer-term evaluations (for example, Spoth et al., 2001). In addition, findings from recent evaluations of these programs are noteworthy. For example, results from several studies have strongly supported the importance of having programs continue into the high school years, rather than truncating them at the end of junior high school, as is done with many programs (for example, Project ALERT, Ellickson et al., 2003; Project Northland, Perry et al., 2002). There is also some evidence of the generalizability of the interventions to nonwhite racial and ethnic groups. For instance, Botvin et al. (2001) originally developed the Life Skills Training (LST) program with predominantly white, middle-class students. In recent studies, a modified version of LST was administered to higher-risk, minority youth. Reductions in binge drinking and positive changes in psychosocial variables at both one- and two-year follow-ups were indicated. These findings suggest that the LST program was effective with both white and minority populations.

In addition, other studies have disaggregated participants based on risk status (such as lower versus higher risk) and conducted evaluations to test the program effectiveness across groups (for example, the Alcohol Misuse Prevention Study, Dielman et al., 1989, and Shope et al., 1992; Project ALERT, Ellickson et al., 2003; Iowa Strengthening Families Program, Spoth et al., 2006). For example, Ellickson et al. reported that the Project ALERT intervention was most effective at reducing alcohol misuse among higher-risk adolescents and less effective at preventing the onset of use and current use among nonusers and experimenters (lower-risk groups). Dielman et al. (1989) and Shope et al. (1992) reported that the Alcohol Misuse Prevention Study intervention was most effective in reducing the rate of increase in alcohol use and misuse behaviors among sixth graders who were exhibiting high-risk behavior (early onset of unsupervised drinking) that potentially put them at risk for later alcohol problems.

Investigators have begun to study *mediators* (specific program components) that are most influential in affecting study outcomes (for example, MacKinnon et al., 1991; Orlando, Ellickson, McCaffrey, & Longshore, 2005; Scheier, Botvin, & Griffin, 2001; Stigler et al., 2006; Wynn et al., 2000). For example, using data from the LST program, Scheier et al. (2001) reported that the LST program significantly increased assertiveness skills (such as drug refusal skills), which in turn prospectively predicted lower alcohol and cigarette use in ninth grade. Thus, the LST program contributed to reductions in later drug use through its impact on an important mediator of adolescents' alcohol use—assertiveness skills.

This brief review of program effects and mediators suggests at least modest success for a number of existing programs. Tobler et al.'s (2000) meta-analysis provided important insights into some of the general characteristics of programs that predict positive changes in outcome variables. Large-scale evaluations of youth participating in prevention programs have indicated the success of these programs in positively affecting substance use behaviors, such as delaying the onset of substance use or decreasing use among those who are current users (for example, Brounstein, Gardner, & Backer, 2006; Springer, Sale, & Sambrano, 2002).

Yet concerns have been raised about the methodological limitations of interventions. For example, Foxcroft, Ireland, Lowe, and Breen (2002) reviewed fifty-six evaluation studies and identified several limitations. Two methodological concerns were (1) in most studies, the unit of allocation was the classroom, school, or community, whereas the unit of analysis was individuals, and (2) high levels of attrition, especially in longer-term follow-up studies, may threaten the validity of the results. In terms of process analyses, Foxcroft et al. cited concern that a number of studies did not control for either implementation fidelity or the number of sessions attended by participants. Although some studies randomly assigned school or study participants to intervention and control or comparison groups, others did not use randomization. Finally, effect sizes for evaluation studies tended to be small, and thus their clinical relevance for reducing substance use was unclear. A number of researchers have recognized these limitations and are addressing them in their evaluation studies, but substantial work remains to improve program effectiveness and to prepare programs for widespread dissemination in real-world contexts.

Substantial work remains to improve program effectiveness and to prepare programs for widespread dissemination in real-world contexts.

There is a need for innovative research designs and methodologies that can redesign prevention programs to become more practitioner-friendly.

Despite the methodological concerns, a number of researchers and policy makers have concluded that the initial step of evaluating and validating the effectiveness of empirically developed teen alcohol and substance use prevention programs has supported their satisfactory effectiveness. It has been suggested that the time is now for widespread dissemination of these programs into schools, clinics, and communities. Consistent with this perspective are Web sites that provide listings of interventions for those interested in identifying empirically based programs appropriate for their needs (for implementation in schools, clinics, or community settings, for example). These Web sites include www.strengtheningfamilies.org, http://nrepp.samhsa.gov, and www.cdc.gov/HealthyYouth/AdolescentHealth/registries.htm.

A recent issue of the journal *Prevention Science* (vol. 5, no. 1, March 2004) was devoted to the discussion of current barriers and challenges to the widespread dissemination of prevention programs into real-world contexts. The articles in this volume addressed future research directions that would facilitate the successful resolution of these barriers. For example, there is a need for innovative research designs and methodologies that can simplify and redesign prevention programs to become more practitioner-friendly (Biglan, 2004; Dusenbury & Hansen, 2004; Kaftarian, Robertson, Compton, Davis, & Volkow, 2004; Pentz, 2004). This endeavor will most certainly require close collaboration between researchers and practitioners (Botvin, 2004). In addition, Spoth, Greenberg, Bierman, and Redmond (2004) discussed the need for *capacity building* among practitioners, so that infrastructures are strengthened and resources provided to support practitioners in their endeavors to effectively implement programs. Finally, the challenges facing practitioners in relation to implementation fidelity versus cultural adaptations were discussed (Castro, Barrera, & Martinez, 2004; Dusenbury & Hansen, 2004; Ringwalt, Vincus, Ennett, Johnson, & Rohrbach, 2004). In sum, while recognizing that there are myriad daunting challenges associated with widespread implementation and dissemination, and that much more research is required to investigate which processes will support successful dissemination and sustainability of these programs on a large scale, there is a growing movement that supports such dissemination.

SUMMARY

Alcohol use among adolescents remains a prominent public health issue. Alcohol use is statistically normative for adolescents and is associated with a broad range of morbidities and mortalities. The three most frequent causes of mortality among adolescents are unintentional injuries (in fatal automobile crashes, for example), homicide, and suicide. The data indicate that although alcohol is not necessarily the direct or the sole cause of these outcomes, high levels of alcohol use are common in the occurrence of these mortalities. Teen alcohol use is also associated with a broad range of health risk behaviors and morbidities, including increased sexually risky behavior (and associated sexually transmitted diseases), co-occurring mental health disorders, and poorer school performance. Progress has been made in the design of interventions to reduce alcohol use and promote better health. However, a number of issues remain with regard to the generalizability of intervention findings to nonwhite populations, the impact of selective dropout on the robustness of intervention findings, and a plethora of demands related to the dissemination of these interventions in real-world contexts. The scientific study of these dissemination processes provides a major challenge to the scientific and practitioner communities, as both strive to encourage better choices by adolescents in reducing their alcohol use and fostering better health.

KEY TERMS

Binge drinking

Capacity building

Current alcohol consumption

Extant programs

Interactive prevention programs

Mediators

Monitoring the Future Survey (MFS)

National Survey of Drug Use and Health (NSDUH)

Noninteractive prevention programs

Social-influence model

Thirty-day use

Universal programs

Youth Risk Behavior Surveillance Survey (YRBSS)

DISCUSSION QUESTIONS

1. Discuss the relationship between teen alcohol use and the leading causes of death among twelve- to twenty-year-olds. Would the causes of mortality be different if alcohol consumption were less prevalent in this age group?

2. Why does the prevalence of alcohol use seem to peak among individuals in their early twenties and not sooner? What are some reasons for this trend?

3. What are the characteristics of an effective alcohol prevention program? Which program types are more efficacious in affecting study outcomes? Interactive or noninteractive? Targeted or universal? Why?

REFERENCES

Bauman, K. E., & Ennett, S. T. (1996). On the importance of peer influence for adolescent drug use: Commonly neglected considerations. *Addiction, 91,* 185–198.

Biglan, A. (2004). Contextualism and the development of effective prevention practices. *Prevention Science, 5,* 15–21.

Botvin, G. J. (2004). Advancing prevention science and practice: Challenges, critical issues, and future directions. *Prevention Science, 5,* 69–72.

Botvin, G. J., Griffin, K. W., Diaz, T., & Ifill-Williams, M. (2001). Preventing binge drinking during early adolescence: One- and two-year follow-up of a school-based preventive intervention. *Psychology of Addictive Behaviors, 15,* 360–365.

Brounstein, P. J., Gardner, S. E., & Backer, T. E. (2006). Research to practice: Efforts to bring effective prevention to every community. *Journal of Primary Prevention, 27,* 91–109.

Castro, F. G., Barrera, M., Jr., & Martinez, C. R., Jr. (2004). The cultural adaptation of prevention interventions: Resolving tensions between fidelity and fit. *Prevention Science, 5,* 41–45.

Centers for Disease Control and Prevention. (2005). YRBSS: Youth Risk Behavior Surveillance System. Retrieved August 30, 2007, from www.cdc.gov/HealthyYouth/yrbs.

Chou, C.-P., Montgomery, S., Pentz, M. A., Rohrbach, L. A., Johnson, C. A., Flay, B. R., & Mac Kinnon, D. P. (1998). Effects of a community-based prevention program on decreasing drug use in high-risk adolescents. *American Journal of Public Health, 88,* 944–948.

Dielman, T. E., Shope, J. T., Leech, S. L., & Butchart, A. T. (1989). Differential effectiveness of an elementary school–based alcohol misuse prevention program. *Journal of School Health, 59,* 255–263.

Dusenbury, L., & Hansen, W. B. (2004). Pursuing the course from research to practice. *Prevention Science, 5,* 55–59.

Ellickson, P. L., McCaffrey, D. F., Ghosh-Dastidar, B., & Longshore, D. L. (2003). New inroads in preventing adolescent drug use: Results from a large-scale trial of Project ALERT in middle schools. *American Journal of Public Health, 93,* 1830–1836.

Foxcroft, D. R., Ireland, D., Lowe, G., & Breen, R. (2002). Primary prevention for alcohol misuse in young people. *Cochrane Database of Systematic Reviews, 3,* 1–71.

Ghosh-Dastidar, B., Longshore, D. L., Ellickson, P. L., & McCaffrey, D. F. (2004). Modifying pro-drug risk factors in adolescents: Results from Project ALERT. *Health Education and Behavior, 31,* 318–334.

Grant, B. (1997). Prevalence and correlates of alcohol use and DSM-IV alcohol dependence in the United States: Results of the National Longitudinal Alcohol Epidemiologic Survey. *Journal of Studies on Alcohol, 58,* 464–473.

Griffin, K. W., Botvin, G. J., Nichols, T. R., & Doyle, M. M. (2003). Effectiveness of a universal drug abuse prevention approach for youth at high risk for substance use initiation. *Preventive Medicine, 36,* 1–7.

Health and Human Services Press Office. (2007, March 6). Acting surgeon general issues national call to action on underage drinking. Retrieved March 22, 2007, from www.hhs.gov/news/press/2007pres/20070306.html.

Johnson, C. A., Pentz, M. A., Weber, M. D., Dwyer, J. H., Baer, N., MacKinnon, D. P., Hansen, W. B., & Flay, B. R. (1990). Relative effectiveness of comprehensive community programming for drug abuse prevention with high-risk and low-risk adolescents. *Journal of Consulting and Clinical Psychology, 58,* 447–456.

Johnston, L. D., O'Malley, P. M., Bachman, J. G., & Schulenberg, J. E. (2006). *Monitoring the Future national survey results on drug use, 1975–2005: Vol. I. Secondary school students* (NIH Publication No. 06–5883). Bethesda, MD: National Institute on Drug Abuse.

Kaftarian, S., Robertson, E., Compton, W., Davis, B. W., & Volkow, N. (2004). Blending prevention research and practice in schools: Critical issues and suggestions. *Prevention Science, 5,* 1–3.

Kumpfer, K. L., Alvarado, R., & Whiteside, H. O. (2003). Family-based interventions for substance use and misuse prevention. *Substance Use and Misuse, 38,* 1759–1787.

Labouvie, E. (1996). Maturing out of substance use. *Journal of Drug Issues, 26,* 457–476.

MacKinnon, D. P., Johnson, C. A., Pentz, M. A., Dwyer, J. H., Hansen, W. B., Flay, B. R., & Wang, E. Y. (1991). Mediating mechanisms in a school-based drug prevention program: First-year effects of the Midwestern Prevention Project. *Health Psychology, 10,* 164–172.

Miller, J. W., Naimi, T. S., Brewer, R. D., & Jones, S. E., (2007). Binge drinking and associated health risk behaviors among high school students. *Pediatrics, 199,* 76–85.

Miller, T. R., Levy, D. T., Spicer, R. S., & Taylor, D. M. (2006). Societal costs of underage drinking. *Journal of Studies on Alcohol, 67,* 519–528.

Miller-Tutzauer, C., Leonard, K. E., & Windle, M. (1991). Marriage and alcohol use: A longitudinal study of "maturing out." *Journal of Studies on Alcohol, 52,* 434–440.

National Academy of Sciences. (2004). Report brief: Reducing underage drinking: A collective responsibility. Retrieved September 5, 2007, from www.iom.edu/CMS/12552/13838/15100.aspx.

Norman, E., & Turner, S. (1993). Adolescent substance abuse prevention programs: Theories, models, and research in the encouraging 80s. *Journal of Primary Prevention, 14,* 3–20.

Orlando, M., Ellickson, P. L., McCaffrey, D. F., & Longshore, D. L. (2005). Mediation analysis of a school-based prevention program: Effects of Project ALERT. *Prevention Science, 6,* 35–46.

Pentz, M. A. (2004). Form follows function: Designs for prevention effectiveness and diffusion research. *Prevention Science, 5,* 23–29.

Pentz, M. A., Dwyer, J. H., MacKinnon, D. P., Flay, B. R., Hansen, W. B., Wang, E. Y., & Johnson, C. A. (1989). A multicommunity trial for primary prevention of adolescent abuse. *Journal of the American Medical Association, 261,* 3259–3266.

Perry, C. L., Williams, C. L., Komro, K. A., Veblen-Mortenson, S., Forster, J. L., Bernstein-Lachter, R., Pratt, L. K., Dudovitz, B., Munson, K. A., Farbakhsh, K., Finnegan, J., & McGovern, P. (2000). Project Northland high school interventions: Community action to reduce adolescent alcohol use. *Health Education and Behavior, 27,* 29–49.

Perry, C. L., Williams, C. L., Komro, K. A., Veblen-Mortenson, S., Stigler, M. H., Munson, K. A., Farbakhsh, K., Jones, R. M., & Forster, J. L. (2002). Project Northland: Long-term outcomes of community action to reduce adolescent alcohol use. *Health Education Research, 17,* 117–132.

Pickrell, T. M. (2006, July). Driver alcohol involvement in fatal crashes by age group and vehicle type. Retrieved August 30, 2007, from www-nrd.nhtsa.dot.gov/pdf/nrd-30/NCSA/RNotes/2006/810598.pdf.

Ringwalt, C. L., Vincus, A., Ennett, S., Johnson, R., & Rohrbach, L. A. (2004). Reasons for teachers' adaptation of substance use prevention curricula in schools with non-white student populations. *Prevention Science, 5,* 61–67.

Scheier, L. M., Botvin, G. J., & Griffin, K. W. (2001). Preventive intervention effects on developmental progression in drug use: Structural equation modeling analyses using longitudinal data. *Prevention Science, 2,* 91–112.

Sher, K. J., & Gotham, H. J. (1999). Pathological alcohol involvement: A developmental disorder of young adulthood. *Development and Psychopathology, 11,* 933–956.

Shope, J. T., Dielman, T. E., Butchart, A. T., Campanelli, P. C., & Kloska, D. D. (1992). An elementary school–based alcohol misuse prevention program: A follow-up evaluation. *Journal of Studies on Alcohol, 53,* 106–121.

Spoth, R., Greenberg, M., Bierman, K., & Redmond, C. (2004). PROSPER Community-University Partnership Model for Public Education Systems: Capacity-building for evidence-based, competence-building prevention. *Prevention Science, 5,* 31–39.

Spoth, R., Shin, C., Guyll, M., Redmond, C., & Azevedo, K. (2006). Universality of effects: An examination of the comparability of long-term family intervention effects on substance use across risk-related subgroups. *Prevention Science, 7,* 209–224.

Spoth, R. L., Redmond, C., & Shin, C. (2001). Randomized trial of brief family interventions for general populations: Adolescent substance use outcomes 4 years following baseline. *Journal of Consulting and Clinical Psychology, 69,* 627–642.

Springer, F., Sale, E., & Sambrano, S. (2002). *The national cross-site evaluation of high-risk youth programs. Monographs series #1—Preventing substance abuse: Major findings from the national cross-site evaluation of high-risk youth programs.* Rockville, MD: Center for Substance Abuse Prevention.

Stigler, M. H., Perry, C. L., Komro, K. A., Cudeck, R., & Williams, C. L. (2006). Teasing apart a multiple component approach to adolescent alcohol prevention: What worked in Project Northland? *Prevention Science, 7,* 269–280.

Subramanian, R. (2006, March). Motor vehicle traffic crashes as a leading cause of death in the United States, 2003. *Traffic Safety Facts Research Note.* Retrieved March 27, 2007, from www-nrd.nhtsa.dot.gov/Pubs/810568.pdf.

Substance Abuse and Mental Health Services Administration, Office of Applied Studies. (2006a). *Results from the 2005 National Survey on Drug Use and Health: National findings.* Retrieved March 27, 2007, from www.drugabusestatistics.samhsa.gov/nsduh/2k5nsduh/2k5Results.pdf.

Substance Abuse and Mental Health Services Administration, Office of Applied Studies. (2006b). *Results from the 2005 National Survey on Drug Use and Health: Detailed tables. Prevalence estimates, standard errors, P values, and sample sizes.* Retrieved March 27, 2007, from www.drugabusestatistics.samhsa.gov/NSDUH/2k5nsduh/tabs/2k5TabsCover.pdf.

Talpert, S. F., & Schweinsburg, A. D. (2005). The human adolescent brain and alcohol use disorders. In M. Galanter (Ed.), *Recent developments in alcoholism, Vol. 17. Alcohol problems in adolescents and young adults* (pp. 177–189). New York: Kluwer Academic/Plenum.

Tobler, N. S., Roona, M. R., Ochshorn, P., Marshall, D. G., Streke, A. V., & Stackpole, K. M. (2000). School-based adolescent drug prevention programs: 1998 Meta-analysis. *Journal of Primary Prevention, 20,* 275–336.

Wechsler, H., Dowdall, G. W., Maenner, G., Gledhill-Hoyt, J., & Lee, H. (1998). Changes in binge drinking and related problems among American college students between 1993 and 1997: Results of the Harvard School of Public Health College Alcohol Study. *Journal of American College Health, 47,* 57–68.

Windle, M. (1999). *Alcohol use among adolescents.* Thousand Oaks, CA: Sage.

Windle, M., Miller-Tutzauer, C., & Domenico, D. (1992). Alcohol use, suicidal behavior, and risky activities among adolescents. *Journal of Research on Adolescence, 2,* 317–330.

Windle, M., & Windle, R. C. (2005). Alcohol consumption and its consequences among adolescents and young adults. In M. Galanter (Ed.), *Recent developments in alcoholism* (Vol. 17, pp. 67–83). New York: Kluwer Academic/Plenum.

Wynn, S. R., Schulenberg, J., Maggs, J. L., & Zucker, R. A. (2000). Preventing alcohol misuse: The impact of refusal skills and norms. *Psychology of Addictive Behaviors, 14,* 36–47.

CHAPTER

SUBSTANCE USE AMONG ADOLESCENTS: RISK, PREVENTION, AND TREATMENT

CHISINA T. KAPUNGU ▪ CHARU THAKRAL ▪ STEFANIE M. LIMBERGER ▪ GERI R. DONENBERG

LEARNING OBJECTIVES

After studying this chapter, you will be able to

- Explore the epidemiology of illicit drug use among adolescents.
- Use the biopsychosocial model to understand risk and protective factors associated with adolescent substance use.
- Evaluate the efficacy of prevention and treatment programs tailored to the gender and culture of adolescent substance users.

Despite gradual declines since the 1990s, adolescent substance use remains a serious problem, and the consequences are devastating for individuals, families, communities, and society. Rates of use and abuse remain high even by historical standards; in 2007, 19 percent of eighth graders, 35.6 percent of tenth graders, and 46.8 percent of twelfth graders reported one or more instances of illicit drug use in their lifetime (Johnston, O'Malley, Bachman, & Schulenberg, 2008), and American high school students report drug involvement that is among the highest in the industrialized world. Surveys predict a resurgence of substances previously on the decline and new drug discoveries that will challenge recent gains.

Several theories exist to explain adolescent substance use. A biopsychosocial model emphasizes several levels of influence, including individual factors, family processes, culture, schools, communities, and society. In this chapter, we review the epidemiology of adolescent illicit drug use, and we present a biopsychosocial framework to understand key risk and protective factors implicated in its development and maintenance. Illicit substance use is defined to encompass both illegal substances (marijuana, hallucinogens, and tranquilizers) and legal substances (prescription medications and inhalants) used to get intoxicated. This chapter presents prevention and treatment programs with documented efficacy and effectiveness, highlighting those tailored for specific populations.

EPIDEMIOLOGY OF ADOLESCENTS' ILLICIT SUBSTANCE USE

National data on the epidemiology of adolescents' illicit *substance use* are derived from several sources, but findings vary depending on the study method. Three surveys are most widely trusted: the National Survey on Drug Use and Health (NSDUH), Monitoring the Future (MTF), and the Youth Risk Behavior Surveillance System (YRBSS). The MTF tracks adolescent substance use trends and related attitudes annually among eighth, tenth, and twelfth graders. The MTF typically reports higher rates of substance use than the NSDUH, likely due in part to underreporting in household settings. From 2002 to 2006, both surveys reported declines in lifetime, past-year, and past-month use of marijuana, ecstasy, and LSD, and no differences in the rates of past-month cocaine and inhalant use. From 2006 to 2007, the MTF reported decreases or leveling off for most substances among eighth, tenth, and twelfth graders, including marijuana, methamphetamine, inhalants, crack or cocaine, sedatives or barbiturates, anabolic steroids, and alcohol (Johnston, O'Malley, Bachman & Schulenberg, 2007a, 2007b). By contrast, prescription drug use rose among high school seniors. In the most recent NSDUH survey, 57.8 percent of respondents reported any illicit drug use before age eighteen.

In the most recent NSDUH survey, 57.8 percent of respondents reported any illicit drug use before age eighteen.

Annual Prevalence

The annual prevalence of drug use—the proportion of adolescents who used a substance in the past twelve months—differs across age groups and specific substances, but rates declined for all three grades overall (Johnston et al., 2008). The proportion of eighth graders who reported any illicit drug use at least once in the past twelve months declined from 24 percent in 1996 to 13 percent in 2007. The decline among tenth graders, from 39 percent in 1997 to 28 percent in 2007, was less than that of eighth graders but more than that of twelfth graders (from 42 percent in 1997 to 36 percent in 2007).

Marijuana continues to be the most widely used illicit drug among teens. Reduced use of marijuana, amphetamines, Ritalin, methamphetamine, and crystal methamphetamine explains the modest declines in overall illicit drug use reported in 2007 (Johnston et al., 2008). By contrast, the prevalence of use for several drugs changed little, including cocaine, crack cocaine, LSD, hallucinogens other than LSD, heroin, and most prescription-type psychoactive drugs used without medical supervision, such as sedatives, tranquilizers, and narcotics other than heroin (namely, OxyContin and Vicodin). Ecstasy (MDMA) is the only drug that appears to be increasing after a sharp decline in the early 2000s.

The abuse of prescription pain medications and other such drugs is among the most concerning new trends among young people. In 2007, 15.4 percent of twelfth graders reported using prescription drugs for nonmedical reasons (Johnston et al., 2008). The most commonly abused pain medications are opioids (morphine, codeine, OxyContin, Davon, Vicodin, Dilaudid, and Demerol), CNS depressants (barbiturates and benzodiazepines), and stimulants. Perceived availability of drugs decreased between 2002 and 2006, but when asked how easy it would be to obtain specific substances, adolescents indicated that it would be "fairly easy" or "very easy" to obtain marijuana (50.1 percent), cocaine (25.9 percent), heroin (14.4 percent), and LSD (14 percent) (Johnston et al., 2008). In 2006, 15.3 percent of adolescents reported being approached by someone selling drugs in the past month, down from the 16.7 percent in 2002 (Substance Abuse and Mental Health Services Administration, 2007).

Gender and Ethnicity

Figure 11.1 displays the rates of substance use for high school boys and girls. Figure 11.2 displays the rates of substance use among White, Black, and Hispanic high school students. Gender and ethnic differences in use vary across drugs and grades (Johnston et al., 2008). Boys' drug use peaked in 1978 (59 percent), and girls' substance use peaked in 1981 (51 percent). In 2006, rates of illicit drug use among males and females declined to 38 percent and 35 percent, respectively. In the NSDUH, rates of current illicit drug use among boys (6.8 percent) and girls (6.4 percent) were similar.

Of the three major ethnic groups, African Americans had the lowest rates of illicit drug use at all three grade levels. Hispanic students reported the highest rates of marijuana, crack, cocaine powder, heroin, and tranquilizer use in eighth grade, and although the gap narrowed over time, Hispanic twelfth graders still reported the highest rate of inhalants, crack, cocaine powder, heroin, heroin with a needle, heroin without a needle, methamphetamine, Rohypnol, and methamphetamine (ice). White twelfth graders reported the highest rate of *any* illicit drug use—and marijuana, LSD, other hallucinogens,

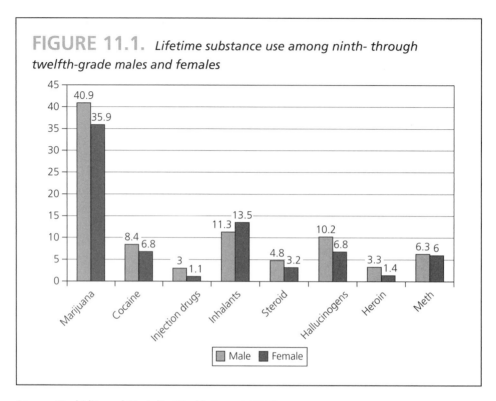

FIGURE 11.1. *Lifetime substance use among ninth- through twelfth-grade males and females*

Source: Morbidity and Mortality Weekly Report (2006).

ecstasy, narcotics other than heroin, OxyContin, Vicodin, amphetamines, Ritalin, sedatives (barbiturates), and tranquilizers.

RISK AND PROTECTIVE FACTORS FOR ADOLESCENT SUBSTANCE ABUSE

The most effective prevention and intervention programs for adolescents target the main risk and protective factors that influence substance use and abuse. *Risk factors* increase the probability of substance use, are additive, and interact over time (Weinberg, 2001). *Protective factors* decrease the likelihood of substance use and can mitigate the impact of risk factors (Burrow-Sanchez, 2006; Newcomb, 1995). Thus, two important goals of substance use prevention and intervention programs are to reduce or eliminate risk factors and increase protective factors.

Consistent with a biopsychosocial framework, research documents a number of risk and protective factors that operate at different stages of development and reflect different domains of influence, including individual mental health, cognition, genetics, sexual abuse, family (parenting style, communication, and parental attitudes), and

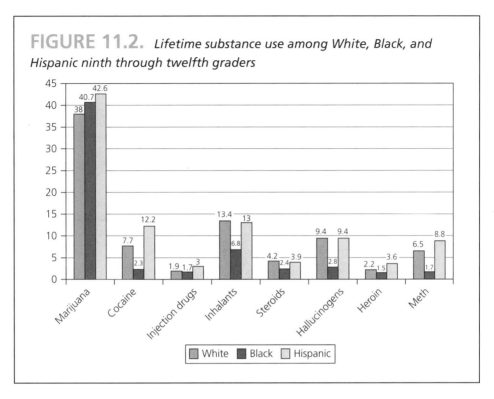

FIGURE 11.2. *Lifetime substance use among White, Black, and Hispanic ninth through twelfth graders*

Source: Morbidity and Mortality Weekly Report (2006).

social processes (at peer, school, community, and society levels; Engel, 1977; Fava & Sonino, 2008; Hawkins, Catalano, & Miller, 1992). The model is comprehensive and provides structure for substance use prevention and intervention program design.

Individual Factors

Individual-level factors related to substance use include mental health problems, genetics, delinquency, history of abuse, and drug-related attitudes and beliefs. Ample evidence supports links between adolescent substance use and psychiatric symptoms or disorders (see Kandel et al., 1997), but comorbid psychiatric disorders are more common for substance dependence than substance use (Roberts, Roberts, & Xing, 2007). The most common mental health problems associated with substance use are mood disorders (Swadi, 1999) and disruptive behavior disorders, namely attention deficit hyperactivity disorder and conduct disorder (Button et al., 2007; Fergusson, Horwood, & Ridder, 2007; Nation & Heflinger, 2006; Weinberg, 2001). Child-onset externalizing disorders predict greater risk for cannabis use disorder (Hayatbakhsh et al., 2008) and other substance use disorders (Fergusson et al., 2007) in early adulthood. Cognitive deficits associated with mental health problems impair decision making in high-risk situations, leading to greater vulnerability to drug use (Gerdes, Hoza, & Pelham, 2003; Hoza, Gerdes, & Hinshaw, 2004; Szobot & Bukstein, 2008). Depression also increases risk for using drugs (Armstrong & Costello, 2002; Costello, Erkanli, Federman, & Angold, 1999; Deykin, Levy, & Wells, 1987; Ingraham & Wender, 1992; Kandel et al., 1997; Rao, 2006; Swadi, 1999), and personality disorders predict later substance use disorders (Cohen, Chen, Crawford, Brook, & Gordon, 2007). Delinquent behavior is related to lifetime and recent illicit drug use; specifically, serious and nonserious adolescent delinquency predates illicit drug use (Doherty, Green, & Ensminger, 2008). Further, adolescents involved in the juvenile justice system report high rates of substance use (Horowitz, Sung, & Foster, 2006; Huizinga, Loeber, Thornberry, & Cothern, 2000).

Ample evidence supports links between adolescent substance use and psychiatric symptoms or disorders.

Childhood physical and sexual abuse are each associated with a greater likelihood of substance use among girls, but the evidence is less clear for boys (Harrison, Fulkerson, & Beebe, 1997; Kilpatrick, Acieno, Resnick, Saunders, & Best, 1997). Perez (2000) explored the relation between adolescent drug use and childhood physical abuse and sexual victimization. Both types of abuse, along with their co-occurrence, were significantly associated with more frequent drug use. In fact, the odds of illicit substance use increased from 50 percent to 80 percent among abused adolescents. Moreover, among drug users, abused teens were significantly younger in mean age of onset for marijuana, cocaine, and uppers.

Drug-related attitudes and beliefs associated with substance use behaviors include perceived risk and harm as a result of using drugs, disapproval of use, and outcome expectations or the costs and benefits of using drugs. Less drug use is related to perceptions of high risk, more negative and harmful consequences, and greater disapproval (Danesco, Kingery, & Coggeshall, 1999; Gonzalez & Haney, 1990; Musher-Eizenman, Holub, & Arnett, 2003). More positive and less negative outcome expectations are related to increased substance use (Musher-Eizenman et al., 2003). More important, changes in attitudes predict changes in behavior. For example, reduced perceptions of harm and disapproval of ecstasy use since 2000 have been linked to increased annual prevalence of use among tenth graders (3.5 percent) and twelfth graders (4.5 percent) in 2007 (Johnston et al., 2008).

Other individual-level factors protect against illicit substance use, including perceptions of social competence, autonomy, self-control, and self-efficacy (Benard, 1991; Kaplan, Martin, & Robbins, 1984; Sale, Sambrano, Springer, & Turner, 2003). Better academic performance is related to less substance use (Eggert & Randell, 2003; Ryan, Miller-Loessi & Nieri, 2007), and adolescents who participate in school-based extracurricular activities report greater academic commitment, higher performance, and lower rates of cigarette, marijuana, and other drug use (Cooper, Valentine, Nye, & Lindsay, 1999; Darling, 2005; Eccles and Barber, 1999). Effective communication to resist drug offers from peers may also protect against use (Ryan et al., 2007).

Family Factors

Family-level factors are consistently implicated in adolescent illicit substance use, namely parental substance use, parenting styles (warmth, monitoring, and supervision), family structure, parental attitudes and behavior (especially drug use), and parent-child communication. Parental substance use increases teens' risk for abuse and dependence (Corsi, Winch, Kwiatowski, & Booth, 2007; McDermott, 1984; Swadi, 1999; Vakalahi, 2001), primarily as a result of dysfunctional parenting. In families where parents use substances, there is typically poor parental monitoring and less stability (Anthony & Petronis, 1995; Corsi et al., 2007, Swadi, 1999). High levels of parental monitoring protect against use by reducing exposure to drugs (Greydanus & Patel, 2005; Kosterman, Hawkins, Guo, Catalano, & Abbott, 2000), and positive parenting (favorable connections between parents and adolescents) is related to less adolescent substance use (Pires & Jenkins, 2007). High parent-adolescent connectedness is associated with low levels of cigarette, alcohol, and marijuana use (Resnick et al., 1997; Vakalahi, 2001), and less drug use is related to high levels of parental involvement along with clear expectations (Brook, Brook, & Pahl, 2006).

Family structures with one parent, divorce, or a stepparent may increase adolescent drug use and more frequent use at earlier ages (Amey & Albrecht, 1998; Butters, 2002; Farrell & Caucasian, 1998; Gil, Vega, Biafora, 1998; Hoffman & Johnson, 1998; Kung & Farrell, 2000; Oman et al., 2007; Paxton, Valois, & Drane, 2007). Parental attitudes and adolescent perceptions of more permissive parental attitudes toward drug use are related to increased use among adolescents (Swadi, 1999; Vakalahi, 2001).

Social Factors

Social-level factors such as peers and communities play a significant role in adolescents' illicit substance use. Teen drug use is related to peer drug use across age groups, gender, and substances (Musher-Eizenman et al., 2003). Three processes may explain how peers influence use (Simons-Morton, 2007; Swadi, 1999). Socialization is the tendency for adolescents to conform to peer attitudes and behaviors (and adopt peer beliefs about drugs), whereas selection occurs when youth seek friends who already have their same beliefs. Substance use can also result from direct and active peer pressure (Swadi, 1999). In essence, associating with peers who use substances increases the availability of and exposure to illicit drugs, facilitates perceptions that drug use is normative, and reinforces use (Kandel, 1996; Musher-Eizenman et al., 2003; Oetting & Beauvais, 1986; Simons-Morton, 2007). Peers can also protect against substance use; adolescents who associate with peers who disapprove of drugs are less likely to use them (Kaplan et al., 1984).

Community-level factors such as disorganization, norms, low attachment, and poor law enforcement are consistently implicated in adolescent drug use. Neighborhood disorder (Jang & Johnson, 2001) and characteristics (particularly abandoned buildings and crime; Hadley-Ives, Stiffman, Elze, Johnson, & Dore, 2000) are associated with increased use (Winstanley et al., 2008), and community norms influence

Community-level factors such as disorganization, norms, low attachment, and poor law enforcement are consistently implicated in adolescent drug use.

the availability and acceptance of drugs in the neighborhood; greater availability predicts increased use (Burrow-Sanchez, 2006). Community norms also affect the perceived level of neighborhood attachment. When residents lack close bonds and do not view themselves as part of the community, there is low neighborhood attachment. Low neighborhood attachment is linked in turn to increased substance use (Van Horn, Hawkins, Arthur, & Catalano, 2007). Lastly, laws govern the sale of drugs, who can buy them, and their age restrictions. Laws also influence the supply and demand for drugs and their cost within a community (Hawkins et al., 1992). When laws and drug enforcement allow drugs to exist and thrive in a community, the negative consequences of substance use seem less serious, and higher rates of use are likely (Lee Van Horn et al., 2007).

In sum, adolescent substance use may be explained by a variety of influences consistent with a biopsychosocial framework comprising individual, family, and social-level factors. Because patterns of drug use, selection, and availability vary by age, gender, and ethnicity, prevention programs must attend to the specific risk and protective factors that are unique to the target population.

PREVENTION OF ADOLESCENTS' ILLICIT SUBSTANCE USE

The prevention of adolescents' illicit substance use has been the focus of extensive efforts. Adolescents who begin drug use at an early age are significantly more likely to intensify use, do poorly in school, and engage in multiple other problem behaviors over time (DuRant, Smith, Kreiter, & Krowchuk, 1999; Lynskey et al., 2002). Thus, programs that prevent, delay, or shift the trajectory of drug use can avert the negative sequelae, such as drunk driving, unsafe sex, and violence. Despite these health concerns, there is little research on preventing illicit drug use among adolescents (with the exception of marijuana), and the prevention efforts that do exist typically co-occur with programs for alcohol and tobacco. Prevention research on inhalant use and ingesting legal products—two emerging concerns—is also limited (Brouette & Anton, 2001; Delva, Spencer, & Lin, 2000). Moreover, reviews of interventions to prevent inhalant abuse (d'Abbs & MacLean, 2000; MacLean & d'Abbs, 2002) report minimal positive effects (Harwood, 1995).

The challenges for adolescent substance use prevention programs are numerous. Programs must address multiple risk and protective factors to prevent the onset of and mitigate the problems associated with drug use. Moreover, implementing programs with high fidelity in school-based settings (where most programs occur) requires extensive teacher training, staff and administration commitment, school resources, and teacher willingness and time to learn the curriculum. Prevention programs often compete with other curricular requirements and administrative priorities.

Three types of prevention programs target drug use among adolescents: school-based, family-based, and community-based (see Table 11.1). *Primary prevention* seeks to prevent initial use. *Secondary prevention* seeks to reduce use and its negative outcomes among already using teens. Lists of exemplary programs are provided by the Office of Juvenile Justice and Delinquency Prevention (Mihalic, Irwin, Elliott, Fagan, & Hansen, 2001) and by the Substance Abuse and Mental Health Services Administration's National Registry of Effective Prevention Programs. In the following sections, we summarize and critically evaluate the empirical evidence for effective school-, family-, and community-based adolescent substance use prevention programs.

School-Based Prevention Programs

School-based drug prevention programs typically address social influences on drug use. Outcome research is mixed; some programs show reduced drug use (Hansen, 1992; Tobler, 1986; Tobler et al., 2000), while others lack rigorous evaluation or reveal minimal change. A comprehensive meta-analysis of 207 school-based prevention programs identified several characteristics of effective alcohol, tobacco, and other drug interventions (Tobler et al., 2000), including interactive delivery methods, experiential activities, meaningful discussions, resistance skills training, a strong theoretical foundation, and an emphasis on comprehensive behavioral life skills and social influences (specifically, handling peer and social pressures and developing resistance skills). Systemwide interventions—those targeting students, peers, families, schools, and communities—were more effective than those targeting adolescents only. The least effective programs were knowledge-only (teaching youth the properties of substances), affective-only (emphasizing self-esteem and values clarification), and a combination of knowledge and affective strategies (Hansen, 1992; Tobler et al., 2000).

Two well-designed programs with documented evidence are noteworthy: LifeSkills Training (LST) and Project ALERT. Both programs are based on social influence, social learning, and life-skills theories. LST was among the first school-based programs to show positive behavioral effects on adolescents' illicit substance use (Botvin & Eng, 1980, 1982). Evaluated extensively with diverse adolescent populations in a series of efficacy studies, findings show reduced marijuana use, polydrug use, and other illicit drug use lasts until the end of high school (Botvin, Baker, Dusenbury, Botvin, & Diaz, 1995; Botvin et al., 2000).

Recent evaluations of LST revealed lower levels of overall illicit drug use, including hallucinogens, inhalants, heroin, polydrugs, and other narcotics among intervention participants relative to controls (Botvin et al., 2000; Botvin, Griffin, Diaz, & Ifill-Williams, 2001; Griffin, Botvin, Nichols, & Doyle, 2003). Effects on drug use were partially mediated by risk-taking and peer norms about drug use (Botvin et al., 2001). Taken together, the results from several large-scale randomized trials provide strong evidence for LST effectiveness with suburban whites and inner-city minorities.

Project ALERT is a two-year, universal drug prevention program for middle school students to motivate them against drug use and develop substance use resistance skills

TABLE 11.1. Adolescent substance use prevention programs

Prevention Setting	Authors	Demographics	Study Design	Outcomes
School-Based Programs				
Project Alert	Longshore, Ellickson, McCaffrey, & St. Clair (2007)	75.9% White; 24.1% nonwhite (N = 1,772)	Randomly assigned to Alert Only (seventh- and eighth-grade curriculum), Alert Plus (booster lessons added in ninth grade), or control condition	At-risk girls in ALERT Plus schools reported significantly lower rates of weekly alcohol and marijuana use compared to controls. Girls reported significantly lower scores on alcohol consequences and high-risk alcohol use. ALERT Only and controls showed no significant differences for at-risk girls or at-risk boys.
LifeSkills Training (LST)	Botvin et al. (2000)	92.3% White, suburban (N = 447)	Randomly assigned to LST (15 sessions in seventh grade, 10 boosters in eighth, and 5 boosters in ninth) or control	Reduced overall illicit drug use; reduced use of hallucinogens, heroin, and other narcotics at 6.5-month follow-up.
	Botvin, Griffin, Diaz, & Ifill-Williams (2001)	61% African American; 22% Hispanic; 6% Asian; 6% White; 5% other; urban (N = 3,621)	Randomly assigned to LST (15 sessions in seventh grade and 10 boosters in eighth) or control	Reduced smoking, drinking, drunkenness, inhalant use, and polydrug use relative to controls. Prevention effects mediated in part by reduced normative expectations, behavioral intentions, and risk taking.

	Authors	Sample	Design	Results
	Griffin, Botvin, Nichols, & Doyle (2003)	58% African American; 29% Hispanic; high-risk, urban (N = 758)	Randomly assigned to LST (15 sessions in seventh grade and 10 boosters in eighth) or control	Reduced smoking, drinking, inhalant use, and polydrug use at the one-year follow-up among subsample of youth at high risk for substance use initiation.
Lions Quest Skills for Adolescence (SFA)	Eisen, Zellman, Massett, & Murray (2002)	33.9% Hispanic; 25.7% White; 17.6% African American; 7.1% Asian American; 14.6% other; urban (N = 7,426)	Randomization to 40-session curriculum or control group	For baseline nonusers, recent cigarette smoking was significantly lower for SFA than controls. Significant treatment group by ethnicity interactions on three drinking behaviors (lifetime alcohol use, recent alcohol use, and recent binge drinking). Hispanics in SFA were less likely to ever or recently drink, and to recently binge drink than Hispanic controls; no treatment differences found among non-Hispanics. For baseline users, there were three significant SFA delays in transition to experimental or recent use of more "advanced" substances: drinking to smoking, drinking to marijuana use, and binge drinking to marijuana.
	Eisen, Zellman, & Murray (2003)	33.9% Hispanic; 25.7% White; 17.6% African American; 7.1% Asian American; 14.6% other; urban (N = 7,426)	Two-year posttest data (one year after intervention)	Lifetime and recent marijuana use were lower in SFA than control schools with pretest usage at two-year posttest (one year post-intervention). Baseline binge drinkers in SFA schools were less likely to report recent binge drinking than students in control schools. Significant treatment effects for increasing students' sense of self-efficacy to refuse offers of marijuana and alcohol in a variety of situations.

(Continued)

TABLE 11.1. (*Continued*)

Prevention Setting	Authors	Demographics	Study Design	Outcomes
Family-Based Programs				
Preparing for the Drug-Free Years (PDFY)	Mason, Kosterman, Hawkins, Haggerty, & Spoth (2003)	White, rural Midwestern (N = 429)	In a randomized block design, schools were assigned to one of three experimental conditions: PDFY, SFP, or minimal-contact control condition	PDFY slowed the rate of increase in polysubstance use during adolescence.
Strengthening Families Program 10–14 (SFP)	Trudeau, Azevedo, Spoth, & Randall (2007)	White, rural Midwestern (N = 383)	In a randomized block design, schools were assigned to one of three experimental conditions: SFP, PDFY, or minimal-contact control condition	Compared to the control group, SFP showed a slower rate of increase in internalizing symptoms and polysubstance use. The intervention slowed the rate of increase in polysubstance use significantly more for girls than for boys.

Program / Author	Sample	Design	Results
Spoth, Clair, Shin, & Redmond (2006)	Study 1: 98% White, rural Midwestern (N = 667) Study 2: White, rural Midwestern (N = 679)	In study 1, schools were assigned to SFP, PDFY, or control condition In study 2, schools were assigned to revised SFP (SFP 10–14) plus LifeSkills SFP Training (SFP 10–14-LST), LST alone, or control condition	In study 1, the SFP past-year methamphetamine rate was significantly different at 0.0% as compared with 3.2% in the control condition at 6.5 years past baseline. In study 2, SFP 10–14-LST showed significant effects on lifetime and past-year use at the 4.5-year follow-up. Both SFP 10–14-LST and LST alone had significant lifetime use effects at the 5.5-year follow-up.

Community-Based Programs

Program / Author	Sample	Design	Results
Midwestern Prevention Project (MPP) Johnson et al. (1990)	76.6% White; 19.2% Black; 2% Hispanic; 1.2% Asian American (N = 1,607)	Randomly assigned to MPP intervention or control group	At the one-year evaluation, students in intervention schools had significantly lower prevalence rates for all three drugs (cigarettes, alcohol, and marijuana) than their counterparts in the comparison schools. Significant reductions at three years in tobacco and marijuana use and equivalent reductions for youth at different levels of risk.
Street Smart Rotheram-Borus et al. (2003)	59% African American; 26% Hispanic; 15% White or other; urban, runaway adolescents (N = 311)	Using a quasi-experimental design, shelters assigned into intervention or control group	Compared to females in the control condition, at two years females in the intervention condition significantly reduced unprotected sexual acts, alcohol use, marijuana use, and number of drugs used over twelve months. Male adolescents in the intervention condition showed significant reductions in marijuana use over six months compared to control youth.

(Ellickson & Bell, 1990; Ellickson, McCaffrey, Ghosh-Dastidar, & Longshore, 2003). The original Project ALERT curriculum was designed for seventh and eighth graders to prevent or reduce marijuana use and was later revised to increase parental involvement. Project ALERT prevented regular and initial use of marijuana among eighth graders at varying levels of risk (Ellickson et al., 2003) and improved perceptions of resistance self-efficacy, drug use prevalence, and peer approval, beliefs, and intentions (Ghosh-Dastidar, Longshore, Ellickson, & McCaffrey, 2004; Orlando, Ellickson, McCaffrey, & Longshore, 2005). Project ALERT was enhanced for ninth graders by adding five booster lessons (to become Project ALERT Plus), and it revealed positive effects; girls but not boys reported less weekly marijuana use and more resistance to social influences and beliefs about the consequences of drug use. There were no significant effects for teens who received the original Project ALERT curriculum (Longshore, Ellickson, McCaffrey, & St. Clair, 2007).

Family-Based Prevention Programs

Family-based programs are designed to reduce or eliminate family-related risk factors associated with adolescent substance use. These programs emphasize family factors implicated in drug use among adolescents, including parenting skills, parent-child communication, and family management. Two family-focused interventions—Preparing for the Drug-Free Years (PDFY) and the Strengthening Families Program: For Parents and Youth 10–14 (SFP 10–14), formerly known as the Iowa Strengthening Families Program—show delayed substance initiation and progression (Redmond, Spoth, Shin, & Lepper, 1999; Spoth, Redmond, & Shin, 2000; Spoth, Redmond, Trudeau, & Shin, 2002). Positive outcomes are sustained over time for both interventions (Spoth, Reyes, Redmond, & Shin, 1999; Spoth, Redmond, & Shin, 2001).

PDFY, guided by the social development model, enhances protective parent-child interactions and reduces risk for early substance use initiation (Catalano, Kosterman, Haggerty, Hawkins, & Spoth, 1999). Results indicate long-term reductions in children's antisocial behavior, improved academic skills, increased prosocial bonding, better family management skills and parenting behavior, and fewer incidents of drug use in school (Kosterman, Hawkins, Haggerty, Spoth, & Redmond, 2001; Mason et al., 2003; Park et al., 2000). Other outcome evaluations reveal less substance and polysubstance use, including inhalants, marijuana, and other illicit drugs following PDFY (Mason et al., 2003; Park et al., 2000; Spoth et al., 1999; Spoth et al., 2001).

SFP is a multicomponent program for elementary, junior, and high school students involving parents and children and emphasizing family skills training (Spoth et al., 2000, 2001). SFP has led to lower levels of substance use for boys and girls and slower increases in polysubstance use for girls, but not boys (Trudeau et al., 2007). When combined with LifeSkills Training, SFP reduces lifetime and past-year methamphetamine use at four-and-a-half-year follow-up (Spoth et al., 2006). SFP has been widely implemented in a variety of settings and with diverse families in the United States, Canada, Australia, Europe, and Central America (Kumpfer &Whiteside, 2000).

Community-Based Prevention Programs

Community-based programs involve an array of influences on teens—from schools and parents to community organizations, media campaigns, and laws—and can reduce adolescent drug use (Donaldson et al., 1996; Ellickson, 1999; Flay, 2000). Unfortunately, most of the outcome research does not evaluate the differential effects of the curricula, schoolwide environmental change, parent training, mass media, or community interventions (Flay, 2000). Thus, it is difficult to identify the most effective and the least effective components. Nevertheless, two especially promising programs are the Midwestern Prevention Project and Street Smart.

The Midwestern Prevention Project (Chou et al., 1998), also known as Project STAR (Students Taught Awareness and Resistance), is a comprehensive, multicomponent, community-based program designed to reduce the prevalence of tobacco, alcohol, and marijuana use among early adolescents and to reduce other illicit drug use among older adolescents (Dwyer et al., 1989; Johnson et al., 1990; MacKinnon et al., 1991; Pentz, MacKinnon, Dwyer, et al., 1989; Pentz, MacKinnon, Flay, et al., 1989; Pentz et al., 1990). The intervention targets school, media, parent, community organizing, and health policy components to help adolescents resist peer pressure to use drugs, counteract pro-smoking influences, and promote positive parent-child communication about substance use prevention. Long-term follow-up studies indicate significant reductions in tobacco and marijuana use and equivalent reductions for adolescents at different levels of risk three years after participation (Johnson et al., 1990).

Illicit substance use is also associated with high-risk sexual behavior (Kingree, Braithwaite, & Woodring, 2000), and for this reason the Centers for Disease Control and Prevention identified prevention interventions that simultaneously decrease sexual and substance use risk. Street Smart is an intensive prevention program delivered in shelters for runaway and homeless adolescents and is designed to reduce substance use, unprotected sex, and number of sex partners. Street Smart participants reported reduced substance use and fewer unprotected sex acts compared to a control group. Females significantly reduced marijuana use and the number of drugs used over twelve months, and males reported reductions in marijuana use over six months (Rotheram-Borus et al., 2003).

Commonalities Across Effective Prevention Programs

Common characteristics of effective prevention programs can serve as guidelines for effective program design and implementation. Most effective programs employ (1) a comprehensive approach that begins early, extends across the life span, addresses multiple risk and protective factors, and generalizes across settings; (2) solid grounding in research and theory; (3) developmental appropriateness; (3) sensitivity to culture and community; (4) a sufficient dosage and follow-up time period; (5) adequate training for prevention program providers; and (6) well-designed evaluation methods (Dusenbury, 2000; National Institute on Drug Abuse, 1997, 2003). In a large meta-analysis, the Center for Substance Abuse Prevention (2002) also identified five program characteristics that showed significant reductions in substance use: (1) emphasis on behavioral life skills; (2) building positive connections with peers and adults through team and interpersonal activities; (3) drawing on prevention theory and research; (4) introspective learning approaches that encourage self-reflection; and (5) intense contact. Programs that delivered behavioral life skills programming were significantly more effective than affective and knowledge-focused programs. Recreation-focused programs that emphasized substance-free leisure and enrichment activities were the second most effective approach. These findings are consistent with other meta-analyses (Tobler et al., 2000).

Evidence-based programs exist to prevent adolescent substance use, but there are several limitations to the current research.

In summary, evidence-based programs exist to prevent adolescent substance use, but there are several limitations to the current research. First, the vast majority of programs are delivered in school settings, where some of the highest-risk teens (such as dropouts, the homeless, and detainees) do not benefit. Programs may prove less effective for these subgroups, and findings may not generalize. Second, information about inhalants and prescription drugs, their storage and potential for misuse and abuse is sparse, despite growing rates of use. Third, the next step in program evaluation should identify the mechanisms for positive or negative outcomes, clarifying what works, for whom, under what conditions, and how outcomes can be sustained. Knowing the differential effects of intervention components will reduce unnecessary resource output and improve cost-effectiveness. Finally, dissemination must occur, and state and local policies must ensure sustainability of empirically validated programs. Engaging communities and agencies early in the development and planning process and encouraging them to take ownership of the programs will enhance dissemination efforts.

Prevention Programs for Minority Populations

Differences in rates of substance use, risk factors, and protective processes across racial and ethnic groups underscore the need for cultural tailoring and evaluating cultural differences of substance use prevention programs (Castro & Alarcon, 2002; Resnicow, Soler, Braithwaite, Ahluwalia, & Butler, 2000). Several models and frameworks for cultural adaptation are available (Castro & Alarcon, 2002; Rosello & Bernal, 1999; Sue, 1998; Sue & Zane, 1987), but little agreement exists about an optimal approach. Several programs have been adapted for gender and minorities, but there is wide inconsistency in their approaches (Huey & Polo, 2008). In most cases, the efficacy of these adaptations has not been examined. We define *cultural sensitivity* as "the extent to which ethnic/cultural characteristics, experiences, norms, values, behavioral patterns, and beliefs of a target population as well as the relevant historical, environmental, and social forces are incorporated in the design, delivery, and evaluation of targeted health promotion materials and programs" (Resnicow et al., 2000, p. 272). Effective *cultural adaptation* attends to both surface and deep structure dimensions (Resnicow, Baranowski, Ahluwalia, & Braithwaite, 1999; Resnicow et al., 2000).

Surface-level changes ensure that program materials match a population's social and behavioral characteristics (such as heritage, language, music, food, and clothing), whereas deeper-level *cultural tailoring* integrates the cultural, social, psychological, environmental, and historical factors of the group that influence health behaviors (Resincow et al., 2000). Though we recognize the heterogeneity within ethnicities, we have combined groups to illustrate common core values and how these are reflected in the tailored programs discussed next.

Native Americans and Alaska Natives. Despite great diversity within this group, Native American tribes share cultural themes of family, community, spirituality, and harmony with nature (Bureau of Indian Affairs, 2003; Hawkins, Cummins, & Marlatt, 2004). Successful substance abuse prevention programs for Native American youth incorporate these themes, involve families and community (such as tribal councils and nontribal agencies), and emphasize bicultural competence skills (Moran & Reaman, 2002).

Schinke, Tepavac, and Cole (2000) developed a prevention program for school-aged Native Americans that incorporated core beliefs, practices, and values, such as tobacco use in traditional ceremonies, spirituality, harmony with nature, integrated holistic concepts of health, and bicultural issues (Botvin, Baker, Dusenbury, Tortu, & Botvin, 1990). The authors compared skills-only, skills-plus-community involvement and support, and a control group. All three groups reported increased tobacco, alcohol, and marijuana use following the intervention, but youth in the skills-only program reported significantly lower rates of smokeless tobacco, alcohol, and marijuana at follow-up.

The Parent, School, Community Partnership Program (Petoskey, Van Stelle, & DeJong, 1998), guided by cognitive-behavioral and community empowerment theories (Freire, 1972), was developed to reduce alcohol, tobacco, and other drug use among Native American adolescents residing on or near reservations. The curriculum incorporated skills and values related to Native American tribal legends and spirituality, and employed cooperative learning techniques and leadership training. Participants reported less past-month marijuana use and less likelihood of accepting marijuana (see Hawkins et al., 2004, and Moran and Reaman, 2002, for reviews on substance use prevention with Native Americans).

Hispanics. Programs for Hispanics integrate core values of *familismo* (strong family ties), *respeto* (respect for parents and elders), *dignidad* (value of self-worth), *caridad* (importance of rituals and ceremonies), fatalism, and *simpatia* (importance of positive social interactions; Castro et al., 2006; Resnicow et al., 2000; Szapocznik, Lopez, Prado, Schwartz, & Pantin, 2006). Acculturation, assimilation, and adaptation are often overlooked in these programs, yet are critically important for several Hispanic subgroups (Vega, Gil, & Kolody, 2002; Warner, Valdez, Canino, de la Rosa, & Turner, 2006). For example, U.S.-born Latinos report higher rates of substance use than immigrants (Vega, Alderete, Kolody, & Aguilar-Gaxiola, 1998; Vega et al., 2002).

Familias Unidas (Pantin et al., 2003) emphasizes the training of parents to prevent substance use among Hispanic adolescents. Implemented in family-centered, multiparent groups, Familias Unidas focuses on parents as change agents by enhancing parent involvement, family support, and parent-child communication. Hispanic cultural beliefs, values, and expectations are integrated into all aspects of the intervention. At one-year follow-up, youth behavior problems decreased and parental investment increased. In combination with Parent Preadolescent Training for HIV Prevention (Krauss et al., 2000; Prado et al., 2007), eighth graders reported less illicit drug use and less unsafe sexual behavior at two-year follow-up.

Keepin' It Real (Hecht et al., 2003; Kulis et al., 2005) also incorporates traditional Hispanic values and cultural practices. In a randomized controlled study, three versions of the curriculum were designed and tested for Mexican Americans, European and African Americans, and a combination of these two groups. Sample size constraints limited analyses to Mexican and Mexican American youth versus a control group. Relative to the controls, intervention participants reported less marijuana, tobacco, and alcohol use, but the Mexican American and multicultural curricula revealed smaller increases in recent marijuana use, decreased intentions to use substances, more positive perceived norms, and greater self-efficacy. Cultural matching of program content with ethnicity did not enhance outcomes. In a follow-up study, Marsiglia, Kulis, Wagstaff, Elek, and Dran (2005) found that Spanish-language preference protected against substance use among Mexican and Mexican American adolescents, underscoring the importance of examining indicators of acculturation in substance use prevention with Hispanic adolescents.

Lions Quest Skills for Adolescence is a school-based comprehensive life-skills prevention program (Eisen et al., 2002) that has been culturally adapted for use in over twenty countries. One-year outcomes indicated lower rates of marijuana use for Hispanic adolescents (see Castro et al., 2006, and Szapocznik et al., 2006, for extensive reviews on substance use prevention with Hispanics).

African Americans. Several effective substance abuse prevention programs integrate African American core values of extended community involvement (communalism), spirituality, expressiveness, respect for verbal communication, connection to ancestors or history, family commitment, promotion of cultural pride or identity, connections with family and community, and intuition and experience (Flay et al., 2004; Resnicow et al., 2000).

Positive Youth Development Collaborative (PYDC), is a comprehensive evidence-based after-school substance abuse program for urban minority middle and high school adolescents (the majority of whom were African American) to promote resilience, build competencies, focus on risk reduction behaviors (Roth & Brooks-Gunn, 2003), provide substance use prevention and health education, and use cultural heritage activities (Tebes et al., 2007). Program content was tailored for urban minority adolescents. PYDC includes African American cultural values of unity, self-determination, and responsibility, as well as culturally consistent teaching approaches such as storytelling and proverbs, and African American history and literature. Participants reported enhanced attitudes and perceptions of drugs as harmful at seven-month follow-up and reduced past-month substance use at one-year follow-up.

Asian Americans. Asians represent a large heterogeneous group of over thirty distinct ethnic groups (Sandhu, 1997) and are the least studied in substance use prevention and treatment. Prevention programs must address Asian cultural attitudes regarding help seeking (such as stigma, shame, and dishonor and a preference for managing conflicts privately within the family), filial piety (obligation or duty to parents), respect for elders, hierarchical family structure, fatalism, moral obligations, extended definition of family, and strong parental expectations for youth academic achievement (Sue & Sue, 2003; Mercado, 2000).

The Competence Through Transitions (CTT) program (Zane, Aoki, Ho, Huang, & Jang, 1998), designed for Chinese, Filipino, Japanese, Korean, and Vietnamese youth, has yielded empirical support. CTT emphasizes skill building and general health issues (HIV and drug education), school and institutional competence (school adjustment, parental rights, responsibilities, and advocacy), social competence, intergenerational family competence (strengthening parent-child relationships), and multicultural competence (strengthening cultural pride). Participants in CTT reported increased knowledge of the negative influences of drugs after the program.

Prevention Programs for Males and Females

Substance use prevention programs generally fail to address gender differences despite different incidence and prevalence rates of substance use in males and females. Blake, Amaro, Schwartz, and Flinchbaugh (2001) reviewed gender-specific programs and identified two worth noting, despite the absence of follow-up data beyond three months.

Girls Incorporated Friendly PEERsuasion (Weiss & Nicholson, 1998) is a secondary school–based substance use prevention program for eleven- to fourteen-year-old girls. After the program, younger (eleven- to twelve-year-olds) but not older girls were more likely to leave situations where peer substance use occurred. Vitaro, Dobkin, and Tremblay (1994) implemented a modified version of the Life-Skills Training (Botvin et al., 1990) for eleven- to twelve-year-old girls, and those who received the intervention reported more negative attitudes toward marijuana and less marijuana use.

Universal programs have also demonstrated gender effects. The Seattle Social Development Project (O'Donnell, Hawkins, Catalano, Abbott, & Day, 1995), which is based on the social development model (Hawkins et al., 1992), focused on school failure, drug abuse, and delinquency in elementary school children. Girls, but not boys, reported marginally lower rates of marijuana use. Moskowitz, Schaps, Schaeffer, and Malvin (1984) delivered a drug education curriculum to seventh graders, and only girls reported improved drug knowledge and perceived peer attitudes toward substance use.

This review presents several culturally adapted substance use programs for minority groups and by gender, but few controlled trials have established their efficacy. Future research will benefit from a consensus on cultural adaptation frameworks and strategies (Huey & Polo, 2008), rigorous outcome evaluations, replication of outcome findings, and greater attention to the moderators and mediators of treatment effects. Finally, the next generation of studies must consider intra-ethnic patterns and contextual factors that influence substance use, such as socioeconomic status, country of origin, immigration history, and acculturation levels (Castro & Alarcon, 2002; Kim, Coletti, Williams, & Hepler, 1995).

TREATMENT OF ADOLESCENT SUBSTANCE ABUSE AND DEPENDENCE

Illicit substance use often co-occurs with other adolescent problem behaviors (Jessor & Jessor, 1977), including violence and criminality, weapons possession, high-risk sexual activity, motor vehicle accidents, and overdoses (Dennis, Dawud-Noursi, Muck, & McDermeit, 2003). Thus, substance abuse treatment programs often target multiple problems simultaneously (Rowe & Liddle, 2003; Waldron, Turner, & Ozechowski, 2006). Research reviews and clinical trials reveal positive short-term outcomes from these programs, but relapse is common (Brown, D'Amico, McCarthy, & Tapert, 2001; Deas & Thomas, 2001; Dennis et al., 2003, 2004; Godley, Godley, Dennis, Funk, & Passetti, 2006; Jainchill, Hawke, De Leon, & Yagelka, 2000; Muck et al., 2001), and empirical data on treatment efficacy among adolescents is relatively sparse. Research is further hampered by the absence of well-designed studies with appropriate comparison groups, small sample sizes, and restricted age ranges. Nevertheless, a few programs are noteworthy.

Only 10 percent of adolescents with substance use disorders receive services, and among those only 25 percent obtain care that is matched to their diverse needs (Center for Substance Abuse Treatment, 2001; National Institute on Drug Abuse, 2001). The goal of substance abuse treatment is to achieve and maintain abstinence and address problems linked to drug use (such as comorbid psychiatric disorders and family functioning). As shown in Table 11.2, the American Academy of Child and Adolescent Psychiatry practice parameters for the treatment of adolescent substance abuse (Bukstein & the Work Group on Quality Issues, 2004) identified nine characteristics of the most effective programs (Brannigan, Schackman, Falco, & Millman, 2004; Drug Strategies, 2003). Unfortunately, an extensive review of 144 highly regarded programs (Brannigan et al., 2004) revealed few that conformed to the academy's nine characteristics. They scored lowest on matched assessment and treatment, engaging and retaining youth, gender and cultural competence, and outcome evaluations. The most common intervention approaches are twelve-step, pharmacologic, student assistance and school-based, behavioral and cognitive-behavioral, and family-based.

Twelve-step programs. Twelve-step programs such as Alcoholics Anonymous (AA) and Narcotics Anonymous (NA) are the most widely practiced approach in inpatient and residential facilities. Twelve-step programs include group therapy, individual and family counseling, lectures, psychoeducation, recreational activities, written assignments, after-care or follow-up treatment, and attending AA or NA meetings. Attendance at twelve-step meetings enhances critical self-regulation, like motivation for abstinence and abstinence-focused coping (Kelly, Myers, & Brown, 2000). Adolescents completing these programs report significantly more abstinence at six-month

TABLE 11.2. **Characteristics of effective substance abuse treatment programs**

Program Characteristic	Description
Matched assessment and treatment	Extensive biopsychosocial evaluation to guide treatment targets
Comprehensive and integrated	Interventions that target multiple domains
Family involvement	Improving parent-child relationships and interactions and parental monitoring to enhance treatment retention and sustain gains
Developmentally appropriate	Materials, activities, content, and language appropriate for teens' biological, social, emotional, and cognitive levels
Engaging and retaining youth	Fostering a strong therapeutic alliance to enhance family engagement and retention
Qualified staff	Culturally competent staff trained in adolescent development, comorbid mental health problems, substance abuse and addiction, and experienced with diverse adolescents, families, and communities
Gender and cultural competence	Program content that is sensitive to gender and culture
Ongoing care	Providing continued services, particularly relapse prevention, after-care planning, and referrals to community agencies
Outcome evaluations	Ongoing assessment of treatment outcomes to measure success, improve services, and identify additional needed resources

follow-up, but results at one and two years are mixed (Winters, Stinchfield, Opland, Weller, & Latimer, 2000).

Pharmacologic interventions. Pharmacological approaches usually focus on a defined problem, such as psychiatric disorders or the neurobiology underlying addictive behavior. The coexistence of psychiatric disorders and adolescent substance abuse has stimulated numerous efforts to treat drug use with psychotropic medications. Unfortunately, the empirical evidence to support pharmacological treatments for adolescent drug use is sparse. Adult pharmacologic strategies to treat withdrawal and cravings have not been tested in adolescents. Pharmacological interventions should be combined with psychosocial and behavioral treatments to increase compliance, address contextual factors related to abuse, and sustain effects.

The empirical evidence to support pharmacological treatments for adolescent drug use is sparse.

Student assistance (SA) and school-based programs. Student assistance and school-based programs have grown in popularity over the past several decades (Wagner, Tubman, & Gil, 2004). A major disadvantage of this approach, however, is that teens must attend school to receive services, and thus these programs do not reach those at greatest risk—dropouts, truants, and homeless youth (McCluskey, Krohn, Lizotte, & Rodriguez, 2002). Two SA programs—Project SUCCESS (Schools Using Coordinated Community Efforts to Strengthen Students) and Residential Assistance Programs—are recognized by the National Registry of Effective Prevention Programs. Early evidence shows significant and sustained reductions in marijuana use among high school students, but few empirical outcome studies exist, and differences in program descriptions, philosophies, and structural procedures make overall conclusions difficult to draw.

One school-based program, Project Towards No Drug Abuse (PTND), was developed for continuation (alternative) high school students at increased risk for serious substance abuse. PTND is based on motivational decision making and emphasizes self-control and communication skills, resisting drug use, healthy decision-making strategies, and motivation against drug use. Findings indicate short- and long-term positive effects on hard drug use but not alcohol (Sun, Skara, Sun, Dent, & Sussman, 2006), tobacco, or marijuana (Dent, Sussman, & Stacy, 2001; Sussman, Dent, & Stacy, 2002).

Behavioral and cognitive-behavioral interventions. Behavioral and cognitive-behavioral treatments of adolescent substance abuse emphasize social skills training, problem solving, anger control, contingency management (CM), and relapse prevention. CM offers incentives and rewards to achieve goals and has yielded positive effects for opiate, cocaine, nicotine, and alcohol dependence (Higgins, Wong, Badger, Ogden, & Dantona, 2000; Higgins et al., 2003; Miller & Wilbourne, 2002; Shoptaw et al., 2002). Voucher-based reinforcement therapy (VBRT), a type of CM, provides "vouchers" in exchange for biological samples (urine or breath) that indicate abstinence. The vouchers have monetary value and can be exchanged for goods and services consistent with the goals of treatment. VBRT has produced significant periods of nondrug use (Higgins, Badger, & Budney, 2000). Relapse prevention programs teach coping strategies to maintain abstinence (Parks, Marlatt, & Anderson, 2004) and view single drug use occurrences ("lapses" or "slips") as learning opportunities, rather than failure. These programs help adolescents anticipate high-risk situations, identify ways to avoid and manage them, and rehearse nondrug responses. Relapse prevention programs effectively treat illicit drug and alcohol use disorders (Carroll, Rounsaville, Nich, & Gordon, 1994; Stephens, Roffman, & Curtin, 2000). Although few empirical studies of CM and relapse prevention exist for teens, both show positive effects for marijuana, cocaine, opiate, and polysubstance use among adults (Dutra, Stathopolou, Leyro, & Otto, 2008).

Family-based programs. Family-based interventions for adolescent substance use are among the most well documented. Some of the more notable types are Multisystemic Therapy (MST; Henggeler, 1999), Brief Strategic Family Therapy (BSFT; Szapocznik, Kurtines, Foote, Perez-Vidal, & Hervis, 1986), Structural Ecosystems Therapy (SET; Robbins, Schwartz, & Szapocznik, 2003), Integrative Family Cognitive Behavior Therapy (IFCBT; Waldron, Slesnick, Brody, Turner, & Peterson, 2001), and Multidimensional Family Therapy (MDFT; Liddle, 2002). Ozechowski and Liddle (2000) evaluated thirteen randomized controlled trials of outpatient family-based treatments. In seven studies, family interventions yielded greater reductions in substance use than alternative treatments, including individual therapy (Azrin et al., 1994; Henggeler et al., 1991; Liddle, 2002; Waldron et al., 2001), adolescent group therapy (Joanning, Quinn, Thomas, & Mullen, 1992; Liddle et al., 2001; Liddle, Rowe, Dakof, Ungaro, & Henderson, 2004), and family psychoeducational drug counseling (Joanning et al., 1992; Lewis, Piercy, Sprenkle, & Trepper, 1990; Liddle et al., 2001).

SUMMARY

Adolescent substance use prevention and treatment research has advanced substantially over the past decade, and yet a large number of those who need services do not receive them or do not benefit from available programs. Better outreach is essential to reach those in need. Programs designed specifically for adolescents lack rigorous outcome evaluations, culturally tailoring, and attention to gender. Substance use is consistently associated with exposure to HIV/AIDS—directly through intravenous drug use and indirectly through impaired decision making and inaccurate condom application. Prevention and treatment efforts should integrate HIV-risk-reduction strategies, as both target similar skills: assertive communication and refusal skills. Treatment intensity and ongoing care predict long-term recovery from drug use, and programs that emphasize engagement and retention maximize positive outcomes and prevent relapse. Comprehensive standardized assessments are critical to accurately evaluate treatment effects, but measures must be sensitive to gender and culture. Future programs will benefit from careful attention to the unique needs and differences within ethnic groups, and with regard to age, gender, comorbid mental illness, and other risk factors. Rigorously designed studies (specifically, randomized clinical trials guided by treatment manuals and evaluated with standardized assessments over time) that identify the most active treatment components will influence resource allocation that is cost-effective and relevant. Careful evaluation of key mediators and moderators of change, predictors of long-term effects, and the impact of individual, family, social, and contextual factors on substance use will guide these efforts. Lastly, evidence-based interventions must be disseminated to relevant treatment settings with assistance in technology transfer through training, resources, and collaboration.

KEY TERMS

Cultural sensitivity

Cultural tailoring

Primary prevention

Protective factors

Risk factors

Secondary prevention

Substance use

DISCUSSION QUESTIONS

1. Describe the most important risk and protective factors involved in adolescent substance use. Use the biopsychosocial framework as a basis for discussion.

2. Discuss how adolescent substance use varies among different racial and ethnic groups. How have prevention programs been tailored to address cultural differences? Provide examples.

3. Envision being a parent of a substance-abusing teen. Given the information provided in this chapter on treatment of adolescent substance use and dependence, which type of treatment program would you prefer your child to attend? Explain your reasoning.

REFERENCES

Amey, C. H., & Albrecht, S. L. (1998). Race and ethnic differences in adolescent drug use: The impact of family structure and the quantity and quality of parental interaction. *Journal of Drug Issues, 28,* 283–298.

Anthony, J. C., & Petronis, K. R. (1995). Early-onset drug use and risk of later drug problems. *Drug and Alcohol Dependence, 40,* 9–15.

Armstrong, T. D., & Costello, E. J. (2002). Community studies on adolescent substance use, abuse, or dependence and psychiatric comorbidity. *Journal of Consulting and Clinical Psychology, 70,* 1224–1239.

Azrin, N. H., McMahon, P. T., Donahue, B., Besalel, V., Lapinski, K. J., Kogan, E., Acierno, R., & Galloway, E. (1994). Behavioral therapy for drug abuse: A controlled treatment outcome study. *Behavioral Research and Therapy, 32*(8), 857–866.

Benard, B. (1991). *Fostering resiliency in kids: Protective factors in the family, school and community*. Portland, OR: Northwest Regional Educational Laboratory, Western Regional Center for Drug-Free Schools and Communities.

Blake, S., Amaro, H., Schwartz, P., & Flinchbaugh, L. (2001). A review of substance abuse prevention interventions for young adolescent girls. *Journal of Early Adolescence, 21,* 294–324.

Botvin, G. J., Baker, E., Dusenbury L., Botvin, E. M., & Diaz, T. (1995). Long term follow-up results of a randomized drug abuse prevention trial in a White middle-class population. *Journal of the American Medical Association, 273,* 1106–1112.

Botvin, G. J., Baker, E., Dusenbury, L., Tortu, S., & Botvin, E. M. (1990). Preventing adolescent drug abuse through a multimodal cognitive-behavioral approach: Results of a 3-year study. *Journal of Consulting and Clinical Psychology, 58,* 437–446.

Botvin, G. J., & Eng, A. (1980). A comprehensive school-based smoking prevention program. *Journal of School Health, 50,* 209–213.

Botvin, G. J., & Eng, A. (1982). The efficacy of a multi-component approach to the prevention of cigarette smoking. *Preventive Medicine, 11,* 199–211.

Botvin, G. J., Griffin, K. W., Diaz T., & Ifill-Williams M. (2001). Drug abuse prevention among minority adolescents: One-year follow-up of a school-based preventive intervention. *Prevention Science, 2,* 1–13.

Botvin, G. J., Griffin, K. W., Diaz, T., Scheier, L. M., Williams, C., & Epstein, J. A. (2000). Preventing illicit drug use in adolescents: Long-term follow-up data from a randomized control trial of a school population. *Addictive Behaviors, 5,* 769–774.

Brannigan, R., Schackman, B. R., Falco, M., & Millman, R. B. (2004). The quality of highly regarded adolescent substance abuse treatment programs: Results of an in-depth national survey. *Archives of Pediatrics and Adolescent Medicine, 158,* 904–909.

Brook, J. S., Brook, D. W., & Pahl, K. (2006). The developmental context for adolescent substance abuse intervention. In H. A. Liddle & C. Rowe (Eds.), *Adolescent substance abuse: Research and clinical advances* (pp. 25–51). New York: Cambridge University Press.

Brouette, T., & Anton, R. (2001). Clinical review of inhalants. *American Journal on Addictions, 10,* 79–94.

Brown, S. A., D'Amico, E. J., McCarthy, D., & Tapert, S. F. (2001). Four-year outcomes from adolescent alcohol and drug treatment. *Journal of Studies on Alcohol, 62,* 381–389.

Bukstein, O. G., & the Work Group on Quality Issues. (2004). *The practice parameter for the assessment and treatment of children and adolescents with substance use disorders*. Washington, DC: American Academy of Child and Adolescent Psychiatry.

Bureau of Indian Affairs. (2003). American Indian population and labor force. Retrieved April 18, 2008, from www.doi.gov/bia/labor.html.

Burrow-Sanchez, J. J. (2006). Understanding adolescent substance abuse: Prevalence, risk factors, and clinical implications. *Journal of Counseling and Development, 84,* 283–290.

Butters, J. (2002). Family stressors and adolescent cannabis use: A pathway to problem use. *Journal of Adolescence, 25,* 645–654.

Button, T. M., Rhee, A. H., Hewitt, J. K., Young, S. E., Corley, R. P., & Stallings, M. C. (2007). The role of conduct disorder in explaining the comorbidity between alcohol and illicit drug dependence in adolescence. *Drug and Alcohol Dependence, 87,* 46–53.

Carroll, K. M., Rounsaville, B. J., Nich, C., & Gordon, L. T. (1994). One-year follow-up of psychotherapy and pharmacotherapy for cocaine dependence: delayed emergence of psychotherapy effects. *Archives General Psychiatry, 51,* 989–997.

Castro, F. G., & Alarcon, E. H. (2002). Integrating cultural variables into drug abuse prevention and treatment with racial/ethnic minorities. *Journal of Drug Issues, 32,* 783–810.

Castro, F. G., Barrera, M., Pantin, H., Martinez, C., Félix-Ortiz, M., Rios, R., Lopez, V.A., & Lopez, C. (2006). Substance abuse prevention intervention research with Hispanic populations. *Drug and Alcohol Dependence, 84S,* S29–S42.

Catalano, R., Kosterman, R., Haggerty, K., Hawkins, D., & Spoth, R. (1999). A universal intervention for the prevention of substance abuse: Preparing for the Drug-Free Years. In R. Ashery, E. Robertson, & K. Kumpfer (Eds.), *NIDA research monograph on drug abuse prevention through family interventions* (pp. 130–159). Rockville, MD: National Institute on Drug Abuse.

Center for Substance Abuse Treatment. (2001). *Treatment episode data set.* Washington, DC: Substance Abuse and Mental Health Services Administration, Department of Health and Human Services. Retrieved April 18, 2008, from www.icpsr.umich.edu/samhda/das.html.

Center for Substance Abuse Prevention. (2002). *Preventing substance abuse: Major findings from the National Cross-Site Evaluation of High-Risk Youth Programs* (Points of Prevention Monograph Series No. 1; DHSS Publication No. SMA-25–01). Rockville, MD: Substance Abuse and Mental Health Services Administration.

Chou, C. P., Montgomery, S., Pentz, M. A., Rohrbach, L. A., Johnson, C. A., Flay, B. R., & MacKinnon, D. P. (1998). Effects of a community-based prevention program in decreasing drug use in high-risk adolescents. *American Journal of Public Health, 88,* 944–948.

Cohen, P., Chen, H., Crawford, T. N., Brook, J. S., & Gordon, K. (2007). Personality disorders in early adolescence and the development of later substance use disorders in the general population. *Drug and Alcohol Dependence, 88,* 71–84.

Cooper, H., Valentine, J. C., Nye, B., & Lindsay, J. J. (1999). Relationships between five after-school activities and academic achievement. *Journal of Educational Psychology, 91,* 369–378.

Corsi, K. F., Winch, P. J., Kwiatkowski, C. F., & Booth, R. E. (2007). Childhood factors that precede drug injection: Is there a link? *Journal of Child and Family Studies, 16,* 808–818.

Costello, E. J., Erkanli, A., Federman, E., & Angold, A. (1999). Development of psychiatric comorbidity with substance abuse in adolescents: Effects of timing and sex. *Journal of Clinical Child Psychology, 28,* 298–311.

d'Abbs, P., & MacLean, S. (2000). *Petrol sniffing in Aboriginal communities: A review of interventions.* Darwin, Australia: Cooperative Research Centre for Aboriginal and Tropical Health.

Danesco, E. R., Kingery, P. M., & Coggeshall, M. B. (1999). Perceived risk of harm from marijuana use among youth in the USA. *School Psychology International, 20,* 39–56.

Darling, N. (2005). Participation in extracurricular activities and adolescent adjustment: Cross-sectional and longitudinal findings. *Journal of Youth and Adolescence, 34*(5), 493–505.

Deas, D., & Thomas, S. E. (2001). An overview of controlled studies of adolescent substance abuse treatment. *American Journal on Addictions, 10,* 178–189.

Delva, J., Spencer, M. S., & Lin, J. K. (2000). Racial/ethnic and educational differences in the estimated odds of recent nitrite use among adult household residents in the United States: An illustration of matching and conditional logistic regression. *Substance Use and Misuse, 35,* 1075–1096.

Dennis, M. L., Dawud-Noursi, S., Muck, R. D., & McDermeit, M. (2003). The need for developing and evaluating adolescent treatment models. In S. J. Stevens & A. R. Morral (Eds.), *Adolescent substance abuse treatment in the United States: Exemplary models from a national evaluation study* (pp. 3–34). Binghamton, NY: Haworth Press.

Dennis, M. L., Godley, S. H., Diamond, G., Tims, F. M., Babor, T., Donaldson, J., Liddle, H., Titus, J. C., Kaminer, Y., Webb, C., Hamilton, N., & Funk, R. (2004). The Cannabis Youth Treatment (CYT) Study: Main findings from two randomized trials. *Journal of Substance Abuse Treatment, 27,* 197–213.

Dent, C. W., Sussman, S., & Stacy, A. W. (2001). Project Towards No Drug Abuse: Generalizability to a general high school sample. *Preventive Medicine, 32*(6), 514–520.

Deykin, E. Y., Levy, J. C., & Wells, V. (1987). Adolescent depression, alcohol and drug abuse. *American Journal of Public Health, 76,* 178–182.

Doherty, E. E., Green, K. M., & Ensminger, M. E. (2008). Investigating the long-term influence of adolescent delinquency on drug use initiation. *Drug and Alcohol Dependence, 93,* 72–84.

Donaldson, S. I., Sussman, S., MacKinnon, D. P., Severson, H. H., Glynn, T., Murray, D. M., & Stone, E. J. (1996). Drug abuse prevention programming: Do we know what content works? *American Behavioral Scientist, 39*(7), 868–883.

Drug Strategies. (2003). *Treating teens: A guide to adolescent drug problems.* Washington, DC: Drug Strategies.

DuRant, R. H., Smith, J. A., Kreiter, S. R., & Krowchuk, D. P. (1999). The relationship between early age of onset of initial substance use and engaging in multiple health risk behaviors among young adolescents. *Archives of Pediatric Adolescent Medicine, 153,* 286–291.

Dusenbury, L. (2000). Family-based drug abuse prevention programs: A review. *Journal of Primary Prevention, 20*(4), 337–352.

Dutra, L., Stathopaulou, G., Leyro, T. M., & Otto, M. W. (2008). A meta-analytic review of psychosocial inter-ventions for substance use disorders. *American Journal of Psychiatry, 165*(2),179–187.

Dwyer, J. H., MacKinnon, D. P., Pentz, M. A., Flay, B. R., Hansen, W. B., Wang, E.Y. I., & Johnson, C. A. (1989). Estimating intervention effects in longitudinal studies. *Journal of Epidemiology, 130,* 781–795.

Eaton, D. K., Kann, L., Kinchen, S., Ross, J., Hawkins, J., Harris, W. A., Lowry, R., McMannus, T., Chyen, D., Shanklin, S., Lim, C., Grunbaum, J., & Wechsler, H. (2005). Youth Risk Behavior Surveillance—United States. *Morbidity and Mortality Weekly Report, 55* (SS05): 1–108.

Eccles, J. S., & Barber, B. L. (1999). Student council, volunteering, basketball, or marching band: What kind of extracurricular involvement matters? *Journal of Adolescent Research, 14,* 10–43.

Eggert, L. L., & Randell, B. P. (2003). *Drug prevention research for high-risk youth.* In Z. Sloboda & W. J. Bukowski (Eds.), *Handbook of drug abuse prevention: Theory, science and practice* (pp. 473–495). New York: Kluwer Academic/Plenum.

Eisen, M., Zellman, G. L., Massett, H. A., & Murray, D. M. (2002). Evaluating the Lions Quest "Skills for Ado-lescence" drug education program: First-year behavior outcomes. *Addictive Behaviors, 27,* 619–632.

Eisen, M., Zellman, G. L., & Murray, D. M. (2003). Evaluating the Lions Quest "Skills for Adolescence" drug education program: Second-year behavior outcomes. *Addictive Behaviors, 28,* 883–897.

Ellickson, P. L. (1999). School-based substance-abuse prevention: What works, for whom, and how? In S. B. Kar (Ed.), *Substance abuse prevention: A multicultural perspective* (pp. 101–128). Amityville, NY: Baywood.

Ellickson, P. L., & Bell, R. M. (1990). Drug prevention in junior high: A multi-site longitudinal test. *Science, 247,* 1299–1305.

Ellickson, P. L., McCaffrey, D. F., Ghosh-Dastidar, B., & Longshore, D. L. (2003). New inroads in preventing adolescent drug use: Results from a large-scale trial of Project ALERT in middle schools. *American Journal of Public Health, 93,* 1830–1836.

Engel, G. L. (1977). The need for a new medical model: A challenge for biomedicine. *Science, 196*(4286), 129–136.

Farrell, A. D., & Caucasian, K. S. (1998). Peer influences and drug use among urban adolescents: Family struc-ture and parent-adolescent relationship as protective factors. *Journal of Counseling and Clinical Psychology, 66,* 248–258.

Fava, G. A., and Sonino, N. (2008). The biopsychosocial model thirty years later. *Psychotherapy and Psychoso-matics, 77,* 1–2.

Fergusson, D. M., Horwood, L. J., & Ridder, E. M. (2007). Conduct and attentional problems in childhood and adolescence and later substance use, abuse, and dependence: Results of a 25-year longitudinal study. *Drug and Alcohol Dependence, 88,* 14–26.

Flay, B. R. (2000). Approaches to substance use prevention utilizing school curriculum plus social environmental change. *Addictive Behaviors, 25,* 861–885.

Flay, B. R., Graumlich, S., Segawa, S., Burns, J. L., Holliday, M. Y., & Aban Aya Investigators. (2004). Effects of two prevention programs on high-risk behaviors among African-American youth: A randomized trial. *Archives of Pediatric and Adolescent Medicine, 158,* 377–384.

Freire, P. (1972). *Pedagogy of the oppressed.* Rickmansworth, England: Penguin.

Gerdes, A. C., Hoza, B., & Pelham, W. E. (2003). Attention-deficit/hyperactivity disordered boys' relationships with their mothers and fathers: Child, mother and father perceptions. *Developmental Psychopathology, 15,* 363–382.

Ghosh-Dastidar, B., Longshore, D., Ellickson, P. L., & McCaffrey, D. F. (2004). Modifying prodrug risk factors in adolescents: Results from Project ALERT. *Health Education and Behavior, 31,* 318–334.

Gil, A. G., Vega, W. A., & Biafora, F. (1998). Temporal influences of family structure and family risk factors on drug use initiation in a multiethnic sample of adolescent boys. *Journal of Youth and Adolescence, 27,* 373–393.

Godley, M. D., Godley, S. H., Dennis, M. L., Funk, R. R., & Passetti, L. L. (2006). The effect of Assertive Con-tinuing Care on continuing care linkage, adherence, and abstinence following residential treatment for adoles-cents with substance use disorders. *Addiction, 102,* 81–93.

Gonzalez, G. M., & Haney, M. L. (1990). Perceptions of risk as predictors of alcohol, marijuana and cocaine use among college students. *Journal of College Student Development, 31,* 313–318.

Greydanus, D. E., & Patel, D. R. (2005). The adolescent and substance abuse: Current concepts. *Current Prob-lems in Pediatric and Adolescent Health Care, 35,* 78–98.

Griffin, K. W., Botvin, G. J., Nichols, T. R., & Doyle, M. M. (2003). Effectiveness of a universal drug abuse pre-vention approach for youth at high risk for substance use initiation. *Preventive Medicine, 36,* 1–7.

Hadley-Ives, E., Stiffman, A. R., Elze, D., Johnson, S. D., & Dore, P. (2000). Measuring neighborhood and school environments: Perceptual and aggregate approaches. *Journal of Human Behavior and Social Environment, 38,* 1–27.

Hansen, W. B. (1992). School-based substance abuse prevention: A review of the state of the art in curriculum, 1980–1990. *Health Education Research, 7*(3), 403–430.

Harrison, P. A., Fulkerson, J. A., & Beebe, T. J. (1997). Multiple substance use among adolescent physical and sexual abuse victims. *Child Abuse and Neglect, 21*(6), 529–539.

Harwood, H. J. (1995). Inhalants: policy analysis of the problem in the United States. In N. J. Kozel, Z. Sloboda, & M. De la Rosa (Eds.), *Epidemiology of inhalant abuse: An international perspective* (pp. 274–304). Rockville, MD: National Institute on Drug Abuse.

Hawkins, E., Cummins, L. H., & Marlatt, G. A. (2004). Preventing substance abuse in American Indian and Alaska Native youth: Promising strategies for healthier communities. *Psychological Bulletin, 130,* 304–323.

Hawkins, J. D., Catalano, R. F., & Miller, J. Y. (1992). Risk and protective factors for alcohol and other drug problems in adolescence and early adulthood: Implications for substance abuse prevention. *Psychological Bulletin, 112,* 64–105.

Hayatbakhsh, M. R., McGee, T. R., Bor, W., Najman, J. M., Jamrozik, K., & Mamun, A. A. (2008). Child and adolescent externalizing behavior and cannabis use disorders in early adulthood: An Australian prospective birth cohort study. *Addictive Behaviors, 33,* 422–438.

Hecht, M. L., Marsiglia, F. F., Elek, E., Wagstaff, D. A., Kulus, S., & Dustman, P. (2003). Culturally grounded substance use prevention: An evaluation of the keepin' it R.E.A.L. curriculum. *Prevention Science, 4,* 233–248.

Henggeler, S. W. (1999). Multisystemic therapy: An overview of clinical procedures, outcomes and policy implications. *Child and Psychology and Psychiatry Review, 4,* 2–10.

Henggeler, S. W., Borduin, C. M., Melton, G. B., Mann, B. J., Smith, L., Hall, J. A., Cone, L., & Fucci, B. R. (1991). Effects of multisystemic therapy on drug use and abuse in serious juvenile offenders: A progress report from two outcome studies. *Family Dynamics of Addiction Quarterly, 1,* 40–51.

Higgins, S. T., Badger, G. J., & Budney, A. J. (2000). Initial abstinence and success in achieving longer term cocaine abstinence. *Experimental and Clinical Psychopharmacology, 8,* 377–386.

Higgins, S. T., Sigmon, S. C., Wong, C. J., Heil, S. H., Badger, G. J., Donham R., Dantona, R. L., & Anthony, S. (2003). Community reinforcement therapy for cocaine-dependent outpatients. *Archives General Psychiatry, 60,* 1043–1052.

Higgins, S. T., Wong, C. J., Badger, G. J., Ogden, D. E., & Dantona, R. L. (2000). Contingent reinforcement increases cocaine abstinence during outpatient treatment and 1 year of follow-up. *Journal of Consulting and Clinical Psychology, 68,* 64–72.

Hoffman, J. P., & Johnson, R. A. (1998). A national portrait of family structure and adolescent drug use. *Journal of Marriage and Family Therapy, 60,* 633–645.

Horowitz, H., Sung, H. E., & Foster, S. E. (2006). The role of substance abuse in juvenile justice systems and populations. *Corrections Compendium Journal, 31,* 24–26.

Hoza, B., Gerdes. A. C., & Hinshaw, S. P. (2004). Self-perceptions of competence in children with ADHD and comparison children. *Journal of Consulting Clinical Psychology, 3,* 382–391.

Huey, S. J., & Polo, A. J. (2008). Evidence-based psychosocial treatments for ethnic minority youth. *Journal of Clinical Child and Adolescent Psychology, 37,* 260–299.

Huizinga, D. H., Loeber, R., Thornberry, T. P., & Cothern, L. (2000). *Co-occurrence of delinquency and other problem behaviors* (National Criminal Justice Reference Service No. 182211). Washington, DC: Office of Justice Programs.

Ingraham, L. J., & Wender, P. H. (1992). Risk for affective disorder and alcohol and other drug abuse in the relatives of affectively ill adoptees. *Journal of Affective Disorders, 26,* 45–51.

Jainchill, N., Hawke, J., De Leon, G., & Yagelka, J. (2000). Adolescents in therapeutic communities: One-year posttreatment outcomes. *Journal of Psychoactive Drugs, 32,* 81–94.

Jang, S. J., & Johnson, B. R. (2001). Neighborhood disorder, individual religiosity and adolescent use of illicit drugs: A test of multilevel hypotheses. *Criminology, 39,* 109–144.

Jessor, R., & Jessor, S. L. (1977). *Problem behavior and psychosocial development: A longitudinal study in youth.* New York: Academic Press.

Joanning, H., Quinn, W., Thomas, F., & Mullen, R. (1992). Treating adolescent drug abuse: A comparison of family systems therapy, group therapy, and family drug education. *Journal of Marital and Family Therapy, 18*, 345–356.

Johnson, C. A., Pentz, M. A., Weber, M. D., Dwyer, J. H., Baer, N., MacKinnon, D. P., Hansen, W. B., & Flay, B. R. (1990). Relative effectiveness of comprehensive community programming for drug abuse prevention with high-risk and low-risk adolescents. *Journal of Consulting and Clinical Psychology, 58,* 447–456.

Johnston, L. D., O'Malley, P. M., Bachman, J. G., & Schulenberg, J. E. (2007a). *Monitoring the Future national survey results on drug use, 1975–2006: Vol. I. Secondary school students* (NIH Publication No. 07–6205). Bethesda, MD: National Institute on Drug Abuse.

Johnston, L. D., O'Malley, P. M., Bachman, J. G., & Schulenberg, J. E. (2007b). *Monitoring the Future national results on adolescent drug use: Overview of key findings, 2006* (NIH Publication No. 07–6202). Bethesda, MD: National Institute on Drug Abuse.

Johnston, L. D., O'Malley, P. M., Bachman, J. G., & Schulenberg, J. E. (2008). *Monitoring the Future national results on adolescent drug use: Overview of key findings, 2007.* Bethesda, MD: National Institute on Drug Abuse.

Kandel, D. B. (1996). The parental and peer contexts of adolescent deviance: An algebra of interpersonal influences. *Journal of Drug Issues, 26*(2), 289–315.

Kandel, D. B., Johnson, J. G., Bird, H. R., Canino, G., Goodman, S. H., Lahey, B. B., Regier, D. A., & Schwab-Stone, M. (1997). Psychiatric disorders associated with substance use among children and adolescents: Findings from the Methods for the Epidemiology of Child and Adolescent Mental Disorders (MECA) Study. *Journal of Abnormal Child Psychology, 25*(2), 121–132.

Kaplan, H. B., Martin, S. S., & Robbins, C. (1984). Pathways to adolescent drug use: Self-derogations, peer influence, weakening of social controls and early substance use. *Journal of Health and Social Behavior, 25,* 270–289.

Kelly, J. F., Myers, M. G., & Brown, S. A. (2000). A multivariate process model of adolescent 12-step attendance and substance use outcome following inpatient treatment. *Psychology of Addictive Behaviors, 14*(4), 376–389.

Kilpatrick, D. G., Acieno, R., Resnick, H. S., Saunders, B. E., & Best, C. L. (1997). A 2-year longitudinal analysis of the relationships between violent assault and substance use in women. *Journal of Consulting and Clinical Psychology, 65*(5), 834–847.

Kim, S., Coletti, S., Williams, C., & Hepler, N. A. (1995). Substance abuse prevention involving Asian/Pacific Islander American communities. In G. J. Botvin, S. Schinke, & M. A. Orlandi (Eds.), *Drug abuse prevention with multiethnic youth* (pp. 295–326). Thousand Oaks, CA: Sage.

Kingree, J. B., Braithwaite, R., & Woodring, T. (2000). Unprotected sex as a function of alcohol and marijuana use among adolescent detainees. *Journal of Adolescent Health, 27,* 179–185.

Kosterman, R., Hawkins, J. D., Guo, J., Catalano, R. F., & Abbott, R. D. (2000). The dynamics of alcohol and marijuana initiation: Patterns and predictors of first use in adolescence. *American Journal of Public Heath, 90,* 360–366.

Kosterman, R., Hawkins, J. D., Haggerty, K. P., Spoth, R., & Redmond, C. (2001). Preparing for the Drug-Free Years: Session-specific effects of a universal parent-training intervention with rural families. *Journal of Drug Education, 31,* 47–68.

Krauss, B. J., Godfrey, C., Yee, D., Goldsamt, L., Tiffany, J., Almeyda, L., Davis, W. R., Bula, E., Reardon, D., Jones, Y., DeJesus, J., Pride, J., Garcia, E., Pierre-Louis, M., Rivera, C., Troche, E., Daniels, T., O'Day, J., & Velez, R. (2000). Saving our children from a silent epidemic: The PATH program for parents and preadolescents. In W. Pequegnat & J. Szapocznik (Eds.), *Working with families in the era of HIV/AIDS* (pp. 89–112). Thousand Oaks, CA: Sage.

Kulis, S., Marsiglia, F. F., Elek, E., Dustman, P., Wagstaff, D. A., & Hecht, M. L. (2005). Mexican/Mexican American adolescents and keepin' in R.E.A.L.: An evidence–based substance use prevention program. *Children and Schools, 27,* 133–145.

Kumpfer, K. L., & Whiteside, H. O. (2000). *Strengthening families program.* Salt Lake City, UT: Department of Health Promotion and Education, University of Utah.

Kung, E. M., & Farrell, A. D. (2000). The role of parents and peers in early adolescent substance use: An examination of mediating and moderating effects. *Journal of Child and Family Studies, 9,* 509–528.

Lee Van Horn, M., Hawkins, J. D., Arthur, M. W. & Catalano, R. F. (2007). Assessing community effects on ado-lescent substance use and delinquency. *Journal of Community Psychology*, 35(8), 925–946.

Lewis, R. A., Piercy, F. P., Sprenkle, D. H., & Trepper, T. S. (1990). Family-based interventions for helping drug-abusing adolescents. *Journal of Adolescent Research, 5,* 82–95.

Liddle, H. A. (2002) Advances in family-based therapy for adolescent substance abuse. In L. S. Harris (Ed), *Problems of drug dependence 2001: Proceedings of the 63rd Annual Scientific Meeting* (pp. 113–115; NIDA Monograph no. 182; NIH Publication no. 02–5097). Bethesda, MD: National Institute on Drug Abuse.

Liddle, H. A., Dakof, G. A., Parker, K., Diamond, G. S., Barrett, K., & Tejeda, M. (2001). Multidimensional fam-ily therapy for adolescent substance abuse: Results of a randomized clinical trial. *American Journal of Drug and Alcohol Abuse, 27,* 651–688.

Liddle, H. A., Rowe, C. L., Dakof, G. A., Ungaro, R. A., & Henderson, C. E. (2004). Early intervention for ado-lescent substance abuse: Pretreatment to posttreatment outcomes of a randomized controlled trial comparing Multidimensional Family Therapy and peer group treatment. *Journal of Psychoactive Drugs, 36*(1), 2–37.

Longshore, D., Ellickson., P. L., McCaffrey, D. F., & St. Clair, P. A. (2007). School-based drug prevention among at-risk adolescents: Effects of ALERT Plus. *Health Education and Behavior, 34*(4), 651–668.

Lynskey, M. T., Heath, A. C., Nelson, E. C., Bucholz, K. K., Madden, P.A.F., Slutske, W. S., Statham, D. J., & Martin, N. G. (2002). Genetic and environmental contributions to cannabis dependence in a national young adult twin sample. *Psychological Medicine, 32,* 195–207.

MacKinnon, D. P., Johnson, C. A., Pentz, M. A., Dwyer, J. H., Hansen, W. B., Flay, B. R., & Wang, E.Y. I. (1991). Mediating mechanisms in a school-based drug prevention program: First-year effects of the Midwestern Pre-vention Project. *Health Psychology, 10,* 164–172.

MacLean, S., & d'Abbs, P. (2002). Petrol sniffing in Aboriginal communities: A review of interventions. *Drug and Alcohol Review, 21,* 51–58.

Marsiglia, F. F., Kulis, S., Wagstaff, D. A., Elek, E., & Dran, D. (2005). Acculturation status and substance use prevention with Mexican and Mexican American youth. *Journal of Social Work Practice in the Addictions, 5,* 85–111.

Mason, W. A., Kosterman, R., Hawkins, J. D., Haggerty, K. P., & Spoth, R. (2003). Reducing adolescents' growth in substance use and delinquency: Randomized trial effects of a preventive parent-training interven-tion. *Prevention Science, 4,* 203–213.

McCluskey, C. P., Krohn, M. D., Lizotte, A. J., & Rodriguez, M. L. (2002). Early substance use and school achieve-ment: An examination of Latino, White, and African-American youth. *Journal of Drug Issues, 32,* 921–943.

McDermott, D. (1984). The relationship of parental drug use and parents' attitude concerning adolescent drug use to adolescent drug use. *Adolescence, 19,* 89–97.

Mercado, M. (2000). The invisible family: Counseling Asian American substance abusers and their families. *Family Journal, 8,* 267–272.

Mihalic, S., Irwin, K., Elliott, D., Fagan, A., & Hansen, D. (2001). *Blueprints for violence prevention*. Washington, DC: Office of Juvenile Justice and Delinquency Prevention.

Miller, W. R., & Willbourne, P. L. (2002). Mesa grande: a methodological analysis of clinical trials of treatments for alcohol disorders. *Addiction, 97,* 265–277.

Moran, J. R., & Reaman, J. A. (2002). Critical issues for substance abuse prevention targeting American Indian youth. *Journal of Primary Prevention, 22,* 201–233.

Moskowitz, J., Schaps, E., Schaeffer, G., & Malvin, J. (1984). Evaluation of a substance abuse prevention pro-gram for junior high school students. *International Journal of the Addictions, 19,* 419–430.

Muck, R., Zempolich, K. A., Titus, J. C., Fishman, M., Godley, M. D., & Schwebel, R. (2001). An overview of the effectiveness of adolescent substance abuse treatment models. *Youth and Society, 33,* 143–168.

Musher-Eizenman, D. R., Holub, S. C., & Arnett, M. (2003). Attitude and peer influences on adolescent sub-stance use: The moderating effect of age, sex and substance. *Journal of Drug Education, 33*(1), 1–23.

Nation, M., & Heflinger, C. A. (2006). Risk factors for serious alcohol and drug use: The role of psychosocial variables in predicting the frequency of substance use among adolescents. *American Journal of Drug and Alcohol Abuse, 32,* 415–433.

National Institute on Drug Abuse. (1997). *Preventing drug abuse among children and adolescents: A research-based guide for parents, educators, and community leaders*. Bethesda, MD: National Institute on Drug Abuse.

National Institute on Drug Abuse. (2001). Monitoring the Future. Rockville, MD: National Institutes of Health. Retrieved April 18, 2008, from www.icpst.umich.edu/SAMHDA/das.html.

National Institute on Drug Abuse. (2003). *Preventing drug abuse among children and adolescents: A research-based guide for parents, educators, and community leaders* (NIH Publication No. 04-4212B). Bethesda, MD: National Institute on Drug Abuse.

Newcomb, M. D. (1995). Identifying high-risk youth: Prevalence and patterns of adolescent drug abuse. In E. Rahdert & D. Chzechowicz (Eds.), *Adolescent drug abuse: Clinical assessment and therapeutic interventions* (National Institute on Drug Abuse Research Monograph 156; DHHS Pub. No. 95-3908).Washington, DC: National Institutes of Health, National Institute on Drug Abuse.

O'Donnell, J., Hawkins, J. D., Catalano, R. F., Abbott, R. D., & Day, L. E. (1995). Preventing school failure, drug use, and delinquency among low-income children: Long-term intervention in elementary schools. *American Journal of Orthopsychiatry, 65,* 87-100.

Oetting, E. R., & Beauvais, F. (1986). Peer cluster theory: Drugs and the adolescent. *Journal of Counseling and Development, 65,* 17-22.

Oman, R. F., Vesely, S. K., Tolma, E., Aspy, C., Rodine, S., & Marshall, L. (2007). Does family structure matter in the relationships between youth assets and youth alcohol, drug and tobacco use? *Journal of Research on Adolescence, 17*(4), 743-766.

Orlando, M., Ellickson, P. L., McCaffrey, D. F., & Longshore, D. (2005). Understanding the impact of a school-based drug prevention program: The role of program-targeted intervening variables. *Prevention Science, 6,* 35-46.

Ozechowski, T. J., & Liddle, H. A. (2000). Family-based therapy for adolescent drug abuse: Knowns and unknowns. *Clinical Child and Family Psychology Review, 3,* 269-298.

Pantin, H., Coatsworth, J. D., Feaster, D. J., Newman, F. L., Briones, E., Prado, G., Schwartz, S. J., & Szapocznik, J. (2003). Familias Unidas: The efficacy of an intervention to promote parental investment in Hispanic immigrant families. *Prevention Science, 4,* 189-201.

Park, J., Kosterman, R., Hawkins, J. D., Haggerty, K. P., Duncan, T. E., Duncan, S. C., & Spoth, R. (2000). Effects of the "Preparing for the Drug-Free Years" curriculum on growth in alcohol use and risk for alcohol use in early adolescence. *Prevention Science, 1,* 125-138.

Parks, G. A., Marlatt, G. A., & Anderson, B. K. (2004). Cognitive-behavioral alcohol treatment. In N. Heather & T. Stockwell (Eds.), *The essential handbook of treatment and prevention of alcohol problems.* Chichester, England: Wiley.

Paxton, R. J., Valois, R. F., & Drane, J. W. (2007). Is there a relationship between family structure and substance use among public middle school students? *Journal of Child and Family Studies, 16,* 593-605.

Pentz, M. A., MacKinnon, D. P., Dwyer, J. H., Wang, E.Y.I., Hansen, W. B., Flay, B. R., & Johnson, C. A. (1989). Longitudinal effects of the Midwestern Prevention Project on regular and experimental smoking in adolescents. *Preventive Medicine, 18,* 304-321.

Pentz, M. A., MacKinnon, D. P., Flay, B. R., Hansen, W. B., Johnson, C. A., & Dwyer, J. H. (1989). Primary prevention of chronic diseases in adolescence: Effects of Midwestern Prevention Project on tobacco use. *American Journal of Epidemiology, 130,* 713-724.

Pentz, M. A., Trebow, E. A., Hansen, W. B., MacKinnon, D. P., Dwyer, J. H., Johnson, C. A., Flay, B. R., Daniels, S., & Cormack, C. (1990). Effects of program implementation on adolescent drug use behavior: The Midwestern Prevention Project (MPP). *Evaluation Review, 14,* 264-289.

Perez, D. M. (2000). The relationship between physical abuse, sexual victimization, and adolescent illicit drug use. *Journal of Drug Issues, 30*(3), 641-662.

Petoskey, E. L., Van Stelle, K. R., & De Jong, J. A. (1998). Prevention through empowerment in a Native American community. *Drugs and Society, 12,* 147-162.

Pires, P., & Jenkins, J. M. (2007). A growth curve analysis of the joint influences of parenting affect, child characteristics and deviant peers on adolescent illicit drug use. *Journal of Youth and Adolescence, 36,* 169-183.

Prado, G., Pantin, H., Briones, E., Schwartz, S., Feaster, D., Huang, S., Sullivan, S., Tapia, M., Sabillon, E., Lopez, B., & Szapocznik, J. (2007). A randomized controlled trial of a parent-centered intervention in preventing substance use and HIV risk behaviors in Hispanic adolescents. *Journal of Consulting and Clinical Psychology, 75,* 914-926.

Rao, U. (2006). Links between depression and substance abuse in adolescents. *American Journal of Preventive Medicine, 31,* 161–174.

Redmond, C., Spoth, R., Shin, C., & Lepper, H. (1999). Modeling long-term parent outcomes of two universal family-focused preventive interventions: One year follow-up results. *Journal of Consulting and Clinical Psychology, 67,* 975–984.

Resnick, M. D., Bearman, P. S., Blum, R. W., Bauman, K. E., Harris, K. M., Jones, J., Tabor, J., Beuhring, T., Sieving, R. E., Shew, M., Ireland, M., Bearinger, L. H., & Udry, J. R. (1997). Protecting adolescents from harm: Findings from the National Longitudinal Study on Adolescent Health. *Journal of the American Medical Association, 278*(10), 823–833.

Resnicow, K., Baranowski, T., Ahluwalia, J. S., & Braithwaite, R. L. (1999). Cultural sensitivity in public health: Defined and demystified. *Ethnicity and Disease, 9,* 10–21.

Resnicow, K., Soler, R., Braithwaite, R. L., Ahluwalia, J. S., & Butler, J. (2000). Cultural sensitivity in substance use prevention: Bridging the gap between research and practice in community-based substance abuse prevention. *Journal of Community Psychology, 28,* 271–290.

Robbins, M. S., Schwartz, S., & Szapocznik, J. (2003). Structural ecosystems therapy with Hispanic adolescents exhibiting disruptive behavior disorders. In J. Ancis (Ed.), *Culturally-responsive interventions for working with diverse populations and culture-bound syndromes* (pp. 71–99). New York: Brunner-Routledge.

Roberts, R. E., Roberts, C. R., & Xing, Y. (2007). Comorbidity of substance use disorders and other psychiatric disorders among adolescents: Evidence from an epidemiologic survey. *Drug and Alcohol Dependence, 88,* 4–13.

Rosello, J., & Bernal, G. (1999). Treatment of depression in Puerto Rican adolescents: The efficacy of cognitive-behavioral and interpersonal treatments. *Journal of Consulting and Clinical Psychology*, *67,* 734–745.

Roth, J. L., & Brooks-Gunn, J. (2003). What exactly is a youth development program? Answers from research and practice. *Applied Developmental Science, 7,* 94–111.

Rotheram-Borus, M. J., Song, J., Gwadz, M., Lee, M. B., Van Rossem, R., & Koopman, C. (2003). Reductions in HIV risk among runaway youth. *Prevention Science, 4,* 179–188.

Rowe, C. L., & Liddle, H. A. (2003). Substance abuse. *Journal of Marital and Family Therapy, 29,* 97–120.

Ryan, L. G., Miller-Loessi, K., & Nieri, T. (2007). Relationships with adults as predictors of substance use, gang involvement, and threats to safety among disadvantaged urban high school adolescents. *Journal of Community Psychology, 35*(8), 1053–1071.

Sale, E., Sambrano, S., Springer, J. F., & Turner, C. W. (2003). Risk, protection, and substance use in adolescents: A multi-site model. *Journal of Drug Education, 33*(1), 91–105.

Sandhu, D. S. (1997). Psychocultural profiles of Asian and Pacific Islander Americans: Implications for counseling and psychotherapy. *Journal of Multicultural Counseling and Development, 25,* 7–22.

Schinke, S. P., Tepavac, L., & Cole, K. D. (2000). Preventing substance use among Native American youth: Three-year results. *Addictive Behaviors, 25,* 387–397.

Shoptaw, S., Rotheram-Fuller, E., Yang, X., Frosch, D., Nahom, D., Jarvik, M. E., Rawson, R. A., & Ling, W. (2002). Smoking cessation in methadone maintenance. *Addiction, 97,* 1317–1328.

Simons-Morton, B. (2007). Social influences on substance use. *American Journal of Health Behavior, 31*(6), 672–684.

Spoth, R. L., Clair, S., Shin, C., & Redmond, C. (2006). Long-term effects of universal preventive interventions on methamphetamine use among adolescents. *Archives of Pediatric Adolescent Medicine, 160,* 876–882.

Spoth, R., Redmond, C., & Shin, C. (2000). Reducing adolescents' aggressive and hostile behaviors: Randomized trial effects of a brief family intervention four years past baseline. *Archives of Pediatrics and Adolescent Medicine, 154,* 1248–1257.

Spoth, R., Redmond, C., & Shin, C. (2001). Randomized trial of brief family interventions for general populations: Adolescent substance use outcomes four years following baseline. *Journal of Consulting and Clinical Psychology, 69,* 627–642.

Spoth, R. L., Redmond, C., Trudeau, L., & Shin, C. (2002). Longitudinal substance initiation outcomes for a universal preventive intervention combining family and school programs. *Psychology of Addictive Behaviors, 16,* 129–134.

Spoth, R., Reyes, M. L., Redmond, C., & Shin, C. (1999). Assessing a public health approach to delay onset and progression of adolescent substance use: Latent transition and loglinear analyses of longitudinal family preventive intervention outcomes. *Journal of Consulting and Clinical Psychology, 67,* 619–630.

Stephens, R. S., Roffman R. A., & Curtin, L. (2000). Comparison of extended versus brief treatments for marijuana use. *Journal of Consulting and Clinical Psychology, 68,* 898–908.

Substance Abuse and Mental Health Services Administration. (2007). *Results from the 2006 National Survey on Drug Use and Health: National findings* (NSDUH Series H-32, DHHS Publication No. SMA 07–4293). Rockville, MD: Office of Applied Studies.

Sue, S. (1998). In search of cultural competence in psychotherapy and counseling. *American Psychologist, 53,* 440–448.

Sue, D. W., & Sue, D. (2003). *Counseling the culturally diverse: Theory and practice* (4th ed.). New York: Wiley.

Sue, S., & Zane, N. (1987). The role of culture and cultural techniques in psychotherapy. *American Psychologist, 42,* 37–45.

Sun, W., Skara, S., Sun, P., Dent, C. W., & Sussman, S. (2006). Project Towards No Drug Abuse: Long-term substance use outcome evaluation. *Preventative Medicine, 42,* 188–192.

Sussman, S., Dent, C. W., & Stacy, A. W. (2002). Project towards no drug abuse: A review of the findings and future directions. *American Journal of Health Behavior, 26*(5), 354–365.

Swadi, H. (1999). Individual risk factors for adolescent substance use. *Drug and Alcohol Dependence, 55,* 209–224.

Szapocznik, J., Kurtines, W. M., Foote, F., Perez-Vidal, A., & Hervis, O. (1986). Conjoint versus one-person family therapy: Further evidence for the effectiveness of conducting family therapy through one person with drug-abusing adolescents. *Journal of Consulting and Clinical Psychology, 54,* 395–397.

Szapocznik, J., Lopez, B., Prado, G., Schwartz, S., & Pantin, H. (2006). Outpatient drug abuse treatment for Hispanic adolescents. *Drug and Alcohol Dependence, 84,* S54–S63.

Szobot, C. M., & Bukstein, O. (2008). Attention hyperactivity disorder and substance use disorders. *Journal of Child and Adolescent Psychiatric Clinics, 17,* 309–323.

Tebes, J. K., Feinn, R., Vanderploeg, J. J., Chinman, M. J., Shepard, J., Brabham, T., Genovese, M., & Connell, C. (2007). Impact of a positive youth development program in urban after-school settings on the prevention of adolescent substance use. *Journal of Adolescent Health, 41*(3), 239–247.

Tobler, N. S. (1986). Meta–analysis of 143 adolescent drug prevention programs: Quantitative outcome results of program participants compared to a control or comparison group. *Journal of Drug Issues, 16,* 537–567.

Tobler, N. S., Roona, M. R., Ochshorn, P., Marshall, D. G., Streke, A. V., & Stackpole, K. M. (2000). School-based adolescent drug prevention programs: 1998 Meta-analysis. *Journal of Primary Prevention, 20,* 275–336.

Trudeau, L., Azevedo, K., Spoth, R., & Randall, G. K. (2007). Longitudinal effects of a universal family-focused intervention on growth patterns of adolescent internalizing symptoms and polysubstance use: Gender comparisons. *Journal of Youth and Adolescence, 36*(6), 740–745.

Vakalahi, H. F. (2001). Adolescent substance use and family-based risk and protective factors: A literature review. *Journal of Drug Education, 31*(1), 29–46.

Van Horn, M. L., Hawkins, J. D., Arthur, M. W., & Catalano, R. F. (2007). Assessing community effects on adolescent substance use and delinquency. *Journal of Community Psychology, 35*(8), 925–946.

Vega, W. A., Alderete, E., Kolody, B., & Aguilar-Gaxiola, S. (1998). Illicit drug use among Mexicans and Mexican Americans in California: The effects of gender and acculturation. *Addiction, 93,* 1839–1850.

Vega, W. A., Gil, A., & Kolody, B. (2002). What do we know about Latino drug use?: Methodological evaluation of state databases. *Hispanic Journal of Behavioral Sciences, 24,* 395–408.

Vitaro, F., Dobkin, P., & Tremblay, R. (1994). A school-based program for the prevention of substance abuse. *International Journal of Psychology, 29,* 431–452.

Wagner, E. F., Tubman, J. G., & Gil, A. G. (2004). Implementing school-based substance abuse interventions: Methodological dilemmas and recommended solutions. *Addiction, 99,* 106–119.

Waldron, H. B., Slesnick, N., Brody, J. L., Turner, C. W., & Peterson, T. R. (2001). Treatment outcomes for adolescent substance abuse at 4- and 7-month assessments. *Journal of Consulting and Clinical Psychology, 69,* 802–813.

Waldron, H. B., Turner, C. W., & Ozechowski, T. J. (2006). Profiles of change in behavioral and family interventions for adolescent substance abuse and dependence. In H. A. Liddle & C. L. Rowe (Eds.), *Adolescent substance abuse: Research and clinical advances* (pp. 357–374). New York: Cambridge University Press.

Warner, L. A., Valdez, A., Canino, G., de la Rosa, M., & Turner, R. J. (2006). Hispanic drug abuse in an evolving cultural context: An agenda for research. *Drug Alcohol Dependence, 84*, S8–S16.

Weinberg, N. Z. (2001). Risk factors of adolescent substance abuse. *Journal of Learning Disabilities, 34*(4), 343–351.

Weiss, F., & Nicholson, H. (1998). Friendly PEERsuasion against substance use: The Girls Incorporated model and evaluation. *Drugs and Society, 12*, 7–22.

Winstanley, E. L., Steinwachs, D. M., Ensminger, M. E., Latkin, C. A., Stitzer, M. L., & Olsen, Y. (2008). The association of self-reported neighborhood disorganization and social capital with adolescent alcohol and drug use, dependence and access to treatment. *Drug and Alcohol Dependence, 92*, 173–182.

Winters, K. C., Stinchfield, R. D., Opland, E., Weller., C., & Latimer, W. W. (2000). The effectiveness of the Minnesota Model approach in the treatment of adolescent drug abusers. *Addiction, 85*, 601–612.

Zane, N., Aoki, B., Ho, T., Huang, L., & Jang, M. (1998). Dosage-related changes in a culturally-responsive prevention program for Asian American youth. *Drugs and Society, 12*, 105–125.

CHAPTER

ADOLESCENT VIOLENCE: RISK, RESILIENCE, AND PREVENTION

SARAH E. KRETMAN ▪ MARC A. ZIMMERMAN ▪ SUSAN MORREL-SAMUELS ▪ DARRELL HUDSON

LEARNING OBJECTIVES

After studying this chapter, you will be able to

▪ Analyze the scope of adolescent violence in the United States.

▪ Consider how and why violence disproportionately affects particular subgroups.

▪ Discover popular frameworks (models) used to study adolescent violence and guide prevention efforts.

Adolescent violence remains a serious public health problem. Despite a relative decrease in the prevalence of violence among adolescents compared with the peak rates of the early 1990s, violence continues to be a major contributor to the premature mortality and morbidity of adolescents and young adults throughout the United States. The Centers for Disease Control and Prevention (CDC, 2004) noted that *adolescent violence* includes aggressive behaviors (such as verbal abuse, bullying, hitting, slapping, or fighting) that do not generally result in serious injury or death, but do have significant consequences on adolescent health nonetheless. Although researchers often conflate violent behavior with verbal abuse, delinquency, and less serious aggressive behavior, this chapter focuses on violent behavior and attitudes that are associated with physical assault.

EPIDEMIOLOGY

According to the CDC, homicide is the second leading cause of death overall for young people aged ten through twenty (CDC, 2007a). In 2005, the CDC documented 2,777 homicides among youth in this age group, an average of over seven murders per day (CDC, 2007b). While most epidemiologic data focus on homicide, violence accounts for a large proportion of injuries among adolescents. In 2005, more than 490,000 youths aged ten to twenty sustained violence-related injuries, and over 47,000 were hospitalized as a result of such injuries (CDC, 2007a).

Adolescents are most frequently victimized by their peers. According to estimates by the Bureau of Justice Statistics (2005), youth aged twelve through twenty years are offenders in approximately 66 percent of all assaults on others of their age group. In 2005, youth aged ten to twenty-four accounted for approximately 44 percent of all violent crime arrests and 50 percent of all murder arrests (Federal Bureau of Investigation [FBI], 2007), although they only accounted for 21 percent of the total population (U.S. Census Bureau, 2006).

Race and ethnicity were not significant predictors of adolescents' violence victimization after controlling for family and community characteristics.

Members of racial and ethnic minorities are at even greater risk of being victims or perpetrators of adolescent violence. Among ten- to twenty-year-olds, homicide is the leading cause of death for African Americans, accounting for just over 40 percent of all deaths (CDC, 2007a). African Americans ages ten through nineteen have homicide victimization rates approximately ten times higher than their white counterparts (Bernard, Paulozzi, & Wallace, 2007). In this age group, homicide has been identified as the second leading cause of death for Hispanics and the third leading cause of death for Native Americans, Alaskan Natives, Asian Pacific Islanders, and Caucasians (CDC, 2007a). Although racial disparities in violence victimization exist, Lauritsen (2003) found that race and ethnicity were not significant predictors of adolescents' violence victimization after controlling for family and community characteristics.

This chapter is supported by two grants from the Centers for Disease Control and Prevention made to the Prevention Research Center of Michigan and Youth Empowerment Solutions.

Differences between genders are also striking, because adolescent violence disproportionately affects males. In 2005, of the 4,717 victims of homicide between the ages of nine and twenty-four, nearly 86 percent were male (FBI, 2007). Overall, homicide is the second leading cause of death among males between the ages of ten and twenty, but the fourth leading cause of death among females of this age group (CDC, 2007a). Males are also more likely to be arrested for violent crimes. In 2005, for example, males accounted for 83 percent of all violent crime arrests and 91 percent of all murder arrests among youth ages ten to twenty-four (FBI, 2007). Males report participating in physical fighting at higher rates (43 percent) than females (28 percent) over a twelve-month period (CDC, 2007c). Males also witness interpersonal violence more frequently than females (CDC, 2004). Many researchers point to differences in the socialization of males and females as one reason for these differences (Graves, 2005).

Recently, much attention has been given to a perceived increase in female violent behavior, but not all researchers agree that this increase has actually occurred. According to arrest data from the FBI (2007) the number of juvenile arrests among both males and females has actually been decreasing. For females under the age of eighteen, the number of arrests for violent crime went down 10 percent over the ten-year period from 1996 through 2005. And over the same period of time, the number of juvenile male violent crime arrests decreased by 27 percent. This difference suggests that violent crime may be declining more slowly for females than males. In the 1990s, the number of females arrested in the United States increased; however, during the same time period their self-reported violent behaviors did not show the same trend. Chesney-Lind and Belknap (2004) argue that females' violent behaviors may not be increasing; rather, they are being arrested more often for the aggressive behaviors that they were already exhibiting. In a qualitative study of violence in high schools, Astor, Meyer, and Behre (1999) found that girls were both the perpetrators and the victims in about half of the violence-related incidents in the schools reported by students, teachers, and administrators participating in the study. They also found that teachers and administrators responded differently to violence perpetrated by males and females and were less likely to take females' violent behavior seriously.

Adolescent violence has significant economic implications as well, and the costs are far broader than simple medical expenditures. The World Health Organization (WHO, 2004) reported that violence-related costs account for about 3 percent of the gross national product for the United States. For those ages fifteen to twenty-four, the total costs of interpersonal violence (including medical costs and lost productivity) are estimated to be more than $13 billion per year (Corso, Mercy, Simon, Finkelstein, & Miller, 2007). It has been estimated that the average assault costs over $8,500 for persons under eighteen years of age who reside in urban areas, while urban victims of murder under age eighteen incur a societal cost that averages over $4 million in combined medical expenses, lost earnings, and diminished quality of life for survivors (Miller, Fisher, & Cohen, 2001).

KEY CONCEPTS

In view of the substantial economic and human costs associated with adolescent violence, effective prevention is vital. Interventions can be implemented in many contexts, such as in schools, homes, neighborhoods, or hospitals. Schools may be an ideal setting for implementation of violence prevention programs, because a large percentage of adolescents spend much of their day in school. Schools are also settings in which violence may occur or where negative social interactions that may precede violence are initiated. Many of the prevention programs related to violence have taken a more traditional, deficit-oriented approach, which focuses on ameliorating risks associated with adolescent violence while largely overlooking opportunities to enhance positive factors in youths' lives. Emerging research on resiliency theory offers an alternative perspective. Application of resiliency theory to the problem of adolescent violence focuses attention on enhancing assets and resources (promotive factors) as a prevention strategy. In this chapter, we discuss both the deficit and the resiliency perspectives on adolescent violence and provide examples of school-based violence prevention interventions based on each perspective.

Schools as a Context for Effective Violence Prevention

In a recent report, the members of the Task Force on Community Preventive Services (a federally funded but independent organization of experts assembled by the CDC) described their meta-analysis studying the effectiveness of universal school-based violence prevention programs. The task force members concluded that there was strong evidence that universal school-based interventions effectively reduce violent behavior across all age groups of school children (resulting in a median of a 15 percent reduction in violent behavior) and that these programs appear to be cost-effective (Hahn et al., 2007a). In their review, the task force members also reported that many of the violence prevention programs had other positive effects, including reductions in drug use and delinquency and improvements in school attendance and achievement.

The task force's findings are supported by Wilson and Lipsey (2007), who reported similar results from their meta-analysis of school-based programs. They found evidence that both universal interventions and selected or indicated interventions (geared toward high-risk students) are effective at reducing violent behavior (with effect sizes of 0.21 and 0.29, respectively). The studies included in Wilson and Lipsey's meta-analysis differ substantially from the studies included in the task force's review, with only about half the studies being included in both meta-analyses. Because of the varying interventions included in each sample, the studies can serve as a sensitivity analysis for each other, and the similarity of their findings provides further evidence for the effectiveness of school-based interventions (Hahn et al., 2007b).

School-based interventions can employ multiple strategies to reduce violence, such as working at an individual level to change behavior or build social skills, working to change the school and/or classroom environment, or offering peer mediation services. The task force members found that all intervention types were effective, but the median effect size for the different types of interventions varied from a 60 percent reduction in violence for peer mediation programs to a 14 percent reduction for cognitive or affective programs (Hahn et al., 2007a). Hahn et al. (2007a) caution, however, that these results are only suggestive of differences in effect sizes because some intervention types had only a few data points (the median effect size for peer mediation interventions was based on only four data points), and no inferential statistical analysis was conducted to compare the effects of the different intervention types. Wilson and Lipsey (2007), in contrast, found no difference in effect sizes among the different intervention modalities in their statistical analysis. They suggest that schools choose the strategy easiest for them to implement with high fidelity.

Notably, Wilson and Lipsey (2007) reported that the comprehensive, multicomponent programs that they included in their review of school-based programs were not associated with a reduction in violent behavior. They pointed out, however, that the comprehensive programs reviewed tended to be long-term, low-frequency programs, and that their lack of effectiveness may be a result of their low intensity compared to the relative high intensity of noncomprehensive programs. Other researchers have reached different conclusions about the effectiveness of comprehensive programs. In their review of the characteristics of effective prevention programs, Nation et al. (2003) found that effective programs were comprehensive and included multiple interventions in multiple settings. The authors of a CDC guide to violence prevention interventions also recommend that violence prevention programs involve multiple components (Thornton, Craft, Dahlberg, Lynch, & Baer, 2002).

The Deficit-Oriented Perspective

Researchers have typically emphasized a *deficit-oriented approach* to adolescent problem behaviors, cataloging risk factors and documenting their adverse effects on healthy adolescent development (Dryfoos, 1990). They have studied risk factors for psychopathology, alcohol and drug abuse, and delinquency, concentrating on identifying vulnerable children. Problem behavior theory (Jessor & Jessor, 1977) and social influence models (Dishion & Loeber, 1985; Huba & Bentler, 1980; Needle et al., 1986) are examples of theories that focus on risk factors associated with negative outcomes for adolescents.

Researchers have traced the antecedents of adolescent violent behavior to a variety of individual, peer, family, and societal risk factors. Adolescents who have exhibited prior antisocial or aggressive behavior are at a higher risk of participating in violent behaviors, as are those who have a history of violence victimization (Dahlberg, 1998; Guerra, Huesmann, Tolan, & Van Acker, 1995; Huesmann, Eron, Lefkowitz, & Walder, 1984; Herrenkohl, Maguin, Hill, Hawkins, Abbott, & Catalano, 2000; Capaldi & Patterson, 1993; Loeber et al., 1993; Ellickson & McGuigan, 2000; Resnick, Ireland, & Borowsky, 2004; Vernberg, Jacobs, & Hershberger, 1999). Engaging in deviant behavior such as substance abuse or gang involvement or associating with peers who engage in deviant behavior also puts youth at a greater risk (Resnick et al., 1997; Saner & Ellickson, 1996; Dukarm, Byrd, Auinger, & Weitzman, 1996; Rainone, Schmeidler, Frank, & Smith, 2006; Herrenkohl et al., 2000). Lower academic and problem-solving skills are also associated with increase in violent behavior (Resnick et al., 1997; Resnick et al., 2004; Pepler & Slaby, 1994). Researchers have also found that normative beliefs about violence are associated with violent behavior. Adolescents who have positive beliefs about violence, who have parents who have favorable attitudes about violence, or who attend schools where students hold positive normative views about violence are also at a higher risk for violence perpetration (Jemmott, Jemmott, Hines, & Fong, 2001; Vernberg et al., 1999; Herrenkohl et al., 2000; Orpinas, Murray, & Kelder, 1999; Fagan & Wilkinson, 1998). Those who have low levels of parental monitoring and involvement, who experience parental conflict, or who witness domestic violence are also more likely to engage in violent behavior (Ary et al., 1999; Orpinas et al., 1999; Herrenkohl, Hill, Hawkins, Chung, & Nagin, 2006; Osofsky, 1999). Researchers have also found that adolescents living in neighborhoods characterized by poverty, unemployment, easy access to weapons, and crowded, deteriorated housing are at a higher risk for engaging in violent behavior (Dahlberg, 1998; Guerra et al., 1995; McLloyd, 1990; Greenberg & Schneider, 1994).

Researchers have traced the antecedents of adolescent violent behavior to a variety of individual, peer, family, and societal risk factors.

Researchers working from the deficit-oriented perspective also focus on risks when creating behavioral interventions to address adolescent problem behavior. Traditional intervention programs generally attempt to reduce risks for a single problem behavior. In violence prevention programs, this often takes the form of teaching skills such as anger management and conflict resolution strategies. The Peacemakers Program, for example, is a universal, school-based program for individual students in grades four to eight (Shapiro, Burgoon, Welker, & Clough, 2002). It is intended to reduce social norms that promote violence and address conflict-related psychosocial skill deficits, reflecting a more traditional risk reduction approach. The program consists of a seventeen-session curriculum delivered by teachers in a classroom setting. Throughout the program, participants learn the application of the golden rule (treat other people the way you want them to treat you). The first few sessions focus on promoting antiviolence norms, and the remaining sessions allow students to learn and practice several conflict-related psychosocial skills, including problem solving, conflict avoidance, assertiveness, communication skills, and specific conflict resolution strategies. The intervention also includes manuals for teachers and school counselors, providing them with strategies for integrating and reinforcing the Peacemakers curriculum throughout the school day.

The evaluation of the Peacemakers Program followed students in four intervention schools (two middle and two elementary schools) and compared them to controls in two schools (one elementary and one middle school). The outcome measures were student self-reports of knowledge of psychosocial skills, self-reports and teacher reports of aggressive behavior, use of mediation services, and school reports of violence- and aggression-related disciplinary actions. These outcomes were assessed at the beginning of the school year, and the program was implemented during the first semester. The outcomes were assessed again during the second semester of the same year, immediately following program implementation. The researchers found that the youth in the intervention schools demonstrated improvements in knowledge of violence-related psychosocial skills and also reported less aggressive behavior. Teachers in the intervention schools also reported less aggressive behavior among the students, and students in the intervention schools were less likely to be involved in aggression-related disciplinary incidents or to receive a suspension for violent behavior. The strongest effects were found for boys and for middle school students (grades six to eight). The fact that the intervention had differential effects for males and females highlights the need to study differences in violence-related processes between the genders. The evaluation, however, only assessed outcomes immediately following implementation; thus, the sustained effects of the intervention remain unknown.

SMART Talk (Students Managing Anger and Resolution Together) is an interactive, multicomponent computer program that teaches sixth-, seventh-, and eighth-grade students anger management, perspective taking, and conflict resolution (Bosworth, Espelange, DuBay, & Daytner, 2000). It is based on social learning theory, developmental theory, and Aggression Replacement Training. The computer program includes interactive interviews, games, and video clips, allowing users to assess their own anger triggers, to consider multiple perspectives in conflict situations, and to learn and practice conflict resolution strategies. Users are able to control which components of the program they utilize. SMART Talk is unique in its interactive, multimedia approach, allowing users to move at their own pace and requiring little training for teachers. Bosworth, Espelange, DuBay, and Daytner (2000) tested the program in a large middle school. At the beginning of the school year, students at the middle school were randomly assigned to teams. Each team consisted of several classes of students, and students from different teams had little interaction with one another during the school day. Teams were randomly assigned to either an intervention or a control group. Sixth-, seventh-, and eighth-grade students in the intervention group had access to the program for thirteen weeks on classroom computers. The computer program tracked each student's use of the intervention. Outcome assessments included student self-reports of beliefs supportive of violence, self-awareness, self-efficacy, intentions to use nonviolent strategies, and aggressive behavior. Students were assessed at baseline and four months after the implementation of the intervention. Students in the intervention condition reported greater reductions in beliefs supportive of violent behavior and increases in intentions to use nonviolent strategies compared to those in the control group. Bosworth et al. (2000), however, did not find any significant differences in aggressive behaviors between the control and intervention conditions. Unfortunately, this evaluation also had limited long-term follow-up and was based on self-reported data from students in one middle school, limiting the generalizability of the results. Both Peacemakers and SMART Talk may be considered deficit-oriented approaches to violence prevention, because they are designed to address skill deficits by teaching students conflict resolution and anger management strategies.

Botvin, Griffin, and Nichols (2006) described another school-based intervention in which a preexisting general skill-building program, Life Skills Training (LST), was adapted to address substance abuse and violent behavior. LST is designed to address demographic, environmental, interpersonal and intrapersonal risk factors associated with violent behavior and substance abuse by teaching cognitive-behavioral skills related to communicating effectively, developing healthy relationships with others, decreasing anxiety, and enhancing self-esteem (Botvin, Baker, Dusenbury, Botvin, & Diaz, 1995; Botvin, Schinke, Epstein, & Diaz, 1994). This adaptation of the LST curriculum included both general life skills taught as part of the traditional LST curriculum and lessons specifically geared toward substance abuse and violence prevention, such as conflict resolution, anger management, and assertiveness skills. When describing the program, Botvin et al. (2006, p. 403) noted that a "common set of demographic environmental, interpersonal and intrapersonal factors appears to be involved in the etiology of drug abuse and violence," and they listed the specific risk factors associated with violence. The LST intervention was designed to address these risk factors. In some ways, the LST curriculum has characteristics of a resiliency-based intervention, as it provides adolescents with skills to help them manage, resist, and avoid violence in their lives. Yet the framework used to design the program was deficit-oriented, because it focused on addressing risks related to violent behavior and substance use.

Botvin et al. (2006) compared sixth-grade students from the intervention schools to students from twenty-one control schools where the usual health curriculum was taught. The students were surveyed before the intervention began and then again three months after it had ended. Students in the intervention group reported less high-frequency fighting and less low- and high-frequency delinquency than their counterparts in the control group. The effects of the intervention were stronger when the researchers looked at a high-fidelity subsample of the intervention group composed only of students who received at least one-half of the intervention sessions, highlighting the importance of implementation fidelity to program effectiveness.

The Resiliency Model: An Alternative Approach

Although most researchers focus on risk factors associated with adolescent violent and other problem behaviors, they are able to explain only a limited amount of variance in these behaviors. Few studies exist that explore why this may be the case. Other investigators estimate that more than half of the youth exposed to risk factors do not end up with negative outcomes associated with these risks (Rutter, 1987; Garmezy, 1991). Researchers have suggested the need for further study of adolescents who possess risk factors but do not engage in problem behavior (Hawkins et al., 1992; Newcomb & Felix-Ortiz, 1992). *Resiliency theory* provides a theoretical framework for this strength-based approach, which helps explain why some youths grow up to be healthy adults in the face of adversity. Over the last two decades the concept of resiliency has received increasing attention in developmental psychology (Cicchetti & Garmezy, 1993; Fergus & Zimmerman, 2005; Luthar & Zelazo, 2003).

Researchers define *resilience* (or resiliency) as successful adaptation in the face of risk (Garmezy, 1991; Masten, 1994; Rutter, 1987; Werner, 1993). It refers to those *promotive factors*—individual assets or social resources—and processes that interrupt the trajectory from risk to problem behaviors or psychopathology. It is critical to note that both one or more risks and one or more promotive factors must be present in order for resiliency to occur. Promotive factors may work through one of several mechanisms to reduce or offset the adverse effects of risk factors (Zimmerman & Arunkumar, 1994). Garmezy, Masten, and Tellegen (1984) have described three basic models of resiliency: the compensatory model, the protective model, and the challenge model.

The *compensatory model* examines how different variables (called compensatory factors) may directly and independently reduce negative outcomes associated with risk factors. *Compensatory factors* are variables that neutralize exposure to risk or operate in a counteractive fashion against the potential negative consequences introduced by a risk (Garmezy et al., 1984; Masten et al., 1988). Both the risk and the compensatory factors contribute additively in the prediction of the outcome (Masten et al., 1988). An analysis of this model would examine the direct main effects of the compensatory factor on the outcome of interest in a linear regression analysis or the direct effects in a structural equation modeling (SEM) approach.

The *protective model,* a second model of resilience, examines whether protective factors modify the effects of risks in an interactive fashion (Rutter, 1985). Although they may have direct effects on outcomes, protective factors act mainly as moderators. Brook, Brook, Gordon, and Whiteman (1990) propose that effects may be associated with a risk-protective mechanism or a protective-protective mechanism. A *risk-protective variable* functions to lessen the negative effect of a risk factor, whereas protective-protective variables enhance the positive effects of promotive factors found to decrease negative outcomes. This model is evaluated by examining the interaction effects of the risk and protective factors using either multiplicative terms in a hierarchical regression analysis or multigroup analysis in SEM using the protective factor to define the groups (for example, median split).

A third model of resilience is the *challenge model* (Garmezy et al., 1984). In this model, the association between a risk factor and an outcome is curvilinear. This suggests that exposure to low levels and high levels of a risk factor are associated with negative outcomes, but moderate levels of the risk are related to less negative (or positive) outcomes (Luthar & Zelazo, 2003). The idea is that adolescents exposed to moderate levels of risk develop skills to overcome it, whereas very high levels of risk may overwhelm their capacity to adapt. Moderate levels of risk may therefore be beneficial, as long as the risk exposure is challenging enough to elicit a coping response, enabling the adolescent to learn from the process of overcoming the risk. In challenge models, the risk and promotive factors studied are the same variable; whether it is a risk or a promotive factor depends on the level of exposure. Too little family conflict, for example, may not give adolescents opportunities to learn how to cope with or solve interpersonal conflicts outside of the home, but too much conflict may be debilitating and lead adolescents to feel hopeless and distressed. A moderate amount of conflict, however, may provide adolescents with enough exposure to learn how to cope with conflict by observing how their family deals with conflicts. Challenge models of resilience are typically tested with polynomial terms in multiple regression (such as

A moderate amount of conflict may provide adolescents with enough exposure to learn how to cope with conflict by observing how their family deals with conflicts.

quadratic or cubic terms) or growth curve modeling (such as hierarchical linear modeling).

Researchers have applied all three models of resiliency when studying promotive factors related to youth violence. Using the compensatory model, they have found that prosocial beliefs have compensated for antisocial socialization (Huang, Kosterman, Catalano, Hawkins, & Abbott, 2001). Adolescent religiosity has compensated for interest in gang involvement, peer substance use, and exposure to violence (Barkin, Kreiter, & Durant, 2001; Howard, Qui, & Boekeloo, 2003). Researchers have also demonstrated the importance of parenting as a promotive factor. Parental support (either maternal or paternal or both) has compensated for exposure to violence, peer violent behavior, and getting into a fight (Zimmerman, Steinman, & Rowe, 1998; Howard et al., 2003). Parental monitoring has also been found to compensate for peer violent and delinquent behavior, risk-taking behavior, and living in a risky neighborhood (Howard et al., 2003; Zimmerman et al., 1998; Griffin et al., 1999). The presence of other adults may also play a role. Adolescents who report having adult mentors are less likely to carry a weapon, hurt others in a physical fight, or report gang membership (Beier, Rosenfeld, Spitalny, Zanzy, & Bontempo, 2000; DuBois & Silverthorn, 2005). Adolescents who participated in the Big Brothers Big Sisters mentoring program were also less likely to hit others when compared to randomly selected controls (Grossman & Tierney, 1998).

Researchers have also found assets and resources that compensate for adolescents' cumulative risk factors for violent behavior. Borowsky, Ireland, and Resnick (2002) found among 13,781 seventh- through twelfth-grade adolescents studied over two years that academic performance, parental presence, parent-family connectedness, and school connectedness—alone and in combination—compensated for the cumulative effects of prior violent behavior, violence victimization, substance use, and school problems on violent behavior. Other researchers have found that cumulative measures of assets and resources compensate for cumulative risk factors (Pollard, Hawkins, & Arthur, 1999; Stouthamer-Loeber, Loeber, Wei, Farrington, & Wikstrom, 2002).

Several researchers studying youth violence have also found support for the protective factor model. In one study, parental support protected adolescents from the risk factors of peer violent behavior, getting in a fight, and exposure to violence (Zimmerman et al., 1998). Other researchers have found that perceived social status was found to protect adolescents from peer delinquent behaviors (Prinstein, Boergers, & Spirito, 2001). Caldwell, Kohn-Wood, Schmeelk-Cone, Chavous, and Zimmerman (2004) found that two dimensions of racial identity—public regard and centrality—protected adolescents against the effects of racial discrimination in a longitudinal study of African American adolescents.

Christiansen and Evans (2005) found support for the challenge model of resilience when studying adolescent violence victimization as an outcome variable. They created a composite risk variable that combined risks for violence victimization; this variable comprised locus of control, anger expression, risky behavior, family conflict, and witnessing violence. Likewise, they also created a composite protective variable consisting of promotive factors. This variable comprised social connectedness, parental monitoring, and social cohesion. After demonstrating main effects for the total risk and protective factors for predicting violence victimization, they added a squared risk term to test its curvilinear effects. They found that those with the lowest levels of risk were more likely to be victimized than those with moderate levels of overall risk, but youth with high levels of risk were much more likely to be victimized. Ostaszewski and Zimmerman (2006) also used a cumulative risk and promotive factor approach and found support for the protective effects of their promotive factor index on externalizing behaviors, including violent behavior.

EXAMPLES OF RESILIENCY-BASED INTERVENTIONS USED IN SCHOOLS

In contrast to a deficit-oriented approach, resiliency-based interventions are designed to enhance promotive factors for adolescents. A resiliency-based program may also work to reduce risk, but the primary focus of the intervention is building assets and resources. Although all the programs described next are based in schools, many of them also reach outside the schools into the surrounding neighborhoods and communities to enhance promotive factors for the participants. Not all programs described here are identified by the researchers as applications of resiliency theory, but we have included them in this brief review because the frameworks used in designing the intervention strategies focus on enhancing promotive factors.

Ngwe et al. (2004) reported on the Aban Aya Youth Project (AAYP), a longitudinal efficacy trial of an intervention designed to reduce risk taking behavior among urban middle-school-aged African American youth that focused on enhancing parental support, developing cultural identity, and building relationships in the community. The program was implemented over a four-year period in grades five through eight. Eligible schools in the Chicago area were stratified according to a risk categorization and then randomly selected and assigned to a control group or to one of two experimental conditions (Flay, Graumlich, Segawa, Burns, & Holliday, 2004). One experimental condition, the school-community program, included a social development curriculum that addressed risk behaviors for violence, substance use, and unsafe sexual behaviors, focusing on individual skill building for problem solving, interpersonal relations, and critical thinking; a parent support group to promote child-parent communication; schoolwide support groups to integrate intervention skills into the school environment; and a community program to establish relationships among parents, schools, and local businesses. The other experimental condition included only the social development curriculum without the parental and school support components or the linkages to the community. The control condition focused on encouraging overall health-enhancing behaviors like physical activity, nutrition, and oral health. Participants were assessed over a four-year period using self-report measures of attitudes about violence, participation in violent behavior, behavioral intentions related to violence, and perceptions of friends' behavior and friends' encouragement to engage in problem behaviors. Ngwe et al. (2004) found that both experimental conditions were more effective than the control condition in reducing an increase in violent behavior among males and that the school-community intervention was more effective than the social development condition alone. Flay et al. (2004) found no intervention effect for females. Using a latent class model, another analysis of the intervention indicated that males in the highest risk group demonstrated the most beneficial outcomes from participating in the intervention. This analysis indicated that the effects for this group of males were three times higher than the effects demonstrated for males overall in the conventional analysis (Segawa, Ngwe, Li, Flay, & Aban Aya coinvestigators, 2005).

Another school-based intervention, the Responding in Peaceful and Positive Ways (RIPP) program, was designed to prevent violence among sixth graders (Farrell, Meyer, Kung, & Sullivan, 2001). Meyer and Farrell (1998) cited resiliency theory when describing the theoretical basis for the development of the RIPP program, stating that resilient adolescents tend to have "social competence, problem-solving skills, autonomy, and a sense of purpose" (p. 9). The RIPP intervention was designed to foster these characteristics by teaching social-cognitive problem solving and violence prevention skills (such as avoiding violent situations). The intervention also included a peer mediation component that was available to all students to help with conflict resolution. Schools were randomly assigned to either the RIPP intervention or a control group. Twenty-five weekly prevention sessions were led by three prevention specialists who were African American, corresponding with the ethnicity of the majority of participants in the intervention group. The fidelity of the intervention was documented using checklists for all the planned procedures and tasks completed by research assistants. Farrell, Meyer, and White (2001) found that adolescents in the control group were 2.2 times more likely to receive disciplinary actions and 5 times more likely to receive in-school suspensions due to violent behaviors than intervention group participants at the first posttest, but these differences did not persist at the twelve-month follow-up. They also found that youth in the intervention condition were 2.5 times less likely to report injuries due to fighting and used the school peer mediation program more often than youth in the control group. Notably, Farrell et al. (2001) found that the program was most effective for students who reported high rates of aggressive behavior prior to entry into the program. These evaluation results suggest that school-based violence prevention programs focusing on high-risk participants may be especially effective.

School-based interventions can also focus on changing the physical environment of the school to prevent violence. Many schools, for example, employ antiviolence strategies such as hiring security guards, installing metal detectors and security cameras, searching students' belongings, and banning backpacks. These can be considered deficit-oriented approaches, but they work to ameliorate risks such as students carrying weapons in schools. Astor et al. (1999) suggested an alternative approach based on their qualitative study of violence in schools. They provided teachers, students, and administrators with maps of their schools and asked them to identify the locations of violent events within the school. The researchers compiled the individual maps to create a single comprehensive map of the violent events in each school. To supplement the information in the maps, they also conducted focus groups with students and interviews with administrators and teachers. They found that violent events occurred most often in what they referred to as "unowned places." These spaces included hallways, parking lots, and cafeterias—areas where teachers and students generally did not feel a sense of ownership or responsibility. In contrast, violence did not occur in owned spaces such as classrooms, where teachers felt directly responsible for the events that occurred.

Astor et al. (1999) suggested that violence prevention interventions should work to decrease the number of unowned places in schools by increasing student and teacher feelings of ownership for those spaces. Astor, Meyer, and Pitner (2001) gave an example of one middle school where teachers devised a positive, friendly way to accomplish this. All the teachers agreed to stand at their doors during the passing period to monitor students while also making an effort to smile and greet as many students as possible by name. Both teachers and students reported that this was a friendly way to increase supervision of students. This strategy is an example of a resiliency approach because it focuses on both increasing teacher supervision and improving teacher-student relationships.

Many interventions make use of adult mentors as a positive means to reduce adolescent risk behaviors, including violent behaviors. These interventions utilize a resiliency approach because they provide adolescents with social resources (in the form of adult mentors) that may help them overcome risks they face. Rollin, Kaiser-Ulrey, Potts, and Creason (2003) described an intervention in three Florida middle schools that connected high-risk adolescents with mentors and internships in the community. Adolescents were considered to be at high risk if they had any of the following characteristics: previous delinquent or violent behavior, high absenteeism at school, or over-age for their grade (nearly all students at each school site met at least one of these inclusion criteria). All adolescents were given an orientation with a teacher at the school and then matched with community mentors according to their career interests. For the duration of the school year, they spent approximately eight hours each week working with one or more mentors. Data were collected at the end of the school year prior to intervention implementation and then again at the end of the school year in which the intervention was implemented. The intervention participants were compared to a control group of students randomly selected from a waiting list for the intervention program. Although they did not directly measure violent behavior, the researchers examined changes in each student across several risk factors for violent behavior, including school absenteeism, number and duration of in-school and out-of-school suspensions, and number of behavioral infractions committed on school property. Rollin et al. (2003) found that the intervention students had greater reductions in number and duration of suspensions and in the number of behavioral infractions committed on school property than the students in the control group.

Youth Empowerment Solutions for Peaceful Communities (YES) provides another example of a resiliency-based program by connecting middle school students with neighborhood organizations to design and carry out community improvement projects (Reischl, Zimmerman, Morrel-Samuels, Franzen, Roberts, & Tyson, 2007). The intervention, based on empowerment and ecological theories (Kelly, 2006; Zimmerman, 1995, 2000) is designed to engage middle-school-aged youth and adults to work together to create environmental changes that promote peaceful neighborhoods. YES is an example of a resiliency approach because it focuses on youth development by creating positive relationships between youth and adults in their community and creating opportunities for adolescents to engage in environmental changes in the community. The students meet regularly throughout the school year, participating in activities designed to develop leadership qualities and to help youth gain a better appreciation of and pride in their cultural history. Additionally, adolescents conduct a community assessment using observational and PhotoVoice techniques (Wang, 2004). They then begin working in intergenerational teams to develop and carry out community improvement projects such as community gardens, neighborhood cleanups, or public artwork (usually murals). Adolescents and neighborhood groups receive technical assistance and material support from local nonprofit organizations. Social marketing is also employed to raise community awareness and investment in the program. The outcome evaluation includes assessments of self-reported attitudes and behaviors among the youth in the two middle schools, crime rates, residents' fear of crime in their neighborhood as recorded in a representative community survey, and police incident reports. The evaluation design includes a comparison neighborhood in the same city with similar demographic characteristics. In addition to comparing intervention and control neighborhoods on the outcome measures, the evaluation also includes pre-post assessments of property parcels (including businesses and homes) in the areas surrounding the community improvement projects in order to assess changes in the quality of each parcel (such as litter or property damage).

Although adolescent violence remains a serious problem, public health interventions have shown promise for reducing its prevalence.

SUMMARY

Although adolescent violence remains a serious problem, public health interventions have shown promise for reducing its prevalence. Schools provide an effective and convenient context in which to implement them, but other settings may also be vital to integrate these programs. Traditionally, violence prevention efforts, like other prevention programs, are interventions based on a deficit approach that focuses on risk reduction or ameliorating the effects of risks. Alternatively, prevention designed to focus on positive factors in adolescents' lives can enhance assets and resources in their schools and in their communities. Researchers are beginning to recognize the need for such strategies, which we have identified as resiliency approaches. In practice, however, the distinction between resiliency-based and deficit-oriented interventions is somewhat blurred. Both types of interventions can employ some of the same strategies, and an intervention can ameliorate deficits and also enhance assets and resources. Yet the underlying framework or theory used for planning and implementing programs may be most vital. A shift in focus from a deficiency to resiliency perspective in the development of interventions may transform adolescent violence prevention from an individual blame orientation to a more ecologically driven, strengths-based approach that involves multiple sectors of communities. Schools provide an especially important context for interventions, but the involvement of families and community organizations in developing the supportive and peaceful environments adolescents require for healthy development is critical for positive development and sustained prevention of violence.

KEY TERMS

Adolescent violence
Challenge model
Compensatory factors
Compensatory model
Deficit-oriented approach

Promotive factors
Protective model
Resilience
Resiliency theory
Risk-protective variable

DISCUSSION QUESTIONS

1. What is resiliency theory, and how can it be applied to understand an adolescent's risk of psychopathology?

2. Use the compensatory model (inclusive of risk and compensatory factors) to discuss why violence may disproportionately affect males and ethnic minority groups in the United States.

3. What is a "deficit-oriented approach" to adolescent problem behavior, and how does it compare to resiliency theory? Which approach or theory do you believe is more advantageous to use as a foundation for creating behavioral interventions to address adolescent violence?

4. In addition to school-based interventions, are there alternative locations where interventions could be developed, adapted, or tailored to prevent violence among adolescents? Discuss your intervention strategy.

REFERENCES

Ary, D. V., Duncan, T. E., Biglan, A., Metzler, C. W., Noell, J. W., & Smolkowski, K. (1999). Development of adolescent problem behavior. *Journal of Abnormal Child Psychology, 12*, 141–150.

Astor, R. A., Meyer, H. A., & Behre, W. J. (1999). Unowned places and times: Maps and interviews about violence in high schools. *American Educational Research Journal, 36*(1), 3–42.

Astor, R. A, Meyer, H. A., & Pitner, R. O. (2001). Elementary and middle school students' perceptions of violence-prone school subcontexts. *Elementary School Journal, 101*(5), 511–528.

Barkin, S., Kreiter, S., & Durant, R. H. (2001). Exposure to violence and intentions to engage in moralistic violence during adolescence. *Journal of Adolescence 24*, 777–789.

Beier, S. R., Rosenfeld, W. D., Spitalny, K. C., Zansky, S. M., & Bontempo, A. N. (2000). The potential role of an adult mentor in influencing high-risk behaviors in adolescents. *Archives of Pediatric and Adolescent Medicine, 154*(4), 327–331.

Bernard, S. J., Paulozzi, L. J., & Wallace, L.J.D. (2007). Fatal injuries among children by race and ethnicity: United States, 1999–2002. *Morbidity and Mortality Weekly Reports, 56*(SS05), 1–16.

Borowski, I. W., Ireland, M., & Resnick, M. D. (2002). Violence risk and protective factors among youth held back in school. *Ambulatory Pediatrics, 2,* 475–484.

Bosworth, K., Espelange, D., DuBay, T., & Daytner, G. (2000). Preliminary evaluation of a multimedia violence prevention program for adolescents. *American Journal of Health Behavior, 24*(4), 268–281.

Botvin, G. J., Baker, E., Dusenbury, L., Botvin, E. M., & Diaz, T. (1995). Long-term follow-up results of a randomized drug abuse prevention trial in a white middle-class population. *Journal of the American Medical Association, 273,* 1106–1112.

Botvin, G. J, Griffin, K. W., & Nichols, T. D. (2006). Preventing youth violence and delinquency through a universal school-based prevention approach. *Prevention Science, 7*(4), 403–408.

Botvin, G. J., Schinke, S. P., Epstein, J. A., & Diaz, T. (1994). The effectiveness of culturally focused and generic skills training approaches to alcohol and drug abuse prevention among minority youths. *Psychology of Addictive Behaviors, 8,* 116–127.

Brook, J. S., Brook, D. W., Gordon, A. S., & Whiteman, M. (1990). The psychosocial etiology of adolescent drug use: A family interactional approach. *Genetic, Social, and General Psychology Monographs, 116,* 111–267.

Bureau of Justice Statistics. (2005). Criminal victimization in the United States: Statistical tables. Retrieved April 3, 2007, from www.ojp.usdoj.gov/bjs/abstract/cvusst.htm.

Caldwell, C. H., Kohn-Wood, L. P., Schmeelk-Cone, K. H., Chavous, T. M., & Zimmerman, M. A. (2004). Racial discrimination and racial identity as risk or protective factors for violent behaviors in African American young adults. *American Journal of Community Psychology, 33,* 91–105.

Capaldi, D. M., & Patterson, G. R. (1993). *The violent adolescent male: Specialist or generalist?* Paper presented at the biennial meeting of the Society for Research in Child Development, New Orleans, LA.

Centers for Disease Control and Prevention. (2004). Youth violence: Fact sheet. Retrieved December 10, 2004, from www.cdc.gov/ncipc/factsheets/yvfacts.htm.

Centers for Disease Control and Prevention. (2007a). Web-Based Injury Statistics Query and Reporting System (WISQARS) [Online]. National Center for Injury Prevention and Control. Retrieved June 4, 2007, from www.cdc.gov/ncipc/wisqars.

Centers for Disease Control and Prevention. (2007b). Youth violence: Fact sheet. Retrieved April 3, 2007, from www.cdc.gov/ncipc/factsheets/yvfacts.htm.

Centers for Disease Control and Prevention. (2007c). *Youth online: Comprehensive results of the Youth Risk Behavior Surveillance System.* National Center for Chronic Disease Prevention and Health Promotion. Retrieved April 3, 2007, from http://apps.nccd.cdc.gov/yrbss.

Chesney-Lind, M., & Belknap, J. (2004) Trends in delinquent girls' aggression and violent behavior. In M. Putallaz & K. L. Bierman (Eds.), *Aggression, antisocial behavior and violence among girls* (pp. 203–220). New York: Guilford Press.

Christiansen, E. J., and Evans, W. P. (2005). Adolescent victimization: Testing models of resiliency by gender. *Journal of Early Adolescence, 25*(3), 298–316.

Cicchetti, D., & Garmezy, N. (1993). Prospects and promises in the study of resilience. *Development and Psychopathology, 5*(4), 497–502.

Corso, P. S., Mercy, J. A., Simon, T. R., Finkelstein, E. A., & Miller, T. R. (2007). Medical costs and productivity losses due to interpersonal and self-directed violence in the United States. *American Journal of Preventative Medicine, 32*(6), 474–482.

Dahlberg, L. L. (1998). Youth violence in the United States: Major trends, risk factors and prevention approaches. *American Journal of Preventive Medicine, 14,* 259–272.

Dishion, T. J., & Loeber, R. (1985). Adolescent marijuana and alcohol use: The role of parents and peers revisited. *American Journal of Drug and Alcohol Abuse, 11*(1–2), 11–25.

Dryfoos, J. G. (1990). *Adolescents at risk: Prevalence and prevention.* New York: Oxford University Press.

DuBois, D. L., & Silverthorn, N. (2005). Natural mentoring relationships and adolescent health: Evidence from a national study. *American Journal of Public Health, 95*(3), 518–524.

Dukarm, C. P., Byrd, R. S., Auinger, P., & Weitzman, M. (1996) Illicit substance use, gender, and the risk of violent behavior among adolescents. *Archives of Pediatrics and Adolescent Medicine, 150*(8), 797–801.

Ellickson, P. L., & McGuigan, K. A. (2000). Early predictors of adolescent violence. *American Journal of Public Health, 90*(4), 566–572.

Fagan, J., & Wilkinson, D. L. (1998) Social contexts and functions of adolescent violence. In D. S. Elliott, B. A. Hamburg, & K. R. Williams (Eds.), *Violence in American schools: A new perspective* (pp. 55–93). New York: Cambridge University Press.

Farrell, A. D., Meyer, A. L., Kung, E. M., & Sullivan, T. N. (2001). Development and evaluation of school-based violence prevention programs. *Journal of Clinical Child Psychology, 30*(2), 207–220.

Farrell, A. D., Meyer, A. L., & White, K. S. (2001). Evaluation of Responding in Peaceful and Positive Ways (RIPP): A school-based prevention program for reducing violence among urban adolescents. *Journal of Clinical Child Psychology, 30*(4), 451–463.

Federal Bureau of Investigation, United States Department of Justice. (2007). *Crime in the United States, 2005.* Retrieved March 29, 2007, from www.fbi.gov/ucr/05cius/index.html.

Fergus, S., & Zimmerman, M. A. (2005). Adolescent resilience: A framework for understanding healthy development in the face of risk. *Annual Review of Public Health, 26*, 399–419.

Flay, B. R., Graumlich, S., Segawa, E., Burns, J. L., & Holliday, M. Y. (2004). Effects of two prevention programs on high-risk behaviors among African American youth. *Archives of Pediatric and Adolescent Medicine, 158*(4), 377–384.

Garmezy, N. (1991). Resiliency and vulnerability to adverse developmental outcomes associated with poverty. *American Behavioral Scientist, 34*(4), 416–430.

Garmezy, N., Masten, A. S., & Tellegen, A. (1984). The study of stress and competence in children: A building block for developmental psychopathology. *Child Development, 55*, 97–111.

Graves, K. N. (2005). Not always sugar and spice: Expanding theoretical and functional explanations for why females aggress. *Aggression and Violent Behavior, 12*(2), 131–140.

Greenberg, M., & Schneider, D. (1994). Violence in American cities: Young black males is the answer, but what was the question? *Social Science and Medicine, 39*(2), 179–187.

Griffin, K. W., Scheier, L. M., Botvin, G. J., Diaz, T., & Miller, N. (1999). Interpersonal aggression in urban minority youth: Mediators of perceived neighborhood, peer, and parental influences. *Journal of Community Psychology, 27*(3), 281–298.

Grossman, J. B., & Tierney, J. P. (1998). Does mentoring work? An impact study of the Big Brothers Big Sisters program. *Evaluation Review, 22*(3), 403–426.

Guerra, N. G., Huesmann, L. R., Tolan, P. H., & Van Acker, R. (1995). Stressful events and individual beliefs as correlates of economic disadvantage and aggression: Implications for preventive interventions among inner-city children. *Journal of Consulting and Clinical Psychology, 63*, 518–528.

Hahn, R., Fuqua-Whitley, D., Wethington, H., Lowy, J., Liberman, A., Crosby, A., Fullilove, M., Johnson, R., Moscicki, E., Price, L., Snyder, S. R., Tuma F., Cory, S., Stone, G., Mukhopadhaya, K., Chattopadhyay, S., Dahlberg, L., Centers for Disease Control and Prevention, & Task Force on Community Preventive Services. (2007a). The effectiveness of school-based programs for the prevention of violent and aggressive behavior. *Morbidity and Mortality Weekly Reports, 56*(RR07), 1–12.

Hahn, R., Fuqua-Whitley, D., Wethington, H., Lowy, J., Liberman, A., Crosby, A., Fullilove, M., Johnson, R., Liberman, A., Moscicki, E., Price, L., Snyder, S., Tuma, F., Cory, S., Stone, G., Mukhopadhaya, K., Chattopadhyay, S., Dahlberg, L., & Task Force on Community Preventive Services. (2007b). The effectiveness of school-based programs to prevent violent and aggressive behavior: A systematic review. *American Journal of Preventive Medicine, 33*(2S), S114–S129.

Hawkins, J. D., Catalano, R. F., Morrison, D., O'Donnell, J., Abbott, R., & Day, L. E. (1992). The Seattle Social Development Project: Effects of the first four years on protective factors and problem behaviors. In J. McCord & R. E. Tremblay (Eds.), *Preventing antisocial behavior: Interventions from birth through adolescence.* New York: Guilford Press.

Herrenkohl, T. I., Hill, K. G., Hawkins, J. D., Chung, I. J., & Nagin, D. S. (2006). Developmental trajectories of family management and risk for youth violent behavior in adolescence. *Journal of Adolescent Heath, 39*(2), 206–213.

Herrenkohl, T., Maguin, E., Hill, K., Hawkins, J., Abbott, R., & Catalano, R. (2000). Developmental risk factors for youth violence. *Journal of Adolescent Health, 26,* 176–186.

Howard, D., Qui, Y., & Boekeloo, B. (2003). Personal and social contextual correlates of adolescent dating violence. *Journal of Adolescent Health, 33,* 9–17.

Huesmann, L., Eron, L., Lefkowitz, M., & Walder, L. (1984). Stability of aggression over time and generations. *Developmental Psychology, 20,* 1120–1134.

Huang, B., Kosterman, R., Catalano, R. F., Hawkins, J. D., & Abbott, R. D. (2001). Modeling mediation in the etiology of violent behavior and adolescence: A test of the social development model. *Criminology, 39,* 75–107.

Huba, G. J., & Bentler, P. M. (1980). The role of peer and adult models for drug taking at different stages in adolescence. *Journal of Youth and Adolescence, 9*(5), 449–465.

Jemmott, J. B., Jemmott, L. S., Hines, P. M., & Fong, G. T. (2001). The theory of planned behavior as a model of intentions for fighting among African American and Latino adolescents. *Maternal and Child Health Journal, 5*(4), 253–263.

Jessor, R., & Jessor, S. L. (1977). *Problem behavior and psychosocial development: A longitudinal study of youth.* New York: Academic Press.

Kelly, J. G. (2006). *Becoming ecological: An expedition into community psychology.* New York: Oxford University Press.

Lauritsen, J. (2003). How families and communities influence youth victimization. *OJJDP Juvenile Justice Bulletin.* Washington, DC: U.S. Department of Justice, Office of Justice Programs, Office of Juvenile Justice and Delinquency Prevention.

Loeber, R., Wung, P., Keenan, K., Giroux, B., Stouthamer-Loeber, M., Van Kammen, W. B., & Maughan, B. (1993). Developmental pathways in disruptive childhood behavior. *Development and Psychopathology, 5,* 103–133.

Luthar, S. S., & Zelazo, L. B. (2003). Research on resilience: An integrative review. In S.S. Luthar (Ed.), *Resilience and vulnerability: Adaptation in the context of childhood adversities* (pp. 510–550). New York: Cambridge University Press.

Masten, A. S. (1994). Resilience in individual development: Successful adaptation despite risk and adversity. In M. Wang & E. Gordon (Eds.), *Risk and resilience in inner city America: Challenges and prospects* (pp. 3–25). Hillsdale, NJ: Erlbaum.

Masten, A. S., Garmezy, N., Tellegen, A., Pelligrini, D. S., Larkin, K., & Larsen, A. (1988). Competence and stress in school children: The moderating effects of individual and family qualities. *Journal of Child Psychology and Psychiatry, 29,* 745–764.

McLoyd, V.C. (1990). The impact of economic hardship on black families and children: Psychological distress, parenting, and socioemotional development. *Child Development, 61*(2), 311–346.

Meyer, A. L., & Farrell, A. D. (1998). Social skills training to promote resilience in urban sixth-grade students: One product of an action research strategy to prevent youth violence in high-risk environments. *Education and Treatment of Children, 21*(4), 461–488.

Miller, T. R., Fisher, D. A., & Cohen, M. A. (2001). Costs of juvenile violence: Policy implications. *Pediatrics, 109*(1), p. e3.

Nation, M., Crusto, C., Wandersman, A., Kumpfer, K. L., Seybolt, D., Morrissey-Kane, E., & Davino, K. (2003). What works in prevention: Principles of effective prevention programs. *American Psychologist, 58*(6/7), 449–456.

Needle, R., McCubbin, H., Wilson, M., Reineck, R., Lazar, A., & Mederer, H. (1986). Interpersonal influences in adolescent drug use: The role of older siblings, parents, and peers. *International Journal of the Addictions, 21*(7), 739–766.

Newcomb, M. D., & Felix-Ortiz, M. (1992). Multiple protective and risk factors for drug use and abuse: Cross-sectional and prospective findings. *Journal of Personality and Social Psychology, 63*(2), 280–296.

Ngwe, J. E., Liu, L. C., Flay, B. R., Segawa, E., & Aban, A. (2004). Violence prevention among African American adolescent males. *American Journal of Health Behavior, 28*(Suppl. 1), S24–S37.

Orpinas, P., Murray, N., & Kelder, S. (1999). Parental influences on students' aggressive behaviors and weapon carrying. *Health Education and Behavior, 26*(6), 774–787.

Osofsky, J. D. (1999). The impact of violence on children. *Future of Children, 9*(3), 33–49.

Ostaszewski, K., & Zimmerman, M. A. (2006). The effects of cumulative risks and promotive factors on urban adolescent alcohol and other drug use: A longitudinal study of resiliency. *American Journal of Community Psychology, 38*(3–4), 237–249.

Pepler, D. J., & Slaby, R. G. (1994). Theoretical and developmental perspectives on youth and violence. In L. D. Eron, J. H. Gentry, & P. Schlegel (Eds.), *Reason to hope: A psychosocial perspective on violence and youth.* (pp. 27–58). Washington, DC: American Psychological Association.

Pollard, J. A., Hawkins, J. D., & Arthur, M. W. (1999). Risk and protection: Are both necessary to understand diverse behavioral outcomes in adolescence? *Social Work Research, 23,* 145–158.

Prinstein, M. J., Boegers, J., & Spirito, A. (2001). Adolescents' and their friends' health-risk behavior: Factors that alter or add to peer influence. *Journal of Pediatric Psychology, 26,* 287–298.

Rainone, G. A., Schmeidler, J. W., Frank, B., & Smith, R. B. (2006). Violent behavior, substance use, and other delinquent behaviors among middle and high school students. *Youth Violence and Juvenile Justice, 4*(3), 247–265.

Reischl, T., Zimmerman, M. A., Morrel-Samuels, S., Franzen, S., Roberts, E. E., & Tyson, Y. (2007, November 6). Youth Empowerment Solutions: Connecting youth with neighborhood organizations to create community change. Scientific session presented at the annual meeting of the American Public Health Association, Washington, DC.

Resnick, M. D., Bearman, P. S., Blum, R. W., Bauman, K. E., Harris, K. M., Jones, J., Tabor, J., Beuhring, T., Sieving, R. E., Shew, M., Ireland, M., Bearinger, L. H., & Udry, J. R. (1997). Protecting adolescents from harm: Findings from the National Longitudinal Study on Adolescent Health. *Journal of the American Medical Association, 278,* 823–832.

Resnick, M. D., Ireland, M., & Borowsky, I. (2004). Youth violence perpetration: What protects? What predicts? Findings from the National Longitudinal Study of Adolescent Health. *Journal of Adolescent Health, 35*(5), 424.e1–424.e10.

Rollin, S. A., Kaiser-Ulrey, C., Potts, I., & Creason, A. H. (2003). A school-based violence prevention model for at-risk eighth grade youth. *Psychology in the Schools, 40*(4), 403–416.

Rutter, M. (1985). Resilience in the face of adversity: Protective factors and resistance to psychiatric disorder. *British Journal of Psychiatry, 147,* 598–611.

Rutter, M. (1987). Psychosocial resilience and protective mechanisms. *American Journal of Orthopsychiatry, 57,* 316–331.

Saner, H., & Ellickson, P. (1996). Concurrent risk factors for adolescent violence. *Journal of Adolescent Health, 19,* 94–103.

Segawa, E., Ngwe, J. E., Li, Y., Flay, B. R., & Aban Aya coinvestigators. (2005). Evaluation of the effects of the Aban Aya Youth Project in reducing violence among African American adolescent males using latent class growth mixture modeling techniques. *Evaluation Review 29*(2), 128–148.

Shapiro, J. P., Burgoon, J. D., Welker, C. J., & Clough, J. B. (2002). Evaluation of the Peacemakers Program: School-based prevention for students in grades four through eight. *Psychology in Schools, 39*(1), 87–100.

Stouthamer-Loeber, M., Loeber, R., Wei, E., Farrington, D. P., & Wikstrom, P.O.H. (2002). Risk and promotive effects in the explanation of persistent serious delinquency in boys. *Journal of Consulting and Clinical Psychology 70,* 111–123.

Thornton, T. N., Craft, C. A., Dahlberg, L. L., Lynch, B. S., & Baer, K. (2002) *Best practices of youth violence prevention: A sourcebook for community action* (rev. ed.). Atlanta: Centers for Disease Control and Prevention, National Center for Injury Prevention and Control.

U.S. Census Bureau, Population Division. (2006, May 10). Annual estimates of the population by sex and five-year age groups for the United States: April 1, 2000, to July 1, 2005 (NC-EST2005-01). Retrieved April 9, 2007, from www.census.gov/popest/estimates.php.

Vernberg, E. M., Jacobs, A. K., & Hershberger, S. L. (1999). Peer victimization and attitudes about violence during early adolescence. *Journal of Clinical Child Psychology, 28*(3), 386–395.

Wang, C. C. (2004). Using PhotoVoice as a participatory assessment and issue selection tool. In M. Minkler & N. Wallerstein (Eds.), *Community-based participatory research for health.* San Francisco: Jossey-Bass.

Werner, E. E. (1993). Risk, resilience, and recovery: Perspectives from the Kauai Longitudinal Study. *Development and Psychopathology, 5,* 503–515.

Wilson, S. J., & Lipsey, M. W. (2007). School-based interventions for aggressive and disruptive behavior. *American Journal of Preventive Medicine, 33*(2S), S130–S143.

World Health Organization. (2004). *The economic dimensions of interpersonal violence.* Geneva, Switzerland.

Zimmerman, M. A. (1995). Psychological empowerment: Issues and illustrations. *American Journal of Community Psychology, 23*, 581–599.

Zimmerman, M. A. (2000). Empowerment theory: Psychological, organizational and community levels of analysis. In J. Rappaport & E. Seidman (Eds.), *Handbook of community psychology* (pp. 43–63). New York: Plenum Press.

Zimmerman, M. A., & Arunkumar, R. (1994). Resiliency research: Implications for schools and policy. *Social Policy Report, 8,* 1–17.

Zimmerman, M. A., Steinman, K. J., & Rowe, K. J. (1998). Violence among urban African American adolescents: The protective effects of parental support. In S. Oskamp & X. B. Arriaga (eds.), *Addressing community problems: Research and intervention.* Newbury Park, CA: Sage.

CHAPTER

13

PREVENTION OF SUICIDAL BEHAVIOR DURING ADOLESCENCE

ANTHONY SPIRITO ▪ QUETZALCOATL HERNANDEZ-CERVANTES

LEARNING OBJECTIVES

After studying this chapter, you will be able to

- Classify attempted and completed suicide by gender and race.
- Catalog possible risk and protective factors for suicide during adolescence.
- Recognize programmatic strengths and shortcomings in school-based suicide awareness and education programs.

Rates of attempted and completed suicide rise precipitously during adolescence (Kessler, Borges, & Walters, 1999). In 2005, approximately 16.9 percent of adolescents in the United States seriously considered attempting suicide, 13 percent developed a suicide plan, 8.4 percent attempted suicide, and 2.3 percent attempted suicide in a manner requiring emergency medical treatment (Centers for Disease Control and Prevention [CDC], 2006). These rates translate into approximately two million attempts per year, of which about 700,000 receive emergency medical treatment (Shaffer & Pfeffer, 2001), resulting in considerable economic burden.

Although there are important differences between those adolescents who attempt and those who complete suicide, a previous suicide attempt is one of the best predictive risk factors for eventual completed suicide by an adolescent. Thus, it is clear that preventing the onset of suicidal behavior, the focus of this chapter, is an important facet of addressing the public health problem of youth suicide.

EPIDEMIOLOGY

In this section we discuss rates of attempted and completed suicide in youth. The primary focus is on rates in the United States. Gender and race differences are also reviewed.

Completed Suicide

Suicide completion is the third leading cause of death for children, adolescents, and young adults (10 to 24 years old) in the United States (CDC, 2007). After puberty, rates of suicide increase with age, until they stabilize in young adulthood. Among the 15 through 24 age group, data collected between 1950 and 2004 indicated a peak in death rates for suicide in 1990 (13.2 per 100,000), decreasing in 2000 (10.2) and not varying significantly afterwards—9.7 in 2003 and 10.3 in 2004 (U.S. Department of Health & Human Services [U.S. DHHS], 2006). The increase in the rate of suicide from the 1970s through the late 1990s has been attributed to rising rates of depression, an increase in substance abuse, and the increased availability of firearms among adolescents (Commission on Adolescent Suicide Prevention, 2005). Indeed, data from the Centers for Disease Control and Prevention (2004) indicate that death by firearms (49 percent) is the leading cause of death for persons between 10 and 19 years of age, followed by suffocation (mostly hanging; 38 percent) and then poisoning (7 percent).

It is unclear why the decrease in suicide rates occurred in the 1990s. Olfson, Marcus, Weissman, and Jensen (2002) note there was a more than threefold increase in antidepressant use by adolescents between 1987 and 1996, which might account for the decrease in suicide. In addition, suicide awareness programs, discussed later in this chapter, were introduced into high schools during the mid-1980s.

Quetzalcoatl Hernandez-Cervantes cowrote this chapter during a postdoctoral summer internship supported by grant UNAM Macroproyecto MP6-11, with supplemental support from the Center for Alcohol and Addiction Studies at Brown University.

Differences by gender in completed suicide in 15- through 29-year-olds are pronounced: 16.8 per 100,000 for males and 3.6 for females in 2004 (U.S. DHHS, 2006). Death rates for suicide among females peaked in 1980 (4.3) and in 1994 for males (23.0). However, in males the trend increased steadily from 1950 (6.5) to its peak in 1994 and began decreasing thereafter to 17.1 per 100,000 in 2004. For females, the trend in suicide rates is much more stable: 2.6 per 100,000 in 1950, and 3.6 in 2004.

Why is this gender difference so pronounced? One possibility is that completed suicide is associated with not just depression but conduct difficulties or aggressive behavior and substance abuse during adolescence, both of which are more common in males than in females. Also, males are much more likely to choose firearms as a suicide method than females. The increase in young male suicide rates in the 1980s and 1990s has also raised interest in whether suicidal behavior is related to masculinity, not only in the United States but in many other countries as well (Hunt, Sweeting, Keoghan, & Platt, 2006).

Rates of death by suicide are highest among Native American males 15 through 24 years old, with a rate of 30.7 per 100,000 in 2004, followed by white (not Hispanic or Latino) males, with a rate of 19.0, and Hispanic or Latino males at 12.8 per 100,000 (U.S. DHHS, 2006). The lowest death rates for suicide in the same age group are found among African American females (2.2), followed by Hispanic or Latino females (2.5), and Asian or Pacific Islander females (2.8). The low rates among African Americans have been attributed to a greater emphasis on religion in African American families. However, the difference in rates of completed suicide between African Americans and whites has decreased over the past few decades.

Attempted Suicide

Rates of attempted suicide rise precipitously during adolescence. Data from the 2005 Youth Risk Behavior Surveillance System (YRBSS) of over 13,000 adolescents indicated that within a twelve-month period, 21.8 percent of females grades nine through twelve and 12 percent of males grades nine through twelve reported suicidal ideation (CDC, 2006). The highest percentages were found among Hispanic or Latino females (24.2 percent), compared to white males, at 12.4 percent. Among females, 10.8 percent reported attempted suicide, with Hispanic or Latino females reporting the highest rate (14.9 percent). Among males, only 6 percent reported attempted suicide, with Hispanic or Latino males having the highest percentage (7.8 percent). This latter trend is also found in students with a suicide attempt requiring medical attention: 2.9 percent were females (with Hispanics or Latinos exhibiting the highest percentage—3.7 percent), and 1.8 percent were males (Hispanics or Latinos with the highest percentage—2.8 percent). Hispanic adolescents consistently report higher rates of suicide attempts than other groups. Data trends from the national YRBSS indicate that seriously considered suicide attempts decreased from 1991 (29 percent) to 2003 (16.9 percent). For attempted

Rates of attempted

suicide rise

precipitously

during

adolescence.

suicide, the rates rose slightly from 1991 (7.3 percent) to 2005 (8.4 percent) (U.S. DHHS, 2006). Medically serious suicide attempts also increased slightly, from 1.7 percent in 1991 to 2.3 percent in 2005.

Why are there such high rates of attempted suicide in Hispanic and Latino families? Disparities between adolescent and parent acculturation, socioeconomic disadvantage, traditional gender-role socialization, and intergenerational conflict create conditions that are believed to lead to adolescent suicidal behavior in Hispanic families (Zayas, Kaplan, Turner, Romano, Gonzalez-Ramos, 2000). Traditionally structured Hispanic families often have restrictive, authoritarian parenting styles, which may affect the development of adolescent females moving toward autonomy, even when the father is absent (Zayas et al., 2000). In addition, the support from extended family members traditionally used to help parents manage these issues is often limited due to immigration. Cuellar and Curry (2007) also note that there is a high occurrence of substance abuse, delinquency, and suicide attempts among a subgroup of adolescent Hispanic females, which may also be related to the high rates of suicidal behavior in this group.

Duarté-Vélez and Bernal (2007) note that in order to identify elements for prevention and treatment of suicidal behavior in Latino youth, studies of specific Latino subgroups should be conducted, such as Latinos from Mexico (64 percent of the Hispanic population in the United States), Puerto Rico (10 percent), the Dominican Republic (3 percent), and Central and South America (3 percent). For example, Fortuna, Perez, Canino, Sribney, and Alegria (2007) examined lifetime suicide attempts in several Latino subgroups in the United States, including Mexicans, Puerto Ricans, Cubans, and others. Although they did not find any differences in rates by these subgroups, they did find that most of the attempts occurred below the age of eighteen years and that one of the associated risk factors was acculturation, even among those without psychiatric morbidity.

Native Americans report the highest rates of attempted suicide during adolescence. The National American Indian Adolescent Health Survey (Borowsky, Resnick, Ireland, & Bloom, 1999) sampled more than 11,000 Native American students in schools on reservations in eight Indian Health Service areas. The overall rate of lifetime suicide attempts was 16.8 percent, and the rate for girls was 21.8 percent. However, the rates also varied considerably across tribes.

Regarding the high rate of suicidal behaviors among American Indian and Alaska Native (AI/AN) communities, Alcántara and Gone (2007) comment that factors such as native identity, social support networks, attitudes toward education, cultural continuity, spirituality, and socioeconomic level affect the suicide epidemiological profile of AI/AN communities. In their review, Alcántara and Gone underscore the protective role of spirituality, positive attitudes toward education, and the presence of cultural continuity, as these were found to be strongly associated with reduced and in some cases nonexistent rates of suicide in certain AI/AN communities.

Walls, Chapple, and Johnson (2007) found that stressors like coercive parenting, caretaker rejection, negative school attitudes and perceived discrimination (surprisingly, mostly from teachers) were related to suicidality among American Indian adolescents from the Midwest and Canada. Walls et al. also found that depressive symptoms and anger mediated the effects of several key predictors of suicidality in American Indian adolescents. Olson and Wahab (2006) note that most risk factors for Native American adolescents are the same as those for other adolescent populations in North America.

The reliability and accuracy of prevalence estimations for adolescent suicide attempts are problematic. It is known that statistics on completed suicide are generally considered to be underestimates of the true incidence, principally because of failure to report and misclassification of unintentional injuries that might be suicides (such as single-car crashes). Similarly, data on nonfatal suicide attempts are typically collected by self-report and thus are subject to definitional vagaries and the adolescent's interpretation of his or her behavior as suicidal or not. Nonetheless, Evans, Hawton, Rodham, and Deeks (2005) reviewed the prevalence of suicidal phenomena in adolescents based on 128 studies from 1963 to 2000. They found that the mean proportion of suicide attempters was 9.7 percent and ideators 29.9 percent. Though the prevalence of suicidal phenomena varies depending on terminology and methodology used, Evans et al. did not find any statistically significant differences attributable to either terminology or methodology in the studies they reviewed, although a higher proportion of suicidal phenomena was reported in studies using anonymous questionnaires versus studies using nonanonymous measures. Thus, the consistency of the findings can lead to some confidence in the general accuracy of these rates.

In summary, completed suicide occurs at a very high rate in adolescents, and the rate increased substantially in the 1980s and 1990s in white males. Native American adolescent males have especially high rates of completed suicide. Attempted suicide is much more common in females than males, with Hispanic females and Native American females from certain tribes demonstrating the highest rates of suicide attempts.

PREVENTION

In the last decade, the field of suicide prevention has benefited from the establishment of the *Evidence-Based Practices Project* (EBPP; Rodgers, Sudak, Silverman, & Litts, 2007). The EBPP is a coalition of the Suicide Prevention Resource Center and the American Foundation for Suicide Prevention, funded by the Substance Abuse and Mental Health Services Administration. The EBPP reviewed suicide prevention programs and created an online registry (www.sprc.org) of evidence-based suicide prevention programs (Rodgers et al., 2007).

The EBPP followed a five-step process to classify programs. The first three steps included a literature review to identify programs, a screening process to eliminate programs that did not meet minimal methodological standards, and ratings by at least three expert reviewers of the twenty-four identified programs. Experts used a 1-to-5 scale to rate each program on ten items: theory, fidelity, design, attrition,

The field of suicide prevention has benefited from the establishment of the Evidence-Based Practices Project.

psychometrics, analysis, threats to validity, safety, integrity, and utility. Programs were classified under "effective" if their ratings on the integrity and utility scores averaged 3.5 or greater, "promising" if the average scores were between 3.0 and 3.5, or "insufficient current support" if either average score fell below 3.0 (Rodgers et al., 2007). Based on this rating scheme, four programs were classified as effective and eight as promising. Two of the four effective programs and six of the eight promising programs targeted adolescents and are discussed below.

Another major effort to review the efficacy of suicide prevention occurred in August 2004, when experts from fifteen countries met in Salzburg, Austria, for a five-day workshop. They reviewed major databases for relevant articles published from 1966 to June 2005 (Mann et al., 2005). This group developed the following classification scheme: awareness and education, screening, means restriction, and media. We follow this same scheme in this chapter. Under each category, as appropriate, we review studies rated as promising or effective by the EBPP, as well as studies cited in the literature, including many noted by the Salzburg project.

Suicide Awareness and Education Programs

Mann et al. (2005) noted that suicide awareness and education are conducted primarily by primary care physicians and by gatekeepers. The gatekeepers for adolescents are based primarily in school settings.

Improving physician recognition of depression and suicide risk is deemed a valuable preventive approach, because many adult suicide victims have contact with their physician in the months prior to their death. Although adolescents' relationships with their doctors are different from those of adults, two studies have examined the effectiveness of primary care physicians in adolescent suicide prevention. Pfaff, Acres, and McKelvey (2001) trained primary care doctors in Australia to recognize and respond to suicidality in their adolescent and young adult patients. Although there was greatly increased identification of suicidal patients, there was no change in physician management or treatment of these individuals. Asarnow et al. (2005) conducted a study in which primary care physicians screened adolescents for depression and then referred them to either standard care or a quality improvement intervention. The latter condition consisted of case managers who supported primary care clinicians in managing the depressed adolescent, cognitive-behavioral therapy provided by the case managers, and education to the physician regarding depression treatment (both psychological and pharmacological). Although not statistically significant, at six-month follow-up suicide attempts dropped from 14.2 percent to 6.4 percent in the quality improvement group, compared to a change from 11.6 percent to 9.5 percent in the usual care group.

The primary venue in which suicide awareness and education programs reach adolescents is schools. The rationale behind school-based programs is that a large proportion of high school students is exposed to peers with suicidal feelings and that adolescents are more likely to tell peers than adults if they have suicidal thoughts. Most programs are designed to increase awareness of suicide warning signs, dispel myths, promote case finding, provide information about availability of mental health resources, provide ways to cope with depression and suicidal feelings, and encourage students to seek help. Kalafat (2003) noted that after an initial surge of interest in school-based suicide prevention programs in schools in the 1980s, interest waned in the mid to late 1990s. However, the Surgeon General's Call to Action to Prevent Suicide (U.S. Public Health Services, 1999) brought renewed interest. Indeed, Objective 4.2 of the National Strategy to Prevent Suicide calls for an increase in the number of evidence-based suicide prevention programs in schools.

The primary venue in which suicide awareness and education programs reach adolescents is schools.

Two major review articles have examined studies in suicide awareness and education programs in the schools: one reviewing studies from 1980 through 1995 (Ploeg et al., 1996) and the other reviewing studies from 1990 through 2002 (Guo & Harstall, 2002). The Ploeg et al. (1996) review concluded that overall knowledge improves with suicide awareness programs, but that attitudes and help seeking are both positively and negatively affected by these programs. Some studies have found that suicide awareness and education programs can have negative effects on boys (Shaffer, Garland, Vieland, Underwood, & Busner, 1991) and a negative effect on adolescents with a history of suicidal behavior (Shaffer, Vieland, Garland, Rojas, Underwood, & Busner, 1990). Guo and Harstall (2002) concluded that these programs improve knowledge and attitudes of participants, but they did not find an effect on suicidal behavior.

The EBPP found two universal suicide awareness and education programs to be promising: the Lifelines program—and its updated version, Lifelines ASAP, which combines material from the Adolescent Suicide Awareness Program (ASAP; Ryerson, 1990)—and the Signs of Suicide (SOS) program (Aseltine & DeMartino, 2004). The latter will be discussed here, as it contains a unique combination of awareness and screening.

SOS is a suicide awareness and education curriculum with a screening program for depression and other risk factors. The educational component of this program teaches adolescents that suicide is directly related to a psychiatric disorder, typically depression, unlike many of the original suicide awareness programs in which suicidal behavior was often described as a reaction to stress. SOS teaches adolescents that mental illness is treatable and that they should respond to a suicidal peer using the ACT technique: acknowledge the signs of suicide, respond with care, and tell a responsible adult. A video dramatization is shown about the signs of suicidality and depression, as well as correct and incorrect ways to respond to a suicidal peer. The screening portion of the SOS program entails completing a seven-item measure of depressed mood. If adolescents meet the clinical cutoff score on this measure, the Columbia Depression Scale, an interpretation sheet attached to the screen encourages them to seek help immediately.

Aseltine and DeMartino (2004) present data from five high schools in Connecticut and Georgia, with over one thousand subjects each in the SOS and control groups. At three-month follow-up, there was a significant improvement in knowledge as well as adaptive attitudes toward depression and suicide. Most important, SOS was the first program to demonstrate a statistically significant reduction in suicide attempts at three

SOS was the first program to demonstrate a statistically significant reduction in suicide attempts at three months: 3.6 percent in SOS versus 5.4 percent in the control group.

months: 3.6 percent in SOS versus 5.4 percent in the control group. The authors noted that a longer-term follow-up is necessary to determine whether this reduction in suicidal behavior persists.

One reason universal suicide awareness and education programs may not be as successful as hoped is that they do not target students at greatest risk for suicide. Selective prevention focuses on groups with known risk factors for suicidal behavior. The EBPP found two suicide awareness and education programs with high-risk youth to be promising and one to be effective. One promising program, Zuni Life Skills Development (LaFromboise & Howard-Pitney, 1995), targets Native American youth who are at high risk for suicide. LifeSkills Training is designed to teach the social competence needed to enhance social and emotional development as well as academic success. The units in the curriculum cover building self-esteem, identifying emotions and stress, increasing communication and problem-solving skills, recognizing and eliminating negative thinking, and setting goals. There is also suicide-specific training. The curriculum was developed so that it would be culturally acceptable to Zuni values and beliefs and was taught by teachers to students. In a randomized controlled trial, adolescents receiving the Zuni LifeSkills curriculum ($N = 69$) reported lower levels of hopelessness and better problem-solving and suicide intervention skills (as assessed by observer report) than the control group ($N = 59$).

The second program categorized by the EBPP as promising was Reconnecting Youth (Eggert, Thompson, Herting, & Nicholas, 1995). The one selective prevention program labeled as effective by the EBPP was Counselors-CARE/Coping and Support Training (Thompson, Eggert, Randell, & Pike, 2001). These two programs were tested by the same research group. Reconnecting Youth is a suicide prevention program for high school students identified as at risk for school dropout. Peers, school staff, and parents were used to deliver four different components of the intervention: school bonding activities, parent involvement, crisis response planning, and a class offered daily for one semester (eighty classes of fifty minutes each). A primary goal of Reconnecting Youth was to enhance feelings of personal control and self-esteem, using skills training to improve decision making, social support from teachers and peers, anger management, and communication. The Eggert et al. (1995) study compared students who screened positive for suicide risk behaviors and who took part in the intervention for one semester ($N = 36$), two semesters ($N = 35$), or who received a comprehensive assessment only ($N = 35$). All three groups demonstrated a reduction in suicidality, depression, hopelessness, and anger at the end of the school year. Only the two intervention groups demonstrated an improvement in level of personal control at follow-up.

The developers followed up their Reconnecting Youth program with a briefer version targeted at potential school dropouts who screened positive on a suicide risk measure. Participants were randomized to one of three conditions. Counselors-CARE (C-CARE) consisted of a two-hour assessment interview followed by a two-hour individual motivational counseling session and social connections intervention designed to link each youth with a school-based case manager, a favorite teacher, or both, as well as a parent. The second condition, Coping and Support Training (CAST) consisted of C-CARE plus a twelve-session coping skills and small-group support program targeting mood management, school performance, and drug use. The third condition was the school's standard of care for at-risk students—a brief assessment, referral to a school counselor, and notification of parents. At nine-month follow-up, both C-CARE and CAST members demonstrated significant improvement in suicidal ideation, depression, and hopelessness compared to the standard care group. CAST was more successful in enhancing personal control and problem solving than the other two conditions.

There are several shortcomings to school-based prevention programs. First, even if a program is effective, confidentiality concerns may limit the number of students who seek help from teachers and other school personnel. Another possible limitation of suicide prevention programs is their specificity. Prevention programs that focus on general mental health skills such as problem-solving, crisis management, mood management, and social skills may be more beneficial to students than programs focusing simply on suicide. Similarly, Kalafat (2003) noted that programs promoting protective factors such as contact with caring adults and a sense of connection with school, family, and community may be preferable to suicide-specific awareness programs. However, these programs are relatively uncommon.

The literature to date has not typically addressed other relevant markers of prevention program effectiveness, such as level of implementation difficulty, cost-effectiveness, and potential for dissemination (Burns & Patton, 2000). One limitation in implementation is lack of fidelity when programs are transported to the community. Kalafat and Ryerson (1999) recommend taking several steps to improve implementation fidelity, including discussing the particulars of the program with key stakeholders in order to address resistance and barriers. In addition, providing additional one-time training has been found to improve helper competency for as long as six months (Chagnon, Houle, Marcoux, & Renaud, 2007). One key to sustainability of these programs is supportive administrators and teachers. Kalafat and Ryerson (1999) noted that identifying core elements that must be retained and others that can be modified or eliminated assists sustainability, but may also impede effectiveness.

Screening

Screening is a method to identify high-risk individuals, rather than populations, who would benefit from further assessment and then possibly referral for treatment. Screening can directly assess suicidality or can address underlying risk conditions, such as depression, associated with suicidal behavior. For adolescents, screening occurs primarily in schools. The most well-researched screening program is the Columbia Teen Screen (McGuire & Flynn, 2003).

The Columbia Teen Screen program consists of multiple stages to identify adolescents at risk for suicide. In the first stage, consent from parents for screening is obtained. In the second stage, the eleven-item Columbia Suicide Screen is administered. This measure assesses symptoms of depression, substance abuse, suicidal ideation, and past suicide attempts. The screen items are embedded within thirty-two general health questions and four items on relationships and family concerns. Administration time is approximately ten minutes. The performance of the teen screen was examined in 1,729 high school students in the New York area. The sensitivity of the screen was 0.75, while specificity was 0.83 (Shaffer et al., 2004). The relatively low specificity indicates the need for a second-stage evaluation to reduce false positives.

Adolescents who screen positive on the Teen Screen are then administered a voice-activated, computerized psychiatric diagnostic interview, the Voice Diagnostic Interview Schedule for Children (Voice-DISC). In the fourth stage, a clinician conducts a brief clinical evaluation based on the diagnostic report provided by the Voice-DISC. If no significant psychiatric difficulty is noted in the interview or the adolescent is already receiving treatment, no further action is required. If the interview reveals significant psychiatric disturbance, the clinician or a case manager contacts the adolescent's parents and a referral is arranged.

McGuire and Flynn (2003) discussed several models of screening being used across the country to implement the Teen Screen program. In one model, a master's-level mental health clinician is hired to work full-time in the school to manage all the steps of the program, from screening to referral. In a second model, a part-time bachelor's-level clinician completes the first stage of the screen and then refers positive screens to the school guidance counselor for further evaluation and referral. In a third model, screening is considered part of the school guidance counselor's responsibilities. In this model, the guidance department conducts all stages of the program. In a variant of this third model, a school-based health center takes the place of the guidance department in implementing the program. In a fourth model, outside personnel are hired to come into a school for a brief period of time to conduct the screen, Voice-DISC, clinical evaluations, and referrals.

There are several limitations to screening model programs like the Columbia Teen Screen. First, there may be resistance to implementation of such programs by school staff. Eckert, Miller, DuPaul, and Riley-Tillman (2003) conducted a survey that exemplifies the need to obtain buy-in from key personnel responsible for implementation of a screening program. The responses of 211 school psychologists to a survey about suicide prevention programs indicated that in-service training and curriculum-based programs were significantly more acceptable than a schoolwide screening program.

One reason for resistance to screening is the fear that asking about suicidality will trigger increased incidences of suicidal ideation and behavior. However, one study found that this was not the case. Gould et al. (2005) conducted a study of students who took part in a two-day screening. Students were randomly assigned to a baseline screen with and without suicide-related questions. Two days after the initial screening, students who had been exposed to questions about suicide were slightly more likely to report suicidal ideation (4.7 percent) than those who were unexposed (3.9 percent).

Resistance can also be related to greater workloads, uneasiness in managing suicidal adolescents, and lack of referral resources. The lack of availability of treatment services for adolescents who screen positive in many communities is particularly problematic. When services are available, adolescents and their families often have difficulty accepting the fact that they need further evaluation and treatment. There are at least two other potential limitations. First, there can be considerable costs involved in the program, and they vary by the model chosen for implementation. Second, there is some concern that screening may not adequately identify minority adolescents at risk of suicide. Kataoka, Stein, Lieberman, and Wong (2003) reviewed the results of a gatekeeper model adolescent suicide prevention program that has been in place in the Los Angeles school system since 1986 and found that Latino students were being underidentified relative to their percentage of the school population.

Means Restriction

A number of approaches have been used to prevent access to lethal means as a suicide reduction strategy. As discussed previously, firearms are the most common method of suicide among adolescents. This is true for males and females, younger and older adolescents, and for all races. Primary prevention of suicide involves reducing access to the means. Brent, Perper, Moritz, Baugher, and Allman (1993) examined the characteristics of suicide in adolescents with no apparent psychopathology and found that the presence of a loaded gun in their homes distinguished these suicides from the comparison groups. They concluded that for suicides in which impulsivity is a major determinant, preventing access to methods might be the most beneficial prevention strategy.

For suicides in which impulsivity is a major determinant, preventing access to methods might be the most beneficial prevention strategy.

Beautrais, Fergusson, and Horwood (2006) compared suicide data for eight years before and ten years after restrictive firearms legislation was introduced in New Zealand. The rate of suicide in youth (fifteen to twenty-four years old) was reduced by 66 percent after legislation was introduced. Brent and Bridge (2003) conclude that restrictive gun regulations contribute to a reduction in youth suicide rates. However, method substitution—leading to an increase in another suicide method such as hanging—has been found in some studies.

The findings discussed above suggest that the dissemination of information to parents about the risk of keeping firearms in the home would be useful. Kruesi, Grossman, Pennington, Woodward, Duda, and Hirsch (1999) provided a three-step intervention called *means restriction* to the parents of adolescents who were seen at an emergency room and who were at risk for suicide. The intervention involved informing parents that their child was at increased risk for suicide, explaining to parents that limiting access to lethal means could reduce risk, and educating parents on ways to limit access to lethal means. At two- to three-month follow-up, the parents in the experimental group were more likely to have taken steps to limit access to lethal means. Five out of eight households that had firearms took actions to limit access to firearms after the program, compared to 0.7 in the control group.

Media

The media can be used in a proactive way to inform people about suicide and to provide education regarding the importance of early detection of risk factors. Suicide prevention programs for the general public typically address depression and the subsequent risk for suicide. Such educational programs may also help decrease the stigma about suicidality, emotional problems, and the use of mental health services. Mann et al. (2005) concluded that these public education programs have modest effects at best on attitudes.

The media can also exacerbate suicide risk by glamorizing suicide. Stack (2005) noted that nonfictional stories about a suicide are more likely than fictional stories to result in imitative suicide. Stack reviewed fifty-five studies and concluded that nonfictional stories about celebrities were 5.27 times more likely to result in imitative suicide, stories on female suicide were 4.89 times more likely to report a copycat effort, and stories reported on television rather than in newspapers were 79 percent less likely to find a copycat effect.

Gould, Jamieson, and Romer (2003) reviewed the literature specifically on adolescents and concluded the evidence is stronger for imitative effects from the news media than from fictional stories. Nonetheless, a few studies have found increased rates of suicide and suicide attempts following television shows about suicide. Gould et al. (2003) concluded that journalists need to be educated about ways to report on suicide to minimize imitation and encourage help seeking. Media guidelines have been prepared by the Centers for Disease Control and Prevention (O'Carroll & Potter, 1994). The CDC's suggestions include limiting the description of the suicide method, limiting the amount of media coverage, providing the telephone numbers of crisis centers or mental health agencies as a public service, and establishing a specific mental health liaison with the media.

SUMMARY

Adolescent suicide as a preventable public health problem is a significant concern, because suicidal behaviors have increased steadily over the last few decades among people aged fifteen to twenty-four, especially males. Social disorganization, developmental-task challenges, migration and mobility, acculturation, family and personal disorganization, diminished moral values, increases in the rate of substance use, access to firearms, and the influence of the media, including exposure to images of violence, have been hypothesized to account for these recent trends in the increase in attempted and completed suicide by adolescents. Prevention of suicidal behavior in the general population of adolescents focuses on general suicide awareness and education, as well as fostering protective factors. These general prevention programs have demonstrated only modest success in changing attitudes toward suicide, with little effect on actual suicidal behavior.

Prevention programs that either screen to identify high-risk individuals or select high-risk groups as the initial focus of a program appear to be more effective in reducing suicidal behavior than awareness and education programs. Thus, universal prevention programs that identify high-risk groups may be the most effective suicide prevention method for adolescents at this time. The cost-effectiveness of screening the general population to identify individuals still needs to be determined and compared to identification of high-risk populations a priori (Mann et al., 2005). Nonetheless, there is sufficient research available now that prevention programs with some evidence can be chosen for implementation. Moderators of effectiveness (such as racial differences) will be important to examine in future research, as well as the best means by which to enhance the protective factors that keep adolescents with high-risk profiles from progressing to suicidal behavior.

KEY TERMS

Evidence-Based Practices Project (EBPP)
Means restriction

Screening

DISCUSSION QUESTIONS

1. What are the benefits and drawbacks of the screening method for identifying high-risk individuals? Do you feel that screening is objective?

2. Discuss possible primary and secondary prevention strategies for suicide among adolescents.

3. Do the media glamorize or sensationalize suicide? How could changes in policy affect the portrayal of suicide within the media?

4. Are there significant differences between adolescents who attempt suicide and those who complete suicide? As an emerging health professional, what do you believe is the best way to prevent the onset of suicidal behavior, thus reducing the rates of completed suicide?

REFERENCES

Alcántara, C., & Gone, J. P. (2007). Reviewing suicide in Native American communities: Situating risk and protective factors within a transactional-ecological framework. *Death Studies, 31*(5), 457–477.

Asarnow, J. R., Jaycox, L. H., Duan, N., LaBorde, A. P., Rea, M. M., Murray, P., Anderson, M., Landon, C., Tang, L., & Wells, K. B. (2005). Effectiveness of a quality improvement intervention for adolescent depression in primary care clinics: A randomized controlled trial. *Journal of the American Medical Association, 293,* 311–319.

Aseltine, R. H., Jr., & DeMartino, R. (2004). An outcome evaluation of the SOS suicide prevention program. *American Journal of Public Health, 94,* 446–451.

Beautrais, A. L., Fergusson, D. M., & Horwood, L. J. (2006). Firearms legislation and reductions in firearm-related suicide deaths in New Zealand. *Australian and New Zealand Journal of Psychiatry, 40,* 253–259.

Borowsky, I., Resnick, M., Ireland, M., & Blum, R. (1999). Suicide attempts among American Indian and Alaska Native youth. *Archives of Pediatric and Adolescent Medicine, 153,* 573–580.

Brent, D. A., & Bridge, J. (2003). Firearms availability and suicide: Evidence, interventions, and future directions. *American Behavioral Scientist, 46,* 1192–1210.

Brent, P. A., Perper, J., Moritz, G., Baugher, M., & Allman, C. (1993). Suicide in adolescents with no apparent psychopathology. *Journal of the American Academy of Child and Adolescent Psychiatry, 32,* 494–500.

Burns, J., & Patton, G. (2000). Preventive interventions for youth suicide: A risk-factor based approach. *Australian and New Zealand Journal of Psychiatry, 34,* 388–407.

Centers for Disease Control and Prevention. (2004). Methods of suicide among persons aged 10–19 years: United States, 1992–2001. *Morbidity and Mortality Weekly Report, 53,* 471–474.

Centers for Disease Control and Prevention. (2006). Youth Risk Behavior Surveillance: United States, 2005. Surveillance Summaries, June 9, 2006. *Morbidity and Mortality Weekly Report 2006, 55*(No. SS–5), 1–108.

Centers for Disease Control and Prevention. (2007). Web-based Injury Statistics Query and Reporting System (WISQARS) [Online]. National Center for Injury Prevention and Control. Retrieved April 3, 2008, from www.cdc.gov/ncipc/wisqars.

Chagnon, F., Houle, J., Marcoux, I., & Renard, J. (2007). Control-group study of an intervention training program for youth suicide prevention. *Suicide and Life-Threatening Behavior, 37,* 135–144.

Commission on Adolescent Suicide Prevention. (2005). *Youth suicide.* In D. L.Evans, E. B. Foa, R. E. Gur, H. Hendin, C. P. O'Brien, M.E.P. Seligman, & B. T. Walsh (Eds.), *Treating and preventing adolescent mental health problems: What we know and what we don't know* (pp. 434–443). New York: Oxford University Press.

Cuellar, J., & Curry, T. R. (2007). The prevalence and comorbidity between delinquency, drug abuse, suicide attempts, physical and sexual abuse, and self-mutilation among delinquent Hispanic females. *Hispanic Journal of Behavioral Sciences, 29,* 68–82.

Duarté-Vélez, Y. M., & Bernal, G. (2007). Suicide behavior among Latino and Latina adolescents: Conceptual and methodological issues. *Death Studies, 31,* 435–455.

Eckert, T., Miller, D., DuPaul, G., & Riley-Tillman, T. C. (2003). Adolescent suicide prevention: School psychologists' acceptability of school-based programs. *School Psychology Review, 32,* 57–76.

Eggert, L. L., Thompson, E. A., Herting, J. R., & Nicholas, L. J. (1995). Reducing suicide potential among high-risk youth: Tests of a school-based prevention program. *Suicide and Life-Threatening Behavior, 25,* 276–296.

Evans, E., Hawton, K., Rodham, K., & Deeks, J. (2005). The prevalence of suicidal phenomena in adolescents: A systematic review of population-based studies. *Suicide and Life-Threatening Behavior, 35,* 239–250.

Fortuna, L. R., Perez, D. J., Canino, G., Sribney, W., & Alegria, M. (2007). Prevalence and correlates of lifetime suicidal ideation and suicide attempts among Latino subgroups in the United States. *Journal of Clinical Psychiatry, 68,* 572–581.

Gould, M., Jamieson, P., & Romer, D. (2003). Media contagion and suicide among the young. *American Behavioral Scientist, 46,* 1269–1284.

Gould, M., Marrocco, F., Kleinman, M., Thomas, G., Mostkoff, K., Cote, J., & Davies, M. (2005). Evaluating iatrogenic risk of youth suicide screening programs: A randomized controlled trial. *Journal of the American Medical Association, 293,* 1639–1643.

Guo, B., & Harstall, C. (2002). *Efficacy of suicide prevention programs for children and youth.* Edmonton, Canada: Alberta Heritage Foundation for Medical Research.

Hunt, K., Sweeting, H., Keoghan, M., & Platt, S. (2006). Sex, gender role orientation, gender role attitudes and suicidal thoughts in three generations: A general population study. *Social Psychiatry and Psychiatric Epidemiology, 41,* 641–647.

Kalafat, J. (2003). School approaches to youth suicide prevention. *American Behavioral Scientist, 43,* 1211–1223.

Kalafat, J., & Ryerson, D. (1999). The implementation and institutionalization of a school-based youth suicide prevention program. *Journal of Primary Prevention, 3,* 157–175.

Kataoka, S., Stein, B., Lieberman, R., & Wong, M. (2003). Suicide prevention in schools: Are we reaching minority youths? *Psychiatric Services, 54,* 11.

Kessler, R., Borges, G., & Walters, E. (1999). Prevalence of and risk factors for lifetime suicide attempts in the National Comorbidity Survey. *Archives of General Psychiatry, 56,* 617–626.

Kruesi, M.J.P., Grossman, J., Pennington, J. M., Woodward, P. J., Duda, D., & Hirsch, J. G. (1999). Suicide and violence prevention: Parent education in the emergency department. *Journal of the American Academy of Child and Adolescent Psychiatry, 38,* 250–255.

LaFromboise, T. D., & Howard-Pitney, B. (1995). The Zuni Life Skills Development Curriculum: Description and evaluation of a suicide prevention program. *Journal of Counseling Psychology, 42,* 479–486.

Mann, J. J., Apter, A., Bertocote, J., Beautrais, A., Currier, D., Haas, A., Hegerl, U., Lonnqvist, J., Malone, K., Marusic, A., Mehlum, L., Patton, G., Phillips, M., Rutz, W., Rihmer, Z., Schmidtke, A., Shaffer, D., Silverman, M., Takahashi, Y., Varnik, A., Wasserman, D., Yip, P., & Hendin, H. (2005). Suicide prevention strategies: A systematic review. *Journal of the American Medical Association, 294,* 2064–2074.

McGuire, L., & Flynn, L. (2003). The Columbia TeenScreen program: Screening youth for mental illness and suicide. *Trends in Evidence-Based Neuropsychiatry, 5,* 56–62.

O'Carroll, P. W., & Potter, L. B. (1994). Suicide contagion and the reporting of suicide: Recommendation from a national workshop. *Morbidity and Mortality Weekly Report, 43*(RR-6), 9–17.

Olfson, M., Marcus, S. C., Weissman, M. M., & Jensen, P. S. (2002). National trends in the use of psychotropic medications by children. *Journal of the American Academy of Child and Adolescent Psychiatry, 41,* 514–521.

Olson, L. M. & Wahab, S. (2006). American Indians and suicide: A neglected area of research. *Trauma, Violence, and Abuse, 7*(1), 19–33.

Pfaff, J. J., Acres, J. G., & McKelvey, R. S. (2001). Training general practitioners to recognize and respond to psychological distress and suicidal ideation in young people. *Medical Journal of Australia, 174,* 222–226.

Ploeg, J., Ciliska, D., Dobbins, M., Hayward, S., Thomas, H., & Underwood, J. (1996). A systematic overview of adolescent suicide prevention programs. *Canadian Journal of Public Health, 87,* 319–324.

Rodgers, P., Sudak, H., Silverman, M., & Litts, D. (2007). Evidence-based practices project for suicide prevention. *Suicide and Life-Threatening Behavior, 37,* 159–164.

Ryerson, D. (1990). Suicide awareness education in schools: The development of a core program and subsequent modifications for special populations or institutions. *Death Studies, 14,* 371–390.

Shaffer, D., Garland, A., Vieland, V., Underwood, M., & Busner, C. (1991). The impact of curriculum-based suicide prevention programs for teenagers. *Journal of the American Academy of Child and Adolescent Psychiatry, 30,* 588–596.

Shaffer, D., & Pfeffer, C. (2001). Practice parameters for the assessment and treatment of children and adolescents with suicidal behavior. *Journal of the American Academy of Child and Adolescent Psychiatry, 40*(Suppl.), 245–515.

Shaffer, D., Scott, M., Wilcox, H., Maslow, C., Hicks, R., Lucas, C. P., Garfinkel, R., & Greenwald, S. (2004). The Columbia Suicide Screen: Validity and reliability of a screen for youth suicide and depression. *Journal of the American Academy of Child and Adolescent Psychiatry, 43,* 71–79.

Shaffer, D., Vieland, V., Garland, A., Rojas, M., Underwood, M., & Busner, C. (1990). Adolescent suicide attempters: Response to suicide-prevention programs. *Journal of the American Medical Association, 264,* 3151–3155.

Stack, S. (2005). Suicide in the media: A quantitative review of studies based on nonfictional stories. *Suicide and Life-Threatening Behavior, 35,* 121–133.

Thompson, E. A., Eggert, L. L., Randell, B. P., & Pike, K. C. (2001). Evaluation of indicated suicide risk prevention approaches for potential high school dropouts. *American Journal of Primary Prevention, 91,* 742–752.

U.S. Department of Health & Human Services. (2006). *Health, United States, 2006, with chartbook on trends in the health of Americans.* Hyattsville, MD: National Center for Health Statistics.

U.S. Public Health Services. (1999). *The Surgeon General's call to action to prevent suicide.* Washington, DC: Author.

Walls, M. L., Chapple, C. L., & Johnson, K. D. (2007). Strain, emotion, and suicide among American Indian youth. *Deviant Behavior, 28*(3), 219–246.

Zayas, L., Kaplan, C., Turner, S., Romano, K., & Gonzalez-Ramos, G. (2000). Understanding suicide attempts in adolescent Hispanic females. *Social Work, 45,* 53–63.

CHAPTER

14

UNINTENTIONAL INJURIES AMONG ADOLESCENTS

DAVID A. SLEET ▪ MICHAEL F. BALLESTEROS

LEARNING OBJECTIVES

After studying this chapter, you will be able to

- Differentiate between injuries and accidents.
- Describe examples of racial disparity according to injury category.
- Evaluate strategies for reducing injury among adolescents.
- Assess how the physical and environmental context affect injury prevalence.

A major health threat facing young people today is unintentional injury. High-risk behaviors contributing to injury continue to threaten the health and the quality of life during adolescence, defined here as ages ten through nineteen. In fact, more adolescents in the United States die from injuries than from all other causes of death combined (Centers for Disease Control and Prevention [CDC], 2008a).

Injuries have plagued adolescents throughout history. U.S. President Theodore Roosevelt, in a letter of admonishment to his young son, Ted, in 1903, cautioned him not to take unnecessary injury risks:

> *I am judging for you as I would for myself. When I was young and rode across country I was light and tough, and if I did, as actually happened, break an arm or a rib, no damage ensued and no scandal was caused. Now I am stiff and heavy, and any accident to me would cause immense talk, and I do not take the chance; simply because it is not worthwhile. On the other hand, if I should now go to war and have a brigade as I had my regiment before Santiago, I should take any chance that was necessary; because it would be worthwhile. In other words, I want to make the risk to a certain accident commensurate with the object gained [Bishop, 1919, pp. 66–67].*

Injuries are a frequent and sometimes devastating outcome of risk taking, but are also inherent in the environment in which adolescents live, work, and play.

Risk taking is a normal part of adolescent life. Managing risks and distinguishing between safe and unsafe risks are important survival skills. Injuries are a frequent and sometimes devastating outcome of risk taking, but are also inherent in the environment in which adolescents live, work, and play (Barrios & Sleet, 2001).

Unintentional injury is responsible for nearly half (45.6 percent) of all deaths to adolescents, killing and crippling young people in the prime of their lives. In 2005, 7,959 U.S. adolescents died from unintentional injuries—the equivalent of twenty-two deaths each day (CDC, 2008a). The majority of unintentional injury deaths (70.3 percent) result from car crashes. What were referred to for decades as *accidents* we now refer to as *injuries*. Injuries are not the result of "accidents" or acts of fate; adolescent injuries result from events that are both predictable and preventable.

One of CDC's public health goals is to help adolescents achieve healthy independence by increasing the number of adolescents who are prepared to be healthy, safe, independent, and productive members of society (CDC, 2007a). CDC's Framework for Adolescent Health focuses on

- Preventing major sources of morbidity and mortality among adolescents
- Preventing key health risk behaviors that contribute to poor health outcomes
- Promoting and establishing healthy adolescent behaviors

Note: The views expressed in this chapter are those of the author and do not necessarily reflect the official views of the U.S. Department of Health and Human Services or the Centers for Disease Control and Prevention.

Injury and *violence* are among the leading health indicators used by the U.S. Department of Health and Human Services (DHHS) to measure the health of the nation by 2010. Injuries were selected as a leading health indicator on the basis of their ability to motivate action, the availability of data to measure progress, and their importance as a public health problem (DHHS, 2000).

Healthy People 2010 (DHHS, 2000) is a well-established and widely accepted source for measures to assess national progress in improving adolescent health. Of the 467 HP 2010 objectives, 107 are relevant for adolescents, and at least 29 are related to unintentional injury.

UNINTENTIONAL INJURIES

An *unintentional injury* is defined as "damage to the body resulting from acute exposure to thermal, mechanical, electrical, or chemical energy or from the absence of such essentials as heat or oxygen" (DHHS, 2000). Unintentional injuries can be further classified by cause and include injuries from motor vehicle crashes, fires and burns, falls, drowning, poisoning, choking, suffocation, and animal bites. Intentional injury (or violence) is discussed in Chapter Twelve.

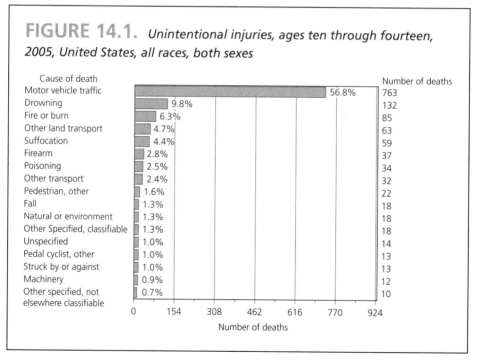

FIGURE 14.1. *Unintentional injuries, ages ten through fourteen, 2005, United States, all races, both sexes*

Cause of death	Percentage	Number of deaths
Motor vehicle traffic	56.8%	763
Drowning	9.8%	132
Fire or burn	6.3%	85
Other land transport	4.7%	63
Suffocation	4.4%	59
Firearm	2.8%	37
Poisoning	2.5%	34
Other transport	2.4%	32
Pedestrian, other	1.6%	22
Fall	1.3%	18
Natural or environment	1.3%	18
Other Specified, classifiable	1.3%	18
Unspecified	1.0%	14
Pedal cyclist, other	1.0%	13
Struck by or against	1.0%	13
Machinery	0.9%	12
Other specified, not elsewhere classifiable	0.7%	10

Note: NEC = not elsewhere classifiable.
Source: CDC (2008a).

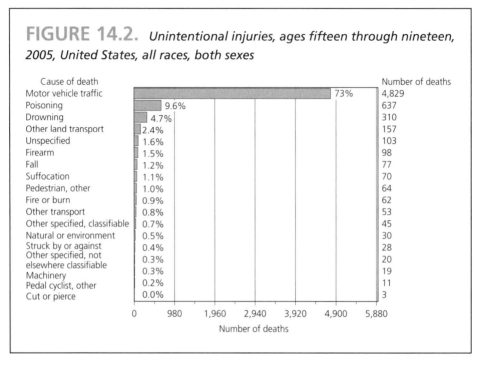

FIGURE 14.2. *Unintentional injuries, ages fifteen through nineteen, 2005, United States, all races, both sexes*

Cause of death	%	Number of deaths
Motor vehicle traffic	73%	4,829
Poisoning	9.6%	637
Drowning	4.7%	310
Other land transport	2.4%	157
Unspecified	1.6%	103
Firearm	1.5%	98
Fall	1.2%	77
Suffocation	1.1%	70
Pedestrian, other	1.0%	64
Fire or burn	0.9%	62
Other transport	0.8%	53
Other specified, classifiable	0.7%	45
Natural or environment	0.5%	30
Struck by or against	0.4%	28
Other specified, not elsewhere classifiable	0.3%	20
Machinery	0.3%	19
Pedal cyclist, other	0.2%	11
Cut or pierce	0.0%	3

Number of deaths: 0, 980, 1,960, 2,940, 3,920, 4,900, 5,880

Note: NEC = not elsewhere classifiable.
Source: CDC (2008a).

Unintentional injuries are the leading cause of death throughout adolescence, and motor vehicle crashes account for 56.8 percent of the unintentional injury deaths to those aged ten through fourteen (see Figure 14.1) and 73.0 percent of the unintentional injury deaths to those aged fifteen through nineteen (see Figure 14.2). Of the five leading causes of death in ages ten through fourteen, unintentional injury is ranked number one, followed by cancers (malignant neoplasms), suicide, homicide, and congenital anomalies (such as birth defects). In ages fifteen through nineteen, unintentional injury is ranked number one, followed by homicide, suicide, malignant neoplasms, and heart disease (Table 14.1).

Fatal injuries for males ages ten through fourteen were almost twice that of females, and more than twice as high among adolescents ages fifteen through nineteen. Fatal injury rates to all those aged fifteen through nineteen was nearly five times the rate of those aged ten through fourteen (see Table 14.2).

Racial disparities in injury are pronounced. Among adolescents, American Indians and Alaska Natives (AI/AN) and blacks consistently had higher total injury death rates than whites (Bernard, Paulozzi, & Wallace, 2007). AI/AN adolescents had the highest rates of motor vehicle traffic deaths (Bernard, Paulozzi, & Wallace, 2007) and are

TABLE 14.1. **Five leading causes of adolescent death, United States, 2005**

Rank	Ages 10–14	Ages 15–19
1	Unintentional injury: 1,343	Unintentional injury: 6,616
2	Malignant neoplasms: 515	Homicide: 2,076
3	Suicide: 270	Suicide: 1,613
4	Homicide: 220	Malignant neoplasms: 731
5	Congenital anomalies: 200	Heart disease: 389

Source: CDC (2008a). (Data from NCHS Vital Statistics System).

reported to have the highest alcohol-related motor vehicle mortality rates among racial/ethnic populations (Voas, Tippetts, & Fisher, 2000).

Deaths are only part of the picture, because for every injury death, there are about twelve injury hospitalizations and 154 emergency department visits (CDC, 2008a). Annually, more than five million adolescents suffer injuries requiring emergency department visits (CDC, 2008a). Costs per injury case for unintentional injuries, on average, were $5,348 for those ten through fourteen and $7,266 for those fifteen through nineteen (Miller, Finkelstein, Zaloshnja, & Hendrie, 2006). Nonfatal unintentional injuries in adolescents show that more than 1.3 million males and 860,723 females (age ten through fourteen) and 1.7 million males and 1.0 million females (aged fifteen through nineteen) were treated in emergency departments for an injury in 2006 (CDC, 2008a). The most common injuries treated in emergency departments for ten- through fourteen-year-olds were struck by or against (being struck by, hit, or crushed or striking against a human, animal, or inanimate object other than a vehicle or machinery), falls, overexertion, cut or pierce (by instruments such as knives, power lawn mowers, power hand tools, and household appliances), and pedal cycle injuries (such as bicycles). For fifteen- through nineteen-year-olds, the most common injuries were struck by or against, falls, motor vehicle occupant, overexertion, and cut or pierce (see Table 14.3).

The leading causes of injury hospitalization to ten- through fourteen-year-olds was falls (7,471), followed by motor vehicle occupant injury (4,514), and for fifteen-through nineteen-year-olds, motor vehicle occupant injury (23,733) followed by falls (7,465) (CDC, 2008a).

TABLE 14.2. **Unintentional adolescent injury deaths and rates per 100,000: United States, 2005**

Age Group	Sex	Number of Deaths	Population	Crude Rate
10–14	Males	866	10,692,773	8.10
	Females	477	10,185,970	4.68
	Subtotal	1,343	20,878,743	6.43
15–19	Males	4,645	10,803,526	43.00
	Females	1,971	10,259,596	19.21
	Subtotal	6,616	21,063,122	31.41
Total		7,959	41,941,865	18.98

Source: CDC (2008a). (Data from NCHS Vital Statistics System for numbers of deaths; Bureau of Census for population estimates.)

Adolescent unintentional injuries are also recognized as a global health problem, with road traffic injuries being the leading cause of death for youth around the world (World Health Organization, 2007). To draw attention to the growing problem of child and adolescent injuries and effective prevention strategies, the World Health Organization (WHO), together with UNICEF, released the *World Report on Child Injury Prevention* (World Health Organization, 2008). To complement the WHO report, CDC released the *CDC Childhood Injury Report* (Borse et al., 2008), which describes patterns of unintentional injuries among newborns through nineteen-year-olds in the United States from 2000 through 2006.

MOTOR VEHICLE INJURIES

Motor vehicle–related injuries are the leading cause of death for adolescents in the United States, accounting for 32 percent of deaths from all causes in this age group and 70 percent of all unintentional injury-related deaths (CDC, 2008a). In 2005,

TABLE 14.3. **Five leading causes of adolescent nonfatal unintentional injuries treated in emergency departments: United States, 2006**

	Age Group	
Rank	**10–14**	**15–19**
1	Struck by or against: 608,658	Struck by or against: 625,205
2	Fall: 602,415	Fall: 476,244
3	Overexertion: 279,148	Motor vehicle occupant: 416,144
4	Cut or pierce: 144,366	Overexertion: 406,699
5	Pedal cyclist: 110,506	Cut or pierce: 227,193

Source: CDC (2008a) data from NEISS All Injury Program operated by the Consumer Product Safety Commission.

5,592 adolescents died in motor vehicle–related crashes. Of these deaths, 2,904 occurred as occupants in motor vehicles. In 2006, 900,589 adolescents were victims of unintentional nonfatal motor vehicle–related injuries (including motorcycle, pedestrian, and bicycle) that resulted in hospital emergency department visits. Of these, over half were drivers or passengers (CDC, 2008a). The likelihood that children and adolescents will suffer fatal injuries in motor vehicle crashes increases when they don't use seat belts or when a driver transporting children or adolescents has been drinking (Quinlan, Brewer, Sleet, & Dellinger, 2000) and when new and inexperienced drivers transport other teenage passengers (Chen, Baker, Braver, & Li, 2000). Road traffic injuries are also the leading cause of death among young people worldwide (Peden et al., 2004).

Injuries to Teen Drivers and Passengers

In 2005, an average of fourteen teenagers a day died in motor vehicle–related crashes, and over 475,000 sustained nonfatal injuries as vehicle occupants (CDC, 2008a). Teenage male driver death rates are about twice that of females (CDC, 2008a).

Although teen-agers drive less than most other drivers, they are involved in a dis-proportionately high number of crashes.

Although teenagers drive less than most other drivers, they are involved in a disproportionately high number of crashes. The crash rate per mile driven for sixteen- through nineteen-year-olds is four times the risk for older drivers, and crash risk is highest at age sixteen. The crash rate per mile driven is twice as high for sixteen-year-olds as it is for eighteen- through nineteen-year-olds (Insurance Institute for Highway Safety, 2008a). Crash risk for both males and females is particularly high during the first months of driving and drops as young drivers accumulate more experience behind the wheel. The comprehensive costs of motor vehicle occupant, bicyclist, and pedestrian injury, including monetized quality-adjusted life years lost, among adolescents aged ten through nineteen years were over $45 billion in 2000 (Miller, Finkelstein, Zaloshnja, & Hendrie, 2006).

Other Traffic-Related Injuries to Teens

Adolescents also suffer injuries as bicyclists, motorcyclists, and pedestrians. Of the 67 million Americans who ride bicycles, half of them are children or teenagers (CDC, 2000). As bicyclists, 139 adolescents were killed in 2005, and in 2006, an estimated 162,808 were treated in emergency departments for bicycle-related nonfatal injuries (CDC, 2008a). Among the bicycle-related deaths, 90 percent are attributed to collisions with motor vehicles (CDC, 2007b). Severe head injuries are responsible for 64 percent to 86 percent of bicycle-related fatalities (Sosin, Sacks, & Webb, 1996), and children aged ten through fourteen years have the highest rate of bicycle-related fatalities. Research has clearly shown that bicycle helmets save lives, yet few adolescents wear a helmet when riding (CDC, 2000). To promote helmet use, the Centers for Disease Control and Prevention (CDC) published and disseminated a set of Bicycle Helmet Recommendations (CDC, 1995) designed for use in planning programs to prevent head injuries among bicyclists through the use of bicycle helmets (Rosenberg & Sleet, 1995; CDC, 1995).

As motorcyclists, 225 males and 24 females aged ten through nineteen were unintentionally killed in 2005. Death rates for males (1.05 per 100,000 population) were nearly nine times that of females (0.12 per 100,000). A total of 54,935 males and 6,675 females were treated in emergency departments for nonfatal motorcycle injuries in 2006. From 2005 to 2006, the rate of hospital emergency department visits per 100,000 population decreased for females (from 40.91 to 32.63) and increased for males (from 231.62 to 255.54) (CDC, 2008a).

As pedestrians, 462 adolescents died unintentionally in 2005. Another 20,403 males and 17,936 females were treated for pedestrian injuries in hospital emergency departments in 2006 (CDC, 2008a). Most pedestrian deaths occur at night—25 percent from 6 PM to 9 PM and 22 percent between 9 PM and midnight (CDC, 2000). Of all pedestrians age sixteen and older killed in nighttime crashes, 55 percent had blood alcohol levels of 0.10 g/dL or higher, higher than the legal limit in every state (CDC, 2000).

Developmental Factors

The high incidence of adolescent traffic-related injury is due in part to lack of experience and in part to lack of maturity. Many months or even years of experience may be needed for adolescents to become proficient in driving (Lonero, Clinton, & Sleet, 2006). Young drivers may also lack experience to recognize, assess, and respond to hazards, and they may be willing to accept higher levels of risks while walking, riding a bike, or driving a car or motorcycle (Irwin, Burg, & Cart, 2002).

In addition, adolescence is a stage of development characterized by increased independence from parents, social pressure from peers, and risk-taking behavior (Sleet & Mercy, 2003). Adolescent alcohol use simply exacerbates these problems. Distracted driving, the use of cell phones while driving, the presence of teen passengers, and the increased use of in-vehicle technologies present additional safety concerns. Technologies such as cell phones, in-vehicle Internet, and on-board navigation systems place additional demands on the adolescent's driver's attention. Research has yet to determine the exact safety consequences of using cell phones and other technologies in combination (Pratt, 2003), and the special risks these devices pose to adolescents who use them while driving.

The high incidence of adolescent traffic-related injury is due in part to lack of experience and in part to lack of maturity.

STRATEGIES FOR REDUCING MOTOR VEHICLE–RELATED INJURIES

A number of effective strategies have been shown to reduce motor vehicle – related injuries to adolescents. Among the most important are graduated licensing and seat belt use. Strategies to reduce the use of alcohol among teens are discussed later in the chapter.

Graduated Driver Licensing

One proven method for helping teens to become safer drivers is *graduated driver licensing* (GDL). Research shows reductions in fatal crashes of 38 percent for sixteen-year-olds under the most comprehensive and strict GDL (Baker, Chen, & Li, 2007). GDL systems work because they directly target the risk factors by giving newly licensed adolescent drivers experience under low-risk driving conditions. GDL systems include restrictions on driving that are lifted as adolescents gain driving experience and competence over a three-staged development process, allowing for time to acquire the skills, maturity, and experience as they prepare for full licensure. Forty-six states and the District of Columbia have enacted at least some components of GDL, but they vary widely from state to state (Jones & Shults, in press). Currently, only twenty-nine states and the District of Columbia have GDL systems that are considered "good" by the Insurance Institute for Highway Safety (IIHS), and even those states rated good do not contain all the elements of an optimal GDL system (IIHS, 2008b).

Other strategies embedded within GDL that will save lives include seat belt use mandates, adhering to speed limits, eliminating the distraction caused by talking or texting on a cell phone, reducing the number of teen passengers, restricting the hours of driving, and zero tolerance for alcohol use when driving. Parents are recognizing their critical role in managing their teen drivers, and many resources are available to assist parent-teen contracts for driving (Simon-Morton, Mickalide, & Olsen, 2006).

Use of Seat Belts and Helmets

Proper use of lap and shoulder belts could prevent approximately 60 percent of deaths to motor vehicle occupants in a crash (National Highway Traffic Safety Administration [NHTSA], 1996). Motorcycle helmets can be 35 percent effective in preventing fatal injuries to motorcyclists and 67 percent effective in preventing brain injuries (NHTSA, 1996). Bicycle helmets could prevent 75 percent of fatal bicycle-related head injuries (Rivara, 1985). Proper use of bicycle helmets can eliminate 65 to 88 percent of bicycle-related brain injuries, and 65 percent of serious injuries to the face (Thompson, Rivara, & Thompson, 1989; Thompson, Nunn, Thompson, & Rivara, 1996; Thompson, Rivara, & Thompson, 1996).

Peer pressure and negative modeling by family members may keep adolescents from using seat belts and bicycle helmets more often.

Adolescents are among the lowest users of seat belts or helmets. Nationwide in 2007, 11.1 percent of high school students claim they never or rarely use seat belts when riding in a car driven by someone else (Jones and Shults, in press). Nonuse was more prevalent in males than females and among black students than white students. Of the 66.8 percent of high school students who had ridden a bicycle in the past twelve months, 85.1 percent had rarely or never worn a bicycle helmet. Significantly more males than females never or rarely wore a helmet (Jones and Shults, in press). Peer pressure and negative modeling by family members may keep adolescents from using seat belts and bicycle helmets more often (Hendrickson, Becker, & Compton, 1997; Liller, Morisset, Noland, & McDermott, 1998).

To complement global efforts to increase helmet use, the World Health Organization has released *Helmets: A Road Safety Manual for Decision-Makers and Practitioners* (WHO, 2006), which explains why helmets are needed, how to assess the problem of nonuse in your community, how to design and implement a helmet program, and how to evaluate a program to determine whether it is working. Building a "culture of safety" for helmet wearing among adolescents will be a necessary ingredient in future efforts to increase adolescent helmet use (Sleet, Dinh-Zarr, & Dellinger, 2007).

HOME AND RECREATION INJURIES

Adolescent injuries occurring in the home and in recreation represent a significant burden in health care costs, injuries, and deaths. Research has demonstrated that many interventions directed at home and recreational environments work to prevent injuries; however, many of these strategies have not gained wide acceptance and use.

Drowning

Unintentional drowning takes a significant toll on adolescents each year, primarily in the summer months. In 2005, there were 442 fatal unintentional adolescent drownings in the United States, averaging almost 8.5 incidents per week (CDC, 2008a). In 2006 an additional 69 died from drowning and other causes in boating-related incidents, and 628 were treated for nonfatal boating-related injuries. Alcohol involvement was the leading contributing factor in fatal boating accidents, contributing to about one in five reported boating deaths (Howland, Mangione, Hingson, Smith, & Bell, 1995; U.S. Coast Guard, 2008). Nonfatal drownings can cause brain damage that may result in long-term disabilities including memory problems, learning disabilities, and permanent loss of basic functioning (a permanent vegetative state).

African American youth had the highest rate of drowning (1.82 per 100,000) in 2005, whereas white youth had the lowest (0.88 per 100,000). Between 2002 and 2005, the fatal unintentional drowning rate for African Americans aged ten through nineteen was 2.28 times that of whites. For American Indians and Alaska Natives, this rate was 1.8 times that of whites. For Asians and Pacific Islanders, the rate was 1.62 times that of whites (CDC, 2008a).

Factors such as the physical environment (access to swimming pools) and a combination of social and cultural issues (developing swimming skills and choosing safe water recreation) may contribute to the racial differences in drowning rates (Branche, Dellinger, Sleet, Gilchrist, & Olson, 2004). The percent of drownings in natural water settings increases with age. Most drownings in those over fifteen years of age occur in natural water settings (Gilchrist, Gotsch, & Ryan, 2004). In survey research, men of all ages, races, and educational levels consistently reported greater swimming ability than women. Men also have much higher drowning rates than women (Gilchrist, Sacks, & Branche, 2000).

Poisonings

A poison is any substance harmful to the body when ingested (eaten), inhaled (breathed), injected, or absorbed through the skin. Any substance can be poisonous if enough is taken. Unintentional poisoning includes the use of drugs or chemicals for recreational purposes in excessive amounts, such as an "overdose." It also includes the excessive use of drugs or chemicals for non-recreational purposes and lead and carbon monoxide poisoning. In 2005, 23,618 (72 percent) of the 32,691 overall poisoning deaths in the United States were unintentional (CDC, 2008a). Unintentional poisoning death rates have been rising steadily since 1992 (CDC, 2004a). Poisoning was second only to motor vehicle crashes as a cause of unintentional injury death in adolescents 15–19 years of age in 2005 (see Figure 14.2; CDC, 2008a).

In 2005, 34 adolescents ages ten through fourteen and 637 adolescents ages fifteen through nineteen died from unintentional poisoning. Poisoning deaths and death rates among both males and females nearly doubled from 2000–2005 in ages fifteen through nineteen (1.74 per 100,000 in 2000; 3.02 per 100,000 in 2005). Only small increases were seen among those ages ten through fourteen. Male rates were three times higher than females in fifteen- through nineteen-year-olds (3.68 versus 1.19), but only slightly higher in males than in females in ages ten through fourteen (0.19 versus 0.15) during the five-year period (CDC, 2008a).

Carbon monoxide (CO) poisoning can also pose a health risk to adolescents. CO is a colorless, odorless, poisonous gas that results from incomplete combustion of fuels (such as natural or liquefied petroleum gas, oil, wood, coal, or other fuels). Common sources include wood- and gas-burning stoves, fireplaces and stoves, space heaters, tobacco smoke, furnaces, generators, and motor vehicle and boat exhaust. During 2004–2006, an average of 20,636 persons per year (of all ages) were treated in hospital emergency departments for non-fire-related CO exposures, and 562 deaths were reported in 2004 (CDC, 2008c; CDC, 2007b). Although males and females were equally likely to visit an emergency department for CO exposure, males were 2.3 times more likely to die.

Fires

Fires and burns are the fifth leading cause of unintentional injury death among adolescents. House fires account for 66 percent of fire-related injuries and 72 percent of fire-related deaths. Although house fire death rates are highest in children and older adults, 147 adolescents lost their lives in fires in 2005, 54,397 were treated in emergency departments, and 566 were hospitalized for fire-related injuries, including burns and smoke inhalation (CDC, 2008a).

Death rates for black and Native American adolescents are more than twice the rate for whites (Warda, Tenenbein, & Moffatt, 1999). House fire deaths occur disproportionately in the Southeast (CDC, 2008a) and in December through February, when more than one-third of house fires occur (U.S. Fire Administration, 2005). The most common causes of residential fires are cooking and heating equipment, and the most common cause of fire-related deaths is cigarette smoking (Ahrens, 2003). Alcohol contributes to approximately 40 percent of deaths in house fires (Smith, Branas, & Miller, 1999).

Alcohol and Injuries

Alcohol is the most commonly used drug among adolescents, and the prevalence and toll of underage drinking in America is widely underestimated. More young people drink alcohol than smoke tobacco or use marijuana (Institute of Medicine [IOM], 2004). Overall in 2001, there were 40,933 injury-related deaths associated with excessive alcohol use or binge drinking among all ages. Of these, over half were unintentional deaths (13,878 traffic deaths and 12,233 nontraffic deaths) (CDC, 2004b).

In 2007, 75 percent of students in grades nine through twelve had ever consumed alcohol in their lifetime, and 44.7 percent reported having at least one drink on at least one occasion during the past month. Twenty-six percent of students engage in episodic heavy drinking—consuming five or more drinks on a single occasion (CDC, 2008b). Underage drinking is not just a problem among older teens: almost one in five eighth graders report recent use (IOM, 2004).

Alcohol's pathway to impairment leading to injury can be biological and psychological, directly affecting adolescent performance by slowing the decision-making process, reducing visual acuity and adaptation to brightness and glare, dividing one's attention, changing perceptions, increasing reaction time, increasing the sense of confidence, inhibiting self-control, and reducing perception of hazards (Lunetta & Smith, 2005). These changes can be particularly pronounced during adolescence, when the brain has yet to fully mature, and experiences in adapting to the effects of alcohol are limited. Alcohol use is associated with 36 percent of fatalities among those aged fifteen to twenty, and 20 percent of fatalities among children less than fifteen years of age (CDC, 1999a). Alcohol use is a factor in more than 30 percent of all drowning deaths (Cummings & Quan, 1999), 14 to 27 percent of all boating-related deaths (Logan, Sacks, Branche, & Ryan, 1999), 34 percent of all pedestrian deaths (CDC, 1999b), and 51 percent of adolescent traumatic brain injuries (Kraus, Rock, & Hemyari, 1990). Alcohol is implicated in deaths due to falls, fire, hypothermia, occupational work, poisoning, and water transport (CDC, 2004b).

Alcohol use is also associated with drug use and delinquency (Wechsler, Dowdall, Davenport, & Castillo, 1995), weapon carrying and fighting (Presley, Meilman, Cashin, & Leichliter, 1997), and motor vehicle crashes (Liu et al., 1997; Sleet, Howat et al., 2009). In 2007, 10.5 percent of high school students reported driving a motor vehicle after drinking alcohol, and 29.1 percent reported they rode in a car in the past thirty days with a driver who had been drinking alcohol (Jones & Shults, in press; CDC, 2008b).

STRATEGIES FOR REDUCING HOME AND RECREATION INJURIES

A number of effective strategies are available to reduce home and recreation injuries such as those related to drowning, poisonings, fires, and alcohol consumption. These strategies will work to protect adolescents, and they are also likely to protect others at risk.

Drowning

To reduce the risk of drowning, environmental protections (such as isolation pool fences and lifeguards) should be adopted; alcohol use should be avoided while swimming, boating, waterskiing, or supervising children; and all participants, caregivers, and supervisors should know water safety skills, be trained in cardiopulmonary resuscitation (CPR), and have access to 911 emergency calls (CDC, 2004c). Adolescents should be supervised when they are in or near water and use personal flotation devices while boating (Quan, Bennett, & Branche, 2006). It is estimated that 423 lives could have been saved in 2006 if all boaters had worn life jackets or personal flotation devices (U.S. Coast Guard, 2008).

Poisonings

Proper maintenance of potential sources of carbon monoxide (CO) poisoning in the home is the best way to avoid unintentional CO poisoning. CO alarms offer an additional layer of protection by sounding a loud noise (much like a smoke alarm) when CO levels reach dangerous levels. The problem of unintentional poisonings is growing among adolescents, and parents and health care providers need to be aware of the potential for improper use of prescription drugs that could escalate into unintentional poisoning. The nationwide toll-free number for Poison Control Centers is available twenty-four hours a day, seven days a week (1-800-222-1222). The centers can provide assistance with poisoning emergencies, answer questions about a specific poison, and provide poison prevention tips.

Fires

A working smoke alarm can reduce the risk of death in a house fire by about 50 percent, and it is cost-effective. An estimated 94 percent of U.S. households have at least one smoke alarm. However, about 25 percent of these do not work because of battery removal or because the batteries are not replaced each year (Warda & Ballesteros, 2007).

Working smoke alarms outside every habitable floor and outside every sleeping area give adolescents and other residents in a burning home enough advance warning to escape nearly all types of fires. Smoke alarms should be tested twice a year and, if possible, equipped with a ten-year, long-life lithium battery. In new construction, smoke alarms can be hardwired and sprinkler systems can be installed for additional protection. Fire escape plans should be a part of every family's disaster plan and should be practiced at least one a year (CDC, 2000).

Alcohol

Injuries related to alcohol use can be reduced by focusing on stronger and more comprehensive laws restricting youth access to alcohol, enhanced law enforcement together with adequate education and publicity targeting teens, training servers and sellers of alcohol, regulation of Internet sales of alcoholic beverages, sobriety checkpoints, and increasing alcohol taxation. Other effective strategies include enforcing the legal minimum drinking age law, reducing alcohol outlet density, zero tolerance laws for young drivers, random breath testing and comprehensive community programs, among others (Sleet, Howat, et al., 2009; Hingson, Swahn, & Sleet, 2007).

SETTINGS FOR ADOLESCENT INJURY

Adolescent injuries can occur in a variety of settings. In addition to those injuries that occur at home, on the road, and in the community, injuries to adolescents also occur at school, while playing sports, and at work.

School-Related Injuries

Approximately 10 to 25 percent of all child and adolescent injuries occur at school, making injury one of the most common health problems treated by school health personnel (Posner, 2000). Fatalities at school are rare; approximately one in four hundred injury-related fatalities among children five to nineteen years of age occur at school (Miller & Spicer, 1998).

In a 2007 nationwide survey among school students in grades nine through twelve who exercised or played sports in the last thirty days, 21.9 percent had to see a doctor or nurse for an injury (CDC, 2008b). In another study, the 15,405,392 injuries to children ages five to nineteen accounted for an estimated 26 percent of visits to the emergency department, of which 16.5 percent (1,859,215 injuries) occurred at school (Linakis, Amanullah, & Mello, 2006).

School injuries can be costly. One study found that in two-thirds of the cases where lawsuits were involved, schools or school districts paid an award to plaintiffs (mean = $562,915; median = $50,000). In most cases, the injured party was male (57.1 percent) and younger than eighteen years of age (79.9 percent). Fractures were the most common type of injury (38.9 percent). Falls were the most common cause of injury (21.9 percent). Among cases of unintentional injury, 74.6 percent involved injury to a student (Barrios, Jones, & Gallagher, 2007).

School-associated injuries are most likely to occur on playgrounds, particularly on climbing equipment, athletic fields, and in gymnasia (Junkins et al., 1999). The most frequent causes of hospitalization from school-associated injuries are falls (43 percent), sports activities (34 percent), and assaults (10 percent) (Di Scala, Gallagher, & Schneps, 1997).

Male students are injured 1.5 times more often than female students (Miller & Spicer, 1998), and males are three times more likely than females to sustain injuries requiring hospitalization (Di Scala et al., 1997). Middle and high school students sustain more school injuries than elementary school students: 41 percent of school injury victims are fifteen to nineteen years of age, 31 percent are eleven to fourteen years of age, and 28 percent are aged five to ten years (Miller & Spicer, 1998).

Schools have a responsibility to prevent injuries from occurring on school property and at school-sponsored events. Schools can teach students the skills necessary to promote safety and prevent unintentional injuries while at home, with friends, at work, at play, and in the community. Prevention is also critical because a wide range of injuries are litigated, and such lawsuits often require schools and school districts to pay costly awards to injured parties (Barrios et al., 2007).

CDC's *School Health Guidelines to Prevent Unintentional Injuries and Violence* (Barrios, Davis, et al., 2001; Barrios, Sleet, & Mercy, 2003) provides a set of recommendations related to the eight aspects of school health efforts. Since publication of these guidelines, school-based injury prevention education has increased. For example, the percentage of districts that required middle schools to teach injury prevention increased from 66.7 percent in 2000 to 80.3 percent in 2006, and the percentage of states that provided funding for staff development on injury prevention increased from 39.6 percent in 2000 to 76 percent in 2006; however, the median number of hours of required instruction decreased from 3.6 hours in 2000 to 1.8 in middle school and from 4.5 hours to 2.4 in high school (Kann, Telljohann, & Wooley, 2007).

Sports-Related Injuries

The risk of injury from recreational activities and sports is greatest during adolescence. In the United States, more than eight million high school students participate in school- or community-sponsored sports annually (CDC, 2000). More than one million serious sports-related injuries occur annually to adolescents aged ten to seventeen years (Bijur et al., 1995), accounting for one-third of all serious injuries in this age group. Sports cause more than 55 percent of nonfatal injuries at school (Scheidt et al., 1995). One study found that one in every fourteen adolescents will be seen in an emergency room or be hospitalized for a sports-related injury every year (Guyer & Gallagher, 1988); however, as many as 40 percent of medically treated injuries may be treated outside of an emergency department (Conn, Annest, & Gilchrist, 2003).

More than one million serious sports-related injuries occur annually to adolescents aged ten to seventeen years, accounting for one-third of all serious injuries in this age group.

Males are twice as likely as females to experience a sports-related injury, probably because males are more likely than females to participate in organized and unorganized sports that carry the greatest risk of injury, such as football, basketball, baseball, and wrestling (Di Scala et al., 1997; Mummery, Spence, Vincenten, & Voaklander, 1998). Among sports with many female participants, gymnastics, track and field, and basketball pose the greatest risk of nonfatal injury (Garrick & Requa, 1978; McLain & Reynolds, 1989). Among sports with male and female teams, such as soccer or basketball, the female injury rate per player tends to be higher than the male injury rate per player (Powell & Barber-Foss, 2000).

In many sports, risk of injury has been reduced by rule changes, conditioning, equipment and surface changes, coaching education, and use of protective gear and clothing (Gilchrist, Saluja, & Marshall, 2007). Changes in personal behavior and the environment in which adolescents play sports can help reduce many injuries (MacKay & Liller, 2006). In addition to implementing what is already known to be effective, some interventions in common practice have not yet been properly evaluated (such as ski helmets), and others are known to be ineffective, but are still used in practice, such as taping normal ankles to prevent sprains (Gilchrist, Saluja, & Marshall, 2007).

Work-Related Injuries

A U.S. General Accounting Office (GAO) study (U.S. GAO, 2002) found that as many as 3.7 million children aged fifteen to seventeen worked in 2001, of which 4 percent were employed illegally. Boys and Hispanic children; children working in construction, agriculture, transportation, and public utilities; and children working in family businesses faced a greater likelihood of being killed than other working children. Compliance with the child labor provisions of the Fair Labor Standards Act was found wanting for these reasons: (1) lack of specific goals for industries in which children have high rates of injuries and fatalities, (2) inadequate methods of measuring compliance success, (3) poor planning and assessment, and (4) inadequate guidance and training of local offices.

On average, adolescents work twenty hours per week for about half the year. Although adolescents who work derive many benefits (such as making money, developing job skills, and building responsibility), potential health and injury risks also result (Dunn, Runyan, Cohen, & Schulman, 1998). In 1992, more than 64,000 adolescents aged fourteen to seventeen years required treatment in a hospital emergency department for injuries sustained at work. Approximately seventy adolescents under eighteen years of age die on the job every year (National Institute for Occupational Safety and Health [NIOSH], 1995). As part of an overall strategy to protect the safety of teens at work, NIOSH has developed and implemented community-based educational strategies to promote the safety of adolescent workers ages fourteen to seventeen (Miara, Gallagher, Bush, & Dewey, 2003).

Nearly two million children and adolescents live or work on farms. Adolescents who work or live on farms are more likely to be exposed to farming-related injury hazards, including tractors, farm machinery, large animals, driving farm vehicles, rotary mowers, and pesticides (Schulman, Evensen, Runyan, Cohen, & Dunn, 1997). Adolescents in rural areas may be exposed to chemicals that are applied in agricultural settings. Seasonal application of pesticides adds to the risk of cumulative exposures. Adolescents can be exposed through the air they breathe, the food they eat, the water they drink, or through a combination of these exposures. Duration and concentration of exposures are important considerations (McDonald, Girasek, & Gielen, 2006).

PREVENTING AND CONTROLLING INJURIES

Opportunities to prevent and control injuries can occur before an injury-causing event (such as avoiding a motor vehicle crash by not drinking and driving), during an injury-causing event (such as wearing a seat belt in a crash), or after an injury-causing event (such as rapid emergency response and care) (Haddon, 1980). Changes in the environment, individual behavior, products, social norms, legislation, and policy can maximize the potential for prevention to work (Cohen & Potter, 1999).

Structural and Behavioral Strategies

Although structural strategies that require little or no action on the part of individuals are often preferred (Wilson & Baker, 1987), they are not always affordable or feasible to implement. Product modifications (such as improving playing fields), environmental changes (such as adding soft surfaces under playground equipment), and legislation (such as mandating bicycle helmet use and implementing graduated licensing laws) often result in the greatest protection to the population, but an adolescent's individual choices and behaviors can, and often do, override these protections (Gielen & Sleet, 2006; Gielen & Girasek, 2001). Therefore, behavioral change should be seen as a necessary component of even the most effective structural, automatic, environmental, or engineering protections (Gielen & Sleet, 2003; Sleet & Gielen, 2007). For example, bicycle and motorcycle helmets that protect against head injury must be fitted properly and worn consistently; automatic braking systems in vehicles require drivers to apply constant pressure on the brake pedal, rather than pumping the brakes; strong laws against speeding and drunk driving must be adopted and also adhered to. Effective injury prevention always involves both educational and environmental countermeasures—it is never an either-or proposition (Schieber & Vegega, 2003; Sleet & Gielen, 2007).

Legislation and Policy

Although adolescent behaviors can be changed by introducing a law or policy that mandates compliance—such as modifying sporting rules to require face protection, requiring protection when operating industrial machinery, or requiring helmet use when riding a bicycle (Shaw & Ogolla, 2006; Dellinger, Sleet, Shults, & Rinehart, 2007)—legislation to influence adolescent behaviors must be supported by the public and employers and enforced by local authorities (Schieber, Gilchrist, & Sleet, 2000). Other injury prevention policy approaches that have proven effective for preventing motor vehicle injuries at a population level are primary seat belt use laws (where one can be cited for nonuse as a primary offense), enhanced police enforcement, 0.08% blood alcohol level laws, minimum legal drinking age laws, sobriety checkpoints, and zero tolerance laws for young and inexperienced drivers (Zaza et al., 2005). Already, policy changes that discourage early adolescent driving, such as rising insurance costs, expensive driving schools, and GDL laws, have reduced the proportion of sixteen-year-olds who hold a driver's license from nearly 43.8 percent in 1998 to 29.8 percent in 2006 (Chapman & Maynard, 2008).

Workplace Protection

In occupational safety, the *Fair Labor Standards Act* (FLSA) is designed to protect youth under age eighteen from hazardous work conditions. They specify minimum ages for different types of work, prohibit work during hazardous times (such as at night), and dictate maximum daily hours of work. Although forty-one states have laws that require young workers age fourteen to seventeen to obtain a work permit, the effectiveness of the permit system on health and safety is not known (Runyan, Schulman, & Ta, 2006). The Teen Drive for Employment Act (Public Law 105-334) is an example of a workplace policy that prohibits all on-the-job driving for sixteen-year-olds and limits the nature and amount of driving permitted for seventeen-year-olds. However, the FLSA does not cover workers aged eighteen and older, who are still in the process of developing driving skills and gaining experience. For these inexperienced young adult drivers, employers should consider adopting strategies similar to those in the graduated licensing laws that grant driving privileges incrementally, such as limiting nighttime, intensive, or high-risk driving until more experience behind the wheel has been gained (Pratt, 2003).

Ecological Approaches

The most effective injury prevention efforts are structured within an ecological framework, addressing individual modifiable factors, family, peer group, worksite, and community and sociocultural factors simultaneously (Allegrante, Marks, & Hanson, 2006; Sleet & Gielen, 2006; Mercy, Sleet, & Doll, 2006). For example, legislation requiring bicycle helmet use should be accompanied by an educational campaign for children and parents, police enforcement in the community, and discounted sales of helmets by local merchants (Abularrage, DeLuca, & Abularrage, 1997; Gilchrist, Schieber, Leadbetter, & Davidson, 2000). Programs addressing the safety of employees can also be extended to focus on the safety of other family members and retirees off the job. Ecological approaches emphasize tailoring specific interventions to the cognitive and physical skills of adolescents and to the social world in which they live.

SUMMARY

The most effective injury prevention efforts are structured within an ecological framework, addressing individual modifiable factors, family, peer group, worksite, and community and sociocultural factors simultaneously.

Injuries are the largest source of premature morbidity and mortality among adolescents and the leading cause of death. Transportation is the largest source of these injuries to young people, primarily due to motor vehicle injuries suffered as drivers and passengers, but also as bicyclists and pedestrians. Other major causes of unintentional injuries to adolescents include drowning, poisonings, and fire and burns. Alcohol is an important contributor to adolescent injuries. The roads, home, school, sports, recreation, and the workplace are settings where injuries commonly occur.

No single solution exists to reduce or prevent adolescent injuries and the disabilities that result. Ecological approaches that consider the importance of the interactions between people and their environment are necessary. Injury policy development, education and skill building, laws and regulation, family, school, community, workplace, home-based strategies, and enforcement are important elements of a comprehensive ecological approach to preventing unintentional injuries. Families and schools, adolescents themselves, community organizations and agencies, and businesses can collaborate to develop, implement, and evaluate interventions to reduce the major sources of injuries among adolescents.

President Theodore Roosevelt was wise in writing letters to his children to caution them against frivolous risk taking, but admonitions alone will not be sufficient to markedly reduce the risk of injuries among adolescents. We need multifaceted approaches that change adolescent and peer behavior, change social norms and expectations, improve environments, and change products. Implementing known and effective prevention strategies such as using seat belts and bicycle and motorcycle helmets, installing residential smoke alarms, reducing drinking and driving, strengthening graduated driver licensing laws, implementing comprehensive school health education programs and policies, promoting the use of safety equipment in sports and leisure, and protecting adolescents at work will all contribute to reducing injuries to young people. The frequency, severity, potential for death and disability, and costs of these injuries, together with the high success potential of prevention strategies, make injury prevention a key public health goal to improve adolescent health in the future.

KEY TERMS

Carbon monoxide (CO)   Injury
Fair Labor Standards Act (FLSA)   Violence
Graduated driver licensing (GDL)   Unintentional injury
Healthy People 2010 (HP 2010)

DISCUSSION QUESTIONS

1. Propose a new policy that could be implemented to reduce unintentional injuries among adolescents.

2. Defend or critique the statement "Effective injury prevention always involves both educational measures and environmental countermeasures."

3. Should more public health dollars be spent on adolescent injury prevention rather than preventing other problems such as teen pregnancy, substance abuse, or sexually transmitted disease? What are the reasons for your choice?

REFERENCES

Abularrage, J. J., DeLuca, A. J., Abularrage, C. J. (1997). Effect of education and legislation on bicycle helmet use in a multiracial population. *Archives of Pediatric and Adolescent Medicine, 151,* 41–44.

Allegrante, J. P., Marks, R., & Hanson, D. W. (2006). Ecological models for the prevention and control of unintentional injury. In A. C. Gielen, D. A. Sleet, and R. DiClemente (Eds.), *Injury and violence prevention: Behavioral science theories, methods, and applications* (pp. 105–126). San Francisco: Jossey-Bass.

Ahrens, M. (2003). The U.S. fire problem overview report: Leading causes and other patterns and trends. Quincy, MA: National Fire Protection Association, Fire Analysis and Research Division.

Baker, S. P., Chen, L., & Li, G. (2007). Nationwide review of graduated driver licensing. Washington, DC: AAA Foundation for Traffic Safety.

Barrios, L., & Sleet, D. A. (2001). Adolescent injuries and violence. In N. J. Smelser & P. B. Baltes (Eds.), *International encyclopedia of the social and behavioral sciences* (pp. 112–116). Amsterdam: Elsevier.

Barrios, L. C., Davis, M. K., Kann, L., Desai, S., Mercy, J. A., Reese, L., E., Sleet, D. A., & Sosin, D. M. (2001, December 7). School health guidelines to prevent unintentional injuries and violence. *MMWR Recommendations and Reports, 50*(RR22), 1–74.

Barrios, L. C., Jones, S. E., & Gallagher, S. S. (2007). Legal liability: The consequences of school injury. *Journal of School Health, 77*(5), 273–279.

Barrios, L. C., Sleet, D. A., & Mercy, J. (2003). CDC school health guidelines to prevent unintentional injuries and violence. *American Journal of Health Education, 34*(5 Suppl.), S18–S22.

Bernard, S. J., Paulozzi, L. J., & Wallace, L.J.D. (2007, May 18). Fatal injuries among children by race and ethnicity: United States, 1999–2002. *MMWR Surveillance Summaries, 56*(SS-5), 1–16.

Bijur, P. E., Trumble, A., Harel, Y., Overpeck, M. D., Jones, D., & Scheidt, P. C. (1995). Sports and recreation injuries in U.S. children and adolescents. *Archives of Pediatric and Adolescent Medicine, 149,* 1009–1016.

Bishop, J. B. (Ed). (1919). *Theodore Roosevelt's letters to his children.* New York: Scribner's.

Borse, N. N., Gilchrist, J., Dellinger, A. M., Rudd, R. A., Ballesteros, M. F., & Sleet, D. A. (2008). CDC childhood injury report: Patterns of unintentional injuries among 0–19 year olds in the United States, 2000–2006. Atlanta, GA: Centers for Disease Control and Prevention, National Center for Injury Prevention and Control.

Branche, C. M., Dellinger, A. M., Sleet, D. A., Gilchrist, J., & Olson, S. J. (2004). Unintentional injuries: The burden, risks and preventive strategies to address diversity. In I. L. Livingston (Ed.), *Praeger handbook of Black American health: Policies and issues behind disparities in health* (2nd ed., pp. 317–327). Westport, CT: Praeger.

Centers for Disease Control and Prevention. (1995). Injury control recommendations: Bicycle helmets. *Morbidity and Mortality Weekly Report, 44*(RR-1).

Centers for Disease Control and Prevention. (1999a). Alcohol involvement in fatal motor-vehicle crashes: United States, 1997–1998. *Morbidity and Mortality Weekly Report, 48*(47), 1086–1087.

Centers for Disease Control and Prevention. (1999b). Pedestrian fatalities: Cobb, DeKalb, Fulton, and Gwinnett counties, Georgia, 1994–1998. *Morbidity and Mortality Weekly Report, 48*(28), 601–605.

Centers for Disease Control and Prevention. (2000). Fact book and state injury profiles: Year 2000. Atlanta: National Center for Injury Prevention and Control.

Centers for Disease Control and Prevention. (2004a). Unintentional and undetermined poisoning deaths: 11 states, 1990–2001. *Morbidity and Mortality Weekly Report, 53,* 233–238.

Centers for Disease Control and Prevention. (2004b). Alcohol attributable deaths and years of potential life lost: United States, 2001. *Morbidity and Mortality Weekly Report, 53*(37), 866–870.

Centers for Disease Control and Prevention. (2004c). Nonfatal and fatal drownings in recreational water settings: United States, 2001 and 2002. *Morbidity and Mortality Weekly Report, 53*(21), 447–452.

Centers for Disease Control and Prevention. (2007a, October 1). Goal action plan for adolescent health (working draft, version 1). Atlanta: Author.

Centers for Disease Control and Prevention. (2007b). Wide-Ranging Online Data for Epidemiologic Research (WONDER) [Online]. Retrieved February 19, 2008, from http://wonder.cdc.gov/mortsql.html.

Centers for Disease Control and Prevention. (2008a). Web-Based Injury Statistics Query and Reporting System (WISQARS) [Online]. National Center for Injury Prevention and Control and NCHS Vital Statistics System. Retrieved April 22, 2008, from www.cdc.gov/ncipc/wisqars.

Centers for Disease Control and Prevention. (2008b). Youth Risk Behavior Surveillance: United States, 2007. *Morbidity and Mortality Weekly Report, 57*(SS-4).

Centers for Disease Control and Prevention. (2008c). Nonfatal, unintentional, non-fire-related carbon monoxide exposures: United States, 2004–2006. *Morbidity and Mortality Weekly Report*, *57*(*33*), 896–899.

Chapman, M. M., & Maynard, M. (2008, February 25). Fewer youths jump behind the wheel at 16. *New York Times.*

Chen, L. H., Baker, S. P., Braver, E. R., & Li, G. (2000). Carrying passengers as a risk factor for crashes fatal to 16- and 17-year-old drivers. *Journal of the American Medical Association, 283*(12), 1578–1582.

Cohen, L. R., & Potter, L. B. (1999). Injuries and violence: risk factors and opportunities for prevention during adolescence. *Adolescent Medicine: State of the Art Reviews, 10*(1), 125–135.

Conn, J. M., Annest, J. L., & Gilchrist, J. (2003). Sports and recreation-related injury episodes in the US population, 1997–99. *Injury Prevention, 9,* 117–123.

Cummings, P., & Quan, L. (1999). Trends in unintentional drowning: The role of alcohol and medical care. *Journal of the American Medical Association, 281*(23), 2198–2202.

Dellinger, A., Sleet, D. A., Shults, R. A., & Rinehart, C. (2007). Interventions to prevent motor vehicle injuries. In L. S. Doll, S. E. Bonzo, J. A. Mercy, & D. A. Sleet (Eds.), *Handbook of injury and violence prevention.* New York: Springer.

Department of Health and Human Services. (2000, January). *Healthy people 2010* (conference edition, in two volumes). Washington, DC: U.S. Department of Health and Human Services.

Di Scala, C., Gallagher, S. S., & Schneps, S. E. (1997). Causes and outcomes of pediatric injuries occurring at school. *Journal of School Health, 67,* 384–389.

Dunn, K. A., Runyan, C. W., Cohen, L. R., & Schulman, M. D. (1998). Teens at work: A statewide study of jobs, hazards, and injuries. *Journal of Adolescent Health, 22,* 19–25.

Garrick, J. G., & Requa, R. K. (1978). Injuries in high school sports. *Pediatrics, 61,* 465–469.

Gielen, A. C., & Girasek, D. C. (2001). Integrating perspectives on the prevention of unintentional injuries. In N. Schneiderman, M. A. Speers, J. M. Silva, H. Tomes, & J. H. Gentry (Eds.), *Integrating behavioral and social sciences with public health.* Washington, DC: American Psychological Association.

Gielen, A. C., & Sleet, D. A. (2003). Application of behavior-change theories and methods to injury prevention. *Epidemiologic Reviews, 25*(1), 65–76.

Gielen, A. C., & Sleet, D. A. (2006). Injury prevention and behavior: An evolving field. In A. C. Gielen, D. A. Sleet, & R. DiClemente (Eds.), *Injury and violence prevention: Behavioral science theories, methods, and applications* (pp. 1–16). San Francisco: Jossey-Bass.

Gilchrist, J., Sacks, J. J., & Branche, C. M. (2000). Self-reported swimming ability in U.S. adults, 1994. *Public Health Reports, 115*(2–3), 110–111.

Gilchrist, J., Saluja, G., & Marshall, S. W. (2007). Interventions to prevent sports and recreation-related injuries. In L. S. Doll, S. E. Bonzo, J. A. Mercy, & D. A. Sleet (Eds.), *Handbook of injury and violence prevention* (pp. 117–136). New York: Springer.

Gilchrist, J., Schieber, R. A., Leadbetter, S., & Davidson, S. C. (2000). Police enforcement as part of a comprehensive bicycle helmet program. *Pediatrics, 106*(1), 6–9.

Guyer, B., & Gallagher, S. (1988). Childhood injuries and their prevention. In H. Wallace, G. Ryan, & A. Oglesby (Eds.), *Maternal and child health practices* (3rd ed.). Oakland, CA: Third Party Publishers.

Haddon, W., Jr. (1980). Options for the prevention of motor vehicle crash injury. *Israel Journal of Medical Sciences, 16*(1), 45–65.

Hendrickson, S. L., Becker, H., & Compton, L. (1997). Collaborative assessment: Exploring parental injury prevention strategies through bicycle helmet use. *Journal of Public Health Management and Practice, 3*(6), 60–70.

Hingson, R.Q.W., Swahn, M. H., & Sleet, D. A. (2007). Interventions to prevent alcohol-related injuries. In L. S. Doll, S. E. Bonzo, J. A. Mercy, & D. A. Sleet (Eds.), *Handbook of injury and violence prevention* (pp. 295–310). New York: Springer.

Howland, J., Mangione, T., Hingson, R., Smith G., & Bell, N. (1995). Alcohol as a risk factor for drowning and other aquatic injuries. In R. R. Watson (Ed.), *Alcohol and accidents—drug and alcohol abuse reviews: Vol 7.* Totowa, NJ: Humana Press.

Institute of Medicine. (2004). *Reducing underage drinking: A collective responsibility.* Washington, DC: National Academies Press.

Insurance Institute for Highway Safety. (2008a). Fatality facts 2006: Teenagers. Retrieved May 10, 2008, from www.iihs.org/research/fatality_facts_2006/teenagers.html.

Insurance Institute for Highway Safety. (2008b). Graduated driver licensing overview. Retrieved May 10, 2008, from www.iihs.org/laws/gdl_full.aspx.

Irwin, C. E., Jr., Burg, S. J., & Cart, C. U. (2002). America's adolescents: Where have we been, where are we going? *Journal of Adolescent Health, 31*(6 Suppl.), 91–121.

Jones, S. E., & Shults, R. A. (in press). Trends and subgroup differences in transportation-related injury risk and safety behaviors among U.S. high school students, 1991–2007. *Journal of School Health.*

Junkins, E. P., Jr., Knight, S., Lightfoot, A. C., Cazier, C. F., Dean, J. M., & Corneli, H. M. (1999). Epidemiology of school injuries in Utah: A population-based study. *Journal of School Health, 69*(10), 409–412.

Kann, L., Telljohann, S. K., & Wooley, S. F. (2007). Health education: Results from the School Health Policies and Programs Study 2006. *Journal of School Health, 77*(8), 408–434.

Kraus, J., Rock, A., & Hemyari, P. (1990). Brain injuries among infants, children, adolescents and young adults. *American Journal of Diseases of Children, 144,* 684–691.

Liller, K. D., Morisset, B., Noland, V., & McDermott, R. J. (1998). Middle school students and bicycle helmet use: Knowledge, attitudes, beliefs, and behaviors. *Journal of School Health, 68*(8), 325–328.

Linakis, J. G., Amanullah, S., & Mello, M. (2006). Emergency department visits for injury in school-aged children in the United States: A comparison of nonfatal injuries occurring within and outside of the school environment. *Academic Emergency Medicine, 13*(5), 567–570.

Liu, S., Siegel, P. Z., Brewer, R. B., Mokdad, A. H., Sleet, D. A., & Serdula, M. (1997). The prevalence of alcohol impaired driving in the U.S.: Results from a national self-reported survey of health behaviors. *Journal of the American Medical Association, 277,* 122–125.

Logan, P., Sacks, J. J., Branche, C. M., & Ryan, G. W. (1999). Alcohol-influenced recreational boat operation in the United States, 1994. *American Journal of Preventive Medicine, 16*(4), 278–282.

Lonero, L. P., Clinton, K. M., & Sleet, D. A. (2006). Behavior change interventions in road safety. In A. C. Gielen, D. A. Sleet, & R. J. DiClemente (Eds.), *Injury and violence prevention: Behavioral science theories, methods, and applications* (pp. 213–233). San Francisco: Jossey-Bass.

Lunetta, P., & Smith, G. A. (2005). The role of alcohol in injury deaths. In R. Preedy & R. Watson (Eds.), *Comprehensive handbook of alcohol-related pathology: Vol. I* (pp. 147–164). New York: Academic Press.

McDonald, E. M., Girasek, D. C., & Gielen, A. C. (2006). Home injuries. In K. D. Liller (Ed.), *Injury prevention for children and adolescents*. Washington, DC: American Public Health Association.

MacKay, M., & Liller, K. (2006). Behavioral considerations for sports and recreational injuries in children and youth. In A. C. Gielen, D. A. Sleet, & R. DiClemente (Eds.), *Injury and violence prevention: Behavioral science theories, methods, and applications* (pp. 257–273). San Francisco: Jossey-Bass.

McLain, L. G., & Reynolds, S. (1989). Sports injuries in a high school. *Pediatrics, 84,* 446–450.

Mercy, J. A., Sleet, D. A., & Doll, L. (2006). Applying a developmental and ecological framework to injury and violence prevention. In K. Liller (Ed.), *Injury prevention for children and adolescents: Research, practice and advocacy* (pp. 1–14). Washington, DC: American Public Health Association.

Miara, C., Gallagher, S., Bush, D., & Dewey, R. (2003). Developing an effective tool for teaching teens about workplace safety. *American Journal of Health Education, 34*(5 Suppl.), S30–S34.

Miller, T. R., Finkelstein, A. E., Zaloshnja, E., & Hendrie, D. (2006). The cost of child and adolescent injuries and the savings from prevention. In K. D. Liller (Ed.), *Injury prevention for children and adolescents: Research, practice, and advocacy* (pp. 15–64). Washington, DC: American Public Health Association.

Miller, T. R., & Spicer, R. S. (1998). How safe are our schools? *American Journal of Public Health, 88*(3), 413–418.

Mummery, W. K., Spence, J. C., Vincenten, J. A., & Voaklander, D. C. (1998). A descriptive epidemiology of sport and recreation injuries in a population-based sample: Results from the Alberta Sport and Recreation Injury Survey. *Canadian Journal of Public Health, 89*(1), 53–56.

National Highway Traffic Safety Administration. (1996, February). Benefits of safety belts and motorcycle helmets: Report to Congress. Washington, DC: U.S. Department of Transportation.

National Institute for Occupational Safety and Health. (1995). NIOSH alert: Request for assistance in preventing deaths and injuries of adolescent workers (DHHS Publication No. 95-125). Washington, DC: U.S. Department of Health and Human Services, Public Health Service, CDC.

Peden, M., Scurfield, R., Sleet, D., Mohan, D., Hyder, A. A., Jarawan, E., & Mathers, C. (Eds.). (2004). World report on road traffic injury prevention. Geneva: World Health Organization.

Posner, M. (2000). *Preventing school injuries: A comprehensive guide for school administrators, teachers, and staff.* New Brunswick, NH: Rutgers University Press.

Powell, J. W., & Barber-Foss, K. D. (2000). Sex-related injury patterns among selected high school sports. *American Journal of Sports Medicine, 28*(3), 385–391.

Pratt, S. G. (2003). Work-related roadway crashes: Challenges and opportunities for prevention (Publication No. 2003-119). Washington, DC: National Institute for Occupational Safety and Health.

Presley, C. A., Meilman, P. W., Cashin, J. R., & Leichliter, J. S. (1997). *Alcohol and drugs on American college campuses: issues of violence and harassment.* Carbondale, IL: Core Institute, Southern Illinois University.

Quan, L., Bennett, E., & Branche, C. (2006). Interventions to prevent drowning. In L. Doll, S. Bonzo, J. Mercy, & D. Sleet (Eds.), *Handbook of injury and violence prevention.* New York: Springer.

Quinlan, K. P., Brewer, R. D., Sleet, D. A., & Dellinger, A. M. (2000). Characteristics of child passenger deaths and injuries involving drinking drivers. *Journal of the American Medical Association, 283*(17), 2249–2252.

Rivara, F. P. (1985). Traumatic deaths in children in the United States: Currently available prevention strategies. *Pediatrics, 75*(3), 456–462.

Rosenberg, M. L., & Sleet, D. A. (1995). Injury control recommendations for bicycle helmets. *Journal of School Health, 65*(4), 133–139.

Runyan, C. W., Schulman, M., & Ta, M. (2006). Adolescent employment: Relationship to injury and violence. In K. D. Liller (Ed.), *Injury prevention for children and adolescents: Research, practice and advocacy*. Washington, DC: American Public Health Association.

Scheidt, P. C., Harel, Y., Trumble, A. C., Jones, D. H., Overpeck, M. D., & Bijur, P. E. (1995). The epidemiology of nonfatal injuries among U.S. children and youth. *American Journal of Public Health, 85*, 932–938.

Schieber, R. A., Gilchrist, J., & Sleet, D. A. (2000). Legislative and regulatory strategies to reduce childhood injuries. *The Future of Children, 10*(1), 111–136.

Schieber, R., & Vegega, M. (2003). Education versus environmental countermeasures: Is it really an either-or proposition? *American Journal of Health Education, 34*(5 Suppl.), S54–S56.

Schulman, M. D., Evensen, C. T., Runyan, C. W., Cohen, L. R., & Dunn, K. A. (1997). Farm work is dangerous for teens: Agricultural hazards and injuries among North Carolina teens. *Journal of Rural Health, 13*, 295–305.

Shaw, F. E., & Ogolla, C. P. (2006). Law, behavior and injury prevention. In A. C. Gielen, D. A. Sleet, & R. DiClemente (Eds.), *Injury and violence prevention: Behavioral science theories, methods, and applications* (pp. 442–466). San Francisco: Jossey-Bass.

Simon-Morton, B. G., Mickalide, A. D., & Olsen, E.C.B. (2006). Preventing motor vehicle crashes and injuries among children and adolescents. In K. D. Liller (Ed.), *Injury prevention for children and adolescents* (pp. 91–122). Washington, DC: American Public Health Association.

Sleet, D. A., Dinh-Zarr, B. T., & Dellinger, A. M. (2007). Traffic safety in the context of public health and medicine. In *Improving traffic safety culture in the United States: The journey forward* (pp. 41–58). Washington, DC: AAA Foundation for Traffic Safety.

Sleet, D. A., & Gielen, A. C. (2006). Injury prevention. In S. S. Gorin & J. Arnold (Eds.), *Health promotion handbook* (2nd ed.). St Louis, MO: Mosby.

Sleet, D. A., & Gielen, A. C. (2007). Behavioral interventions for injury and violence prevention. In L. Doll, S. Bonzo, J. Mercy, & D. Sleet (Eds.), *Handbook of injury and violence prevention*. New York: Springer.

Sleet, D. A., Howat, P., Elder, R., Maycock, B., Baldwin, G., & Shults, R. (2009). Interventions to reduce impaired driving and traffic injury. In J. C. Verster, S. R. Pandi-Perumal, J. G. Ramaekers, & J. J. de Gier (Eds.), *Drugs, driving, and traffic safety*. Basel, Switzerland: Birkhauser Verlag.

Sleet, D. A., & Mercy, J. A. (2003). Promotion of safety, security, and well-being. In M. H. Bornstein, L. Davidson, C.L.M. Keyes, K. A. Moore, & the Center for Child Well-Being (Eds.), *Well-being: Positive development across the life course*. Mahwah, NJ: Erlbaum.

Smith, G. S., Branas, C., & Miller, T. R. (1999). Fatal nontraffic injuries involving alcohol: A meta-analysis. *Annals of Emergency Medicine, 33*(6), 659–668.

Sosin, D. M., Sacks, J. J., & Webb, K. W. (1996). Pediatric head injuries and deaths from bicycling in the United States. *Pediatrics, 98*(5), 868–870.

Thompson, D. C., Nunn, M. E., Thompson, R. S., & Rivara, F. P. (1996). Effectiveness of bicycle safety helmets in preventing serious facial injury. *Journal of the American Medical Association, 276*(24), 1974–1975.

Thompson, R. S., Rivara, F. P., & Thompson, D. C. (1989). A case-control study of the effectiveness of bicycle safety helmets. *New England Journal of Medicine, 320*(21), 1361–1367.

Thompson, D. C., Rivara, F. P., & Thompson, R. S. (1996). Effectiveness of bicycle safety helmets in preventing head injuries: A case-control study. *Journal of the American Medical Association, 276*(24), 1968–1973.

U.S. Coast Guard, Department of Homeland Security. (2008). Boating statistics, 2006 [Online]. Retrieved March 26, 2008, from www.uscgboating.org/statistics/Boating_Statistics_2006.pdf.

U.S. Fire Administration. (2005). Fatal fires. *Topical Fire Research Series, 5*(1), 1–6.

U.S. General Accounting Office. (2002). Child labor: Labor can strengthen its efforts to protect children who work (Report to the Chairman, Subcommittee on Labor, Health and Human Services, and Education, Committee on Appropriations, U.S. Senate). Retrieved March 26, 2008, from www.gao.gov/new.items/d02880.pdf.

Voas, R. B., Tippetts, A. S., & Fisher, D. A. (2000). Ethnicity and alcohol related fatalities: 1990 to 1994 (NHTSA Report No. DOT HS 809 068). Landover, MD: Pacific Institute for Research and Evaluation.

Warda, L., Tenenbein, M., & Moffatt, M. E. (1999). House fire injury prevention update. Part I: A review of risk factors for fatal and non-fatal house fire injury. *Injury Prevention, 5*(2), 145–150.

Warda, L. J., & Ballesteros, M. F. (2007). Interventions to prevent residential fire injury. In L. S. Doll, S. E. Bonzo, J. A. Mercy, & D. A. Sleet (Eds.), *Handbook of injury and violence prevention* (pp. 97–115). New York: Springer.

Wechsler, H., Dowdall, G. W., Davenport, A., & Castillo, S. (1995). Correlates of college student binge drinking. *American Journal of Public Health, 85,* 921–926.

World Health Organization. (2006). *Helmets: A road safety manual for decision-makers and practitioners.* Geneva: Author.

World Health Organization. (2007). *Youth declaration for road safety.* Geneva: Author.

World Health Organization. (2008). *World report on child injury prevention.* Geneva: Author.

Wilson, M., & Baker, S. (1987). Structural approach to injury control. *Journal of Social Issues, 43*(2), 73–86.

Zaza, S., Sleet, D. A., Shults, R. A., Elder, R. W., Dinh-Zarr, T., Nichols, J. L., & Thompson, R. S. (2005). Reducing injuries to motor vehicle occupants. In S. Zaza, P. Briss, & K. Harris (Eds.), *The guide to community preventive services: What works to promote health?* (pp. 329–384). New York: Oxford University Press.

CHAPTER

15

SEXUALLY TRANSMITTED DISEASE TRANSMISSION AND PREGNANCY AMONG ADOLESCENTS

LAURA F. SALAZAR ▪ JOHN S. SANTELLI ▪ RICHARD A. CROSBY ▪ RALPH J. DICLEMENTE

LEARNING OBJECTIVES

After studying this chapter, you will be able to

- Explain the epidemiology of sexually transmitted disease transmission and pregnancy among adolescents.
- Investigate the socioecological antecedents of adolescent sexual risk taking that relate to sexually transmitted disease acquisition and teen pregnancy.
- Identify both proximal and distal determinants of adolescent risk-taking behavior.

In the United States the related epidemics of teen pregnancy and sexually transmitted disease (STD) among persons under the age of twenty-five continue to be a focal point in public health. In a nation that does not universally embrace comprehensive sex education, some adolescents may not be fully prepared to navigate the social and emotional challenges that accompany intimate relationships. Likewise, teens need to learn to negotiate whether they will have sex, with whom they will have sex, and the use of reliable contraception and STD prophylaxis (condoms). The "costs" of adolescents' unprotected sexual activity can be measured in physical, mental, social, and economic terms.

The economic costs of teens giving birth are substantial. Recent estimates suggest that on average the annual cost associated with a child born to a teen mother is $1,430; however, this cost increases dramatically to about $4,000 annually when the teen mother is seventeen years of age or younger. Between 1991 and 2004, the estimated cumulative public cost of teen childbearing during this time period was $161 billion (Hoffman, 2006).

The consequences of STD acquisition among adolescents can also be quite significant. Infertility in females and sterility in males may be a consequence of repeated infections with gonorrhea and chlamydia acquired during adolescence (Centers for Disease Control and Prevention, 2006; Eng & Butler, 1997). Infection with *Trichomonas vaginalis* and human papilloma virus is also common among teens. Many adolescents who are diagnosed with an STD incur feelings of self-blame, depression, anxiety, and lowered self-esteem (Fortenberry et al., 2002; Gardner, Frank, & Amankwaa, 1998; Salazar et al., 2006), which may in turn contribute to protracted delays in seeking care (DiClemente, Salazar, Crosby, & Rosenthal, 2005). Unfortunately, the costs of STDs among U.S. adolescents now include the devastating effects of HIV/AIDS.

Economic lifetime costs per case for acquiring an STD (such as HIV, HPV, genital herpes, hepatitis B, chlamydia, gonorrhea, trichomoniasis, or syphilis) range from a high of about $200,000 per person for HIV to a low of $18 per person for trichomoniasis (Chesson, Blandford, Gift, Tao, & Irwin, 2004). Economists using STD incidence data among U.S. adolescents aged fifteen through twenty-four for the year 2000 determined that the total estimated burden for the eight aforementioned STDs was about $6.5 billion.

On average, almost thirteen years elapse between the time adolescents become fertile and their sexual feelings intensify, and the time they marry (Guttmacher Institute, 2002; U.S. Census Bureau, 2004). Figure 15.1 shows how dramatically the median age of first marriage in the United States has risen since 1960, reaching about 25.3 years for females and 27.1 years for males in the year 2000. This trend creates a long period during which adolescents need to avoid unintended pregnancy and avert STD acquisition through either abstinence from sex or reliable contraception and condom use. The long time between median age for initiation of sexual intercourse and median age at marriage (in 2002) means that teens are at risk for most of the period between maturation and marriage. Many teenagers do not use contraceptives correctly and consistently, thereby placing themselves at risk of pregnancy and STDs (Abma, Chandra, Mosher, Peterson, & Piccinino, 1997; Crosby et al., 2005a; Crosby et al., 2005b).

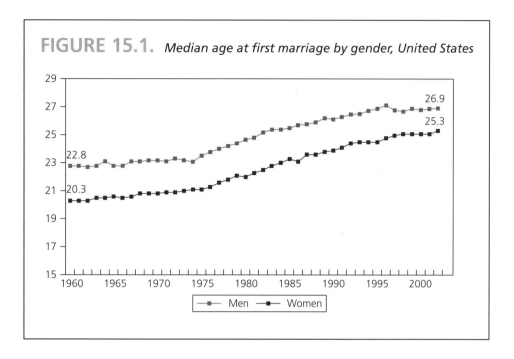

FIGURE 15.1. *Median age at first marriage by gender, United States*

Moreover, multiple consecutive or concurrent sexual partnerships are common during this period before marriage, increasing the risk for sexually transmitted diseases.

EPIDEMIOLOGY

In general, epidemiology refers to the study of the rates and determinants of disease in populations. Although teen pregnancy and teen birth are not diseases per se, in the next section we present the rates for teen pregnancy and teen births in addition to teen STD rates in the United States to reveal the extent of the problems. Because teen pregnancy and teen birth are not considered infectious diseases that can be transmitted, we present the incidence of both. Incidence refers to the number of new cases over a specified time interval (such as yearly). Because STDs vary qualitatively (viral versus bacterial, curable versus incurable, or long survival period versus short-lived if treated), depending on the type it may be meaningful to examine both incidence and prevalence patterns in teen STD rates. Moreover, we present the rates of pertinent behavioral determinants underlying STD acquisition and transmission.

Teen Pregnancy and Birth Rates

From 1991 through 2005, despite significant decreases by about a third in teen pregnancy and birth rates, the United States still maintained the highest rates in the industrialized world. In fact, rates of teen pregnancy in the United States are two to six times higher than those in most of Western Europe, including France, Holland, Denmark, and Sweden, and two times higher than Canada (Hoffman, 2006). In 2002, among all females aged fifteen through nineteen, there were over 760,000 pregnancies, which amounts to about 75 per 1,000 (Guttmacher Institute, 2006). Rates among minority teens are much higher than rates for their Caucasian counterparts, at about 134 per 1,000 for African Americans and 132 per 1,000 for Hispanics, as compared to 48 per 1,000 for non-Hispanic Whites (Guttmacher Institute, 2006). More than 30 percent of girls in the United States become pregnant before twenty years of age, and many become pregnant a second time before this age (National Campaign to Prevent Teen Pregnancy, 2006). In 2001, about 82 percent of teen pregnancies were unintended (Finer & Henshaw, 2006). Consistent with the very high U.S. teen pregnancy rate is its very high teen birth rate.

Although the United States still has one of the highest teen pregnancy rates of the industrialized nations, recent declines have been well documented. Pregnancy rates among fifteen- to nineteen-year-olds declined 35 percent from 1990 to 2004 (Ventura, Abma, Mosher, & Henshaw, 2008), and birth rates dropped 34 percent between 1991 and 2005 (Martin, Hamilton, Sutton, et al., 2007). An important question stemming from these declines is, Why did they occur? Findings from a recent study suggest that declines in adolescent pregnancy rates (from 1995 and 2002) resulted primarily from improved contraceptive use (Santelli, Lindberg, Finer, & Singh, 2007). This varied by age, with the decline in pregnancy risk among eighteen- and nineteen-year-olds being entirely attributable to increased contraceptive use. Among those fifteen to seventeen years of age, decreased sexual activity was responsible for about one-quarter (23 percent) of the decline, and increased contraceptive use was responsible for the remaining 77 percent. Improved contraceptive use included increases in the use of many individual methods, increases in the use of multiple methods, and substantial declines in nonuse.

Although the United States still has one of the highest teen pregnancy rates of the industrialized nations, recent declines have been well documented.

In view of these downward trends in sexual risk behaviors and teen birth rates, many were surprised and disappointed by the 3 percent increase in teen birth rate in 2006, the most recent year for which data are available (Hamilton, Martin, & Ventura, 2007). The largest increase (5 percent) was among African American teens—the group that previously had experienced the largest declines. Using representative data from the Youth Risk Behavior Surveillance System (YRBSS), researchers revealed that teens' use of condoms and contraception declined from 2003 to 2007, which may have contributed to the increase in birth rates in 2006 (Santelli, Orr, & Lin, 2007).

Sexually Transmitted Disease

Although persons aged fifteen through twenty-four represent 25 percent of the sexually active population, they account for about half of all new cases of STD (Weinstock, Berman, & Cates, 2004). This means that nearly four million cases of STD occur annually among teens and over six million cases occur among people aged twenty to twenty-four (American Social Health Association, 1998). In addition, an estimated one-third of all sexually active young people become infected by an STD by age twenty-four (American Social Health Association, 1998). Female adolescents are disproportionately affected; a recent study by the CDC found that one in four (26 percent) young women between the ages of fourteen and nineteen in the United States—or 3.2 million teenage girls—is infected with at least one of the most common sexually transmitted diseases: human papilloma virus (HPV), chlamydia, herpes simplex virus, and trichomoniasis (Forhan et al., 2008).

A vast racial disparity persists in the incidence of STDs among adolescents. Rates of STDs are typically much higher for African American adolescents compared to all other adolescents. For example, in 2005 the rates of chlamydia and gonorrhea among fifteen- to nineteen-year-old African American adolescents were about 14 and 35 times higher, respectively, than rates for their white counterparts (Centers for Disease Control and Prevention, 2006).

In 2004 alone, the rate of new AIDS cases among African American adolescent males (fifteen to twenty-four years of age) was 283 per 100,000, compared to 97 among same-age Hispanic males, and 18 among same-age white males. Although African American males have the highest rate of AIDS, other trends can be seen in data

Although persons aged fifteen through twenty-four represent 25 percent of the sexually active population, they account for about half of all new cases of STD.

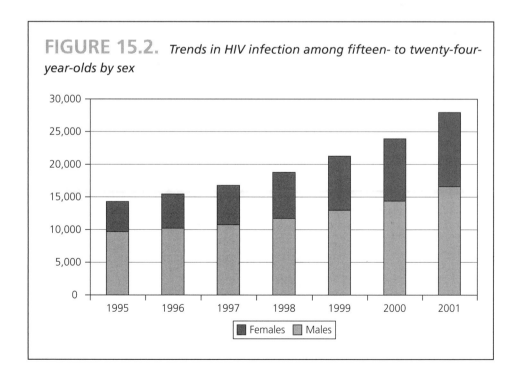

FIGURE 15.2. *Trends in HIV infection among fifteen- to twenty-four-year-olds by sex*

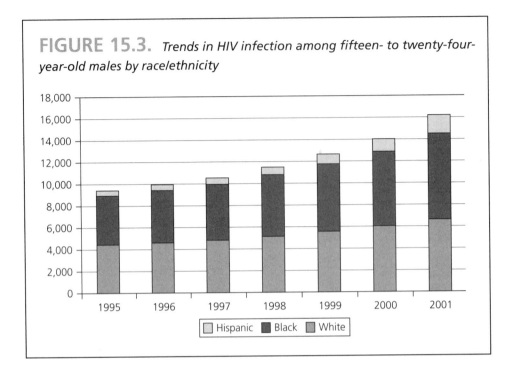

FIGURE 15.3. *Trends in HIV infection among fifteen- to twenty-four-year-old males by race/ethnicity*

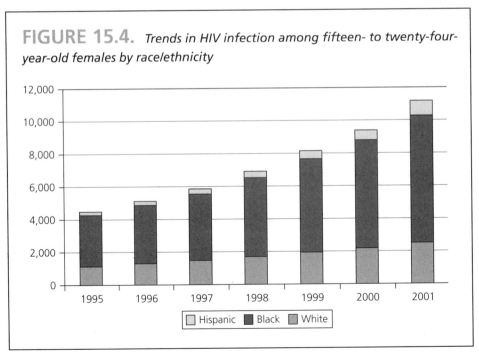

FIGURE 15.4. *Trends in HIV infection among fifteen- to twenty-four-year-old females by race/ethnicity*

that use reportable HIV infection cases from the years leading up to 2004. As shown in Figure 15.2, overall males still constitute a majority of the cases among adolescents ages fifteen to twenty-four; however, the percentages for females among HIV reported infections (all races and ethnicities) have increased from about 32 percent of the total in 1995 to about 40 percent of the total number of reported cases.

Given the disproportionate percentages of African American male adolescents who are living with AIDS, it is not surprising that black males represented a significant number of the HIV infection cases among males (about 48 percent in 2001) (see Figure 15.3). Even more alarming is the disproportionate percentage of black females, who represented about 68 percent of the HIV infection cases among all females (see Figure 15.4).

The racial disparity in HIV/AIDS can also be seen in Figures 15.5 and 15.6, which show race/ethnicity population percentages next to race/ethnicity percentages for adolescents diagnosed with HIV/AIDS in the year 2005. As indicated, although Hispanic population percentages are proportional to their HIV/AIDS percentages for both age groups—15 percent compared to 15 percent (fifteen- to nineteen-year-olds) and 16 percent compared to 18 percent (twenty- to twenty-four-year-olds)—Black non-Hispanics are disproportionately affected by HIV/AIDS. Black non-Hispanic adolescents constitute 17 percent and 16 percent of the population for fifteen- to nineteen-year-olds and for twenty- to twenty-four-year-olds respectively, yet they represent 69 percent and 58 percent of reported HIV/AIDS cases for 2005.

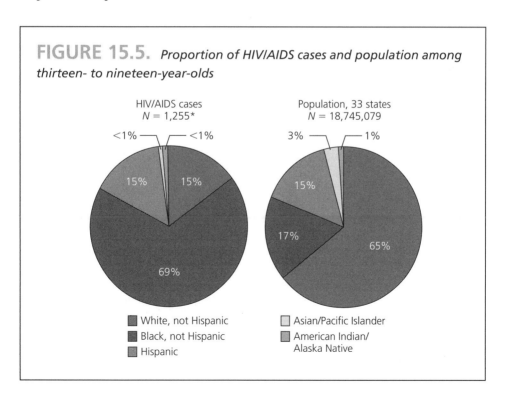

FIGURE 15.5. *Proportion of HIV/AIDS cases and population among thirteen- to nineteen-year-olds*

HIV/AIDS cases
N = 1,255*

Population, 33 states
N = 18,745,079

■ White, not Hispanic
■ Black, not Hispanic
■ Hispanic
□ Asian/Pacific Islander
▨ American Indian/ Alaska Native

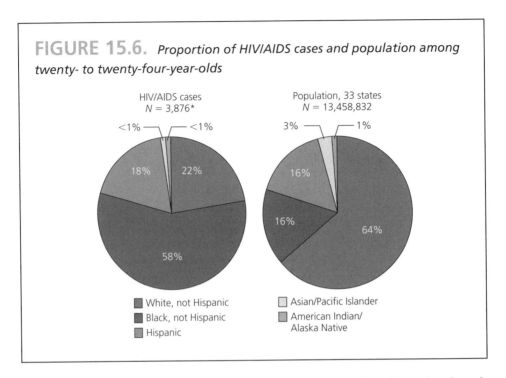

FIGURE 15.6. *Proportion of HIV/AIDS cases and population among twenty- to twenty-four-year-olds*

Three risk behaviors are especially important to consider when discussing the epidemiology of STDs: sex unprotected by condoms, sex with multiple partners, and concurrency of sexual partners. Findings from the YRBSS indicate that a significantly greater proportion of adolescent females (55 percent) reported condom use at last sex in 2007, compared to 46 percent in 1991 (Balaji et al., 2008). Significant increases were also observed for adolescent males (from 55 percent in 1991 to 69 percent in 2007). Condom use peaked in 2003 and declined nonsignificantly through 2007. Although these trends are noteworthy, it is important to note that data regarding the proportion of a population using condoms is much different from a measure capturing *frequency* of condom use.

Data from the same study also indicate that the percent of adolescent females reporting sex with multiple partners has remained relatively constant. For example, in 1991 adolescent females were equally likely to report having more than four lifetime sexual partners (13.8 percent) compared to those assessed in 1997 (14.1 percent) (Brener, Kann, Lowry, Wechsler, & Romero, 2006). Further, significant differences in the proportion reporting multiple partners in 1999 (13.1 percent) and 2005 (12.0 percent) were not observed. Conversely, for males a significant decrease in the proportion reporting they had sex with two or more partners was observed between 1991 (38 percent) and 1997 (34 percent), whereas a significant decrease between 1999 (38 percent) and 2005 (35 percent) was not observed (Santelli, Orr, et al., 2007).

Concurrency (multiple concurrent sexual partners) is a concept drawn from the study of *sexual networks,* which is not well described by statistics on the number of sexual partners. The basic premise of sexual network theory is that STIs are transmitted most efficiently (at a high reproductive rate) in a population when networks are highly interactive and when large numbers of microstructures (small but highly interactive subgroups) are present as well as when the geographic distance between members is short (Cunningham et al., 2004; Koumans et al., 2001; Rosenberg, Gurvey, Adler, Dunlop, & Ellen, 1999). Indeed, in one poignant research example it was shown that each of these factors favored transmission during a syphilis epidemic and declined (thereby not favoring an accelerated reproductive rate) as the epidemic declined (Cunningham et al., 2004). The essence of this approach to understanding repeat STD acquisition is that disease transmission occurs within a social milieu that may sometimes greatly increase risk.

KEY CONCEPTS AND RESEARCH FINDINGS

Factors related to sexual risk behaviors range from intrapersonal and interpersonal (social interactions with family, intimate partners, and peers) to characteristics of school, community, and society. Some factors can be considered distal determinants, while others are proximal determinants. *Distal influences* refer to those factors that do not always have a direct or immediate effect on the health behavior and whose causal pathway is not always known. *Proximal influences,* on the other hand, may demonstrate an immediate and noticeable influence on health behavior, but also may be caused by or mediate the effect of distal influences (Anderson, 2004).

Factors related to sexual risk behaviors range from intrapersonal and interpersonal to characteristics of school, community, and society.

Although ostensibly it makes sense for sexual risk reduction interventions for adolescents to combine adolescent pregnancy and adolescent STD-acquisition as outcomes, it is important to note that the actual risk behaviors that underlie these two outcomes vary somewhat. Pregnancy is averted by the consistent and correct use of reliable contraceptive methods (such as oral contraception and Depo Provera), whereas STDs are averted by only one type of contraceptive device (condoms) and the odds of acquisition are greatly magnified by multiple partnerships, the prevalence of STDs in the sexual networks of selected partners, and the shape of sexual networks. Thus, the antecedents for teen pregnancy and STD acquisition are presented separately.

Antecedents of Teen Pregnancy

With the socioecological model as a framework, this next section delineates the relevant factors that have been shown empirically to be related to teen pregnancy and teen birth rates.

Societal Characteristics Social policies on sex education (such as abstinence-only education versus comprehensive sex education), accessibility to family planning services, and affordability of contraceptives are each examples of *macrosystem* factors that may influence teen pregnancy and birth rates (Kirby, 2002; Santelli, 2007). The societal constructs of gender and race/ethnicity are also critically important macrolevel factors. Gender and race/ethnicity are deemed as societal characteristics rather than individual characteristics because of the ways society constructs and attaches culture-bound conventions and roles. Gender and racial/ethnic roles vary across a continuum and within and across societies. Thus, when we discuss gender and race/ethnicity in this section, we are referring to the sociological constructs, rather than the biological.

As described previously, major racial and ethnic disparities persist in pregnancy and birth rates and contraceptive use. Black and Hispanic youth are disproportionately affected compared to whites. Rates of contraceptive use also vary significantly as a function of race/ethnicity. 2005 YRBSS data show that although black female adolescents had higher rates of condom use at last sexual encounter (62 percent) versus white (56 percent) or Hispanic (50 percent) female adolescents, they had a lower incidence of using the pill (11 percent) than white (27 percent), but not Hispanic female adolescents (9 percent), who had the lowest. Hispanic female adolescents had the highest incidence of not using any method at last sexual encounter (28 percent) versus black adolescents (19 percent) or white adolescents (14 percent), who had the lowest (Santelli, Orr, & Lin, 2007).

Understanding reasons why African American and Hispanic teens have lower oral contraceptive use, higher nonuse of any methods, and thus higher pregnancy rates than white teens may involve cultural and socioeconomic differences. Some minority groups view teen pregnancy as a positive occurrence versus something deviant (Orshan, 1996). In a culture that honors young motherhood, teens may gain status by becoming pregnant. In one study 25 percent of African American female adolescents revealed a desire to become pregnant and that desire for childbearing was related to inconsistent condom use (Davies et al., 2003). Crosby et al. found that among a sample of pregnant teens recruited from a prenatal clinic, almost half (49.2 percent) indicated that the pregnancy was not unplanned (Crosby, DiClemente, Wingood, Rose, & Lang, 2003b). Other research supports the idea that some teen pregnancies may be intentional (Frost & Oslak, 1999). It is important to note that although intentions of or a desire for childbearing is associated with teen pregnancy among both adolescent Latinas and African Americans (Bryant, 2006; East, Khoo, & Reyes, 2006; Frost & Oslak, 1999), the majority of Latina and African American teens do not become teenage mothers.

Teen pregnancy may also be perceived as a pathway to adulthood or to obtaining status, especially when opportunities for social mobility are blocked (Franklin, 1993; Frost & Oslak, 1999). Much research has shown that teens who reside in neighborhoods where a significant proportion of households are below the poverty level are at greater risk of becoming pregnant and giving birth (Barnett, Papini, & Gbur, 1991; Crosby & Holtgrave, 2006; Frost & Oslak, 1999; Hogan & Kitagawa, 1985; Kirby, Coyle, & Gould, 2001; Klein & Committee on Adolescence, 2005; Klerman, 1994; Mersky & Reynolds, 2007; Miller, 1992; Singh, Darroch, & Frost, 2001).

Another societal characteristic that plays a distinct role in shaping cultural norms and influencing behaviors is the media (Strasburger, 1995). Teens are exposed to more than eight hours of mass media daily (Roberts, Foehr, Rideout, & Brodie, 1999). Media play a significant role in the socialization of adolescents (Thornburgh & Lin, 2002) and may strongly influence sexual behavior. For example, the higher the ratio of exposure to extreme sexual content (particularly to pornographic content), the more likely teens are to have had sex and to not use a condom at last sexual encounter (Salazar, DiClemente, Wingood, Daluga, & Lang, 2008).

Peer and Community Characteristics   It is not surprising that peer influence is a critical factor in teen engagement in sexual risk behaviors, their use of contraceptives, and their risk of pregnancy (Meade & Ickovics, 2005; Vesely et al., 2004). Teens having friends who are sexually active or who become pregnant are more likely to be sexually active, to become pregnant, or have a repeat pregnancy (Bearman & Bruckner, 1999; East, Felice, & Morgan, 1993; Gibson & Kempf, 1990; Gillmore, Lewis, Lohr, Spencer, & White, 1997; Miller et al., 1997; Raneri & Wiemann, 2007; Small & Luster, 1994). In one longitudinal study, results suggested that teen motherhood and teen fatherhood are related to associating with peers who are physically aggressive, low academic achievers, low in popularity, and older (Xie, Cairns, & Cairns, 2001). Yet when teens have quality peer role models (such as friends who participate in extracurricular activities), they are less likely to engage in sexual intercourse, and those who are sexually active are more likely to use birth control (Vesely et al., 2004) and less likely to become pregnant (Dogan-Ates & Carrion-Basham, 2007; Xie et al., 2001).

Characteristics of teens' communities are also important. Living in a racially segregated community, regardless of socioeconomic status (Ku, Sonenstein, & Pleck, 1993; Sucoff & Upchurch, 1998), and living in neighborhoods characterized by poverty (Dryfoos, 1990; Hayes, 1987), fewer economic opportunities coupled with high unemployment rates (Bunting & McAuley, 2004; Ku, Sonenstein, & Pleck, 1993), high crime rates (Kirby, 2003), disadvantage, and disorganization (Hogan & Kitagawa 1985; Miller 2002; Miller, Benson, & Galbraith, 2001) are all associated with increased risk of adolescent pregnancy. Some of these negative neighborhood attributes could potentially be offset by the level of cohesion and/or social capital present in the neighborhood to the extent adult neighbors interact with teens and provide outside support and informal control (Crosby & Holtgrave, 2006; Crosby, Holtgrave, DiClemente, Wingood, & Gayle, 2003; Denner, Kirby, Coyle, & Brindis, 2001; Moore & Chase-Lansdale, 2001). In fact, perceived social support from neighbors and nonparental adult role models and having more working adults in social networks have been associated with reduced risk of teen pregnancy (Ku, Sonenstein, & Pleck, 1993; Moore & Chase-Lansdale, 2001; Vesely et al., 2004).

Avoiding risky sexual behavior and consequent teen pregnancy may be motivated to a large degree by the level of involvement teens have with their schools, social group affiliations, extracurricular activities, and church (Raneri & Wiemann, 2007). Positive characteristics of schools and teachers such as a sense of connectedness (see Chapter Eighteen) can enhance teens' academic motivation and thus be protective against teen pregnancy (Dogan-Ates & Carrion-Basham, 2007; Kasen, Cohen, & Brook, 1998). When teens feel motivated to achieve academically and feel engaged, they tend to think about their future life and career aspirations and are less likely to

Avoiding risky sexual behavior and consequent teen pregnancy may be motivated to a large degree by the level of involvement teens have with their schools, social group affiliations, extracurricular activities, and church.

become pregnant or to impregnate someone (Fergusson & Woodward, 2000; Kasen et al., 1998; Manlove, 1998; Small & Luster, 1994). Even when a teen becomes pregnant, if she can stay in school then she will be less likely to have a repeat pregnancy (Linares, Leadbeater, Kato, & Jaffe, 1991; Manlove, Mariner, & Papillo, 2000).

There is some research to support that when teens have an attachment to a faith community, they are less likely to engage in premarital sex, thus reducing their risk of pregnancy—especially when the faith community espouses norms disapproving of premarital sex such as Catholic or fundamentalist Protestant churches (Kirby, 2003).

Family Characteristics Parents who are involved and who consistently maintain knowledge of their children's day-to-day activities are said to be "monitors" of their children's whereabouts. Parental monitoring has been found to be associated robustly with reduced rates of adolescent pregnancy (Barnett et al., 1991; Miller et al., 2001; Scaramella, Conger, Simons, & Whitbeck, 1998). Furthermore, parental attitudes and attributes also play a role. Adolescents whose parents hold attitudes disapproving toward adolescent sex, are supportive of their teens, have high educational expectations of their teens, communicate frequently and with "warmth," have quality interactions with teens, and provide clear sanctions against teenage sexual activity are less likely to engage in risky sexual behavior and become teen parents (Barnett et al., 1991; Gibson & Kempf, 1990; Hanson, Myers, & Ginsburg, 1987; Khaleque & Deperry, 2005; Markham et al., 2003; Metzler, Noell, Biglan, Ary, & Smolkowski, 1994; Miller et al., 2001; Resnick et al., 1997; Russell, 2002; Velez-Pastrana, Gonzalez-Rodriguez, & Borges-Hernandez, 2005). Reduced risk taking may be explained by the results of one study that found several of these familial factors were related to delaying the timing of first sexual intercourse and to a greater likelihood of using contraceptives (Hogan, Sun, & Cornwell, 2000; Vesely et al., 2004).

Other research strongly implicates parental inactions as risk factors for teen pregnancy. For example, adolescents who perceive that their parents (or parental figures) *infrequently* monitor their behaviors, whose parents *do not engage* in frequent or good communication, whose parents are *unsupportive* of them and whose parents are *not disapproving* of sex are more likely to become pregnant (Barnett et al., 1991; Crosby, DiClemente, et al., 2002a; Gillmore et al., 1997; Hogan & Kitagawa, 1985; Luster & Small, 1994; Raneri & Wiemann, 2007) or more likely to report that their pregnancy was unplanned and unwanted (Crosby, DiClemente, Wingood, Rose, & Lang, 2003).

The structure of the family also plays a role (see Chapter Nineteen). Teens raised in single-parent households are at increased risk of teen pregnancy (Barnett et al., 1991; Fagot, Pears, Capaldi, Crosby, & Leve, 1998; Langille, Flowerdew, & Andreou, 2004; Miller et al., 2001; Powers, 2005; Robbins, Kaplan, & Martin, 1985). The absence of the father in households with a female teen was significantly related to teen pregnancy in one study, even after controlling for other related familial factors (Ellis et al., 2003). Family poverty has also been strongly linked with teenage pregnancy (Miller et al., 2001; Robbins, Kaplan, & Martin, 1985; Russell, 2002; Woodward, Fergusson, & Horwood, 2001). Kirby, (2003) posited that teens whose parents have lower levels of education and income do not place as much emphasis on obtaining an education, pursuing a career, or avoiding early childbearing, perhaps because they do not have as many resources to support these goals as their higher educated and income-earning counterparts.

Relational Characteristics Multiple findings suggest that adolescent females who perceive that their sex partner desired pregnancy may be substantially more likely to become pregnant (Crosby, DiClemente, et al., 2002b; Frost & Oslak, 1999; Stevens-Simon, Sheeder, & Harter, 2005). Teen females having sex with male partners who are several years older also have an elevated risk of pregnancy (Kirby, 2002; Raneri & Wiemann, 2007). Teen females reporting long-term relationships with their male partners are more likely to become pregnant (Gillmore et al., 1997; Kalmuss & Namerow, 1994; Koniak-Griffin, Lesser, Uman, & Nyamathi, 2003).

Individual Characteristics A study of African American teen females found that those reporting they had acquired at least four sex partners in their lifetime were significantly more likely to become pregnant than those acquiring fewer partners (Crosby, DiClemente, et al., 2002b). Of note, the behavior of acquiring multiple sex partners may be an important indicator of co-occurring risk rather than a proximal antecedent to pregnancy. Another example of co-occurrence is substance use. Marijuana use, for example, has been associated with elevated risk of teen pregnancy (Crosby, DiClemente, et al., 2002b; Gest, Mahoney, & Cairns, 1999; Gillmore et al., 1997; Luster & Small, 1994; Small & Luster, 1994; Yamaguchi & Kandel, 1987). Physical aggression may also be a behavior that co-occurs with teen pregnancy (Gest et al., 1999; Small & Luster, 1994; Xie et al., 2001). Similarly, cognitive deficits, low educational achievement, and conduct disorders have been associated with teen pregnancy (Gest et al., 1999; Xie et al., 2001).

Several psychological factors may be important proximal antecedents of teen pregnancy (Kirby, 2001). For example, self-efficacy to avoid sex in general (Young, Martin, Young, & Ting, 2001) and risky sex in particular (Sionean et al., 2002) may also be important.

Antecedents of STD and HIV Acquisition

Following the same socioecological framework used to organize the antecedents of teen pregnancy, this section will delineate the relevant factors associated not only with STD acquisition but also with the pertinent sexual risk behaviors that underlie STD acquisition.

Societal Characteristics Media may influence adolescents' sexual behaviors and increase the risk of STD Acquisition. One study found that greater exposure to rap music videos was related to aggressive behavior, being arrested, multiple sex partners, drug use, and testing positive for an STD (Wingood et al., 2003), and an association between exposure to X-rated movies and negative condom attitudes, having multiple sex partners, more frequent sexual intercourse, not using contraception during last intercourse, and testing positive for chlamydia was also found (Wingood et al., 2001).

Peer and Community Characteristics As mentioned previously, an important developmental aspect of adolescence is the increasing importance of peer influences. Peer pressure to smoke, drink alcohol, and engage in sexual intercourse increases with age (Brown, Clasen, & Eicher, 1986). Adolescents and young adults who perceive that their friends are having unprotected sex and engaging in other types of risky sex are more likely to adopt their friends' behaviors (Bachanas et al., 2002; Boyer et al., 2000; Crosby et al., 2000; DiClemente et al., 1996; Doljanac & Zimmerman, 1998; Millstein & Moscicki, 1995). Perceived social support from peers has been related to STD diagnosis (Salazar et al., 2007). In contrast, perceived peer norms supportive of STD-protective behaviors can have a significant influence on their adoption and maintenance of preventive behaviors (Boyer et al., 2000; Crosby et al., 2000; DiClemente et al., 1996; Doljanac & Zimmerman, 1998; Millstein & Moscicki, 1995).

Community characteristics can also influence adolescents' adoption of STD-protective behaviors. Adolescents' affiliations with social organizations (Crosby, DiClemente, Wingood, Harrington, Davies, & Malow, 2002), adolescents' perception of higher levels of social support (St. Lawrence, Brasfield, Jefferson, Alleyne, & Shirley, 1994), and positive school environments may serve as protective factors. For example, among a nationally representative sample of adolescents, a sense of belonging to a school (that is, their feeling of being positively connected to peers, teachers, and other members of the school) was associated with delaying sexual intercourse (Resnick et al., 1997; see also Chapter Eighteen). Interestingly, the mere fact that an adolescent is enrolled in school appears to be a protective factor against testing positive for an STD and those risk factors contributing to an STD (Crosby et al., 2007).

Adolescents who have better availability of and access to condoms tend to have higher rates of condom use (Furstenberg, Geitz, Teitler, & Weiss, 1997; Guttmacher et al., 1997) without an increase in overall rates of sexual activity (Kirby, 2001).

An emerging line of inquiry suggests that another community characteristic—*social capital*—may also influence adolescents' risk behaviors. Social capital in this context refers to the connections adolescents have to other adolescents within their social network and between their social network and other social networks. One study demonstrated that social capital was *inversely* correlated with AIDS case rates, as well as the incidence of chlamydia, gonorrhea, and syphilis among adults (Holtgrave & Crosby, 2003). More recent research has shown that adolescents residing in states with greater levels of social capital were less likely to engage in selected sexual risk behaviors (Crosby, Holtgrave, et al., 2003).

Other aspects of communities may also affect adolescents' risk of STD acquisition. "Communities that have high rates of STDs among adults may pose a heightened risk for adolescents." Recent research suggests that the disproportionate incidence of STDs among African American adolescents may be a consequence of residing in communities that have high rates of STDs, rather than the adolescents' behavioral characteristics (Ellen, Aral, & Madger, 1998; Jennings & Ellen, 2003).

Family Characteristics Perceived family support, parent-family connectedness, family structure, family cohesiveness, parental monitoring, and parent-adolescent communication about sex help prevent adolescents from engaging in many risky sexual behaviors (Crosby, DiClemente, Wingood, Cobb, et al., 2001; Crosby, DiClemente, Wingood, Sionean, et al., 2001; DiClemente, Crosby, & Salazar, 2006; DiClemente, Wingood, Crosby, Cobb, et al., 2001; DiClemente, Wingood, Crosby, Sionean, Cobb, et al., 2001; DiIorio, Kelley, & Hockenberry-Eaton, 1999; Dittus & Jaccard, 2000; Dittus, Jaccard, & Gordon, 1999; Dutra, Miller, & Forehand, 1999; Ramirez-Valles, Zimmerman, & Newcomb, 1998; Resnick et al., 1997; Romer et al., 1999; Small & Luster, 1994). Parental monitoring is a particularly important familial factor. Emerging evidence suggests that adolescents who perceive that their parents (or parental figure) know where they are and who they are with outside of school or work are substantially less likely to engage in sexual risk behaviors and to have a STD diagnosis (Bettinger et al., 2004; Crosby, DiClemente, Wingood, Lang, & Harrington, 2003; DiClemente, Wingood, Crosby, Sionean, Cobb, et al., 2001; Li, Stanton, & Feigelman, 2000; Romer et al., 1999). Even among detained youth, parental monitoring has been shown to be a protective factor against STD infection (Crosby et al., 2006). Moreover, parents' influence can also buffer adolescents against the influence of negative peer norms that encourage risky sexual behaviors.

> *Perceived family support, parent-family connectedness, family structure, family cohesiveness, parental monitoring, and parent-adolescent communication about sex help prevent adolescents from engaging in many risky sexual behaviors.*

Relational Characteristics Relationship characteristics also play a pivotal role in influencing adolescents' risky behavior and their likelihood of acquiring an STD. Although commonalities occur across gender, some differences also exist. Among adolescent females, lack of relationship control (Crosby et al., 2000), longer length of relationship (Crosby et al., 2000; Fortenberry, Tu, Harezlak, Katz, & Orr, 2002, Plichta, Weisman, Nathanson, Ensminger, & Robinson, 1992), fear of condom use negotiation (Sionean et al., 2002), less frequent partner communication about sexually related topics (Catania, Coates, Greenblatt, & Dolcini, 1989; Sieving et al., 1997), and having older sex partners (Begley, Crosby, DiClemente, Wingood, & Rose, 2003) have each been associated with greater likelihood of engaging in STD risk behaviors or acquiring STDs. Other relational risk factors include perceptions of partner control over STD acquisition (Rosenthal et al., 1999), perception of low partner support of condoms (Weisman, Plichta, Nathanson, Ensminger, & Robinson, 1991), being a date rape victim (Valois, Oeltmann, Waller, & Hussey, 1999), and being a victim of dating violence (Silverman, Raj, Mucci, & Hathaway, 2001; Valois et al., 1999; Wingood et al., 2001). In one recent study, researchers found that among a sample of 715 African American female adolescents, experiencing gender-based violence was associated with STD-related sexual risk behaviors (Sales, Salazar, DiClemente, Wingood, & Crosby, 2008). Similar associations have been found for having a new partner (Bunnell et al., 1999) and having a risky partner (Katz, Fortenberry, Tu, Harezlak, & Orr, 2001).

For males, partner communication about sexually related topics (Lindberg, Ku, & Sonenstein, 1998; Wilson, Kastrinakis, D'Angelo, & Getson, 1994), belief in male responsibility for contraception (Lindberg, Ku, & Sonenstein, 1998), being in early stage of relationship (Ku, Sonenstein, & Pleck, 1994; Lindberg, Ku, & Sonenstein, 1998), and perceptions of partners' sexual inexperience (Ku, Sonenstein, & Pleck, 1994) have been associated with increased condom use. Furthermore, suspicion of partners' *high risk* for an STD (Ku, Sonenstein, & Pleck, 1994), perceived partners' negative attitude toward condom use (Pendergrast, DuRant, & Gaillard, 1992), and being a dating violence victim (Valois et al., 1999) have been related to unprotected intercourse and an increased number of sexual intercourse partners.

Individual Characteristics A broad spectrum of intrapersonal characteristics has been examined in the literature to better understand which critical factors underlie condom use and other STD-related behaviors, including STD acquisition (DiClemente & Crosby, 2003; DiClemente, Salazar, & Crosby, 2007; Crosby & Miller, 2002; DiClemente & Crosby, 2003; Jemmott et al., 2000; Santelli, DiClemente, Miller, & Kirby, 1999). Perceived susceptibility, a cornerstone of the health beliefs model (Rosenstock, 1974), has been shown to be associated with sexual risk behaviors. For example, studies suggest that adolescents who perceive that they are at risk for pregnancy and STDs tend to engage in less risky sexual behaviors than those who do not have these perceptions (Boyer et al., 2000; Sieving et al., 1997; Zimet et al., 1992). Self-efficacy is another individual characteristic shown to be a consistent protective factor for adolescents. Adolescents who feel confident in using condoms (Bandura, 1994; Jemmott III, Jemmott, Spears, Hewitt, & Cruz-Collins, 1992; Rosenthal, Moore, & Flynn, 1991; Sieving et al., 1997; Sionean et al., 2002), in their ability to negotiate condom use with their partners (DiClemente, Wingood, Crosby, Cobb, et al., 2001; Sionean et al., 2002), in their ability to say no to sexual intercourse not protected by a condom (Rosenthal, Moore, & Flynn, 1991), and in their ability to discuss sexual matters such as previous partners and sexual histories (Catania et al., 1989; Crosby, DiClemente, Wingood, Cobb, et al., 2002; DiClemente, Wingood, Crosby, Cobb, et al., 2001, 2001; Weisman, Nathanson, & Ensminger, 1989; Sieving et al., 1997) tend to use condoms more often and have lower rates of STDs (Crosby, DiClemente, Wingood, Sionean, et al., 2001).

Adolescents are undergoing a general process of self-discovery that facilitates transition to adulthood. This process may entail taking more risks as compared to other life periods, but some risk taking is not considered atypical during adolescence (Gullone, Moore, Moss, & Boyd, 2000). Those adolescents who are high risk takers, have high levels of impulsivity, or have a proclivity for sensation-seeking behavior may place themselves at greater risk for STD acquisition (Brown, DiClemente, & Park, 1992; Donohew et al., 2000; Kahn, Kaplowitz, Goodman, & Emans, 2002; Kowaleski-Jones & Mott, 1998; Stanton, Li, Cottrell, & Kaljee, 2001; Spitalnick et al., 2007). For example, Pack, Crosby, and St. Lawrence, (2001) found impulsivity was robustly associated with sexual risk behaviors across four samples of youth living in the southern United States. Also, Kahn and colleagues, (2002) found that greater impulsivity was associated with a greater frequency of sexual risk behavior and a history of chlamydia infection among a sample of adolescent females.

Individual characteristics such as low self-esteem, psychological distress, and depression also place many adolescents at risk for engaging in STD-associated sexual behaviors (DiClemente, Wingood, Crosby, Sionean, Brown, et al., 2001; Kowalski-Jones & Mott, 1998; Shrier, Harris, Sternberg, & Beardslee, 2001; Shrier, Harris, & Beardslee, 2002; Spencer, Zimet, Aalsma, & Orr, 2002). Depression has been shown to predict STD diagnosis in a recent prospective study (Shrier, Harris, & Beardslee, 2002) and also has been associated prospectively with a host of STD-related risk behaviors (DiClemente, Wingood, Crosby, Sionean, Brown, et al., 2001). Self-esteem has been found to distinguish between positive and negative STD diagnoses among female adolescent clinic attendees (Gardner, Frank, & Amankwaa, 1998).

Adolescents who are high risk takers, have high levels of impulsivity, or have a proclivity for sensation-seeking behavior may place themselves at greater risk for STD acquisition.

Not surprising, adolescents who engage in unprotected intercourse tend to perceive more barriers toward condom use (Crosby et al., 2000; Sieving et al., 1997), believe that using condoms results in less pleasure (Catania et al., 1989; Hingson et al., 1990; Jemmott et al., 1992; Sieving et al., 1997; Weisman, Nathanson, & Ensminger 1989), hold more negative attitudes toward using condoms (Fisher, Fisher, & Rye, 1995; Norris & Ford, 1994), and perceive low susceptibility to STD and HIV infection (Hingson et al., 1990; Zimet et al., 1992).

Other types of behaviors have also been shown to co-occur with risky sexual behaviors where research has revealed significant associations between adolescents' sexual risk behaviors and alcohol or drug use (Bachanas et al., 2002; Doljanac & Zimmerman, 1998; Millstein & Moscicki, 1995; Shafer & Boye, 1991; Sieving et al., 1997) and antisocial behaviors (Doljanac & Zimmerman, 1998). Moreover, many of these same behavioral factors are related to STD acquisition (Boyer, Tschann, & Shafer,, 1999; Boyer et al., 2000; Liau et al., 2002; Millstein & Moscicki 1995; Schwarcz et al., 1992; Shafer & Boyer, 1991; Shrier et al., 1999; Shrier, Harris, & Beardsleek 2002; Sieving et al., 1997; Strunin & Hingsonm 1992), as well as having multiple sex partners (Boyer et al., 2000; Fortenberry et al., 1999; Johnson, Neas, Parker, Fortenberry, & Cowan, 1993; Lewis, Melton, Succop, & Rosenthal, 2000; Millstein & Moscicki, 1995; Rosenthal, Biro, Succop, Bernstein, & Stanberry, 1997).

SUMMARY

Averting pregnancy and sexually transmitted diseases among teens represents an enormous challenge. The challenge may best be met by locating prevention efforts at multiple levels of causation—from societal, community, and peer levels to family, relational, and individual levels. Further, traditional medical counseling can be used as a complement to this approach. However, an important perspective of an ecological approach is that risk behavior should not be conceptualized as stemming strictly from "individual deficits." Ultimately, understanding the complex interplay between these omnipresent levels of influences will be critical to designing more effective and sustainable prevention interventions.

As a practical guide to intervention development, Table 15.1 lists relatively common antecedents to teen pregnancy and STD acquisition. Of note, the listing represents those antecedents with the greatest potential to be influenced by intervention efforts. As shown in Table 15.1 and as described in this chapter, each antecedent applies to both pregnancy and STD acquisition. Thus, the table illustrates an important concept: interventions to prevent teen pregnancy and those designed to avert teens' acquisition of STDs may comprise similar objectives. Many of the antecedents identified in the table are indeed targeted by current approaches to pregnancy and STD prevention for teens. The next chapter (Chapter Sixteen) provides an in-depth examination of interventions designed to avert teen pregnancy and STD acquisition.

TABLE 15.1.   Common and modifiable antecedents of teen pregnancy and STD acquisition

Antecedent	Corresponding Intervention Objective
Exposure to sexual imagery via media	Provide teens with alternate media or reduce their consumption of sexual imagery in media
Peer influences favoring risky sex	Change teens' faulty perceptions and promote healthy peer norms
Lack of perceived social support	Provide teens with strong social support mechanisms
Lack of positive aspirations for the future	Promote optimism for the future among teens and structure success in their goals
Lack of Connection to school	School programs should accommodate the psychosocial needs of all teens
Lack of parental monitoring	Intervene with parents to promote their increased vigilance in monitoring teens
Lack of parental disapproval of sex	Intervene with parents to help them express their values about sex to their teens

Antecedent	Corresponding Intervention Objective
Lack of parental communication about sex	Intervene with teens and with parents to foster open communication about sex
Underdeveloped self-efficacy for refusing sex	Teach teens skills that will enhance sex refusal self-efficacy
Underdeveloped self-efficacy for negotiating safer sex	Teach teens skills necessary to negotiate safer sex with their partners
Underdeveloped self-efficacy for condom use	Teach teens how to negotiate condom use and how to use condoms
Long length of relationship with one partner	Develop learning techniques for teens in long-standing relationships that promote continued safer sex practices
Impulsivity	Develop learning techniques that teach teens how to recognize the signs of "losing sexual control"

 ## KEY TERMS

Concurrency   Proximal influences
Distal influences   Sexual networks
Macrosystem   Social capital

 ## DISCUSSION QUESTIONS

1. Although teen births in the United States have generally declined over the last five years, pregnancy and birth among particular ethnic groups remain consistently high. Discuss possible psychosocial factors that may influence higher risk-taking behavior in certain subgroups.

2. Clarify the concept of concurrency as it relates to STD transmission among adolescents. Should concurrency be addressed within prevention interventions?

3. How are the antecedents of adolescent pregnancy similar to those of STD acquisition? Which antecedents have the greatest potential to be influenced by intervention efforts? Why?

REFERENCES

Abma, J., Chandra, A., Mosher, W., Peterson, L., & Piccinino, L. (1997). Fertility, family planning, and women's health: New data from the 1995 National Survey of Family Growth. *Vital and Health Statistics, 23*(19), DHHS Publication No. PHS 97–1995.

American Social Health Association. (1998). *Sexually transmitted diseases in America: How many and at what cost?* Menlo Park, CA: Kaiser Family Foundation.

Anderson, N. B. (2004). *Encyclopedia of health and behavior.* Thousand Oaks, CA: Sage.

Bachanas, P. J., Morris, M. K., Lewis- Gess, J. K., Sarett- Cuasay, E. J., Sirl, K., Ries, J. K., & Sawyer, M. K. (2002). Predictors of risky sexual behavior in African American adolescent girls: Implications for prevention interventions. *Journal of Pediatric Psychology, 27*(6), 519–530.

Balaji, A., Lowry, R., Brener, N., Kann, L., Romero, L., & Wechsler, H. (2008). Trends in HIV- and STD-related risk behaviors among high school students: United States 1991–2007. *Morbidity and Mortality Weekly Report, 57*(30), 817–822.

Bandura, A. (1994). Social cognitive theory and exercise of control over HIV infection. In R. J. DiClemente & J. L. Peterson (Eds.), *Preventing AIDS: Theories and methods of behavioral interventions* (pp. 25–59). New York: Springer.

Barnett, J. K., Papini, D. R., & Gbur, E. (1991). Familial correlates of sexually active pregnant and nonpregnant adolescents. *Adolescence, 26*(102), 457–472.

Bearman, P., & Bruckner, H. (1999). *Power in numbers: Peer effects on adolescent girls' sexual debut and pregnancy.* Washington, DC: National Campaign to Prevent Teen Pregnancy.

Begley, E., Crosby, R. A., DiClemente, R. J., Wingood, G. M., & Rose, E. (2003). Older partners and STD prevalence among pregnant African American teens. *Sexually Transmitted Diseases, 30*(3), 211–213.

Bettinger, J. A., Celentano, D. D., Curriero, F. C., Adler, N. E., Millstein, S. G., & Ellen, J. M. (2004). Does parental involvement predict new sexually transmitted diseases in female adolescents? *Archives of Pediatrics and Adolescent Medicine, 158*(7), 666–670.

Boyer, C. B., Shafer, M., Wibbelsman, C. J., Seeberg, D., Teitle, E., & Lovell, N. (2000). Associations of sociodemographic, psychosocial, and behavioral factors with sexual risk and sexually transmitted diseases in teen clinic patients. *Journal of Adolescent Health, 27*(2), 102–111.

Boyer, C. B., Tschann, J. M., & Shafer, M. A. (1999). Predictors of risk for sexually transmitted diseases in ninth grade urban high school students. *Journal of Adolescent Research, 14*(4), 448–465.

Brener, N. D., Kann, L., Lowry, R., Wechsler, H., & Romero, L. (2006). Trends in HIV-related risk behaviors among high school students: United States 1991–2005. *Morbidity and Mortality Weekly Report, 55*(31), 851–854.

Brown, B. B., Clasen, D. R., & Eicher, S. A. (1986). Perceptions of peer pressure, peer conformity dispositions, and self-reported behavior among adolescents. *Developmental Psychology, 22*(4), 521–530.

Brown, L. K., DiClemente, R. J., & Park, T. (1992). Predictors of condom use in sexually active adolescents. *Journal of Adolescent Health, 13*(8), 651–657.

Bryant, K. D. (2006). Update on adolescent pregnancy in the Black community. *Association of Black Nursing Faculty Journal, 17*(4), 133–136.

Bunnell, R. E., Dahlberg, L., Rolfs, R., Ransom, R., Gershman, K., Farshy, C., Newhall, W. J., Schmid, S., Stone, K., & St. Louis, M. (1999). High prevalence and incidence of sexually transmitted diseases in urban adolescent females despite moderate risk behaviors. *Journal of Infectious Diseases, 180,* 1624–1631.

Bunting, L., & McAuley, C. (2004). Research review: Teenage pregnancy and parenthood—the role of fathers. *Child and Family Social Work, 9* (3), 295–303.

Catania, J. A., Coates, T. J., Greenblatt, R. M., & Dolcini, M. M. (1989). Predictors of condom use and multiple-partnered sex among sexually active adolescent women: Implications for AIDS-related health interventions. *Journal of Sex Research, 26* (4), 514–524.

Cates, J. R., Herndon, N. L., Schulz, S. L., & Darroch, J. E. (2004). *Our voices, our lives, our futures: Youth and sexually transmitted diseases.* Chapel Hill, NC: University of North Carolina, Chapel Hill.

Centers for Disease Control and Prevention. (2006). *Trends in reportable sexually transmitted diseases in the United States 2005.* Atlanta, GA: Author.

Chesson, H. W., Blandford, J. M., Gift, T. L., Tao, G., & Irwin, K. L. (2004). The estimated direct medical cost of sexually transmitted diseases among American youth 2000. *Perspectives on Sexual and Reproductive Health, 36* (1), 11–19.

Crosby, R. A., DiClemente, R. J., Wingood, G. M., Cobb, B. K., Harrington, K., Davies, S. L., Hook, E. W., III, & Oh, M. K. (2001). HIV/STD-protective benefits of living with mothers in perceived supportive families: A study of high-risk African American female teens. *Preventive Medicine, 33* (3), 175–178.

Crosby, R. A., DiClemente, R. J., Wingood, G. M., Cobb, B. K., Harrington, K., Davies, S. L., Hook, E. W., III, & Oh, M. K. (2002). Condom use and correlates of African American adolescent females' infrequent communication with sex partners about preventing sexually transmitted diseases and pregnancy. *Health Education and Behavior, 29* (2), 219–231.

Crosby, R. A., DiClemente, R. J., Wingood, G. M., Sionean, C., Cobb, B. K., & Harrington, K. (2000). Correlates of unprotected vaginal sex among African American female adolescents: Importance of relationship dynamics. *Archives of Pediatrics and Adolescent Medicine, 154* (9), 893–899.

Crosby, R., DiClemente, R. J., Wingood, G. M., Sionean, C., Cobb, B. K., Harrington, K., Davies, S., Hook, E. W., III, & Oh, M. K. (2001). Correct condom application among African American adolescent females: The relationship to perceived self-efficacy and the association to confirmed STDs. *Journal of Adolescent Health, 29* (3), 194–199.

Crosby, R. A., DiClemente, R. J., Wingood, G. M., Harrington, K., Davies, S., Hook, E. W., III, & Oh, M. K. (2002a). Low parental monitoring predicts subsequent pregnancy among African-American adolescent females. *Journal of Pediatric and Adolescent Gynecology, 15* (1), 43–46.

Crosby, R. A., DiClemente, R. J., Wingood, G. M., Harrington, K., Davies, S., Hook, E. W., III, & Oh, M. K. (2002b). Psychosocial predictors of pregnancy among low-income African-American adolescent females: A prospective analysis. *Journal of Pediatric and Adolescent Gynecology, 15* (5), 293–299.

Crosby, R. A., DiClemente, R. J., Wingood, G. M., Harrington, K., Davies, S., & Malow, R. (2002). Participation by African-American adolescent females in social organizations: Associations with HIV-protective behaviors. *Ethnicity and Disease, 12* (2), 186–192.

Crosby, R. A., DiClemente, R. J., Wingood, G. M., Lang, D. L., & Harrington, K. (2003). Infrequent parental monitoring predicts sexually transmitted infections among low-income African American female adolescents. *Archives of Pediatrics and Adolescent Medicine, 157* (2), 169–173.

Crosby, R. A., DiClemente, R. J., Wingood, G. M., Rose, E., & Lang, D. (2003). Correlates of unplanned and unwanted pregnancy among African-American female teens. *American Journal of Preventive Medicine, 25* (3), 255–258.

Crosby, R. A., DiClemente, R. J., Wingood, G. M., Salazar, L. F., Rose, E., Levine, D., Brown, L., Lescano, C., Pugatch, D., Flanigan, T., Fernandez, I., Schlenger, W., & Silver, B. J. (2005a). Condom failure among adolescents: Implications for STD prevention. *Journal of Adolescent Health, 36* (6), 534–536.

Crosby, R. A., DiClemente, R. J., Wingood, G. M., Salazar, L. F., Rose, E., Levine, D., Brown, L., Lescano, C., Pugatch, D., Flanigan, T., Fernandez, I., Schlenger, W., & Silver, B. J. (2005b). Correlates of condom failure among adolescent males: An exploratory study. *Preventive Medicine, 41*(5–6), 873–876.

Crosby, R. A., DiClemente, R. J., Wingood, G. M., Salazar, L. F., Rose, E., & Sales, J. M. (2007). The protective value of school enrollment against sexually transmitted disease: A study of high-risk African American adolescent females. *Sexually Transmitted Infections, 83* (3), 223–227.

Crosby, R. A., DiClemente, R. J., Wingood, G. M., Sionean, C., Cobb, B. K., Harrington, K. F., Davies, S., Hook, E. W., III, & Oh, M. K. (2001). Correlates of casual sex among African-American female teens. *Journal of HIV/AIDS Prevention & Education for Adolescents and Children, 4* (4), 55–67.

Crosby, R. A., & Holtgrave, D. R. (2006). The protective value of social capital against teen pregnancy: A state-level analysis. *Journal of Adolescent Health, 38* (5), 556–559.

Crosby, R. A., Holtgrave, D. R., DiClemente, R. J., Wingood, G. M., & Gayle, J. A. (2003). Social capital as a predictor of adolescents' sexual risk behavior: A state-level exploratory study. *AIDS and Behavior, 7*(3), 245–252.

Crosby, R. A., & Miller, K. S. (2002). *Family influences on adolescent females' sexual health.* In G. M. Wingood & R. J. DiClemente (Eds.), *Handbook of women's sexual and reproductive health* (pp. 113–127). New York: Kluwer Academic/Plenum.

Crosby, R.A., Voisin, D., Salazar, L. F., DiDiClemente, R. J., Yarber, W. L., & Caliendo, A. M. (2006). Family influences and biologically confirmed sexually transmitted infections among detained adolescents. *American Journal of Orthopsychiatry, 76* (3), 389–394.

Cunningham, S. D., Michaud, J. M., Johnson, S. M., Rompalo, A., & Ellen, J. M. (2004). Phase-specific network differences associated with the syphilis epidemic in Baltimore city 1996–2000. *Sexually Transmitted Diseases, 31,* 611–615.

Davies, S. L., DiClemente, R. J., Wingood, G. M., Harrington, K. F., Crosby, R. A., & Sionean, C. (2003). Pregnancy desire among disadvantaged African American adolescent females. *American Journal of Health Behavior, 27* (1), 55–62.

Denner, J., Kirby, D., Coyle, K., & Brindis, C. (2001). The protective role of social capital and cultural norms in Latino communities: A study of adolescent births. *Hispanic Journal of Behavioral Sciences, 23*(1), 3–21.

DiClemente, R. J., Lodico, M., Grinstead, O. A., Harper, G., Rickman, R. L., Evans, P. E., & Coates, T. J. (1996). African-American adolescents residing in high-risk urban environments do use condoms: Correlates and predictors of condom use among adolescents in public housing developments. *Pediatrics, 98,* 269–278.

DiClemente, R. J., & Crosby, R. A. (2003). Sexually transmitted diseases among adolescents: Risk factors, antecedents, and prevention strategies. In G. R. Adams & M. D. Berzonsky (Eds.), *Blackwell handbook of adolescence* (pp. 573–605). Malden, MA: Blackwell Publishing.

DiClemente, R. J., Crosby, R. A., & Salazar, L. F. (2006). Family influences on adolescents' sexual health: Synthesis of the research and implications for clinical practice. *Current Pediatric Reviews, 2* (4), 369–373.

DiClemente, R. J., Salazar, L. F., & Crosby, R. A. (2007). A review of STD/HIV preventive interventions for adolescents: Sustaining effects using an ecological approach. *Journal of Pediatric Psychology, 32*(8), 888–906.

DiClemente, R. J., Salazar, L. F., Crosby, R. A., & Rosenthal, S. L. (2005). Prevention and control of sexually transmitted diseases among adolescents: The importance of a socio-ecological perspective—A commentary. *Public Health, 119,* 825–836.

DiClemente, R. J., Wingood, G. M., Crosby, R., Cobb, B. K., Harrington, K., & Davies, S. L. (2001). Parent-adolescent communication and sexual risk behaviors among African American adolescent females. *Journal of Pediatrics, 139* (3), 407–412.

DiClemente, R. J., Wingood, G. M., Crosby, R. A., Sionean, C., Brown, L. K., Rothbaum, B., Zimand, E., Cobb, B. K., Harrington, K., & Davies, S. (2001). A prospective study of psychological distress and sexual risk behavior among black adolescent females. *Pediatrics, 108* (5), p. e85.

DiClemente, R. J., Wingood, G. M., Crosby, R. A., Sionean, C., Cobb, B. K., Harrington, K., Davies, S., Hook, E. W., III, & Oh, M. K. (2001). Parental monitoring: Association with adolescents' risk behaviors. *Pediatrics, 107* (6), 1363–1368.

DiIorio, C., Kelley, M., & Hockenberry-Eaton, M. (1999). Communication about sexual issues: Mothers, fathers, and friends. *Journal of Adolescent Health, 24* (3), 181–189.

Dittus, P. J., & Jaccard, J. (2000). Adolescents' perceptions of maternal disapproval of sex: Relationship to sexual outcomes. *Journal of Adolescent Health, 26* (4), 268–278.

Dittus, P. J., Jaccard, J., & Gordon, V. V. (1999). Direct and nondirect communication of maternal beliefs to adolescents: Adolescent motivations for premarital sexual activity. *Journal of Applied Social Psychology, 29*(9), 1927–1963.

Dogan-Ates, A., & Carrion-Basham, C. Y. (2007). Teenage pregnancy among Latinas: Examining risk and protective factors. *Hispanic Journal of Behavioral Sciences, 29* (4), 554–569.

Doljanac, R. F., & Zimmerman, M. A. (1998). Psychosocial factors and high-risk sexual behavior: Race differences among urban adolescents. *Journal of Behavioral Medicine, 21* (5), 451–467.

Donohew, L., Zimmerman, R., Cupp, P. S., Novak, S., Colon, S., & Abell, R. (2000). Sensation seeking, impulsive decision-making, and risky sex: Implications for risk-taking and design of interventions. *Personality and Individual Differences, 28* (6), 1079–1091.

Dryfoos, J. G. (1990). *Adolescents at risk: Prevalence and prevention.* New York: Oxford University Press.

Dutra, R., Miller, K. S., & Forehand, R. (1999). The process and content of sexual communication with adolescents in two-parent families: Associations with sexual risk-taking behavior. *AIDS and Behavior, 3*(1), 59–66.

East, P. L., Felice, M. E., & Morgan, M. C. (1993). Sisters' and girlfriends' sexual and childbearing behavior: Effects on early adolescent girls' sexual outcomes. *Journal of Marriage and the Family, 55,* 953–963.

East, P. L., Khoo, S. T., & Reyes, B. T. (2006). Risk and protective factors predictive of adolescent pregnancy: A longitudinal, prospective study. *Applied Developmental Science, 10* (4), 188–199.

Ellen, J. M., Aral, S. O., & Madger, L. S. (1998). Do differences in sexual behaviors account for the racial/ethnic differences in adolescents' self-reported history of a sexually transmitted disease? *Sexually Transmitted Diseases, 25* (3), 125–129.

Ellis, B. J., Bates, J. E., Dodge, K. A., Fergusson, D. M., Horwood, L. J., Pettit, G. S., & Woodward, L. (2003). Does father absence place daughters at special risk for early sexual activity and teenage pregnancy? *Child Development, 74* (3), 801–821.

Eng, T. R., & Butler, W. T. (Eds.). (1997). *The hidden epidemic: Confronting sexually transmitted diseases.* Washington, DC: National Academies Press.

Fagot, B. I., Pears, K. C., Capaldi, D. M., Crosby, L., & Leve, C. S. (1998). Becoming an adolescent father: Precursors and parenting. *Developmental Psychology, 34* (6), 1209–1219.

Fergusson, D. M., & Woodward, L. J. (2000). Teenage pregnancy and female educational under-achievement: A prospective New Zealand birth cohort. *Journal of Marriage and the Family, 62*, 147–161.

Finer, L. B., & Henshaw, S. K. (2006). Disparities in rates of unintended pregnancy in the United States 1994 and 2001. *Perspectives on Sexual and Reproductive Health, 38* (2), 90–96.

Fisher, W. A., Fisher, J. D., & Rye, B. J. (1995). Understanding and promoting AIDS-preventive behavior: Insights from the theory of reasoned acti*on. Health Psychology, 14* (3), 255–264.

Forhan, S. E., Gottlieb, S. L., Sternberg, M. R., Xu, F., Datta, S. D., Berman, S., & Markowitz, L. E. (2008). Prevalence of sexually transmitted infections and bacterial vaginosis among female adolescents in the United States: Data from the National Health and Nutrition Examination Survey (NHANES), 2003–2004. Oral presentation at the National STD Prevention Conference, Chicago, IL.

Fortenberry, J. D., Brizendine, E. J., Katz, B. P., Wools, K. K., Blythe, M. J., & Orr, D. P. (1999). Subsequent sexually transmitted infections among adolescent women with genital infection due to Chlamydia trachomatis, Neisseria gonorrhoeae, or Trichomonas vaginalis. *Sexually Transmitted Diseases, 26* (1), 26–32.

Fortenberry, J. D., McFarlane, M., Bleakley, A., Bull, S., Fishbein, M., Grimley, D. M., Malotte, C. K., & Stoner, B. P. (2002). Relationships of stigma and shame to gonorrhea and HIV screening. *American Journal of Public Health, 92* (3), 378–381.

Fortenberry, J. D., Tu, W., Harezlak, J., Katz, B. P., & Orr, D. P. (2002). Condom use as a function of time in new and established adolescent sexual relationships: Unveiling the hidden epidemic of sexually transmitted diseases. *American Journal of Public Health, 92* (2), 211–213.

Franklin, D. L. (1993). *Early childbearing patterns among African Americans: A socio-historical perspective.* New Brunswick, NJ: Rutgers University Press.

Frost, J. J., & Oslak, S. (1999). *Teenagers' pregnancy intentions and decisions: A study of young women in California choosing to give birth.* New York: Guttmacher Institute.

Furstenberg, F. F., Jr., Geitz, L. M., Teitler, J. O., & Weiss, C. C. (1997). Does condom availability make a difference? An evaluation of Philadelphia's health resource centers. *Family Planning Perspectives, 29*(3), 123–127.

Gardner, L. H., Frank, D., & Amankwaa, L. I. (1998). A comparison of sexual behavior and self-esteem in young adult females with positive and negative tests for sexually transmitted diseases. *Association of Black Nursing Faculty Journal, 9* (4), 89–94.

Gest, S. D., Mahoney, J. L., & Cairns, R. B. (1999). A developmental approach to prevention research: Configural antecedents of early parenthood. *American Journal of Community Psychology, 27* (4), 543–565.

Gibson, J. W., & Kempf, J. (1990). Attitudinal predictors of sexual activity in Hispanic adolescent families. *Journal of Adolescent Research, 5* (4), 414–430.

Gillmore, M. R., Lewis, S. M., Lohr, M. J., Spencer, M. S., & White, R. D. (1997). Repeat pregnancies among adolescent mothers. *Journal of Marriage and the Family, 59*(3), 536–550.

Gullone, E., Moore, S., Moss, S., & Boyd, C. (2000). The Adolescent Risk-Taking Questionnaire: Development and psychometric evaluation. *Journal of Adolescent Research, 15* (2), 231–250.

Guttmacher Institute. (2002). *In their own right: Addressing the sexual and reproductive health needs of American men.* New York: Author.

Guttmacher Institute. (2006). *U.S. teenage pregnancy statistics: National and state trends and trends by race and ethnicity.* New York: Author.

Guttmacher, S., Lieberman, L., Ward, D., Freudenberg, N., Radosh, A., & Des Jarlais, D. (1997). Condom availability in New York City public high schools: Relationships to condom use and sexual behavior. *American Journal of Public Health, 87* (9), 1427–1433.

Hamilton, B. E., Martin, J. A., & Ventura, S. J. (2007). Births: Preliminary data for 2006. National Vital Statistics Report (Vol. 56). Atlanta: National Center for Health Statistics.

Hanson, S. L., Myers, D. E., & Ginsburg, A. L. (1987). The role of responsibility and knowledge in reducing teenage out-of-wedlock childbearing. *Journal of Marriage and the Family, 49* (2), 241–256.

Hayes, C. D. (Ed.). (1987). *Risking the future: Adolescent sexuality, pregnancy, and childbearing.* Washington, DC: National Research Council.

Hingson, R. W., Strunin, L., Berlin, B. M., & Heeren, T. (1990). Beliefs about AIDS, use of alcohol and drugs, and unprotected sex among Massachusetts adolescents. *American Journal of Public Health, 80* (3), 295–299.

Hoffman, S. D. (2006). *By the numbers: The public costs of adolescent childbearing.* Washington, DC: National Campaign to Prevent Teen Pregnancy.

Hogan, D. P., & Kitagawa, E. M. (1985). The impact of social status, family structure, and neighborhood on the fertility of Black adolescents. *American Journal of Sociology, 90* (4), 825–855.

Hogan, D. P., Sun, R., & Cornwell, G. T. (2000). Sexual and fertility behaviors of American females aged 15–19 years: 1985, 1990, and 1995. *American Journal of Public Health, 90* (9), 1421–4125.

Holtgrave, D., & Crosby, R. A. (2003). Social capital, poverty, and income inequality as predictors of gonorrhea, syphilis, chlamydia and AIDS case rates in the United States. *Sexually Transmitted Infections, 79,* 62–64.

Jemmott, J. B., III, Jemmott, L. W., Spears, H., Hewitt, N., & Cruz-Collins, M. (1992). Self-efficacy, hedonistic expectancies, and condom-use intentions among inner-city black adolescent women: A social cognitive approach to AIDS risk behavior. *Journal of Adolescent Health, 13*(6), 512–519.

Jemmott, L. S., Outlaw, F. H., Jemmott, J. B., Brown, E. J., Howard, M., & Hopkins, B. H. (2000). Strengthening the bond: The mother-son health promotion project. In W. Pequegnat & J. Szapocznik (Eds.), *Working with families in the era of HIV/AIDS* (pp. 133–154). Thousand Oaks, CA: Sage.

Jennings, J. M., & Ellen, J. M. (2003). Does sex partner concurrency and geographic context affect STI risk for female adolescents and their main sex partners? *Journal of Adolescent Health, 32*(2), 127–128.

Johnson, J., Neas, B., Parker, D. E., Fortenberry, J. D., & Cowan, L. D. (1993). Screening for urethral infection in adolescent and young adult males. [See comment]. *Journal of Adolescent Health, 14* (5), 356–361.

Kahn, J. A., Kaplowitz, R. A., Goodman, E., & Emans, S. J. (2002). The association between impulsiveness and sexual risk behaviors in adolescent and young adult women. *Journal of Adolescent Health, 30* (4), 229–232.

Kalmuss, D. S., & Namerow, P. B. (1994). Subsequent childbearing among teenage mothers: The determinants of a closely spaced second *birth. Family Planning Perspectives, 26* (4), 149–153.

Kasen, S., Cohen, P., & Brook, J. S. (1998). Adolescent school experiences and dropout, adolescent pregnancy, and young adult deviant behavior. *Journal of Adolescent Research, 13* (1), 49–72.

Katz, B. P., Fortenberry, J. D., Tu, W., Harezlak, J., & Orr, D. P. (2001). Sexual behavior among adolescent women at high risk for sexually transmitted infections. *Sexually Transmitted Diseases, 28* (5), 247–251.

Khaleque, A., & Deperry, A. A. (2005). Parent-adolescent relationships, premarital sex, and teen pregnancy in America: A multi-ethnic perspective. *Psychological Studies, 50* (4), 355–358.

Kirby, D. (2001). *Emerging answers: Research findings on programs to reduce teen pregnancy.* Washington, DC: National Campaign to Reduce Teen Pregnancy.

Kirby, D. (2002). Antecedents of adolescent initiation of sex, contraceptive use and pregnancy. *American Journal of Health Behavior, 26* (6), 473–485.

Kirby, D. (2003). Risk and protective factors affecting teen pregnancy and the effectiveness of programs designed to address them. In D. Romer (Ed.), *Reducing adolescent risk: Toward an integrated approach* (pp. 265–283). Thousand Oaks, CA: Sage.

Kirby, D., Coyle, K., & Gould, J. B. (2001). Manifestations of poverty and birthrates among young teenagers in California zip code areas. *Family Planning Perspectives, 33* (2), 63–69.

Klein, J. D., & Committee on Adolescence. (2005). Adolescent pregnancy: current trends and issues. *Pediatrics, 116* (1), 281–286.

Klerman, L. V. (1994). The association between adolescent parenting and childhood poverty. In A. C. Huston, (Ed.), *Children in poverty: Child development and public policy* (pp. 79–104). New York: Cambridge University Press.

Koniak-Griffin, D., Lesser, J., Uman, G., & Nyamathi, A. M. (2003). Teen pregnancy, motherhood, and unprotected sexual activity. *Research in Nursing and Health, 26* (1), 4–19.

Koumans, E. H., Farley, T. A., Gibson, J. J., Langley, C., Ross, M. W., McFarlane, M., Braxton, J., & St Louis, M. E. (2001). Characteristics of persons with syphilis in areas of persisting syphilis in the United States: Sustained transmission associated with concurrent partnerships. *Sexually Transmitted Diseases, 28*(9), 497–503.

Kowaleski-Jones, L., & Mott, F. L. (1998). Sex, contraception and childbearing among high-risk youth: Do different factors influence males and females? *Family Planning Perspectives, 30* (4), 163–169.

Ku, L., Sonenstein, F. L., & Pleck, J. H. (1993). Neighborhood, family, and work: Influences on the premarital behaviors of adolescent males. *Social Forces, 72* (2), 479–503.

Ku, L., Sonenstein, F. L., & Pleck, J. H. (1994). The dynamics of young men's condom use during and across relationships. *Family Planning Perspectives, 26* (6), 246–251.

Langille, D. B., Flowerdew, G., & Andreou, P. (2004). Teenage pregnancy in Nova Scotia communities: Associations with contextual factors. *Canadian Journal of Human Sexuality, 13* (2), 83–94.

Lewis, L. M., Melton, R. S., Succop, P. A., & Rosenthal, S. L. (2000). Factors influencing condom use and STD acquisition among African American college women. *Journal of American College Health, 49* (1), 19–23.

Li, X., Stanton, B., & Feigelman, S. (2000). Impact of perceived parental monitoring on adolescent risk behavior over 4 years. *Journal of Adolescent Health, 27* (1), 49–56.

Liau, A., DiClemente, R. J., Wingood, G. M., Crosby, R. A., Williams, K. M., Harrington, K., Davies, S. L., Hook, E. W., III, & Oh, M. K. (2002). Associations between biologically confirmed marijuana use and laboratory-confirmed sexually transmitted diseases among African American adolescent females. *Sexually Transmitted Diseases, 29* (7), 387–390.

Linares, L. O., Leadbeater, B. J., Kato, P. M., & Jaffe, L. (1991). Predicting school outcomes for minority group adolescent mothers: Can subgroups be identified? *Journal of Research on Adolescence, 1* (4), 379–400.

Lindberg, L. D., Ku, L., & Sonenstein, F. L. (1998). Adolescent males' combined use of condoms with partners' use of female contraceptive methods. *Maternal and Child Health Journal, 2* (4), 201–209.

Luster, T., & Small, S. A. (1994). Factors associated with sexual risk-taking behaviors among adolescents. *Journal of Marriage and the Family, 56* (3), 622–632.

Manlove, J. (1998). The influence of high school dropout and school disengagement on the risk of school-age pregnancy. *Journal of Research on Adolescence, 8* (2), 187–220.

Manlove, J., Mariner, C., & Papillo, A. R. (2000). Subsequent fertility among teen mothers: Longitudinal analyses of recent national data. *Journal of Marriage and the Family, 62* (2), 430–448.

Markham, C. M., Tortolero, S. R., Escobar-Chaves, S. L., Parcel, G. S., Harrist, R., & Addy, R. C. (2003). Family connectedness and sexual risk-taking among urban youth attending alternative high schools. *Perspectives on Sexual and Reproductive Health, 35* (4), 174–179.

Martin, J. A., Hamilton, B. E., Sutton, P. D., Ventura, S. J., Menacker, F., Kirmeyer, S., & Munson, M. L. (2007). Births: Final data for 2005. *National Vital Statistics Reports, 56* (6).

Meade, C. S., & Ickovics, J. R. (2005). Systematic review of sexual risk among pregnant and mothering teens in the USA: Pregnancy as an opportunity for integrated prevention of STD and repeat pregnancy. *Social Science and Medicine, 60* (4), 661–678.

Mersky, J. P., & Reynolds, A. J. (2007). Predictors of early childbearing: Evidence from the Chicago longitudinal study. *Children and Youth Services Review, 29* (1), 35–52.

Metzler, C. W., Noell, J., Biglan, A., Ary, D., & Smolkowski, K. (1994). The social context for risky sexual behavior among adolescents. *Journal of Behavioral Medicine, 17* (4), 419–438.

Miller, B. C. (1992). Adolescent parenthood, economic issues, and social policies. *Journal of Family and Economic Issues, 13* (4), 467–475.

Miller, B. C. (2002). Family influences on adolescent sexual and contraceptive behavior. *Journal of Sex Research, 39* (1), 22–26.

Miller, B. C., Benson, B., & Galbraith, K. A. (2001). Family relationships and adolescent pregnancy risk: A research synthesis. *Developmental Review, 21* (1), 1–38.

Miller, B. C., Norton, M. C., Curtis, T., Hill, E. J., Schvaneveldt, P., & Young, M. H. (1997). The timing of sexual intercourse among adolescents: Family, peer, and other antecedents. *Youth and Society, 29,* 54–83.

Millstein, S. G., & Moscicki, A.-B. (1995). Sexually transmitted disease in female adolescents: Effects of psychosocial factors and high risk behaviors. *Journal of Adolescent Health, 17* (2), 83–90.

Moore, M. R., & Chase-Lansdale, P. L. (2001). Sexual intercourse and pregnancy among African American girls in high-poverty neighborhoods: The role of family and perceived community environment. *Journal of Marriage and the Family, 63* (4), 1146–1157.

National Campaign to Prevent Teen Pregnancy. (2006). *How is the 3 in 10 statistic calculated?* Washington, DC: Author.

Norris, A. E., & Ford, K. (1994). Associations between condom experiences and beliefs, intentions, and use in a sample of urban, low-income, African-American and Hispanic youth. *AIDS Education and Prevention, 6* (1), 27–39.

Orshan, S. A. (1996). Acculturation, perceived social support, and self-esteem in primigravida Puerto Rican teenagers. *Western Journal of Nursing Research, 18* (4), 460–473.

Pack, R. P., Crosby, R. A., & St. Lawrence, J. S. (2001). Associations between adolescents' sexual risk behavior and scores on six psychometric scales: Impulsivity predicts risk. *Journal of HIV/AIDS Prevention and Education for Adolescents and Children, 4* (1), 33–47.

Pendergrast, R. A., Jr., DuRant, R. H., & Gaillard, G. L. (1992). Attitudinal and behavioral correlates of condom use in urban adolescent males. *Journal of Adolescent Health, 13* (2), 133–139.

Plichta, S., Weisman, C., Nathanson, C. A., Ensminger, M. E., & Robinson, J. C. (1992). Partner-specific condom use among adolescent women clients of a family planning clinic. *Journal of Adolescent Health, 13* (6), 506–511.

Powers, D. A. (2005). Effects of family structure on the risk of first premarital birth in the presence of correlated unmeasured family effects. *Social Science Research, 34* (3), 511–537.

Ramirez-Valles, J., Zimmerman, M. A., & Newcomb, M. D. (1998). Sexual risk behavior among youth: Modeling the influence of prosocial activities and socioeconomic factors. *Journal of Health and Social Behavior, 39* (3), 237–253.

Raneri, L. G., & Wiemann, C. M. (2007). Social ecological predictors of repeat adolescent pregnancy. *Perspectives on Sexual and Reproductive Health, 39* (1), 39–47.

Resnick, M. D., Bearman, P. S., Blum, R. W., Bauman, K. E., Harris, K. M., Jones, J., Tabor, J., Beuhring, T., Sieving, R. E., Shew, M., Ireland, M., Bearinger, L. H., & Udry, J. R. (1997). Protecting adolescents from harm: Findings from the National Longitudinal Study on Adolescent Health. *Journal of the American Medical Association, 278* (10), 823–832.

Robbins, C., Kaplan, H. B., & Martin, S. S. (1985). Antecedents of pregnancy among unmarried adolescents. *Journal of Marriage and the Family, 43* (3), 339–348.

Roberts, D. F., Foehr, U. G., Rideout, V. J., & Brodie, M. (1999). *Kids & media @ the new millennium.* Menlo Park, CA: Kaiser Family Foundation.

Romer, D., Stanton, B., Galbraith, J., Feigelman, S., Black, M. M., & Li, X. (1999). Parental influence on adolescent sexual behavior in high-poverty settings. *Archives of Pediatrics and Adolescent Medicine, 153* (10), 1055–1062.

Rosenberg, M. D., Gurvey, J. E., Adler, N., Dunlop, M. B., & Ellen, J. M. (1999). Concurrent sex partners and risk for sexually transmitted diseases among adolescents. *Sexually Transmitted Diseases, 26* (4), 208–212.

Rosenstock, I. M. (1974). Historical origins of the health belief model. *Health Education Monographs, 2,* 328–335.

Rosenthal, S. L., Biro, F. M., Succop, P. A., Bernstein, D. I., & Stanberry, L. R. (1997). Impact of demographics, sexual history, and psychological functioning on the acquisition of STDs in adolescents. *Adolescence, 32* (128), 757–769.

Rosenthal, S. L., Cohen, S. S., DeVellis, R. F., Biro, F. M., Lewis, L. M., Succop, P. A., & Stanberry, L. R. (1999). Locus of control for general health and STD acquisition among adolescent girls. *Sexually Transmitted Diseases, 26* (8), 472–475.

Rosenthal, D., Moore, S., & Flynn, I. (1991). Adolescent self-efficacy, self-esteem, and sexual risk-taking. *Journal of Community and Applied Social Psychology, 1* (2), 77–88.

Russell, S. T. (2002). Childhood developmental risk for teen childbearing in Britain. *Journal of Research on Adolescence, 12* (3), 305–324.

Salazar, L. F., Crosby, R. A., DiClemente, R. J., Wingood, G. M., Rose, E., Sales, J. M., & Caliendo, A. M. (2007). Personal, relational and peer-level risk factors for laboratory confirmed STD prevalence among low-income African American females. *Sexually Transmitted Diseases, 34* (10), 761–766.

Salazar, L. F., DiClemente, R. J., Wingood, G. M., Crosby, R. A., Lang, D. L., & Harrington, K. (2006). Biologically confirmed sexually transmitted infection and depressive symptomatology among African-American female adolescents. *Sexually Transmitted Infections, 82* (1), 55–60.

Salazar, L. F., DiClemente, R. J., Wingood, G. M., Daluga, N., & Lang, D. L. (2008). Teens' exposure to pornography and its relation to STD/HIV-associated risk behaviors. Unpublished raw data.

Sales, J. M., Salazar, L. F., DiClemente, R. J., Wingood, G. M., Rose, R., & Crosby, R. A. (2008). The mediating role of partner communication skills on HIV/STD-associated risk behaviors in African American female adolescents with a history of gender-based violence. *Archives of Pediatric and Adolescent Medicine, 162*(5), 432–438.

Santelli, J. S. (2007, December 14). Knocked up. *The Guardian* (London). Retrieved April 14, 2008, from www .guardian.co.uk/commentisfree/2007/dec/14/knockedup.

Santelli, J. S., DiClemente, R. J., Miller, K. S., & Kirby, D. (1999). Sexually transmitted diseases, unintended pregnancy, and adolescent health promotion. *Adolescent Medicine, 10,* 87–108.

Santelli, J. S., Lindberg, L. D., Finer, L. B., & Singh, S. (2007). Explaining recent declines in adolescent pregnancy in the United States: The contribution of abstinence and improved contraceptive use. *American Journal of Public Health, 97* (1), 150–156.

Santelli, J. S., Orr, M., & Lin, A. J. (2007). *Trends in sexual behaviors and contraceptive use in US high school students 1991–2005: Are positive trends faltering?* Paper presented at the American Public Health Association 135th Annual Meeting and Expo, Washington, DC.

Scaramella, L. V., Conger, R. D., Simons, R. L., & Whitbeck, L. B. (1998). Predicting risk for pregnancy by late adolescence: A social contextual perspective. *Developmental Psychology, 34* (6), 1233–1245.

Schwarcz, S. K., Bolan, G. A., Fullilove, M., McCright, J., Fullilove, R., Kohn, R., & Rolfs, R. T. (1992). Crack cocaine and the exchange of sex for money or drugs: Risk factors for gonorrhea among black adolescents in San Francisco. *Sexually Transmitted Diseases, 19* (1), 7–13.

Shafer, M. A., & Boyer, C. B. (1991). Psychosocial and behavioral factors associated with risk of sexually transmitted diseases, including human immunodeficiency virus infection, among urban high school students. *Journal of Pediatrics, 119* (5), 826–833.

Shrier, L. A., Harris, S. K., & Beardslee, W. R. (2002). Temporal associations between depressive symptoms and self-reported sexually transmitted disease among adolescents. *Archives of Pediatric Adolescent Medicine, 156* (6), 599–606.

Shrier, L. A., Harris, S. K., Sternberg, M., & Beardslee, W. R. (2001). Associations of depression, self-esteem, and substance use with sexual risk among adolescents. *Preventive Medicine, 33* (3), 179–189.

Sieving, R., Resnick, M. D., Bearinger, L., Remafedi, G., Taylor, B. A., & Harmon, B. (1997). Cognitive and behavioral predictors of sexually transmitted disease risk behavior among sexually active adolescents. *Archives of Pediatric Adolescent Medicine, 151* (3), 243–251.

Silverman, J. G., Raj, A., Mucci, L. A., & Hathaway, J. E. (2001). Dating violence against adolescent girls and associated substance use, unhealthy weight control, sexual risk behavior, pregnancy, and suicidality. *Journal of the American Medical Association, 286* (5), 572–579.

Singh, S., Darroch, J. E., & Frost, J. J. (2001). Socioeconomic disadvantage and adolescent women's sexual and reproductive behavior: The case of five developed countries. *Family Planning Perspectives, 33*(6), 251–258.

Sionean, C., DiClemente, R. J., Wingood, G. M., Crosby, R., Cobb, B. K., Harrington, K., Davies, S. L., Hook, E. W., III, & Oh, M. K. (2002). Psychosocial and behavioral correlates of refusing unwanted sex among African-American adolescent females. *Journal of Adolescent Health, 30* (1), 55–63.

Small, S. A., & Luster, T. (1994). Adolescent sexual activity: An ecological, risk-factor approach. *Journal of Marriage and the Family, 56* (1), 181–192.

Spencer, J. M., Zimet, G. D., Aalsma, M. C., & Orr, D. P. (2002). Self-esteem as a predictor of initiation of coitus in early adolescents. *Pediatrics, 109* (4), 581–584.

Spitalnick, J., DiClemente, R. J., Wingood, G. M., Crosby, R. A., Milhausen, R., Sales, J. M., McCarty, F., Rose, E., & Younge, S. (2007). Brief report: Sexual sensation seeking and its relationship to risky sexual behaviour among African-American adolescent females. *Journal of Adolescence, 30* (1), 165–173.

St. Lawrence, J. S., Brasfield, T. L., Jefferson, K. W., Alleyne, E., & Shirley, A. (1994). Social support as a factor in African-American adolescents' sexual risk behavior. *Journal of Adolescent Research, 9,* 292–310.

Stanton, B., Li, X., Cottrell, L., & Kaljee, L. (2001). Early initiation of sex, drug-related risk behaviors, and sensation-seeking among urban, low-income African-American adolescents. *Journal of the National Medical Association, 93* (4), 129–138.

Stevens-Simon, C., Sheeder, J., & Harter, S. (2005). Teen contraceptive decisions: Childbearing intentions are the tip of the iceberg. *Women and Health, 42*(1), 55–73.

Strasburger, V. C. (1995). *Adolescents and the media: Medical and psychological impact.* Thousand Oaks, CA: Sage.

Strunin, L., & Hingson, R. W. (1992). Alcohol, drugs, and adolescent sexual behavior. *International Journal of the Addictions, 27* (2), 129–146.

Sucoff, C. A., & Upchurch, D. M. (1998). Neighborhood context and the risk of childbearing among metropolitan-area Black adolescents. *American Sociological Review, 63* (4), 571–585.

Thornburgh, D., & Lin, H. S. (Eds.). (2002). *Youth, pornography, and the Internet*. Washington, DC: National Academies Press.

U.S. Census Bureau. (2004). Annual social and economic supplement: 2003 Current population survey (table MS-2). Current Population Reports, P20–553.

Valois, R. F., Oeltmann, J. E., Waller, J., & Hussey, J. R. (1999). Relationship between number of sexual intercourse partners and selected health risk behaviors among public high school adolescents. *Journal of Adolescent Health, 25,* 328–335.

Velez-Pastrana, M. C., Gonzalez-Rodriguez, R. A., & Borges-Hernandez, A. (2005). Family functioning and early onset of sexual intercourse in Latino adolescents. *Adolescence, 40* (160), 777–791.

Ventura, S. J., Abma, J., Mosher, W., & Henshaw, S. K. (2008). Estimated pregnancy rates by outcome for the United States 1990–2004. *National Vital Statistics Report, 56* (15), 1–25, 28.

Vesely, S. K., Wyatt, V. H., Oman, R. F., Aspy, C. B., Kegler, M. C., Rodine, S., Marshall, L., & McLeroy, K. R. (2004). The potential protective effects of youth assets from adolescent sexual risk behaviors. *Journal of Adolescent Health, 34* (5), 356–365.

Weinstock, H., Berman, S., & Cates, W. (2004). Sexually transmitted diseases among American youth: Incidence and prevalence estimates. *Perspectives on Sexual and Reproductive Health, 36* (1), 6–10.

Weisman, C., Plichta, S., Nathanson, C., Ensminger, M., & Robinson, J. C. (1991). Consistency of condom use for disease prevention among adolescent users of oral contraceptives. *Family Planning Perspectives, 23,* 71–74.

Wilson, M. D., Kastrinakis, M., D'Angelo, L. J., & Getson, P. (1994). Attitudes, knowledge, and behavior regarding condom use in urban black adolescent males. *Adolescence, 29* (113), 13–26.

Wingood, G. M., DiClemente, R. J., Bernhardt, J. M., Harrington, K., Davies, S. L., Robillard, A., & Hook, E. W., III. (2003). A prospective study of exposure to rap music videos and African American female adolescents' health. *American Journal of Public Health, 93* (3), 437–439.

Wingood, G. M., DiClemente, R. J., Harrington, K., Davies, S., Hook, E. W., III, & Oh, M. K. (2001). Exposure to X-rated movies and adolescents' sexual and contraceptive-related attitudes and behaviors. *Pediatrics, 107* (5), 1116–1119.

Woodward, L., Fergusson, D. M., & Horwood, L. J. (2001). Risk factors and life processes associated with teenage pregnancy: Results of a prospective study from birth to 20 years. *Journal of Marriage and the Family, 63* (4), 1170–1184.

Xie, H., Cairns, B. D., & Cairns, R. B. (2001). Predicting teen motherhood and teen fatherhood: Individual characteristics and peer affiliations. *Social Development, 10* (4), 488–511.

Yamaguchi, K., & Kandel, D. (1987). Drug use and other determinants of premarital pregnancy and its outcome: A dynamic analysis of competing life events. *Journal of Marriage and the Family, 49* (2), 257–270.

Young, T. M., Martin, S. S., Young, M. E., & Ting, L. (2001). Internal poverty and teen pregnancy. *Adolescence, 36* (142), 289–304.

Zimet, G. D., Bunch, D. L., Anglin, T. M., Lazebnik, R., Williams, P., & Krowchuck, D. P. (1992). Relationship of AIDS-related attitudes to sexual behavior changes in adolescents. *Journal of Adolescent Health, 13* (6), 493–498.

CHAPTER

16

INTERVENTIONS TO PREVENT PREGNANCY AND SEXUALLY TRANSMITTED DISEASES, INCLUDING HIV INFECTION

DOUGLAS KIRBY ▪ RICHARD A. CROSBY ▪ JOHN S. SANTELLI ▪ RALPH J. DICLEMENTE

LEARNING OBJECTIVES

After studying this chapter, you will be able to

- Analyze adolescent intervention programs that have affected adolescent sexual behavior within the last two decades.

- Discover common characteristics of efficacious adolescent intervention programs.

The high endemic rates of pregnancy and sexually transmitted diseases (STDs) among adolescents in the United States warrant substantial efforts to prevent them. Such efforts should be designed to change those sexual behaviors that place youth at risk of either unwanted pregnancy or STDs. In particular, programs should delay the initiation of sex, and among adolescents who do have sex, reduce the frequency of sex, reduce the number of sexual partners, increase condom use, or increase other contraceptive use (see Chapter Fifteen). To change these sexual behaviors and thereby reduce unintended pregnancy or STDs, programs must address those risk and protective factors that they can markedly change and in turn have a marked impact on one or more of these sexual behaviors (see Chapter Fifteen).

Over the last three decades, people have developed innumerable and extremely diverse programs to reduce teen pregnancy and STDs. Some programs have focused only on abstinence, while others have focused much more on increasing condom or contraceptive use. Some have tried to increase knowledge about the consequences of sexual behavior and methods of preventing pregnancy and STDs, while others have tried to change attitudes, perceptions of norms, skills, and intentions, and still others have tried to improve access to condoms and other contraceptives. Some have focused on teens themselves, while others have focused on their families or entire communities. Some have focused on *sexual* risk and protective factors, while others have addressed more distal factors that do not involve sexuality at all, such as connection to school or family, belief in the future, or employment opportunities.

Because unintended teen pregnancy and STDs are important problems and because resources to address them are always limited, it is important to determine which types of programs and which specific programs are most effective at changing behaviors that place youth at risk. Accordingly, researchers have conducted numerous analyses and meta-analyses of programs to reduce sexual risk (Corcoran & Pillai, 2007; Herbst et al., 2006; Scher & Maynard, 2006; Underhill, Montgomery, & Operario, 2007; Underhill, Operario, & Montgomery, 2007). In general, their results are somewhat encouraging, demonstrating that some approaches do have reasonably strong evidence that some types of programs are effective.

Financial support for this chapter was provided by the William and Flora Hewlett Foundation. The views reflected in this paper do not necessarily reflect those of the William and Flora Hewlett Foundation. This paper is based in part on the publication *Emerging Answers 2007,* published by the National Campaign to Prevent Unplanned and Teen Pregnancy (available at www.thenc.org).

This chapter reviews the evidence for the impact on sexual behavior of a wide variety of programs. It differs from most other reviews because it covers a wider variety of types of programs, reviews a greater number of studies, and is more recent (also see *Emerging Answers 2007: Research Findings on Programs to Reduce Teen Pregnancy and Sexually Transmitted Diseases,* on which this chapter is based.) In addition, it is not a formal statistical meta-analysis, but rather a more in-depth analysis of the programs.

METHODS USED IN THIS REVIEW

Given the huge number and great variety of programs that have been developed and the hundreds of evaluations that have been conducted of these programs, criteria must first be specified for the inclusion of studies before they can be selected. To be included in this chapter, studies had to meet the following criteria. The intervention program had to

- Focus on adolescents of middle school or high school age (or their parents)

- Be implemented in the United States

    The research methods had to

- Include a reasonably strong experimental or quasi-experimental design with well-matched intervention and comparison groups and both pretest and posttest data collection

- Have a sample size of at least one hundred

- Measure program impact on one or more of the following sexual behaviors: initiation of sex, frequency of sex, number of sexual partners, use of condoms or contraception more generally, composite measures of sexual risk (such as frequency of unprotected sex), pregnancy rates, birth rates, and STD rates

- Measure impact on those behaviors that can change quickly (frequency of sex, number of sexual partners, use of condoms, and use of contraception or sexual risk taking) for at least three months or measure impact on those behaviors or outcomes that change less quickly (initiation of sex and pregnancy rates or STD rates) for at least six months

Finally, the study had to be completed or published in 1990 or thereafter. (To be as inclusive as possible, we did not require studies to be published in peer-reviewed journals, but nearly all were.) The methods for identifying and coding these and other studies are described elsewhere (Kirby, 2007). This chapter does not include all the studies meeting these criteria. For example, it excludes studies of early childhood development, studies of welfare reform, and a few other studies. However, it does include nearly all of them.

CURRICULUM-BASED SEX AND STD/HIV EDUCATION PROGRAMS

As noted earlier, many different types of programs have been developed. The first two types of programs shown in Exhibit 16.1—abstinence and comprehensive sex and STD/HIV education programs—are based on written curricula and are implemented with groups of young people (as opposed to one-on-one interaction between individuals). These programs are particularly well designed for implementation in schools, where they can potentially reach large numbers of youth, yet they can also be implemented in other clinic and community settings where they can reach other youth, including potentially higher-risk youth who have dropped out of school. Because abstinence and comprehensive sex education programs differ from one another, their studies are presented separately.

EXHIBIT 16.1. **Programs focusing primarily on sexual risk and protective factors**

Curriculum-based sexuality education programs in any setting
   Abstinence education programs
   Sexuality and HIV education programs
Sex and HIV education programs for parents and their families
Stand-alone video-based and computer-based interventions
Clinic-based programs designed to provide reproductive health care or to improve access to condoms or other contraceptives
   Family planning services
   Protocols for clinic appointments and supportive activities
   Advance provision of emergency contraception
   Other clinic characteristics and programs
School-based health centers, school-linked reproductive health clinics, and school condom availability programs
Community-wide pregnancy or STD/HIV prevention initiatives with multiple components
Programs Focusing Primarily on Nonsexual Factors
Youth development programs for adolescents
   Service-learning programs
   Vocational education and employment programs
   Other youth development programs
Programs Focusing on Both Sexual and Nonsexual Factors
   Programs to address substance abuse, violence, and sexual risk
   Very intensive long-term programs

Abstinence Programs

In this chapter, *abstinence programs* are defined as those that encourage only abstinence and not condom or other contraceptive use. They are not the same as *comprehensive programs*, which emphasize abstinence as the safest behavior but also encourage condom or other contraception use for those who do have sex.

As shown in Table 16.1, there were only eight studies of nine different abstinence programs meeting the selection criteria for this chapter (Kirby, 2007; Weed, Ericksen, Lewis, Grant, & Wibberly, 2008). One of these studies measured the impact of two different abstinence programs. It is a particularly important study, because it was very rigorous and it evaluated abstinence programs carefully selected because they were believed to be effective. The results from this study demonstrated no effects on initiation of sex, age of initiation of sex, abstinence in the previous twelve months, number of sexual partners or use of condoms or other contraceptives during sex. The lack of behavioral results was quite compelling.

TABLE 16.1. **Curriculum-based sex and STD/HIV education programs: Number of studies reporting effects on different sexual behaviors and outcomes**

Outcomes Measured	Abstinence Education Programs (*N* = 9)	Comprehensive Programs (*N* = 48)
Delay sex	(*N* = 9)	(*N* = 32)
Delayed initiation	2	15
No significant results	7	17
Hastened initiation	0	0
Reduce frequency of sex	(*N* = 6)	(*N* = 21)
Reduced frequency	2	6
No significant results	4	15
Increased frequency	0	0
Reduce number of partners	(*N* = 5)	(*N* = 24)
Reduced number	1	11
No significant results	4	12
Increased number	0	1
Increase condom use	(*N* = 5)	(*N* = 32)
Increased use	0	15
No significant results	5	17
Reduced use	0	0

(Continued)

TABLE 16.1. *(Continued)*

Outcomes Measured	Abstinence Education Programs (*N* = 9)	Comprehensive Programs (*N* = 48)
Increase contraceptive use	(*N* = 4)	(*N* = 9)
Increased use	0	4
No significant results	4	4
Reduced use	0	1
Reduce sexual risk taking	(*N* = 3)	(*N* = 24)
Reduced risk	0	15
No significant results	3	9
Increased risk	0	0
Reduce pregnancy: self-report	(*N* = 4)	(*N* = 6)
Reduced number	0	2
No significant results	3	4
Increased number	1	0
Reduce pregnancy: laboratory test	(*N* = 0)	(*N* = 2)
Reduced number	0	0
No significant results	0	2
Increased number	0	0
Reduce childbirth: self-report	(*N* = 3)	(*N* = 1)
Reduced number	0	1
No significant results	3	0
Increased number	0	0
Reduce STDs: self-report	(*N* = 4)	(*N* = 2)
Reduced number	0	0
No significant results	3	2
Increased number	1	0
Reduce STDs: laboratory test	(*N* = 0)	(*N* = 4)
Reduced number	0	2
No significant results	0	2
Increased number	0	0

Of the seven other abstinence studies, only two delayed sexual initiation (Weed et al., 2008). Both were based on quasi-experimental designs and had other limitations, thus providing only weak evidence for their positive effects.

Of the six studies that measured impact on frequency of sex among those who had previously had sex, two reduced the frequency of sex and the other four had no significant impact. Finally, one of five programs reduced the number of sexual partners, and the other four had no significant impact. In regard to sexual risk, none of the five studies that measured use of condoms found a significant impact on condom use. Similarly, the four studies that measured impact on contraceptive use did not find an impact.

Comprehensive Sex and STD/HIV Education Programs

Forty-eight studies of comprehensive programs were identified (Kirby, 2007). These programs promoted both abstinence and use of condoms or other forms of contraception.

Across all these comprehensive studies, 47 percent delayed the initiation of sex and none hastened initiation; 6 out of 21 (29 percent) reduced frequency, and none increased frequency; 11 out of 24 (46 percent) reduced number of sexual partners, and only 1 increased the number of sexual partners. Nearly half (47 percent) increased condom use, 4 out of 9 (44 percent) increased contraceptive use, but 1 decreased it. Finally, 69 percent had a significant positive impact on one or more behaviors, and 38 percent had a positive impact on two or more behaviors. For example, the Safer Choices intervention delayed the initiation of sex among Hispanic youth and increased both condom and contraceptive use among both boys and girls of all races/ethnicities (Kirby et al., 2004).

These findings were remarkably robust. Programs were effective in different communities and cultures throughout the country. For example, programs were effective with youth in low- and middle-income communities and in rural and urban areas. They were effective in school, clinic, and community settings. They were effective with both males and females, both younger and older youth, and both sexually experienced and inexperienced youth. Not every program was effective with every group, but one or more programs were effective with each of these groups.

The curricula continued to be effective when they were implemented with fidelity by others in different communities.

Robustness was also demonstrated in replication studies. A critically important question is whether or not a program that has been found to be effective in one community and study will subsequently be effective in other communities when implemented and evaluated by others. Four curricula have been evaluated two or more times, and those studies demonstrated that the curricula continued to be effective when they were implemented with fidelity by others in different communities. They were *less* likely to remain effective if

1. They were shortened considerably

2. Activities for increasing condom use were omitted

3. They were designed for and evaluated in community settings, but were subsequently implemented in classroom settings

Program Effects on Psychosocial Mediators

Although the preceding summary provides strong evidence that a majority of the programs had an impact on sexual risk behaviors, without the results of the impact on the mediating mechanisms, that summary does not explain *how or why* these programs had an impact. Those questions can be partially answered by examining programmatic impact on the risk and protective factors that programs attempted to change in order to change behavior. At least 50 percent of the studies that measured impact on each of the following factors actually found a statistically significant positive impact:

- Knowledge about HIV and STDs (including methods of preventing STD/HIV and pregnancy)

- Perceived risk of HIV or STDs

- Values and attitudes regarding several sexual topics, such as abstinence and condoms

- Self-efficacy to refuse sex, to obtain and use condoms, and to avoid risk

- Motivation to avoid sex or restrict the number of sex partners

- Intention to use a condom

- Intention to avoid risk

- Communication with partner about STDs

- Communication with parents about sex, condoms, and contraception

- Avoiding situations that could lead to sex

All these factors have been demonstrated empirically to be related to sexual behaviors (Kirby, Lepore, & Ryan, 2005). Thus, it appears likely that changes in these factors contributed to the changes in sexual risk-taking behaviors.

Common Characteristics of Efficacious Programs

An analysis of the effective curricula and a smaller number of ineffective curricula led to the identification of seventeen common characteristics of effective programs. The methods used to identify these characteristics are presented in Table 16.2 (as described by Kirby, Laris, & Rolleri, 2007). A tool to assess whether or not curricula incorporate these characteristics has also been developed (Kirby, Rolleri, & Wilson, 2007). The seventeen characteristics of effective curricula describe their development, content, and implementation. The large majority of the effective programs incorporated most of the seventeen characteristics of successful curriculum-based programs identified in this chapter. Also, programs that incorporated these characteristics were much more likely to change behavior positively than programs that did not incorporate many of these characteristics.

TABLE 16.2. The seventeen characteristics of effective curriculum-based sex and STD/HIV education programs

The Process of Developing the Curriculum	The Contents of the Curriculum Itself	The Process of Implementing the Curriculum
1. Involved multiple people with different backgrounds in theory, research, and sex and STD/HIV education to develop the curriculum	*Curriculum goals and objectives* 6. Focused on clear health goals—the prevention of STD/HIV and/or pregnancy	14. Secured at least minimal support from appropriate authorities, such as departments of health or education, school districts, or community organizations
2. Assessed relevant needs and assets of target group	7. Focused narrowly on specific behaviors leading to these health goals (such as abstaining from sex or using condoms or other contraceptives), gave clear messages about these behaviors, and addressed situations that might lead to them and how to avoid them	15. Selected educators with desired characteristics (whenever possible), trained them, and provided monitoring, supervision, and support
3. Used a logic model approach that specified the health goals, the behaviors affecting those health goals, the risk and protective factors affecting those behaviors, and the activities addressing those risk and protective factors	8. Addressed multiple sexual psychosocial risk and protective factors that affect sexual behavior (such as knowledge, perceived risks, values, attitudes, perceived norms, and self-efficacy) *Activities and teaching methodologies*	16. If needed, implemented activities to recruit and retain youth and overcome barriers to their involvement (such as publicizing the program, offering food, or obtaining consent)
4. Designed activities consistent with community values and available resources (such as staff time, staff skills, facility space, and supplies)	9. Created a safe social environment for youth to participate 10. Included multiple activities to change each of the targeted risk and protective factors	17. Implemented virtually all activities with reasonable fidelity
5. Pilot-tested the program	11. Employed instructionally sound teaching methods that actively involved the participants, helped participants personalize the information, and were designed to change each group of risk and protective factors	
	12. Employed activities, instructional methods, and behavioral messages that were appropriate to the youths' culture, developmental age, and sexual experience	
	13. Covered topics in a logical sequence	

Programs that were effective consistently gave a clear message about behavior. Most commonly, that message was some version of the following: "You should always avoid unprotected sex. Abstinence is the safest and best choice. If you have sex, always use protection against pregnancy and STD."

The teams of people who developed the effective curricula appeared to develop *logic models* when they developed their curricula—that is, they specified (1) the health goals they wished to achieve (such as reductions in teen pregnancy or STD), (2) the behaviors they wanted to change in order to achieve these health goals, (3) the risk and protective factors (or mediating factors) that have a causal impact on these behaviors, and (4) activities that would markedly improve those risk and protective factors. They often used health and *sociopsychological theories* (such as social cognitive theory, the theory of planned behavior, the health belief model, and other theories) to identify the important *mediating factors* (such as knowledge, attitudes, perception of norms, self-efficacy, and intentions) that in turn affect behavior. Sometimes they also used instructional theory to determine what types of activities would produce positive change in these mediating factors.

Effective curricula incorporated multiple activities designed to improve each of the important mediating factors. These activities actively involved adolescents and helped them personalize the information. For example, they used games to increase students' knowledge, role playing exercises to improve their skills to say no to sex or to insist on using condoms or contraception, and anonymous voting activities about what sexual behaviors are right for them (such as abstinence or having sex with protection) in order to change perception of peer norms. Effective curricula had adolescents describe the characteristics of the situations that might lead to unwanted, unintended sex or unprotected sex and then had them describe strategies for avoiding these situations. Effective programs also included activities that were appropriate to the adolescents' gender, age, and level of sexual experience. If programs were implemented in schools, then they were typically quite long (eleven or more sessions) in order to include enough activities to change the mediating factors and behavior. Effective programs, especially school-based programs, provided training to the educators, received parental consent, and often included homework assignments to talk with parents about assigned topics.

Programs for Families

Most parents and their children have remarkably few conversations about sexual topics, often because both parents and their teens feel uncomfortable doing so. To help alleviate this problem, educational programs have been designed to increase parent-child communication. These include programs for parents only (sometimes fathers only and sometimes mothers only), programs for parents and their children together, homework assignments in school sex education classes requiring communication with parents, and video programs with written materials to be completed at home. Nearly all of them included multiple sessions, lasting as long as forty-nine hours over many weeks.

Several studies suggest that few parents are willing or able to participate in special parent programs. With remarkable consistency, however, many studies also indicate that when parents participate, they do increase their communication with their children about sexuality in the short term, as well as their comfort with that communication (Kirby & Miller, 2002). However, those positive effects on communication seem to dissipate over time.

Because a simple relationship between parent-child communication and adolescent sexual and contraceptive behavior does not exist, a handful of studies have also examined the programs' effects on adolescents' sexual behavior (Kirby, 2007). See Table 16.3.

Overall, the results are somewhat encouraging, particularly regarding condom use. Although only one of five programs succeeded in delaying the initiation of sex, and one of one reduced the frequency of sex, all four of the four studies that measured impact on condom use found a significant increase in condom use. Notably, those studies that included rather intensive programs for adolescents as well as their parents were especially likely to show significant effects. This result is not surprising because the programs for adolescents by themselves might have been effective even without the parent component. Finally, two of the studies suggest that increasing parental involvement and monitoring may also have an impact.

When parents participate, they increase their communication with their children about sexuality in the short term, as well as their comfort with that communication.

Video and Computer-Based Programs

For decades videos have been incorporated into facilitator-led group sessions, either to provide accurate information or to serve as teasers to generate group discussion. However, with the rapid changes in media and computer technology during the last decade, stand-alone video or computer programs have been developed. Adolescents increasingly have access to computers on which they view the enormous numbers of videos that their peers and others put online. Many enjoy and are completely comfortable with this interactive computer video technology. Multiple studies suggest that interactive video and computer programs can improve knowledge and attitudes about sexuality (Robinson et al., 2002; Thompson, Simonson, & Hargrave, 1996). Three different studies have measured the impact of videos, interactive videos, or computer-based interventions on behavior (Kirby, 2007). Their results are mixed. One video was based on theory, strived to increase perceived risk of STD/HIV, and used dialogue, music, images, and stories that would appeal to the adolescents. However, it was short (fourteen minutes), was not interactive, and did not have a significant impact on behavior.

The second video was a stand-alone interactive video used in clinics. The video included a section on sexual situations (negotiation behaviors to reduce STD risk), risk reduction (getting and using condoms and condom efficacy), reproductive health,

TABLE 16.3. **Programs for parents and their families: Number of studies reporting effects on different sexual behaviors and outcomes**

Outcomes Measured	Parent Programs ($N = 7$)
Delay sex	($N = 5$)
Delayed initiation	1
No significant results	4
Hastened initiation	0
Reduce frequency of sex	($N = 1$)
Reduced frequency	1
No significant results	0
Increased frequency	0
Increase condom use	($N = 4$)
Increased use	4
No significant results	0
Reduced use	0
Increase contraceptive use	($N = 1$)
Increased use	0
No significant results	1
Reduced use	0
Reduce sexual risk taking	($N = 2$)
Reduced risk	0
No significant results	2
Increased risk	0
Reduce pregnancy: self-report	($N = 1$)
Reduced number	1
No significant results	0
Increased number	0
Reduce STDs: self-report	($N = 1$)
Reduced number	1
No significant results	0
Increased number	0

and sexually transmitted disease. The study demonstrated that the video reduced the percent of girls who had sex during the first three months after the first exposure to the video and reduced the reported STD rate at six months.

The last of the three studies compared the relative effects in alternative schools of a computerized intervention based on Project LIGHT (Living in Good Health Together), a small-group intervention, and a control group. At three months, adolescents participating in the computerized intervention were less likely to have had sex the previous three months than those receiving instruction in the small groups. Adolescents in the computerized group also had fewer sexual partners than the control group.

Of note, a six-session computer-based intervention completed online appeared to delay the initiation of sex and possibly reduce the number of subsequent sexual partners ($p = .055$). However, it only measured impact for five months. In addition, a different computer-based interactive program was designed for college students. It was based on the information-motivation-behavioral skills model of health behavior and also motivational interviewing. A randomized trial measured its impact for only one month and found that it increased condom use during that month.

Programs Based on Family Planning Services

According to the 2002 National Survey of Family Growth, an estimated 3.9 million fifteen- to nineteen-year-old females—nearly 40 percent of all females in that age group—made one or more visits to a clinic or private medical source for a family planning service in a single year (Martinez, Mosher, Abma, & Jones, 2005). The primary objective of family planning clinics (or family planning services offered within other health settings) is to provide clients with contraception and other reproductive health services and with the knowledge and skills to use them. According to a 1995 national survey of publicly funded family planning agencies, these agencies typically provided special services for teens (Frost & Bolzan, 1997). About 87 percent of them encouraged counselors to spend more time with teenagers than with other clients, and 69 percent had at least one special program serving teens. For example, 30 percent had special clinics for teens and 49 percent provided education or outreach in schools or youth centers. According to a more recent national survey of publicly funded family planning clinics conducted in 2003, 91 percent of clinics counseled teens under eighteen about abstinence, and 89 percent encouraged teens under eighteen to discuss issues related to sex with their parents (Lindberg, Frost, Sten, & Dailard, 2006). They also counseled older adolescents to do the same. About 42 to 45 percent of the clinics also had educational programs for teens on these topics.

The estimated number of adolescent pregnancies averted by family planning services depends greatly on the assumptions made about the prevalence of teen sexual and contraceptive activity if prescription contraceptives were not available. If one assumes that adolescents would use over-the-counter methods of contraception if prescription methods were not available, then the estimated number of additional teen pregnancies averted per year ranges from 40,000 to 160,000 nationally, depending on possible changes in sexual activity (Kahn, Brindis, & Glei, 1999).

Unfortunately, the research on the impact of family planning services is limited. Although several studies have examined the effects of family planning clinics on pregnancy or birth rates (Kirby, 2007), the strength of their conclusions is greatly weakened by conflicting results among studies and by several severe methodological limitations. Thus, the actual impact on adolescent pregnancy rates of either family planning services generally or subsidized family planning clinics specifically has not been accurately estimated. However, data from California have been used to assess the impact on teen pregnancy rates of making reproductive health services more available to teens.

In 1997, California implemented Family PACT, a program to prevent unintended pregnancy by providing comprehensive clinical services for family planning and reproductive health at no cost to low-income adolescents and adults. For teens, income was based on their personal income, not on their parents' income. Thus, the vast majority of teens were eligible. Eligibility was quickly assessed at point of service and teens did not have to go elsewhere (such as to a Medicaid office) to become eligible. Parental consent was not required, and patients were assured of the confidentiality of their visits. In addition, Family PACT expanded the number of clinic providers by including private for-profit providers as well as nonprofit providers. Consequently, the number of providers increased from about 450 clinic sites in 1995–1996 to more than 1,900 sites in 2000–2001 (Brindis et al., 2003). Family PACT also increased the fee paid by the state for each service. Finally, the state Office of Family Planning strongly encouraged state-funded community teen pregnancy programs to inform youth about the availability of reproductive health services and to make referrals to Family PACT clinics. Evaluation data indicate that many adolescents received these referrals and attended the clinics.

During 2002, Family PACT prevented tens of thousands of unintended teen pregnancies.

What was the impact of these changes on teen use of state-funded family planning services? Clinic records reveal that the number of adolescent clients served annually by state-supported family planning services increased from 99,739 before Family PACT was instituted to more than 300,000 per year during the following six years (Brindis et al., 2003; California Department of Health Services, 2006). This threefold increase suggests that when free confidential reproductive health services are made more readily available, many more teens will use them. A subsequent study estimated that during 2002, Family PACT prevented tens of thousands of unintended teen pregnancies (Foster et al., 2006). If Family PACT actually succeeded in doing this, then it would have substantially reduced the overall teen pregnancy rate throughout the state. In this regard, it should be noted that Family PACT was implemented during a period of time when California birth rates were declining more rapidly than birth rates in nearly all other states. Although many factors probably contributed to this rapid decline, Family PACT may have been one of the important ones.

Protocols for Clinic Appointments and Supportive Activities

Six studies have examined program changes in one-on-one interactions within the clinics—interactions prescribed by clinic protocols (Kirby, 2007). All six studies evaluated interventions that were part of longer medical appointments. Remarkably, all six had positive effects on sexual behavior (Table 16.4). The fact that all six of these studies found positive effects on behavior is very encouraging, and the fact that several of them were effective, even with brief, modest interventions, is also encouraging. It should be noted that all six of the interventions focused on sexual and contraceptive behavior, gave clear messages about appropriate sexual and contraceptive behavior, and included one-on-one consultation about the client's behavior.

At the very least, these studies suggest that such approaches should be further developed and rigorously evaluated. The results should also encourage medical providers to review their instructional protocols and spend more time talking with adolescents about their sexual and contraceptive activity. It should also be remembered that some of the sex and STD/HIV education programs that were curriculum- and group-based and were discussed previously in this chapter were implemented in clinic settings and found to be effective. For example, when activities from Be Proud! Be Responsible!, Making a Difference, and Making Proud Choices were integrated into a four-hour curriculum and implemented in a clinic setting, it reduced unprotected sex, number of sexual partners, and STD rates at twelve months (Jemmott, Jemmott, Braverman, & Fong, 2005). Similarly, Sistering, Informing, Healing, Loving, and Empowering is a group-based program implemented in an STD clinic for adolescent females that reduced the number of partners, increased condom use, decreased pregnancy rates, and decreased STD rates at six or twelve months (DiClemente et al., 2004).

Advance Provision of Emergency Contraception

One of the most common reasons that teens say they didn't use contraception is that they didn't expect to have sex. Emergency contraception is the only method of contraception that can be used up to seventy-two hours after sex and dramatically reduce the chances of pregnancy. Thus, in theory it has the potential to significantly reduce teen pregnancy. Four studies measured the impact of providing emergency contraception in advance to adolescents (Kirby, 2007; see Table 16.4). Some of these studies included adolescents up through age twenty-four. All four found that providing emergency contraception in advance significantly increased the use of emergency contraception at least in the short run. This is consistent with studies of advance provision of emergency contraception to adults in the United States and in other countries. Furthermore, these studies of teens and young adults found few significant effects on use of other forms of contraception or condom use, and the few results that were significant were mixed—both positive and

TABLE 16.4. **Clinic-based interventions: Number of studies reporting effects on different sexual behaviors and outcomes**

Outcomes Measured	Protocols for Clinic Appointments (N = 6)	Advance Provision of Emergency Contraception (N = 4)	Other Clinic Characteristics (N = 2)
Delay sex	(N = 1)	(N = 0)	(N = 1)
Delayed initiation	0	0	0
No significant results	0	0	1
Hastened initiation	1	0	0
Reduce frequency of sex	(N = 3)	(N = 2)	(N = 1)
Reduced frequency	1	0	0
No significant results	2	2	1
Increased frequency	0	0	0
Reduce number of partners	(N = 2)	(N = 1)	(N = 0)
Reduced number	1	0	0
No significant results	1	1	0
Increased number	0	0	0
Increase condom use	(N = 4)	(N = 4)	(N = 0)
Increased use	3	1	0
No significant results	1	3	0
Reduced use	0	0	0
Increase contraceptive use	(N = 2)	(N = 3)	(N = 2)
Increased use	2	0	0
No significant results	0	2	2
Reduced use	0	1	0
Increase emergency contraceptive use	(N = 0)	(N = 4)	(N = 0)
Increase use	0	4	0
No significant results	0	0	0
Decrease use	0	0	0

Outcomes Measured	Protocols for Clinic Appointments (*N* = 6)	Advance Provision of Emergency Contraception (*N* = 4)	Other Clinic Characteristics (*N* = 2)
Reduce sexual risk taking	(*N* = 2)	(*N* = 4)	(*N* = 0)
Reduced risk	2	0	0
No significant results	0	3	0
Increased risk	0	1	0
Reduce pregnancy: self-report	(*N* = 2)	(*N* = 1)	(*N* = 2)
Reduced number	1	0	0
No significant results	1	1	2
Increased number	0	0	0
Reduce pregnancy: laboratory test	(*N* = 0)	(*N* = 2)	(*N* = 0)
Reduced number	0	0	0
No significant results	0	2	0
Increased number	0	0	0
Reduce STDs: self-report	(*N* = 4)	(*N* = 1)	(*N* = 0)
Reduced number	0	0	0
No significant results	4	1	0
Increased number	0	0	0
Reduce STDs: laboratory test	(*N* = 0)	(*N* = 2)	(*N* = 0)
Reduced number	0	0	0
No significant results	0	2	0
Increased number	0	0	0
Reduce childbirth: self-report	(*N* = 0)	(*N* = 0)	(*N* = 1)
Reduced number	0	0	0
No significant results	0	0	1
Increased number	0	0	0

negative on use of other forms of contraception or unprotected sex. Although these mixed effects require further investigation, it appears likely that providing emergency contraception to teens does not have negative effects overall, just as it does not have negative effects among adult women.

Three of the studies measured the impact of the advance provision of emergency contraception on pregnancy rates. None found a statistically significant effect, although one of them reported a programmatically meaningful impact. Because emergency contraception is not designed to be used repeatedly, any given individual is likely to use it only a couple of times a year. Given that the chances of pregnancy resulting from one or two acts of unprotected sex are quite small, the use of emergency contraception once or twice over an entire year will only reduce the chance of becoming pregnant during that year by a small amount. Thus, much larger samples sizes are needed to detect the impact on pregnancy.

Other Clinic Characteristics and Programs

Two studies investigated other characteristics of clinic structure or protocols (Kirby, 2007; see Table 16.4). The first evaluated the effect of a citywide effort to improve family planning services for young people. That initiative, called Responsible Education on Sexuality and Pregnancy for Every Community's Teens, involved nine existing clinics that initiated or expanded after-school or evening hours, began teenage walk-in hours, decreased the average waiting time for appointments, and increased the hours reserved for teenagers only. The program also trained staff to work with teens. In addition, the program included school and community activities, as well as a media campaign. This study differed from most others in this review by assessing effects of a citywide effort on all adolescents rather than on those who actually used the clinic. This is a far more demanding challenge, but it was appropriate given the initiative's goal to expand services and its communitywide efforts. However, a comparison of changes over time between the catchment area and a comparison area revealed no significant changes in contraceptive use, pregnancy, or childbearing rates.

The second study examined two different interventions, both of which were very modest. During a clinic visit, patients either were invited to bring their parents to six subsequent visits or received two to six telephone calls from the clinic staff regarding their use of the contraceptives method(s) they had chosen. Only 36 percent of the teens in the first group attended any subsequent visits with their parents, but most adolescents in the second group (84 percent) did receive the phone calls. The program failed to have an effect on adolescents' use of contraception or pregnancy.

School-Based Provision of Contraception

School-based health centers are clinics located on school grounds that offer services to students. In contrast, school-linked clinics are located near schools and provide similar services. The purpose of both types of clinics is to provide primary health care services that are affordable and accessible to students who otherwise might not have ongoing access to such services. In 2001–2002, there were at least 1,378 school-based health centers throughout the country, and 77 percent of these served students in grades seven through twelve (National Assembly on School-Based Health Care, 2002).

Although more than 80 percent of clinics serving adolescents provided at least one reproductive health service (such as gynecologic exams, birth control counseling, pregnancy testing, and STD diagnosis and treatment), only about one-fourth of these clinics dispensed hormonal contraceptives (National Assembly on School-Based Health Care, 2002). About one-fourth also dispensed condoms.

When school-based and school-linked clinics are well-staffed and well-run and dispense contraceptives, they show many qualities of ideal adolescent reproductive health providers—their location is convenient to the students, they reach both females and males, they provide comprehensive health services, they are confidential, their staff are selected and trained to work with adolescents, they can easily conduct follow-up, their services are free, and they integrate education, counseling, and medical services.

When school-based clinics make contraception available, many adolescents obtain it from the clinics. For example, in a study of four clinics that provided prescriptions or actually dispensed contraceptives, the proportion of sexually experienced females who obtained contraceptives through the clinic varied from 23 percent to 40 percent.

Four studies have examined the effects of school-based health centers (Kirby, 1991; Kirby et al., 1993; Newcomer, Duggan, & Toczek, 1999; Ricketts & Guernsey, 2006) and a fifth study examined the impact of a *school-linked* reproductive health clinic (Zabin, Hirsch, Smith, Streett, & Hardy, 1986; see Table 16.5). Three of the five studies examined school-based or school-linked clinics in three or more schools. These studies measured population effects—the effects on the entire school population and not just on those students who actually used the clinics for family planning services.

One study evaluated a school-based clinic in Norfolk, Virginia. That clinic did not focus on reproductive health, and it prescribed but did not dispense contraception. It did not affect the onset or frequency of sexual intercourse or increase contraceptive use or reduce pregnancy or birth rates in that school (Kirby, 1991).

These results are consistent with the results of two other studies of school-based clinics in six and nineteen schools, respectively, that employed very weak quasi-experimental designs and are therefore not included in Table 16.5. Those two studies consistently found that the clinics did not increase sexual behavior. Although their results for contraceptive use were mixed, overall they found little impact on contraceptive use one way or the other. However, the first study clearly found substitution effects—even though many adolescents obtained contraception from the clinics, most would have obtained contraception elsewhere if the clinics had not been there.

TABLE 16.5. **School-based clinics and condom availability programs: Number of studies reporting effects on different sexual behaviors and outcomes**

Outcomes Measured	School-Based or -Linked Clinics (N = 5)	School Condom Availability (N = 1)
Delay sex	(N = 2)	(N = 1)
Delayed initiation	1	0
No significant results	1	1
Hastened initiation	0	0
Reduce frequency of sex	(N = 1)	(N = 1)
Reduced frequency	0	0
No significant results	1	1
Increased frequency	0	0
Increase condom use	(N = 0)	(N = 1)
Increased use	0	0
No significant results	0	1
Reduced use	0	0
Increase contraceptive use	(N = 2)	(N = 0)
Increased use	1	0
No significant results	1	0
Reduced use	0	0
Reduce sexual risk taking	(N = 0)	(N = 1)
Reduced risk	0	0
No significant results	0	1
Increased risk	0	0
Reduce pregnancy: self-report	(N = 2)	(N = 0)
Reduced number	1	0
No significant results	1	0
Increased number	0	0

Outcomes Measured	School-Based or -Linked Clinics (*N* = 5)	School Condom Availability (*N* = 1)
Reduce childbirth: self-report	(*N* = 1)	(*N* = 0)
Reduced number	0	0
No significant results	1	0
Increased number	0	0
Reduce childbirth: public records	(*N* = 3)	(*N* = 0)
Reduced number	1	0
No significant results	2	0
Increased number	0	0

Three additional studies examined clinic impact on birth rates and found mixed results. Two studies found that they did not affect birth rates, though a study of Denver-based clinics that did not prescribe contraception found that the clinics may have reduced birth rates among blacks.

In contrast to these school-*based* health centers that were located on the school grounds and that provided primary health care services, the Self Center in Baltimore was located across the street from a high school and four blocks away from a junior high school and provided *only* reproductive health services (Zabin et al., 1986). More specifically, it provided educational, counseling, and reproductive health services in the clinic, as well as educational and counseling services in the two schools. In both schools, the staff implemented a peer education program and after-school group discussions, while in the clinic the staff provided individual counseling, group counseling, and contraceptive services. Survey data collected from the two program schools and two matched comparison schools suggest there was a delay in the intervention schools in the onset of sexual intercourse among those youth who had not yet initiated sex and an increase in the use of contraception among those who had ever had sex. In addition, there was an apparent decrease in pregnancy rates in the program schools two years after the Self Center opened.

School Condom Availability Programs

Given the threat of AIDS, other STDs, and pregnancy, more than three hundred schools without school-based clinics have made condoms available through school counselors, nurses, teachers, vending machines, or baskets (Kirby & Brown, 1996). In addition to these, more than two hundred schools make condoms available to students through school-based clinics.

When available in schools, the number of condoms obtained per student from schools varied greatly from program to program (Kirby & Brown, 1996). In general, students in smaller alternative schools obtained many more condoms per student than students in larger schools or students in mainstream schools. In addition, when schools made multiple brands of condoms available in baskets in convenient and private locations and without any restrictions, students obtained many more condoms than when there were restrictions (such as when students could obtain only a small number of condoms from school personnel at specified times after brief counseling). Finally, students obtained many more condoms in schools that had clinics.

Only one study meeting the criteria for this review presented results on the behavioral effects of condom availability programs in schools (Table 16.5). That study measured the impact of making condoms available in baskets in nine Philadelphia schools (Furstenberg, Geitz, Teitler, & Weiss, 1997). Students in those schools could receive reproductive health information, condoms, and general health referrals. Neither sexual behavior nor condom use was significantly affected. These results were similar to a study in Seattle that also showed a substitution effect but no impact on sexual behavior and no positive impact on condom use (Kirby et al., 1999).

YOUTH DEVELOPMENT PROGRAMS

Research suggests that improving young women's performance in school, their plans for their futures and their connection to their families, schools, and faith communities all reduce their pregnancy and birth rates (Kirby, Lepore, & Ryan, 2005). In the United States between the mid-1950s and the mid-1970s, increasingly large percentages of young women pursued higher education and more challenging professional careers and postponed marriage and childbearing. During these years, the teen birth rate declined markedly (Guttmacher Institute, 1994). Observing these trends, some professionals working with adolescents believed that two of the most promising approaches to reducing teen pregnancy were to improve educational and career opportunities through youth development programs and to increase their connection with responsible adults and institutions.

Vocational Education and Employment Programs

Vocational education and employment programs typically include academic instruction (or an educational requirement) and either vocational education or actual jobs. Three different studies evaluated such programs, all in multiple sites (Kirby, 2007; see Table 16.6). The Summer Training and Education Program (STEP) included academic remediation, life skills education, half-time summer employment, and personal support, but had no significant impact on either sexual behavior or contraceptive use. Similarly, the Job Corps and JOBSTART combined remedial, academic, and vocational education and to varying degrees other support services, including life skills education, health education, health care, and job placement assistance. Neither program affected pregnancy or birth rates.

Service-Learning Programs

By definition, *service-learning programs* include (1) voluntary or unpaid service in the community (such as tutoring, working as a teacher's aide, working in nursing homes,

TABLE 16.6. **Youth development programs that focus on nonsexual risk and protective factors: Number of studies reporting effects on different sexual behaviors and outcomes**

Outcomes Measured	Vocational Education (N = 3)	Service Learning (N = 4)	Other Youth Development (N = 3)
Delay sex	(N = 1)	(N = 1)	(N = 1)
Delayed initiation	0	1	1
No significant results	1	0	0
Hastened initiation	0	0	0
Reduce frequency of sex	(N = 1)	(N = 1)	(N = 0)
Reduced frequency	0	1	0
No significant results	1	0	0
Increased frequency	0	0	0
Reduce number of partners	(N = 0)	(N = 0)	(N = 2)
Reduced number	0	0	2
No significant results	0	0	0
Increased number	0	0	0
Increase condom use	(N = 0)	(N = 0)	(N = 1)
Increased use	0	0	0
No significant results	0	0	1
Reduced use	0	0	0
Increase contraceptive use	(N = 1)	(N = 0)	(N = 0)
Increased use	0	0	0
No significant results	1	0	0
Reduced use	0	0	0
Reduce pregnancy: self-report	(N = 1)	(N = 3)	(N = 1)
Reduced number	0	3	1
No significant results	0	0	0
Increased number	1	0	0

(Continued)

TABLE 16.6. (*Continued*)

Outcomes Measured	Vocational Education (*N* = 3)	Service Learning (*N* = 4)	Other Youth Development (*N* = 3)
Reduce childbirth: self-report	(*N* = 3)	(*N* = 0)	(*N* = 2)
Reduced number	0	0	1
No significant results	2	0	1
Increased number	1	0	0
Reduce STDs: self-report	(*N* = 0)	(*N* = 0)	(*N* = 1)
Reduced number	0	0	0
No significant results	0	0	1
Increased number	0	0	0

or helping fix up parks and recreation areas) and (2) structured time for preparation and reflection before, during, and after service (through group discussions, journal writing, or papers). Sometimes the service is voluntary, but other times it is prearranged as part of a class. Often, but not always, the service is linked to academic instruction in the classroom.

Strong evidence suggests that service-learning programs reduce actual teen pregnancy rates.

Strong evidence suggests that service-learning programs reduce actual teen pregnancy rates. Four different studies, three of which evaluated programs in multiple locations, have consistently indicated that service learning reduces either sexual activity or teen pregnancy (Kirby, 2007; see Table 16.6). The Teen Outreach Program (TOP), the Learn and Serve programs, and service learning added to a health education program all were effective. However, for the first two programs, the effects were demonstrated only for the academic year in which youth were involved.

Several explanations for observed effects of service learning programs have been suggested: participants developed ongoing relationships with caring program facilitators; some may have developed greater autonomy and felt more competent in their relationships with peers and adults; some may have been heartened by the realization that they could make a difference in the lives of others; some were encouraged by their volunteer experiences to think more about their futures—all of which might have increased motivation to avoid pregnancy. It may also be that both supervision and alternative activities simply reduced the opportunity for participants to engage in unprotected sex. After all, these programs were time intensive—the mean numbers of hours that youth spent in TOP and Learn and Serve programs during the academic year were forty-six hours and seventy-seven hours, respectively.

The study of TOP found that the kinds of volunteer service varied considerably from site to site, but TOP appeared to be most effective when young people had some control over where they volunteered. The effectiveness of TOP was *not* dependent on the fidelity of the implementation of the TOP curriculum, which suggests that the service itself is the most important component of the programs.

Other Youth Development Programs

Other youth development programs have also demonstrated positive effects on pregnancy or childbearing (Table 16.6). For example, the Quantum Opportunities Program (Hahn, Leavitt, & Aaron, 1994) provided adolescents with educational activities (such as tutoring and computer-based instruction), community service activities, and development activities (such as arts and career and college planning). Findings from the experimental study evaluating this program suggested that it might have reduced birth rates, but only at the .10 level of statistical significance.

Similarly, the Seattle Social Development Program (Hawkins, Catalano, Kosterman, Abbott, & Hill, 1999; Lonczak, Abbott, Hawkins, Kosterman, & Catalano, 2002) was designed to increase children's attachment to school and family by improving teaching strategies (such as cooperative learning), parenting skills, and students' social skills (such as decision making and refusal skills). When the grade school students were followed to age eighteen, those receiving the intervention were less likely to report a pregnancy than the comparison group. They were also more attached to school, got higher grades, and engaged in fewer delinquent acts. When the same students were followed to age twenty-one, those receiving the intervention reported initiating sex at a later age, having fewer sexual partners, and being more likely to have used a condom at last sex than students in the control group.

The New Beginnings Program was designed to prevent mental health problems among children of divorced parents (Wolchik et al., 2002). This program for mothers focused on methods of improving the quality of the mother-child relationship, the use of effective discipline, access to the father, and avoidance of interparent conflict. The program for mothers and their children also focused on effective coping strategies, improving parent-child relationships, and addressing stressors related to divorce. Programs had significant positive effects on mental health problems, substance use, and number of sexual partners.

INTENSIVE PROGRAMS COMBINING YOUTH DEVELOPMENT AND REPRODUCTIVE HEALTH

Of all the programs evaluated, perhaps the most intensive and long-term program was the Children's Aid Society–Carrera Program (CAS-Carrera Program; Philliber, Kaye, Herring, & West, 2002). It recruited adolescents when they were about thirteen to fifteen years old and encouraged them to participate throughout high school. During those school years, it operated five days a week. Some programs had regularly scheduled special events, education programs, and entrepreneurial activities. During the summer months, paid employment, including entrepreneurial activities, was emphasized, along with evening maintenance programs. Adolescents spent an average of sixteen hours per month in the program during the first three years. The CAS-Carrera Program used a holistic approach, providing the following multiple services: (1) family life and sex education, (2) an education component that included individual academic assessment, tutoring, help with homework, preparation for standardized exams, and assistance with college entrance, (3) a work-related intervention that included a job club, stipends, individual bank accounts, employment, and career awareness, (4) self-expression through the arts, and (5) individual sports. In addition, the program provided mental health care and comprehensive medical care, including reproductive health and contraception when needed. In all of these areas, staff tried to create close caring relationships with the participants. Although the program focused on adolescents, it also provided services for their parents and other adults in the community.

The evaluation study of the CAS-Carrera Program included twelve sites (six New York City sites and six sites elsewhere in the country). The study found that for girls the program significantly delayed the initiation of sexual intercourse, increased the use of condoms along with another highly effective method of contraception, and reduced pregnancy rates for three years. However, the favorable results for initiation of sex and avoiding sexual risk among girls were found only in the six New York City sites and not in the six sites elsewhere in the country (Scher & Maynard, 2006). For boys, the program had no significant positive behavioral effects in any of the sites. The study did have one unexpected finding: boys in the programs were significantly *less* likely to report using both condoms and another highly effective contraception method at last sex than boys in the comparison group. This result was found among boys who had initiated sexual activity prior to the program.

Some of the challenges of implementing the CAS-Carrera Program arose in a serious attempt to replicate the program in three communities in Florida (Kirby, Rhodes, & Campe, 2005). The Florida staff earnestly tried to implement all the CAS-Carrera Program components, but they did so without the benefit of the training and support from the CAS-Carrera staff. They faced challenges in recruiting adolescents, keeping them involved, and retaining staff. Adolescents participated less frequently and for shorter periods of time in these programs than in the original CAS-Carrera Program, and those assigned to the control group ended up participating in other somewhat similar activities (such as school sports) offered by the communities. There were no significant positive effects on the large majority of outcomes, including sexual behaviors.

COMMUNITYWIDE PREGNANCY OR STD/HIV PREVENTION PROGRAMS

During the last two decades, there has been a growing recognition that it might take more than just single programs focusing on discrete populations of teens to change teen pregnancy or STD/HIV rates markedly. Thus, some communities have developed communitywide collaboratives with the goal of reducing teen pregnancy and STD rates.

Eight studies have examined the impact of six different communitywide programs; three studies evaluated the impact of a single program (Kirby, 2007). See Table 16.7. These community initiatives and their impact differed considerably. Nevertheless, these studies confirm that community initiatives focusing on pregnancy or STD/HIV prevention do not hasten or increase sexual activity, even when they focus primarily on condom or contraceptive use. None of the studies found any significant negative effects. With regard to delay in sex, condom, or other contraceptive use or pregnancy or birth rates, these studies are encouraging. Four found significant effects on one or more these outcomes. This is particularly impressive because most of these studies measured impact on communitywide outcomes, not on outcomes measured only among those most directly involved. One or more programs found positive effects on initiation of sex, number of sexual partners, condom use, and pregnancy rates, suggesting that the effects of these programs are not limited to any particular behavior.

There has been a growing recognition that it might take more than just single programs focusing on discrete populations of teens to change teen pregnancy or STD/HIV rates markedly.

TABLE 16.7. **Communitywide pregnancy or STD/HIV prevention initiatives with multiple components: Number of studies reporting effects on different sexual behaviors and outcomes**

Outcomes Measured	Community-Based Initiatives (N = 6)
Delay sex	(N = 4)
Delayed initiation	3
No significant results	1
Hastened initiation	0
Reduce frequency of sex	(N = 2)
Reduced frequency	0
No significant results	2
Increased frequency	0
Reduce number of partners	(N = 1)
Reduced number	1
No significant results	0
Increased number	0

(Continued)

TABLE 16.7. *(Continued)*

Outcomes Measured	Community-Based Initiatives (*N* = 6)
Increase condom use	(*N* = 2)
Increased use	1
No significant results	1
Reduced use	0
Increase contraceptive use	(*N* = 1)
Increased use	0
No significant results	1
Reduced use	0
Reduce pregnancy: self-report	(*N* = 1)
Reduced number	0
No significant results	1
Increased number	0
Reduce pregnancy: public records	(*N* = 3)
Reduced number	2
No significant results	1
Increased number	0
Reduce childbirth: self-report	(*N* = 1)
Reduced number	0
No significant results	1
Increased number	0
Reduce childbirth: public records	(*N* = 1)
Reduced number	0
No significant results	1
Increased number	0

By far the most intensive program, the one in Denmark, South Carolina, might also have been the most effective in terms of reducing pregnancy, although this is difficult to determine for sure (Koo, Dunteman, George, Green, & Vincent, 1994; Vincent, Clearie, & Schluchter, 1987; Vincent, Drane, Joshi, Shankarnarayan, & Nimmons, 2004). After the program was implemented, the pregnancy rate for fourteen- to seventeen-year-olds declined significantly for several years. After parts of the program ended—for example, some of the community efforts declined in intensity, the school nurse resigned and her links to family planning clinics and her distribution of condoms ended, some teachers left the school, and more generally program momentum declined—the pregnancy rate returned to preprogram levels. From the existing data, it is not clear which of the program components or other unknown factors produced the changes over time in pregnancy rates.

In 1995–1996, the School/Community Program hired three additional health educators, and in 1998 the program hired yet another three (Vincent et al., 2004). These six health educators provided a large amount of sex education in the classroom and even met individually about reproductive health issues with nearly every Medicaid-eligible student (86 percent of the student body) twice a month. After this program component was implemented, the pregnancy rate again declined markedly. Again it cannot be known with confidence whether these six educators caused the pregnancy rate to decline or other factors produced that decline.

SUMMARY

More than one hundred studies have measured the impact of programs designed to reduce teen pregnancy and STD rates. These studies support the following conclusions:

- Professionals concerned with teen pregnancy and STD rates have developed a wide variety of programs to reduce sexual risk taking among teens. These can be divided into multiple groups of programs, each with common characteristics.

- Nearly all the groups include studies that found some significant positive effects on sexual behavior. Thus, there are multiple approaches to reducing adolescent risk.

- Curriculum-based comprehensive sex and STD/HIV education programs have been evaluated for the longest period of time and the most frequently. Currently, they have the most consistently positive effects on sexual behavior. Programs that incorporate seventeen characteristics are particularly likely to change behavior (they focus on sexual behavior, give a clear message about sexual behavior, discuss and practice ways to avoid unwanted or unprotected sex, teach skills, and are interactive).

- Well-designed one-on-one clinic programs have strong evidence of impact, especially when they incorporate as many of the seventeen characteristics as possible in a short time interval.

- Intensive service-learning programs have good evidence for reducing teen pregnancy. That impact may last during the academic year in which youth are involved.

On the other hand, other youth development programs, such as JobStart and Job-Corps, did not have positive effects.

- Intensive interactive videos or computer programs are producing quite promising results.

- Across all these programs, results demonstrate that it is possible to emphasize both abstinence and condoms or other forms of contraception without increasing sexual behavior or reducing protection.

- None of these programs is a complete answer; none dramatically reduced sexual risk to an acceptable level. However, some reduced sexual risk taking by about one-third and have the potential to help reduce pregnancy and STD rates if widely implemented.

These results are more positive than the results ten years ago, and those in turn are more positive than earlier results. Programs are continually evolving and are continually becoming more effective. This is a very encouraging and important trend.

One of the reasons programs have continued to become more effective is because of the interplay among theory, program development, and program evaluation. For at least three decades, people have developed programs to reduce sexual risk, using a variety of theories to increase their effectiveness, and researchers have evaluated the impact of these programs not only on the sexual behaviors, but also on the risk and protective factors that were targeted in order to change the behaviors. This research not only provided an increasing amount of evidence about what types of programs changed the targeted risk and protective factors and sexual behaviors, it also provided much more evidence on which potentially important risk and protective factors actually affected sexual behavior. Thus, this research continually improved theory about what factors changed behavior. And then, in a virtuous cycle, as this theory improved, program developers used that improved theory to develop more effective programs, which were in turn evaluated. For example, thirty years ago, many people concerned with teen pregnancy believed that knowledge about contraception and access to contraceptives largely affected contraceptive use. Thus, some sex education programs strived to increase knowledge, and some school-based clinics strived to increase access to contraception. However, early research showed that these programs did increase knowledge and did improve access to contraception, but they did not markedly increase contraceptive use. Other factors not fully understood at the time were very important. Fortunately, over time these other factors have become more fully understood, and programs have become more effective.

A second evolution in the field is the recognition that there is not only one effective approach to reducing sexual risk behavior, and no single approach will be completely effective. Although most of the effective programs do strive to change sexual psychosocial risk and protective factors, other programs such as youth development and service-learning programs target other factors and end up having a positive impact on behavior. Similarly, studies have demonstrated that programs can be effective in different settings, such as schools, clinics, youth-serving agencies, and communities, and with different groups such as teens themselves or their families. On the other hand, as noted earlier, none of these programs completely eliminates sexual risk. To have a dramatic impact on teen pregnancy and STD rates, communities and organizations within them will probably need to implement programs in a variety of settings, and different types of programs may need to address different risk and protective factors, so that collectively they can address a greater number of important factors affecting the sexual behavior of youth.

KEY TERMS

Abstinence programs
Comprehensive programs
Logic models
Mediating factors
School-based health centers

Service learning programs
Sociopsychological theories
Vocational education and employment programs

DISCUSSION QUESTIONS

1. Which types of program do you feel are likely to be most effective at reducing adolescent sexual risk behavior? Why?

2. Should there be a standardized way to measure intervention efficacy across programs? Is standardization feasible?

3. Compare and contrast program characteristics across different intervention venues discussed within this chapter (school, clinic, and community). Does the venue help determine the level of program efficacy?

REFERENCES

Brindis, C. D., Llewelyn, L., Marie, K., Blum, M., Biggs, A., & Maternowska, C. (2003). Meeting the reproductive health care needs of adolescents: California's family planning access, care and treatment program. *Journal of Adolescent Health, 32*(S), 79–90.

California Department of Health Services, Office of Family Planning. (2006). *Fact sheet on adolescent services.* Sacramento: Author.

Corcoran, J., & Pillai, V. K. (2007). Effectiveness of secondary pregnancy prevention programs: A meta-analysis. *Research on Social Work Practice, 17,* 5–18.

DiClemente, R. J., Wingood, G. M., Harrington, K. F., Lang, D. L., Davies, S. L., Hook, E. W., III, Oh, M. K., Crosby, R. A., Hertzberg, V. S., Gordon, A. B., Hardin, J. W., Parker, S., & Robillard, A. (2004). Efficacy of an HIV prevention intervention for African American adolescent girls: A randomized controlled trial. *Journal of the American Medical Association, 292*(2), 171–179.

Foster, D., Biggs, M., Amaral, G., Brindis, C., Navarro, S., Bradsberry, M., & Stewart, F. (2006). Estimates of pregnancies averted through California's family planning waiver program in 2002. *Perspectives on Sexual and Reproductive Health, 38*(3), 126–131.

Frost, J., & Bolzan, M. (1997). The provision of public-sector services by family planning agencies in 1995. *Family Planning Perspectives, 29*(1), 6–14.

Furstenberg, F. F., Geitz, L. M., Teitler, J. O., & Weiss, C. C. (1997). Does condom availability make a difference? An evaluation of Philadelphia's health resource centers. *Family Planning Perspectives, 29*(3), 123–127.

Guttmacher Institute. (1994). *Sex and America's teenagers.* New York: Author.

Hahn, A., Leavitt, T., & Aaron, P. (1994). *Evaluation of the Quantum Opportunities Program (QOP): Did the program work?* Waltham, MA: Brandeis University, Center for Human Resources.

Hawkins, J. D., Catalano, R. F., Kosterman, R., Abbott, R., & Hill, K. G. (1999). Preventing adolescent health-risk behaviors by strengthening protection during childhood. *Archives of Pediatrics and Adolescent Medicine, 153*(3), 226–234.

Herbst, J., Kay, L., Passin, W., Lyles, C., Crepaz, N., & Marin, B. (2006). A systematic review and meta-analysis of behavioral interventions to reduce HIV risk behaviors of Hispanics in the United States and Puerto Rico. *AIDS and Behavior, 11*(1), 25–47.

Jemmott, J., III, Jemmott, L., Braverman, P., & Fong, G. (2005). HIV/STD risk reduction interventions for African American and Latino adolescent girls at an adolescent medicine clinic. *Archives of Pediatric Adolescent Medicine, 159,* 440–449.

Kahn, J. G., Brindis, C. D., & Glei, D. A. (1999). Pregnancies averted among U.S. teenagers by the use of contraceptives. *Family Planning Perspectives, 31*(1), 29–34.

Kirby, D. (1991). *An evaluation of the Lake Taylor High School Health Center.* Scotts Valley, CA: ETR Associates.

Kirby, D., Baumler, E., Coyle, K., Basen-Enquist, K., Parcel, G., Harrist, R., & Banspach, S. W. (2004). The "Safer Choices" intervention: Its impact on the sexual behaviors of different subgroups of high school students. *Journal of Adolescent Health, 35*(6), 442–452.

Kirby, D., Brener, N. D., Brown, N. L., Peterfreund, N., Hillard, P., & Harrist, R. (1999). The impact of condom distribution in Seattle schools on sexual behavior and condom use. *American Journal of Public Health, 89*(2), 182–187.

Kirby, D., & Brown, N. (1996). School condom availability programs in the United States. *Family Planning Perspectives, 28*(5), 196–202.

Kirby, D., Laris, B., & Rolleri, L. (2007). The impact of sex and HIV education programs in schools and communities on sexual behaviors among adolescents and young adults. *Journal of Adolescent Health, 40*(3), 206–217.

Kirby, D., Lepore, G., & Ryan, J. (2005). *Sexual risk and protective factors: Factors affecting teen sexual behavior, pregnancy, childbearing and sexually transmitted disease. Which are important? Which can you change?* Washington, DC: National Campaign to Prevent Teen Pregnancy.

Kirby, D., & Miller, B. (2002). Interventions designed to promote parent-teen communication about sexuality. In S. Feldman & D. Rosenthal (Eds.), *Parent-adolescent communication on sexual issues. New Directions for Child and Adolescent Development.* no. 97. San Francisco: Jossey-Bass.

Kirby, D., Resnik, M. D., Downes, B., Kocher, T., Gunderson, P., Pothoff, S., Zelterman, D., & Blum, R. W. (1993). The effects of school-based health clinics in St. Paul upon school-wide birth rates. *Family Planning Perspectives, 25*(12), 12–16.

Kirby, D., Rolleri, L., & Wilson, M. M. (2007). *Tool to assess the characteristics of effective sex and STD/HIV education programs.* Washington, DC: Healthy Teen Network.

Kirby, D. B. (2007). *Emerging answers 2007: Research findings on programs to reduce teen pregnancy and sexually transmitted diseases.* Washington, DC: National Campaign to Prevent Teen and Unwanted Pregnancy.

Kirby, D. B., Rhodes, T., & Campe, S. (2005). *The implementation of multi-component youth programs to prevent teen pregnancy modeled after the Children's Aid Society–Carrera Program.* Scotts Valley, CA: ETR Associates.

Koo, H. P., Dunteman, G. H., George, C., Green, Y., & Vincent, M. (1994). Reducing adolescent pregnancy through school and community-based education: Denmark, South Carolina, revised 1991. *Family Planning Perspectives, 26*(5), 206–217.

Lindberg, L. D., Frost, J. J., Sten, C., & Dailard, C. (2006). Provision of contraceptive and related services by publicly funded family planning clinics, 2003. *Perspectives on Sexual and Reproductive Health, 38*(3), 139–147.

Lonczak, H. S., Abbott, R. D., Hawkins, D., Kosterman, R., & Catalano, R. F. (2002). Effects of the Seattle Social Development Project on sexual behavior, pregnancy, birth, and sexually transmitted disease outcomes by age 21 years. *Archives of Pediatrics and Adolescent Medicine, 156*(5), 438–447.

Martinez, C., Mosher, W., Abma, J., & Jones, J. (2005). Fertility, family planning, and reproductive health of U.S. women: Data from the 2002 National Survey of Family Growth. *Vital and Health Statistics, 23*(25), 1–160.

National Assembly on School-Based Health Care. (2002). *School-based health center census 2001–2002.* Washington, DC: National Assembly on School-Based Health Care.

Newcomer, S., Duggan, A., & Toczek, M. (Eds.). (1999). *Do school-based clinics influence adolescent birth rates?* Paris: International Union for the Scientific Study of Population.

Philliber, S., Kaye, J. W., Herring, S., & West, E. (2002). Preventing pregnancy and improving health care access among teenagers: An evaluation of the Children's Aid Society–Carrera Program. *Perspectives on Sexual and Reproductive Health, 34*(5), 244–251.

Ricketts, S. A., & Guernsey, B. P. (2006). School-based health centers and the decline in black teen fertility during the 1990s in Denver, Colorado. *American Journal of Public Health, 96*(9), 1588–1592.

Robinson, B., Uhl, G., Miner, M., Bockting, W., Scheltema, K., Rosser, B., & Rossover, B. (2002). Evaluation of a sexual health approach to prevent HIV among low income, urban, primarily African American women: Results of a randomized controlled trial. *AIDS Education and Prevention, 14*(3 Suppl. A), 81–96.

Scher, L. S., & Maynard, R. (2006). *Interventions intended to reduce pregnancy-related outcomes among adolescents*: Campbell Collaboration Social Welfare Group.

Thompson, A., Simonson, M., & Hargrave, C. (1996). *Educational technology: A review of the research.* Washington, DC: Association for Educational Communications and Technology.

Underhill, K., Montgomery, P., & Operario, D. (2007). Sexual abstinence only programmes to prevent HIV infection in high income countries: Systematic review. *British Medical Journal, 335,* 248.

Underhill, K., Operario, D., & Montgomery, P. (2007). Systematic review of abstinence-plus HIV prevention programs in high-income countries. *PLoS Medicine, 4*(9), e275.

Vincent, M., Clearie, A., & Schluchter, M. (1987). Reducing adolescent pregnancy through school and community-based education. *Journal of the American Medical Association, 257*(24), 3382–3386.

Vincent, M., Drane, W., Joshi, P., Shankarnarayan, S., & Nimmons, M. (2004). Sustained reduction in adolescent pregnancy rates through school and community-based education, 1982–2000. *American Journal of Health Education, 35*(2), 76–83.

Weed, S. E., Ericksen, I. H., Lewis, A., Grant, G. E., & Wibberly, K. H. (2008). An abstinence program's impact on cognitive mediators and sexual initiation. *American Journal of Health Behavior, 32*(1), 60–73.

Wolchik, S., Sandler, I., Millsap, R., Plummer, B., Greene, S., Anderson, E., Dawson-McClure, S. R., Hipke, K., & Haine, R. A. (2002). Six-year follow-up of preventive interventions for children of divorce: A randomized controlled trial. *Journal of the American Medical Association, 288*(15), 1874–1881.

Zabin, L. S., Hirsch, M. B., Smith, E. A., Streett, R., & Hardy, J. B. (1986). Evaluation of a pregnancy prevention program for urban teenagers. *Family Planning Perspectives, 18*(3), 119–126.

PART

3

POPULATIONS, POLICY, AND PREVENTION STRATEGIES

CHAPTER

17

INCARCERATED AND DELINQUENT YOUTH

NICHOLAS FREUDENBERG

LEARNING OBJECTIVES

After studying this chapter, you will be able to

- Describe the scope of adolescent incarceration within the criminal justice system.
- Evaluate the health and service needs of incarcerated youth.
- Compare how health professionals and policy makers work within the justice system to ensure proper care of adolescent offenders.

In 2004, an estimated 800,000 young people under age twenty spent time in correctional or juvenile justice facilities in the United States, a number that has increased dramatically in recent decades and gives this country the highest rate of youth incarceration in the developed world (Harrison & Beck, 2005; Harrison & Beck, 2006; Sickmund, Sladky, & Kang, 2005). In 2003, law enforcement agencies arrested 2.2 million young people under the age of eighteen (Snyder & Sickmund, 2006), further increasing the number of young people who come into contact with the criminal or juvenile justice systems.

*For some youth,
incarceration or
arrest is a single
experience with
limited conse-
quences, but for
many it is the
starting point for
ongoing criminal
justice system
contact.*

For some youth, *incarceration* or arrest is a single experience with limited consequences, but for many it is the starting point for ongoing criminal justice system contact. Since incarceration is associated with a disproportionate burden of infectious and chronic diseases, substance abuse, mental health problems, violence, unemployment, school dropout, and discrimination (Freudenberg, 2001; National Commission on Correctional Health Care, 2005; Re-Entry Policy Council, 2005), finding ways to help incarcerated or detained youth improve their lives and avoid reincarceration is an important health goal. In addition, youth who are incarcerated disproportionately engage in health risk behaviors before being incarcerated and the experience of incarceration may contribute to subsequent risk behavior (Valois, MacDonald, Bretous, Fischer, & Drane, 2002). Although researchers differ on the pathways by which antisocial and criminal behavior influence sexual and drug risks (Chung, Hawkins, Gilchrist, Hill, & Nagin, 2002; Jessor & Jessor, 1978), the reciprocal relationships among these problem behaviors provide an important entry point for health interventions.

Adolescents are incarcerated in juvenile justice facilities, prisons, or jails. Since states vary in their definition of the age and criminal charges that lead to assignment to the adult criminal justice system, the focus in this chapter is on youth under the age of twenty who are being held in juvenile, adult correctional facilities, or other components of the criminal justice system. In the 1980s and 1990s, the number of inmates under eighteen years of age held in state prisons and jails in the United States doubled (Strom, 2000). Since 1999, however, the under-eighteen jail and prison population has declined (Snyder & Sickmund, 2006). As a result of its criminal justice and drug policies, however, the United States continues to lead the world in the number and proportion of juveniles it holds in jails and prisons.

In 2004, an estimated 125,000 youth under the age of eighteen were admitted to U.S. jails (Harrison & Beck, 2005; Beck, 2006). After we account for multiple admissions, this represents 89,000 unique individuals. In addition, at least 600,000 eighteen- and nineteen-year-olds were admitted to U.S. jails. Another 100,000 teens were admitted to juvenile justice facilities that year (Sickmund, Sladky, & Kang, 2005). These youth were overwhelmingly male, low-income, and African American or Latino, ensuring that the impact of incarceration would have disproportionate effects by gender, class, and race/ethnicity.

The vast majority of incarcerated adolescents return to their community within days, weeks, or months. Studies show that between half and three-quarters of adolescent offenders are rearrested in the year after release (Freudenberg, Daniels, Crum, Perkins, & Richie, 2005; Fagan, 1996). This "churning" (Taxman, Byrne, & Pattavina, 2005) between detention and neighborhoods disrupts individuals, families, and communities. For the individual, it contributes to school failure or dropout and reduced employment prospects (Holzer, Offner, & Sorenson, 2005). For families, it contributes to increased family conflict, economic dependence, or housing eviction (Travis, Soloman, & Waul, 2005). For communities, it contributes to more crime (Clear, Rose, Waring, & Scully, 2003) and reduced community cohesion, associated with increases in violence and infectious diseases (Sampson, Raudenbush, & Earls, 1997; Cohen et al., 2000; Thomas & Torrone, 2006). For municipalities, high rates of recidivism contribute to spiraling criminal justice costs (annual incarceration costs for adolescents can reach $100,000 per adolescent, and as many as 70 percent are reincarcerated within a year), and reduced public resources for education and health care (Re-Entry Policy Council, 2005). Finally, youth reentry is complicated by pervasive negative attitudes toward young black and Latino men, attitudes often shaped by mass media, politicians, and researchers (Diiulio, Bennett, & Walters, 1996; Hutchinson, 1997).

Studies show that between half and three-quarters of adolescent offenders are rearrested in the year after release.

Reducing the number of young people who are incarcerated and improving the conditions of confinement for those who are can also benefit population health. For inmates, time spent in a correctional facility can increase the risk of tuberculosis, violence, and psychological conditions (Bellin, Fletcher, & Safyer, 1993; Wolff, Blitz, Shi, Bachman, & Siegel, 2006), and high rates of incarceration may contribute to or exacerbate socioeconomic and racial/ethnic disparities in health (Freudenberg, 2002; Gaiter, Potter, & O'Leary, 2006; Iguchi, Bell, Ramchand, & Fain, 2005).

COMPARISONS

In assessing the health behaviors, problems, and needs of incarcerated and delinquent youth, several types of comparison are useful, each contributing unique insights. First, incarcerated and delinquent youth can be compared to the general population of young people. Most studies show that young people involved with the criminal and juvenile justice systems engage in more risk behaviors and are at higher risk of poor health outcomes, even when they are compared with demographically similar nonincarcerated young people.

A second comparison is between incarcerated youth and incarcerated adults. For example, one study compared adult males incarcerated in New York City jails to incarcerated adult females and adolescent males (Freudenberg et al., 2005) and found gender similarities between adult and adolescent males, as well as developmental differences between these two groups. These types of studies generally show that young people have significantly lower prevalence of most health problems than adults behind

Most studies show that young people involved with the criminal and juvenile justice systems engage in more risk behaviors and are at higher risk of poor health outcomes, even when they are compared with demographically similar nonincarcerated young people.

bars. Thus, by keeping more young people out of correctional facilities, it may be possible to prevent the lifetime health problems associated with incarceration.

A third useful comparison is between incarcerated young people with different characteristics, such as race/ethnicity, gender, or sexual orientation. Socioeconomic and racial/ethnic comparisons show the disproportionate burden of incarceration and its adverse health sequelae on disadvantaged youth. These studies highlight the importance of matching health services to the needs of specific adolescent populations. For example, health problems and needs vary significantly by gender, making gender-specific services especially important for both young women and young men.

Finally, cross-national comparisons show the impact of policy differences on the role of incarceration among nations (Panel on Juvenile Crime, 2001) and illustrate the extent to which the United States is an outlier in its reliance on locking up young people.

KEY CONCEPTS: HEALTH CONDITIONS AND HEALTH BEHAVIOR

Youth at risk of incarceration or detention encounter the same health problems as other young people, especially other low-income and disadvantaged youth. This section summarizes available evidence on various health conditions selected for their higher prevalence or severity among young people involved with the juvenile or criminal justice systems or for the attention they attract within detention facilities. Several recent reviews provide additional information on the health needs of this population (Staples-Horne, Duffy, & Rorie, 2007; Gallagher & Dobrin, 2007; Golzari, Hunt, & Anoshiravani, 2006).

Sexual, Drug-Related, and Violent Behavior

Young people involved in justice systems are more likely to report risky sexual behavior, substance use, and to be victims or perpetrators of violence than their nonincarcerated peers. These behaviors can put them at risk of sexually transmitted infections, unwanted pregnancy, or sexual assault; dependence or social problems related to substance use, especially tobacco, heavy marijuana and alcohol use; and injury, homicide, and posttraumatic stress disorder.

Several studies show high rates of sexual risk behavior, including low prevalence of consistent condom use, multiple partners, and sexual activity while high on drugs or alcohol among incarcerated or detained youth (Romero, Teplin, McClelland, Abram, Welty, & Washburn, 2007; Teplin, Mericle, McClelland, & Abram, 2003). For example, a study of fifteen- to twenty-nine-year-old men who visited STD clinics in Newark, New Jersey, found that men with gonorrhea were more than twice as likely to have a history of incarceration as those without this infection (Mertz et al., 2000). Another study comparing young arrestees to nonarrestees in three states found that the arrestees reported more alcohol and drug use, substance use during sex, unprotected sex acts, and STD diagnoses than nonarrestees (Tolou-Shams, Brown, Gordon, & Fernandez, 2007). Recent studies also show high rates of chlamydia among incarcerated male adolescents (Pathela et al., 2007).

Not surprisingly, a significant proportion of adolescent female inmates have been pregnant, and many adolescent males have contributed to a pregnancy. One study found that about a third of one sample of detained adolescent girls had been pregnant (Crosby, Salazar, DiClemente, Yarber, Caliendo, & Staples-Horne, 2004); in another study, 17 percent of adolescent males reported they had fathered a child (Freudenberg, Mosely, Labriola, Daniels, & Murrill, 2007).

While HIV and hepatitis C infection rates among incarcerated adolescents are much lower than among incarcerated adults, they are higher than among other nonincarcerated youth (Romero et al., 2007; Templeton, 2006).

Drugs of choice among incarcerated and delinquent youth are generally alcohol and marijuana, and some studies show high rates of heavy use of these substances (Malow, Dévieux, Rosenberg, Samuels, & Jean-Gilles, 2006; Freudenberg et al., 2005). Rates of cocaine and heroin use are much lower than among adult inmates (Freudenberg et al., 2007). While some marijuana use is common among U.S. adolescents, the heavy use among many incarcerated youth is associated with school and work problems and risk of reincarceration (Foley, 2006). Anecdotal evidence indicates high rates of tobacco use among incarcerated young people, a predictor of lifetime health problems, but few studies have examined this issue systematically.

Young people involved with the juvenile or criminal justice system are at much higher risk of being victims or perpetrators of violence than their nonincarcerated peers. Both male and female inmates report high rates of physical and sexual abuse as children (Browne, Miller, & Maguin, 1999; Johnson, Ross, Taylor, Williams, Carvajal, & Peters, 2006), setting the stage for subsequent victimization and perpetration. Juvenile offenders are also more likely to carry guns than their peers (Ash, Kellermann, Fuqua-Whitley, & Johnson, 1996).

Juvenile offenders are also at higher risk of injury and death. One study found that young people involved in the Chicago juvenile justice system were more than four times more likely to die an early violent death than noninvolved young people (Teplin, McClelland, Abram, & Mileusnic, 2005). Other studies show a high prevalence of trauma-related injuries both prior to and during incarceration (Staples-Horne et al., 2007).

Other Infectious Diseases and Chronic Conditions

Other infectious diseases prevalent in correctional facilities include tuberculosis, hepatitis B and C, methicillin-resistant staphylococcus aureus, influenza, pneumonia, and meningitis. In general, adolescents have lower rates of these conditions than adult inmates, in part because of lower rates of compromised immunity and chronic health conditions. Adequate infection control measures are essential to prevent disease outbreaks (Bick, 2007).

Chronic conditions that affect incarcerated youth include asthma, diabetes, and other respiratory conditions (Anderson & Farrow, 1998; Feinstein, Lampkin, Lorish, Klerman, Maisiak, & Oh, 1998; Golzari et al., 2006). Since many young people lack a regular source of medical care prior to incarceration, and few correctional systems offer chronic disease management programs, some inmates may experience preventable exacerbations of preexisting chronic illness.

Mental Health

More than two-thirds of detained youth have one or more psychiatric disorders (Wasserman, McReynolds, Lucas, Fisher, & Santos, 2002). Rates of mild, moderate, and severe mental illness, from anxiety to posttraumatic stress disorders to psychosis, are generally higher among incarcerated than nonincarcerated youth (Abram et al., 2007; Teplin, Abram, McClelland, Dulcan, & Mericle, 2002), and minority youth report higher levels of unmet needs than white youth (Rawal, Romansky, Jenuwine, & Lyons, 2004). In many cases, substance use presents as a comorbid condition with other mental health problems, further complicating treatment and prevention efforts.

In many cases, substance use presents as a comorbid condition with other mental health problems, further complicating treatment and prevention efforts.

Juvenile and adult justice systems struggle to meet the mental health needs of their populations (Thomas & Penn, 2002), in part because of inadequate resources, lack of trained staff, and punitive attitudes toward young people with behavioral or psychological problems. Preventing suicide is often a significant challenge for correctional officials, and incarcerated adolescents appear to have higher rates of attempted and successful suicides than their nonincarcerated peers (Penn, Esposito, Schaeffer, Fritz, & Spirito, 2003).

Dental Conditions

Incarcerated adolescents commonly report untreated dental problems, leading to pain and discomfort (Bolin & Jones, 2006). Dental problems can also contribute to employment discrimination or other forms of discrimination due to missing teeth (Treadwell, Northridge, & Bethea, 2007). Several surveys of incarcerated adolescents show that dental problems are among the most common health complaints (Staples-Horne et al., 2007).

ROLES FOR HEALTH PROFESSIONALS

Health professionals, health policy makers, and health researchers can play important roles in improving the health of young people involved with the criminal and juvenile justice system. This section considers three different levels of responsibility for health professionals, correctional and health policy makers, and researchers: (1) protection from harm, (2) early intervention and treatment, and (3) health promotion. Table 17.1

TABLE 17.1. Roles for health professionals within adolescent correctional facilities

Roles for Health and Other Professionals	Health Conditions or Other Outcomes	Selected Types of Intervention
Protect from harm within criminal justice system	Suicide	Suicide watch, mental health screening, mortality reviews, special housing
	Physical or sexual assault	Training and supervision for correctional staff, facility design, educational and vocational programs, post assault treatment programs
	Deliberate indifference to medical needs	Quality assurance programs, legal and advocacy monitoring of correctional health services, adequate funding for correctional health services
	Uncontrolled serious mental illness	Mental health screening at intake, quality assurance programs for mental health services, strong linkages with alternative to incarceration programs
	Hazardous conditions or programs (such as extreme heat or cold, abusive staff, or dangerous programs)	Clear accountability for facility conditions, legal and advocacy monitoring of facility, emergency preparedness plans

TABLE 17.1. *(Continued)*

Roles for Health and Other Professionals	Health Conditions or Other Outcomes	Selected Types of Intervention
Early intervention and treatment	HIV infection	Easy availability of rapid HIV screening and counseling, condom availability programs, ongoing HIV prevention counseling and education, facility-based treatment for HIV positives, linkages with community providers for postrelease care, adequate formulary to provide needed HIV medications
	Other sexually transmitted infections	Intake screening and treatment for gonorrhea, syphilis, chlamydia, and other infections as appropriate
	Other communicable diseases	Screening and treatment for tuberculosis, hepatitis C, and others as appropriate
	Asthma	Facility-based self-management programs, acute care for asthmatic episodes
	Diabetes	Nutrition counseling, diabetes management programs, glucose monitoring

Dental problems	Dental assessment, treatment for identified conditions
Psychiatric conditions	Symptom screening and psychiatric history, referrals for identified conditions, safe housing for those with psychiatric conditions
Drug, alcohol, and tobacco use	Intake screening for substance use; age-, gender-, and substance-appropriate treatment options inside facility and after release, smoking cessation programs
Violence	Acute medial care for facility-based injuries, screening and treatment for posttraumatic stress disorder, referrals for facility-based and postrelease conflict resolution, and anger management programs
Health promotion	
Safer sexual behavior	Sex education, condom availability, reproductive health services, including access to abortion and prenatal care
Safer and reduced drug, alcohol, and tobacco use	Peer education prevention programs, harm reduction services, wide range of facility-based and postrelease service options
Improved diet and more physical activity	Healthy food service, reduced access to unhealthy foods, weight loss programs, options for age- and gender-appropriate physical activities, safe and usable recreation facilities

TABLE 17.1. *(Continued)*

Roles for Health and Other Professionals	Health Conditions or Other Outcomes	Selected Types of Intervention
	Increased positive social support	Opportunities for connections to caring adults, family and friend visitation programs, structured facility-based programs to create prosocial environment
	Higher school achievement	Facility-based school, GED, ESL, and basic education programs; educational assessment; assessment and referrals for learning and behavioral problems; placement in postrelease educational program
	Improved employment opportunities	Facility-based and postrelease vocational training, facility-based work programs geared to local economy, employment counseling
	Linked to regular source of medical care	Electronic medical records to ensure continuity of care and to reduce duplication of services, emphasis on preventive services within correctional health program, secure linkages and referrals to community-based providers
	More alternatives to violence	Safe physical environment, training for correctional staff, anger management programs, educational and vocational programs

lists some of the activities within each level of responsibility. While no youth correctional facility is currently fulfilling all the tasks listed in this table, every facility carries out some of these responsibilities, and all can use this list as a tool to consider strengthening their capacity to improve the health of the young people in their custody.

First, at a minimum health professionals have an ethical obligation to protect young people from being harmed by the process of incarceration, correctional and health policy makers have an obligation to ensure that policies and practices do not encourage or condone such harm, and researchers can both document harm and evaluate interventions designed to protect health. The ethical foundations for these activities are both the medical principle of Do No Harm and the legal responsibility of the justice system to act in loco parentis for minor youth and to protect from harm all inmates in their custody. On the legal side, according to the Supreme Court decision in *Estelle* v. *Gamble* (1976), "deliberate indifference" by prison workers to an inmate's serious illness or injury violates the Eighth Amendment to the U.S. Constitution, which bans cruel and unusual punishment. The court held that deliberate indifference could be "manifested by prison doctors in their response to the prisoner's needs or by prison guards in intentionally denying or delaying access to medical care or intentionally interfering with the treatment once prescribed." Key issues in this domain include prevention of suicide and sexual or physical assault, acute medical and psychiatric care, and at least some preparation for community reentry after incarceration.

At the second level, health professionals can assess the health needs of incarcerated individuals and populations, identify those with problems, take action to either treat the identified condition or make an appropriate, ethical, and effective referral, and provide acute medical or psychiatric care for emergent health conditions. Policy makers can design policies and programs that facilitate such services, and researchers can elucidate the barriers to effective early identification and treatment and evaluate interventions. The underlying value that supports these activities is that health professionals, whether inside a correctional facility or in the community, have an ethical responsibility to identify and treat conditions that could jeopardize future health. Key health conditions in this domain include sexually transmitted infections and other communicable diseases, chronic conditions, psychiatric conditions, substance use, dental disease, and other health behaviors (such as sexual activity, nutrition, physical activity, or violence) that can jeopardize current or future health.

Fortunately, evidence that demonstrates the benefits or promise of various interventions is available to guide health officials and policy makers in selecting programs to prevent these health conditions. Several recent reviews summarize this literature (Chapman, Desai, & Falzer, 2006; Dowden & Latimer, 2006, National Institutes of

Health professionals have an ethical obligation to protect young people from being harmed by the process of incarceration, correctional and health policy makers have an obligation to ensure that policies and practices do not encourage or condone such harm, and researchers can both document harm and evaluate interventions designed to protect health.

Evidence that demonstrates the benefits or promise of various interventions is available to guide health officials and policy makers in selecting programs to prevent these health conditions.

Health, 2004; Staples-Horne et al., 2007; Underwood & Knight, 2006; Zack, 2007).

Finally, at the third level health professionals have an opportunity to promote the health of incarcerated young people and to prepare them for successful life after release. Health policy makers can create the institutional and political climate in which health promotion can thrive within correctional settings, and researchers can provide the evidence base needed to develop health-promoting programs and policies. In this case, the ethical foundations for this level are twofold. On the one hand, no person deserves to be punished after release by having his or her health compromised by the process of incarceration or release. On the other hand, by improving the health of people released from incarceration, we also improve the health of their family, their sex and drug partners, and the community as a whole. Thus, on both the levels of individual and population health, health professionals and policy makers working with young people in the juvenile and adult correctional systems have both the opportunity and the obligation to take action to improve lifetime health.

THE HEALTH-PROMOTING CORRECTIONAL FACILITY

In recent years, some public health, correctional health, and criminal justice professionals have promulgated the concept of a "health-promoting" jail or prison (Gatherer, Moiler, & Hayton, 2005; World Health Organization, 2006; Ramaswamy & Freudenberg, 2007). A few have applied some of these concepts to youth facilities (Greene, Lucarelli, & Shocksnider, 1999). A variety of organizations and documents provide the foundation for expanding correctional health care from meeting the minimum standards of avoiding "deliberate indifference" to medical needs to a more holistic approach that seeks to promote the well-being of inmates and the communities to which they return. Following are some of these organizations:

- American Public Health Association's (2003) Standards for Health Services in Correctional Facilities

- National Commission on Correctional Health Care's Clinical Guidelines (2003; 2001)

- Re-Entry Policy Council Policy Statements on Physical Health Care (2005)

- In Europe, the Health in Prisons Project, sponsored by the World Health Organization (2006; Gatherer, Moiler, & Hayton, 2005; Whitehead, 2006)

- American Academy of Pediatrics' (2001) Recommendations for Health Care in Juvenile Justice Systems

- Consensus Report of the Mental Health Assessments in Juvenile Justice Project (Wasserman et al., 2003)

Although these organizations and documents provide a strong foundation for standards for health care in correctional facilities and reentry services for young people, evidence suggests that few systems fully meet these emerging standards. For example, one study found that despite the recommendation of the American Academy of Pediatrics, just 53 of the approximately 3500 juvenile justice residential facilities in the United States have received voluntary accreditation for facility health care from the National Commission on Correctional Health Care (Gallagher & Dobrin, 2007). After reviewing two national censuses of 726 juvenile justice facilities in the United States, Gallagher and Dobrin (2007) concluded that "very few detention centers meet a minimum standard of care."

These deficiencies suggest two parallel courses of action. On the one hand, advocates for improved health for young people involved in the justice system need to continue to articulate a comprehensive vision of approaches to justice and health that promote rather than undermine health and to mobilize the constituencies that can help to realize such a vision. On the other hand, health professionals, researchers, and policy makers also need to develop a pragmatic approach to achieving the incremental improvements that can help set the stage for more transformative change. In this section, I consider the former, and in the conclusion I suggest steps toward the latter.

What constitutes a health-promoting correctional facility? According to the World Health Organization (1986), *health promotion* describes the "process of enabling people to increase control over and to improve their health." Health promotion seeks to bring about changes in individuals, groups, institutions, and policies in order to improve population health. The Ottawa Charter for Health Promotion, adopted by the WHO in 1986, identifies five critical activities for health promotion: developing personal skills for health, creating supportive environments, strengthening community action for health, reorienting health services, and building healthy public policy (WHO, 1986). Each of these domains of activity provides opportunities for promoting health within correctional facilities for young people, as summarized in Table 17.2. Once again, though no correctional facility yet provides all these services, each element has been implemented somewhere and every setting has the potential to expand or improve its services in at least a few of these domains.

SUMMARY

This chapter has presented evidence that young people caught up in the juvenile or adult justice systems face a variety of health and social needs and that few systems currently address these needs adequately. A key challenge for health professionals, policy makers, and researchers involved in justice systems for young people is to find the right balance between the incremental changes that make modest improvements in the short run and the transformative changes that are needed to end the harm imposed by current practices and policies. Only transformation can reverse decades of increasing rates of youth incarceration, inadequate correctional health services, and punitive policies that demonize low income young people of color. Yet only incremental

TABLE 17.2. Elements of a comprehensive correctional health promotion program for young people

Health Promotion Priority	Selected Activities and Approaches in Jails or Prisons	Selected Health and Social Outcomes: Inmates	Selected Health and Social Outcomes: Correctional Facilities	Selected Health and Social Outcomes: Society as a Whole
Develop personal skills	Offer sex education, chronic disease management, family planning, parenting, violence prevention, harm reduction and other health programs	Improved asthma, reduced STDs, lower health care costs, better chances for successful reentry	Reduced asthma episodes, lower health care costs, lower recidivism	Reduced transmission of infectious diseases and reliance on health care system for emergency care; reduced violence
Create supportive environments	Reduce overcrowding, improve sanitary conditions, encourage positive social support, reduce physical and sexual assault and intimidation, provide access to healthy food and opportunities for physical activity, encourage family visits	Reduced transmission of infectious diseases, reduced anxiety and depression, lower violence rates, improved diet, reduced obesity, better family functioning postrelease	No overcrowding, lower violence rates and incidences of sexual assault in jails and prisons, lowered anxiety for corrections staff	Reduced transmission of infectious diseases, lower violence rates, including domestic violence, better outcomes for spouses and children of inmates

Strengthen community action for health	Establish linkages with community organizations, faith organizations, and youth services providers, organize community coalitions to advocate for health-promoting policies	Increased access to health care and promotion, access to higher quality health care	Greater infrastructure and resources for health care and promotion, less reliance on funding from corrections departments and time from staff to provide services	Increased social cohesion in high incarceration communities and, as a result, less violence and STDs
Reorient health services	Shift from acute episodic treatment to health promotion disease management and prevention, develop continuity of care inside and after release, train providers to promote health	Improved control of chronic conditions, lower health care costs after release	Greater infrastructure for providing health care and promotion, lower health care costs, greater efficiency through health promotion	Better community health outcomes, reliance on health care system for emergency care, more seamless medical care inside and upon release
Build healthy public policy	Advocate policies that provide substance abuse, mental health, and other services during incarceration and after release, reduce stigma against people returning, provide job training and education inside and after release	Increased access to and use of substance abuse treatment services and mental health services, increased ability to find employment and reduce dependency after release	Greater infrastructure for substance abuse and mental health treatment and promotion	Lower unemployment rates and illegal activity

Source: Adapted from Ramaswamy and Freudenberg (2007).

changes that can improve the daily living conditions and health of young people currently incarcerated are likely to be achieved in the current political climate.

I conclude with four recommendations for finding this balance. First, health and criminal justice researchers can document the health, social, and financial costs of failing to reduce youth incarceration rates or better prepare young people for reentry. Policy makers who may not be moved by moral or public health arguments may respond better to economic arguments. When annual per capita costs for incarceration of young people approach $100,000 per year and recidivism rates are often as high as 70 percent, the financial case for alternative approaches is compelling.

Second, a strong evidence base for effective health programs exists. Researchers can do more to synthesize this evidence and translate it into practice guidelines, and policy makers can do more to bring successful programs to scale and find funding streams that can institutionalize support. Too many health interventions within justice programs for young people never move beyond demonstration project, a sign of the need for stronger leadership within the field and for additional stable funding streams. Health providers can ensure that the programs in their facilities follow evidence-based practice guidelines and document their successes and limitations in achieving their objectives. More systematic evaluation will help others to learn from the wide range of existing practice.

Third, health professionals, including pediatricians, nurses, social workers, and public health workers, need to make the case that all young people, whether incarcerated, homeless, or living in a wealthy suburb, deserve a single standard of care. Making the services that promote health a basic human right, especially for young people who have a life in front of them, corresponds to a variety of international covenants, including the United Nations Convention on the Rights of Children, the Universal Declaration of Human Rights, and to the spirit of American democracy and social justice.

Fourth, health providers, researchers, and policy makers engaged in providing health services for incarcerated young people need to mobilize a variety of constituencies to achieve both the incremental and transformative changes necessary to improve health. These constituencies include faith-based organizations, civil and human rights groups, organizations of health providers, criminal justice reformers, community organizations within high-incarceration communities, and young people caught up in the justice system and their families. By framing the issue of health for incarcerated youth broadly—as a health, social, moral, economic, and political issue—it may be possible to bring new players onto the field and thus achieve policy changes not possible with the current stakeholders engaged.

Prior to the recent decline, several decades of increasing adolescent incarceration have highlighted the adverse consequences of this policy for young people, their families, and for society as a whole. As the costs of this policy become more apparent, as adolescent crime rates fall, and as a body of evidence on alternative approaches accumulates, health professionals can play a critical role in creating health services and youth justice systems that support rather than undermine health.

KEY TERMS

Health promotion   Incarceration

DISCUSSION QUESTIONS

1. What types of adverse health outcomes are associated with spending time in correctional facilities? Discuss policy or public health implications.

2. Compare and contrast the service needs and health problems of incarcerated adolescents to those of incarcerated adults. Do problems appear to be shared among groups or differ between groups?

3. This chapter considers three levels of responsibility for health professionals involved in the criminal and juvenile justice system: protection from harm, early intervention and treatment, and health promotion. Which of these three responsibilities is *most* important when trying to improve the health of young people in custody? Why?

4. What is meant by the concept of a "health-promoting" jail or prison? How does the interpretation of this concept measure up to the reality of the jails and prisons in this country?

REFERENCES

Abram, K. M., Washburn, J. J., Teplin, L. A., Emanuel, K. M., Romero, E. G., & McClelland, G. M. (2007). Post-traumatic stress disorder and psychiatric comorbidity among detained youths. *Psychiatric Services, 58,* 1311–1316.

American Academy of Pediatrics, Committee on Adolescent Health. (2001). Health care for children and adolescents in the juvenile correctional care system. *Pediatrics, 107,* 799–803.

American Public Health Association. (2003). *Standards for health services in correctional institutions* (3rd ed.). Washington, DC: Author.

Anderson, B., & Farrow, J. A. (1998). Incarcerated adolescents in Washington State: Health services and utilization. *Journal of Adolescent Health, 221,* 363–367.

Ash, P., Kellermann, A. L., Fuqua-Whitley, D., & Johnson A. (1996). Gun acquisition and use by juvenile offenders. *Journal of the American Medical Association, 275*(22), 1754–1758.

Beck, A. (2006, June). *The importance of successful reentry to jail population growth.* Paper presented at the Jail Reentry Roundtable, Washington, DC. Retrieved from www.urban.org/projects/reentry-roundtable/upload/beck.PPT.

Bellin, E. Y., Fletcher, D. D., & Safyer, S. M. (1993). Association of tuberculosis infection with increased time in or admission to the New York City jail system. *Journal of the American Medical Association, 269*(17), 2228–2231.

Bick, J. A. (2007). Infection control in jails and prisons. *Clinical Infectious Diseases, 45,* 1047–1055.

Bolin, K., & Jones, D. (2006). Oral health needs of adolescents in a juvenile detention facility. *Journal of Adolescent Health, 38,* 755–757.

Browne, A., Miller, B., & Maguin, E. (1999). Prevalence and severity of lifetime physical and sexual victimization among incarcerated women. *International Journal of Law and Psychiatry, 22*(3–4), 301–322.

Chapman, J. F., Desai, R. A., & Falzer, P. R. (2006). Mental health service provision in juvenile justice facilities: Pre- and postrelease psychiatric care. *Child and Adolescent Psychiatry Clinics of North America, 15*(2), 445–458.

Chung, I. J., Hawkins, J. D., Gilchrist, L. D., Hill, K. G., & Nagin, D. S. (2002). Identifying and predicting offending trajectories among poor children. *Social Services Review, 76*(4), 663–685.

Clear, T., Rose, D. R., Waring, E., & Scully, K. (2003). Coercive mobility and crime: A preliminary examination of concentrated incarceration and social disorganization. *Justice Quarterly, 20,* 33–64.

Cohen, D., Spear, S., Scribner, R., Kissinger, P., Mason, K., & Wildgen, J. (2000). Broken windows and the risk of gonorrhea. *American Journal of Public Health, 90,* 230–236.

Crosby, R., Salazar, L. F., DiClemente, R. J., Yarber, W. L., Caliendo, A. M., & Staples-Horne, M. (2004). Health risk factors among detained adolescent females. *American Journal of Preventive Medicine, 27*(5), 404–410.

Dowden, C., & Latimer, J. (2006). Providing effective substance abuse treatment for young-offender populations: What works! *Child and Adolescent Psychiatry Clinics of North America, 15*(2), 517–537.

Diiulio, J., Bennett, W. J., & Walters, J. P. (1996). *Body count: Moral poverty . . . and how to win America's war against crime and drugs.* New York: Simon and Schuster.

Estelle v. *Gamble,* 429 U.S. 97 (1976).

Fagan, J. (1996). The comparative advantage of juvenile versus criminal court sanctions on recidivism among adolescent felony offenders. *Law and Policy, 18*(1–2), 77–114.

Feinstein, R. A., Lampkin, A., Lorish, C. D., Klerman, L. V., Maisiak, R., & Oh, M. K. (1998). Medical status of adolescents at time of admission to a juvenile detention center. *Journal of Adolescent Health, 22,* 190–196.

Foley, J. D. (2006). Adolescent use and misuse of marijuana. *Adolescent Medicine Clinics, 7,* 319–334.

Freudenberg, N. (2001). Jails, prisons, and the health of urban populations: A review of the impact of the correctional system on community health. *Journal of Urban Health, 78,* 214–235.

Freudenberg, N. (2002). Adverse effects of US jail and prison policies on the health and well-being of women of color. *American Journal of Public Health, 92*(12), 1895–1899.

Freudenberg, N., Daniels, J., Crum, M., Perkins, T., & Richie, B. E. (2005). Coming home from jail: The social and health consequences of community reentry for women, male adolescents, and their families and communities. *American Journal of Public Health, 95,* 1725–1736.

Freudenberg, N., Moseley, J., Labriola, M., Daniels, J., & Murrill, C. (2007). Comparison of health and social characteristics of people leaving New York city jails by age, gender, and race/ethnicity: Implications for public health interventions. *Public Health Reports, 122,* 733–743.

Gaiter, J. L., Potter, R. H., & O'Leary, A. (2006). Disproportionate rates of incarceration contribute to health disparities. *American Journal of Public Health, 96*(7), 1148–1149.

Gallagher, C. A., & Dobrin, A. (2007) Can juvenile justice detention facilities meet the call of the American Academy of Pediatrics and National Commission on Correctional Health Care? A national analysis of current practices. *Pediatrics, 119,* 991–1001.

Gatherer, A., Moiler, L., & Hayton, P. (2005). The World Health Organization European Health in Prisons Project after 10 years: Persistent barriers and achievements. *American Journal of Public Health, 95,* 1696–1700.

Golzari, M., Hunt, S. J., & Anoshiravani, A. (2006). The health status of youth in juvenile detention facilities. *Journal of Adolescent Health, 38,* 776–782.

Greene, E., Lucarelli, P., & Shocksnider, J. (1999). Health promotion and education in youth correctional facilities. *Pediatric Nursing, 25,* 312–314.

Harrison, P. M., & Beck, A. J. (2005). Prison and jail inmates at midyear 2004 (Publication No. NCJ 208801). Washington, DC: Department of Justice.

Harrison, P. M., & Beck, A. J. (2006). Prison and jail inmates at midyear 2005 (Publication No. NCJ 213133). Washington, DC: Department of Justice.

Holzer, H. J., Offner, P., & Sorenson, E. (2005). Declining employment prospects among young black less-educated men: The role of incarceration and child support. *Journal of Policy Analysis and Management, 24,* 329–350.

Hutchinson, E. O. (1997). *The assassination of the black male image.* New York: Simon and Schuster.

Iguchi, M. Y., Bell, J., Ramchand, R. N., & Fain, T. (2005). How criminal system racial disparities may translate into health disparities. *Journal of Health Care for the Poor and Underserved, 16*(4 Suppl. B), 48–56.

Jessor, R., & Jessor, S. L. (1978). Theory testing in longitudinal research on marijuana use. In D. Kandel (Ed.), *Longitudinal research on drug use* (pp. 41–71). Washington, DC: Hemisphere.

Johnson, R. J., Ross, M. W., Taylor, W. C., Williams, M. L., Carvajal, R. I., & Peters, R. J. (2006). Prevalence of childhood sexual abuse among incarcerated males in county jail. *Child Abuse and Neglect, 30,* 75–86.

Malow, R. M., Dévieux, J. G., Rosenberg, R., Samuels, D. M., & Jean-Gilles, M. M. (2006). Alcohol use severity and HIV sexual risk among juvenile offenders. *Substance Use and Misuse, 41,* 1769–1788.

Mertz, K. J., Finelli, L., Levine, W. C., Mognoni, R. C., Berman, S. M., Fishbein, M., Garnett, G., & St Louis, M. E. (2000). Gonorrhea in male adolescents and young adults in Newark, New Jersey: Implications of risk factors and patient preferences for prevention strategies. *Sexually Transmitted Diseases, 27,* 201–207.

National Commission on Correctional Health Care. (2001). Clinical guides. Retrieved from www.ncchc.org/resources/clinicalguides.html.

National Commission on Correctional Health Care. (2003). *Standards for health services in jails.* Chicago: Author.

National Commission on Correctional Health Care. (2005). *The health status of soon-to-be-released inmates, 2002.* Chicago: Author.

National Institutes of Health. (2004). State-of-the-science conference statement on preventing violence and related health-risking social behaviors in adolescents. *NIH Consensus Statements and Scientific Statements, 21*(2), 1–34.

Panel on Juvenile Crime. (2001). *Juvenile crime, juvenile justice.* Washington, DC: National Academies Press.

Pathela, P., Hennessy, R. R., Blank, S., Parvez, F., Franklin, W., & Schillinger, J. A. (2007). The contribution of a urine-based jail screening program to citywide male chlamydia and gonorrhea case rates in New York city. *Sexually Transmitted Diseases.* (Epub ahead of print.)

Penn, J. V., Esposito, C. L., Schaeffer, L. E., Fritz, G. K., & Spirito, A. (2003). Suicide attempts and self-mutilative behavior in a juvenile correctional facility. *Journal of the American Academy of Child and Adolescent Psychiatry, 42,* 762–769.

Ramaswamy, M., & Freudenberg, N. (2007). Health promotion in jails and prisons: An alternative paradigm for correctional health services. In R. Griefinger (Ed.), *Public health behind bars: From prisons to communities* (pp. 229–248). New York: Springer.

Rawal, P., Romansky, J., Jenuwine, M., & Lyons, J. S. (2004). Racial differences in the mental health needs and service utilization of youth in the juvenile justice system. *Journal of Behavioral Health Services and Research, 31,* 242–254.

Re-Entry Policy Council. (2005). Report of the Re-Entry Policy Council: Charting the safe and successful return of prisoners to the community. New York: Author.

Romero, E. G., Teplin, L. A., McClelland, G. M., Abram, K. M., Welty, L. J., & Washburn, J. J. (2007). A longitudinal study of the prevalence, development, and persistence of HIV/sexually transmitted infection risk behaviors in delinquent youth: Implications for health care in the community. *Pediatrics, 119*(5), 1126–1141.

Sampson, R. J., Raudenbush, S. W., & Earls, F. (1997). Neighborhoods and violent crime: A multilevel study of collective efficacy. *Science, 277*(5328), 918–924.

Sickmund, M., Sladky, T. J., & Kang, W. (2005). Census of juveniles in residential placement databook. Retrieved from http://ojjdp.ncjrs.org/ojstatbb/cjrp.

Snyder, H. N., & Sickmund, M. (2006). Juvenile offenders and victims: 2006 National report. Washington, DC: U.S. Department of Justice, Office of Justice Programs, Office of Juvenile Justice and Delinquency Prevention.

Staples-Horne, M., Duffy, K., & Rorie, M. T. (2007). Juvenile corrections and public health collaborations: Opportunities for improved outcomes. In R. Griefinger (Ed.), *Public health behind bars: From prisons to communities* (pp. 304–319). New York: Springer.

Strom, K. J. (2000). Profile of state prisoners under age 18, 1985–97: Special report (Publication No. NCJ 176989). Washington, DC: United States Department of Justice, Bureau of Justice Statistics.

Taxman, F. S., Byrne, J. M., & Pattavina, A. (2005). Racial disparity and the legitimacy of the criminal justice system: Exploring consequences for deterrence. *Journal of Health Care for the Poor and Underserved, 16*(4), 57–77.

Templeton, D. J. (2006). Sexually transmitted infection and blood-borne virus screening in juvenile correctional facilities: A review of the literature and recommendations for Australian centres. *Journal of Clinical Forensic Medicine, 13*(1), 30–36.

Teplin, L. A., Abram, K. M., McClelland, G. M., Dulcan, M. K., & Mericle, A. A. (2002). Psychiatric disorders in youth in juvenile detention. *Archives of General Psychiatry, 59,* 1133–1143.

Teplin, L. A., McClelland, G. M., Abram, K. M., & Mileusnic, D. (2005). Early violent death among delinquent youth: A prospective longitudinal study. *Pediatrics, 115,* 1586–1593.

Teplin, L. A., Mericle, A. A., McClelland, G. M., & Abram, K. M. (2003). HIV and AIDS risk behaviors in juvenile detainees: Implications for public health policy. *American Journal of Public Health, 93,* 906–912.

Thomas, C. R., & Penn, J. V. (2002). Juvenile justice mental health services. *Child and Adolescent Psychiatric Clinics of North America, 11,* 731–748.

Thomas, J. C., & Torrone, E. (2006). Incarceration as forced migration: Effects on selected community health outcomes. *American Journal of Public Health, 96,* 1762–1765.

Tolou-Shams, M., Brown, L. K., Gordon, G., & Fernandez, I. (Project SHIELD Study Group). (2007). Arrest history as an indicator of adolescent/young adult substance use and HIV risk. *Drug and Alcohol Dependence, 88,* 87–90.

Travis, J., Soloman, A. L., & Waul, M. (2005). *From prison to home: The dimensions and consequences of prisoner reentry.* Washington, DC: Urban Institute.

Treadwell, H. M., Northridge, M. E., & Bethea T. N. (2007). Building the case for oral health care for prisoners: Presenting the evidence and calling for justice. In R. Griefinger (Ed.), *Public health behind bars: From prisons to communities* (pp. 333–344). New York: Springer.

Underwood, L. A., & Knight, P. (2006). Treatment and postrelease rehabilitative programs for juvenile offenders. *Child and Adolescent Psychiatry Clinics of North America, 15*(2), 539–556.

Valois, R. F., MacDonald, J. M., Bretous, L., Fischer, M. A., & Drane, J. W. (2002). Risk factors and behaviors associated with adolescent violence and aggression. *American Journal of Health Behavior, 26*(6), 454–464.

Wasserman, G. A., McReynolds, L. S., Lucas, C. P., Fisher, P., & Santos, L. (2002). The voice DISC-IV with incarcerated male youths: Prevalence of disorder. *Journal of the American Academy of Child and Adolescent Psychiatry, 41*(3), 314–321. (Erratum in 2003, *42*(2), 260.)

Wasserman, G. A., Jensen, P., Ko, S., Cocozza, J., Trupin, E., Angold, A., Cauffman, E., & Grisso, T. (2003). Mental health assessments in juvenile justice: Report on consensus conference. *Journal of the American Academy of Child and Adolescent Psychiatry, 42*(7), 752–761.

Whitehead, D. (2006). The health promoting prison (HPP) and its imperative for nursing. *International Journal of Nursing Studies, 43*(1), 123–131.

Wolff, N., Blitz, C. L., Shi, J., Bachman, R., & Siegel, J. A. (2006). Sexual violence inside prisons: Rates of victimization. *Journal of Urban Health, 83*(5), 835–848.

World Health Organization. (1986, November). Ottawa Charter for Health Promotion. First International Conference on Health Promotion, Ottawa, Canada.

World Health Organization. (2006). Health in Prisons Project. World Health Organization Regional Office for Europe. Retrieved from www.euro.who.int/prisons.

Zack, B. (2007). HIV prevention: Behavioral interventions in correctional settings. In R. Griefinger (Ed.), *Public health behind bars: From prisons to communities* (pp. 156–173). New York: Springer, 2007.

CHAPTER

18

DEPRESSION AND SEXUAL RISK BEHAVIOR IN ADOLESCENTS

LYDIA A. SHRIER

LEARNING OBJECTIVES

After studying this chapter, you will be able to

- Recognize that depressive symptoms are common during adolescence and vary by gender.
- Demonstrate an understanding of the bidirectional relationship between adolescent depression and sexual risk behavior.
- Translate possible mechanisms for the depression–sexual risk association in adolescence.
- Identify gaps within the literature and determine future directions for mental health intervention.

The epidemics of sexually transmitted infections (STIs) and unplanned pregnancy in adolescents demand increased understanding of factors that contribute to adolescent sexual risk behavior in order to develop more effective preventive interventions. Studies of adolescents in a variety of settings have indicated that elevated depressive symptomatology and emotional distress correlate with higher rates of sexual activity, sexual risk behaviors, and STIs. Although relatively few studies have examined temporal associations suggestive of causality, age cohort and other longitudinal studies with adolescents and young adults indicate that the relationship between depressive symptoms and risk behaviors may be bidirectional. Research on affect and sexual thoughts and behaviors suggest possible mechanisms for the depression–sexual risk link. The implications of the association between depression and sexual risk behavior are discussed in the context of clinical care, research, and interventions.

EPIDEMIOLOGY OF HIV, STIS, AND PREGNANCY IN ADOLESCENTS

The rates of STIs and pregnancy among adolescents are alarmingly high. Annually, an estimated one-half of all new HIV infections (Office of National AIDS Policy, 1996; Rosenberg, Biggar, & Goedert, 1994) and almost one-half of all new cases of STIs occur in adolescents and young adults (Weinstock, Berman, & Cates, 2004). Although rates have been declining, the U.S. teenage pregnancy and birth rates continue to be the highest among Western industrialized countries (Guttmacher Institute, 2006). Compared with adult mothers, adolescent mothers may be less likely to graduate from high school (Hofferth, Reid, & Mott, 2001), and their children may be more likely to use drugs, belong to gangs, be unemployed, and become young parents themselves (Pogarsky, Thornberry, & Lizotte, 2006).

One of the developmental tasks for young people is to emerge from adolescence as sexually healthy adults able to sustain intimate relationships. For some youth, this challenge is met through sexual behavior, some of which places them at increased risk for STIs and pregnancy. Behavioral risk factors for adverse outcomes of sexual intercourse include early age at first intercourse, having multiple sexual partners, engaging in unprotected sex, and having partners who are at high risk for having STIs. According to the 2005 Youth Risk Behavior Surveillance System (YRBSS), 46.8 percent of high school students have had sexual intercourse (6.2 percent before the age of thirteen years), and 14.3 percent have had more than four sexual partners (Eaton et al., 2006). Of the students who had sexual intercourse in the previous three months (33.9 percent), only 62.8 percent reported condom use during last intercourse (Eaton et al., 2006). Because heterosexual behaviors occur more frequently and confer greater risk of both STIs and unplanned pregnancy than same-sex behaviors, they will be the focus of discussion in this chapter.

DEPRESSIVE SYMPTOMS, MOOD DISORDERS, AND EMOTIONAL DISTRESS IN ADOLESCENTS

Depressive symptoms (Eaton et al., 2006), major depression, *dysthymia* (chronic depression), and other mood disorders (Lewinsohn, Hops, Roberts, Seeley, & Andrews, 1993; Saluja, Iachan, Scheidt, Overpeck, Sun, & Giedd, 2004) are common in adolescents. The lifetime prevalence of depression in adolescence has been estimated to range from 12.0 percent to 25.3 percent (Birmaher, Ryan, Williamson, Brent, & Kaufman, 1996; Lewinsohn et al., 1993). Data from the 1988–1994 National Health and Nutrition Examination Survey III revealed that 12.2 percent of fifteen- to nineteen-year-olds have dysthymia or major depressive disorder (Riolo, Nguyen, Greden, & King, 2005); a school-based survey of younger teens found depressive symptoms in 18 percent (Saluja et al., 2004). According to the 2005 YRBSS, 28.5 percent of high school students felt so sad or hopeless almost every day for at least two weeks in the previous twelve months that they stopped doing some usual activities, and 16.9 percent seriously considered suicide (Eaton et al., 2006).

Twenty-nine percent of high school students felt so sad or hopeless almost every day for at least two weeks that they stopped doing some usual activities, and 16.9 percent seriously considered suicide.

Evidence of the Association Between Depression and Sexual Risk

There is a large body of empirical literature suggesting that depression may play a key role in the development and maintenance of sexual risk behaviors and acquisition of STIs (DiClemente & Ponton, 1993; DiClemente et al., 2001; Ethier et al., 2006; Lehrer, Shrier, Gortmaker, & Buka, 2006; Pao et al., 2000; Shrier, Braslins, et al., 2003; Shrier, Harris, & Beardslee, 2002; Shrier, Harris, Sternberg, & Beardslee, 2001; Stiffman, Dore, Earls, & Cunningham, 1992). First, surveys of adult STI clinic clients have found high rates of clinically significant depressive symptoms. For example, using a gender-specific Beck Depression Inventory (BDI) score cutoff, 23 percent of male and 14 percent of female STI clinic clients were depressed (Hutton, Lyketsos, Zenilman, Thompson, & Erbelding, 2004); 11.9 percent of the sample met diagnostic criteria for major depression (Erbelding, Hutton, Zenilman, Hunt, & Lyketsos, 2004).

Second, in sexually active young people, depressive symptoms and disorders have been linked to increased sexual risk behaviors and elevated rates of STIs. Almost one-third of a community and clinical sample of sexually active young women ages fifteen through twenty-four years had a score on the Center for Epidemiologic Studies Depression (CES-D) Scale of twenty-four or higher, consistent with a diagnosis of depression (Mazzaferro et al., 2006). Women in this study who were depressed—especially the teenagers—were more likely than nondepressed women to report having multiple partners and using condoms inconsistently in the past year. Among 173 young African

American women attending urban health centers, depressive symptoms were associated with having multiple partners, an IV drug–using partner, and a partner with an STI (Orr, Celentano, Santelli, & Burwell, 1994). However, the association is not consistently observed; in a clinic-based sample of 158 African American female adolescents, depressive symptoms assessed on the BDI were not associated with sexual risk behaviors (Bachanas et al., 2002). Variability in sample size and composition, rates of depression and sexual risk behaviors, and data collection and analysis methods may contribute to differences in the presence and strength of the associations.

Third, compared to young people without psychiatric disorders, those with severe mental illness engage in increased sexual risk behavior, including early onset of sexual activity, more sexual partners, and less condom use (Brown, Danovsky, Lourie, & DiClemente, 1997; DiClemente & Ponton, 1993; Smith, 2001; Valois, Bryant, Rivard, & Hinkle, 1997). Limited research has been done in which depressive disorders are specifically examined in relation to sexual risk. In a New Zealand birth cohort ($N =$ 930), young adults (age twenty-one) with depressive disorders had increased risk of reporting sexual intercourse under the age of sixteen (risk ratio [RR] 1.3), a lifetime history of STI (RR 1.6), and multiple partners and inconsistent condom use (RR 2.2) (Ramrakha, Caspi, Dickson, Moffitt, & Paul, 2000).

Fourth, in longitudinal studies, depressive symptoms have been associated with subsequent sexual risk behavior (Brown et al., 2006; DiClemente et al., 2001; Lehrer, Shrier, Gortmaker, & Buka, 2006; Shrier, Harris, & Beardslee, 2002; Stiffman et al., 1992) and high rates of incident STIs (Shrier et al., 2001). Stiffman et al. (1992) found that depressive symptoms (as well as other psychiatric problems) during adolescence predicted sexual risk behaviors in young adulthood and that improvement in symptoms over time was associated with lower risk. In another study, almost one-half of 522 sexually active African American girls ages fourteen through eighteen were classified as psychologically distressed (score of seven or lower on the eight-item CES-D) (DiClemente et al., 2001). At six months, those who were distressed at baseline had higher odds than those who were not of having unprotected sex (adjusted odds ratio [AOR] 2.1), having nonmonogamous sex partners (AOR 1.7), not using contraception (AOR 1.5), and being pregnant (AOR 2.0). Among 415 male and female African American adolescents, those with depressive symptoms (on five items from Brief Symptom Inventory depression subscale) at baseline reported more inconsistent condom use at six months (AOR 3.9), compared to nondepressed adolescents (Brown et al., 2006).

The association between depression and sexual risk appears to be bidirectional. Analyses of National Longitudinal Study of Adolescent Health (Add Health) data revealed that patterns of sexual behavior predicted high levels of depressive symptoms one year later, especially for girls (Hallfors, Waller, Bauer, Ford, & Halpern, 2005). Other Add Health analyses found that both boys and girls who were diagnosed with an STI in the past year were at increased risk of having very high levels of depressive symptoms by one year later (Shrier, Harris, & Beardslee, 2002). Other studies have suggested that being diagnosed with an STI has psychological sequelae in adolescents (Biro & Rosenthal, 1992; Rosenthal, Biro, Cohen, Succop, & Stanberry, 1995).

Possible Mechanisms for the Depression–Sexual Risk Associations

There are many possible explanations for the empirical links between depression, sexual risk behavior, and STIs. This section will focus on how depression may be associated with sexual behavior through cognitive, behavioral, and relational processes. With regard to the reverse relationship, for some adolescents diagnosis of an STI may be the initiating event in the development of a depressive episode (Lewinsohn, Hoberman, Teri, & Hautzinger, 1985). However, some adolescent girls with a history of STI have lower emotional distress, perhaps owing to increased counseling or medical attention associated with identification of the STI (Ethier et al., 2006). Although research suggests a causal relationship of sexual risk behavior and STI with subsequent depression, it is possible that sexual risk indicates psychological, social, or environmental problems that also lead to depression. Low socioeconomic status is associated with increased risk for depression (Lorant et al., 2003) and sexual behaviors, including initiating intercourse and not using a condom (Santelli, Lowry, Brener, & Robin, 2000), although the relations are not consistent or always linear (Santelli et al., 2000). *Social capital* (social connectedness) and parental and school connectedness are protective against both depression and sexual risk behavior (Fitzpatrick, Piko, Wright, & LaGory, 2005; Resnick et al., 1997).

Prolonged depressed mood is the hallmark of depression; 90 to 95 percent of adolescents and young adults with major depressive disorder report depressed mood for at least two weeks (the rest meet the *Diagnostic and Statistical Manual of Mental Disorders,* fourth edition, 1994, criteria for major depressive disorder with the symptom of anhedonia—the inability to find pleasure in normally pleasurable activities) (Lewinsohn, Petit, Joiner, & Seeley, 2003). Depressed mood may be associated with subsequent sexual behavior through several cognitive processes. Compared to nondepressed adolescents, those who are depressed may have less knowledge or understanding about STI and pregnancy prevention (Katz, Mills, Singh, & Best, 1995), perhaps as a result of impaired ability to assimilate new information or missed school days related to their mental illness. Depressed mood can impair the ability to judge or accurately perceive risk of STI or unintended pregnancy and lower self-efficacy and motivation to engage in safer sex behaviors. For example, compared with their less affected peers, adolescent girls with more depressive symptoms at baseline reported at six-month follow-up greater fear about adverse consequences of negotiating condom use (AOR 2.0), more perceived barriers to condom use (AOR 2.2), lower self-efficacy to negotiate condom use (AOR 1.6), and more perceived norms that did not support healthy relationships (AOR 1.7; DiClemente et al., 2001). In Add Health, positive perceptions of sex were associated with initiating sexual intercourse in nondepressed, but not in depressed adolescent girls (Rink, Tricker, & Harvey, 2007).

Efforts to regulate depressed mood may also result in engaging in sexual intercourse and in unsafe sexual behaviors. Sexually active adolescents report their highest positive affect when thinking about sex (Shrier, Shih, Hynes, Mariano, & Beardslee, 2003) and experience improved positive and negative affect both before (Shrier &

Efforts to regulate depressed mood may also result in engaging in sexual intercourse and in unsafe sexual behaviors.

de Moor, 2006) and after sex (Shrier, Shih, Hacker, & de Moor, 2007). These findings suggest that efforts to reduce sexual risk may conflict with thoughts and behaviors that produce desirable mood. However, condom use has been associated with lower levels of negative mood (Fortenberry et al., 2005), and other research has found no association between negative affect and condom use (Shrier et al., 2007). Adolescents who report having sex to cope with negative emotions engage in increased sexual risk behaviors, such as having multiple partners (Cooper, Shapiro, & Powers, 1998). Psychiatric distress, including depressive symptoms, is associated with substance use (Rao, Daley, & Hammen, 2000; Shrier, Harris, Kurland, & Knight, 2003), which is linked to increased sexual risk behavior and STIs (Shrier, Emans, Woods, & DuRant, 1997; Tapert, Aarons, Sedlar, & Brown, 2001).

The role of sexual relationships in self-validation, demonstrating the capacity for intimacy, and creating pleasurable experiences in response to depressed mood must also be considered (Bancroft et al., 2003). However, depression may result in having dysfunctional social interactions (Brown et al., 1997; Kalichman, Kelly, Johnson, & Bulto, 1994; Smith, 2001). Compared to their nondepressed peers, depressed youth may feel less in control of their relationships (DiClemente et al., 2001) and more likely to engage in unsafe sexual practices to gratify or placate their partners (Cooper et al., 1998). Although limited research has been done with young heterosexual couples, there is indirect evidence that youth who are depressed may choose partners who are also depressed, thereby compounding their sexual risk. Planalp (2003) has suggested that because differences in emotion are not comfortable, couples may attempt to coordinate their feelings. In a study of same-sex undergraduate dyads, Locke and Horowitz (1990) found that similarity in dysphoria predicted satisfaction with the interpersonal interaction, which may motivate assortive coupling (meaning each of the two individuals in a couple may experience depression) among depressed individuals. In a study of 136 high-risk young heterosexual couples, if at least one partner was depressed, approximately one-half of the time the other partner was also depressed (Shrier et al., 2008). These doubly depressed couples had the greatest risk of reporting recent substance use around the time of sexual intercourse.

Gender Differences in Depression and Sexual Risk

There are gender differences in both depression and sexual behavior. Female adolescents are more likely than male adolescents to report depressive symptoms (Paxton, Valois, Watkins, Huebner, & Drane, 2007) and to not use condoms consistently (Brown et al., 2006; Eaton et al., 2006). Male adolescents are more likely to have initiated sexual intercourse at a young age and report more lifetime partners compared with their female peers (Eaton et al., 2006). Further, gender differences exist in the association between depressive symptoms and sexual risk. In Add Health, depressive symptoms at baseline predicted condom nonuse at last sex, birth control nonuse at last sex, substance use at last sex (Lehrer et al., 2006), and being diagnosed with STI (Shrier, Harris, & Beardslee, 2002) over the next year for boys, but depression predicted only substance use at last sex for girls (Lehrer et al., 2006). In contrast, cross-sectional analyses of the baseline Add Health data found that adolescent girls engaging in low and moderate sexual behavior and substance use reported more depressive symptoms than adolescent boys engaging in similar behaviors (Waller et al., 2006). Other research has also found stronger associations between depressive symptoms and sexual risk behaviors for girls as compared to boys. For example, in a study of high-risk adolescents and young adults, a high level of depressive symptomatology was associated with an increased risk of gonorrhea among young women but not young men, who reported decreased coital frequency in the previous thirty days (Shrier, Braslins, et al., 2003).

There are several possible explanations for the differences in sexual risk between male and female adolescents who are depressed. Relative to depressed young women, young men who are depressed may have decreased opportunities for social interactions that could lead to sexual intercourse, perhaps owing to social stigma associated with male depression. College freshmen were more likely to rate a depressed male roommate negatively than a depressed female roommate (Siegel & Alloy, 1990). Depressed male adolescents may be less likely than depressed female adolescents to have sex to manage their affect (Dawson, Shih, de Moor, & Shrier, 2008), perhaps owing to an increased likelihood of rejection (Joiner, Alfano, & Metalsky, 1992).

Depressive-style coping has been used by girls in response to an STI diagnosis. Compared to their coping with an interpersonal stressor, adolescent girls were less likely to use functional coping strategies and more likely to use self-blame in response to being diagnosed with an STI (Baker et al., 2001). Similar research has not been conducted in adolescent boys. Emotional distress following STI diagnosis may differ depending on the nature of the STI (an incurable viral infection such as herpes versus a curable bacterial infection such as gonorrhea). There may also be gender differences in psychological sequelae because young women are at greater risk of physical adverse outcomes from STIs, including infertility and ectopic pregnancy.

Low self-esteem is highly correlated with depression (Orvaschel, Beeferman, & Kabacoff, 1997) and predictive of depression (Roberts, Gotlib, & Kassel, 1996). Self-esteem may play a role in the association between sexual risk behavior and subsequent depression, particularly for adolescent girls, for whom social norms discourage sexual activity. Engaging in early sexual behavior and having multiple or risky partners may contribute to low self-esteem, which in turn may contribute to the development of depression in girls (Ethier et al., 2006). In a longitudinal study of 188 young adolescents (with a mean age of 12.5 years), girls with *lower* self-esteem and boys with *higher* self-esteem at baseline were more likely than their gender-matched peers to initiate sexual intercourse within the subsequent two years (Spencer, Zimet, Aalsma, & Orr, 2002).

INTERVENTIONS

Relatively few studies have tested safer sex interventions among youth with mental illness, and none has specifically targeted depressed adolescents. A literature review on HIV risk in adolescents with severe mental illness (Smith, 2001) identified three prevention studies for these youth (Brown, Reynolds, & Lourie, 1997; Ponton, DiClemente, &

McKenna, 1991; Slonim-Nevo, Ozawa, & Auslander, 1991). Slonim-Nevo et al. (1991) evaluated the effects of a ninety-minute group education and discussion intervention on HIV knowledge, attitudes, and behaviors of youth ages ten through eighteen years living in residential centers; thirty youth in two centers received the intervention, and twenty-four youth in one center were the control group. The intervention did not result in changes in HIV knowledge, attitudes, or risk behavior assessed at one-month follow-up. The authors acknowledged that the brief, single-session intervention did not include components that may be related to intervention effectiveness, including clarifying participants' values and aspirations as a means of establishing that they deserve to be protected against HIV, supporting positive attitudes toward HIV prevention, and developing skills for preventative behaviors.

Two more comprehensive cognitive behavioral HIV prevention programs were tested in adolescent psychiatric inpatients. Evaluation of an eight-session group program showed no differences between pre- and immediately postintervention assessments of HIV risk knowledge or perceived risk, although participants did have lower misconceptions about transmission risk from casual contact and lower intentions to engage in risk behaviors after the program (Ponton et al., 1991). The authors did not report the sociodemographic characteristics or psychiatric diagnoses of the participants, limiting readers' ability to generalize the findings or to determine whether there were particular subgroups of participants for whom the intervention was most effective. Brown et al. (1997) found improvement in HIV knowledge, tolerance of people with AIDS, and self-efficacy for safer sex behaviors improved immediately following a ten-session cognitive-behavioral program. However, by the three-month follow-up, these cognitive improvements were no longer evident; the study did not assess any sexual behavior outcomes.

In a recent study of fifty thirteen- to nineteen-year-olds with major depressive disorder, a nonnicotine substance use disorder, and conduct disorder who were receiving outpatient substance use treatment, receipt of one individual cognitive-behavioral therapy session on HIV risk reduction was associated with increased HIV knowledge and improved beliefs about condoms (Thurstone, Riggs, Klein, & Mikulich-Gilbertson, 2007). As with the studies by Ponton et al. (1991) and Brown et al. (1997), this study did not include a control group, so the improved outcomes could not be clearly attributed to the intervention.

For the most part, studies have not examined the effects of depression on response to interventions in psychiatrically impaired or general adolescent samples. Limited sample size to look at effect modification has been cited as one reason for this omission (Thurstone et al., 2007). Cognitive, social, and behavioral dysfunction in depression may attenuate the effectiveness of safer sex interventions. Alternatively, as suggested by others (Compton, Cottler, Ben-Abdallah, Cunningham-Williams, & Spitznagel, 2000), depressed youth may be more motivated than nondepressed youth to change their behaviors because they hope to reduce their levels of distress. Lightfoot, Tevendale, Comulada, and Rotheram-Borus (2007) found that young people living with HIV who had high levels of depression increased the proportion of protected sex acts with HIV-negative partners over time. Youth were randomized to an eighteen-session telephone intervention, an eighteen-session in-person intervention, or a delayed intervention. Although overall the in-person condition was associated with the greatest reductions in HIV transmission risk behaviors (Rotheram-Borus et al., 2004), for youth who were emotionally distressed the telephone condition was more effective (Lightfoot et al., 2007). Similarly provocative findings were seen among 333 heterosexually active, drug-using adult women who were randomized to a four-session enhanced motivation condition, a four-session enhanced negotiation condition, or a standard education control condition (Sterk, Theall, & Elifson, 2006). Persistently high levels of depression were associated with higher rates of drug use and sexual risk behaviors. Although women in both enhanced intervention arms reported lower sexual and drug risk behaviors than women in the control arm, women who received the motivation intervention reported lower levels of depression at six-month follow-up. The authors postulated that depressed women benefited most from assignment to the motivation condition because that intervention focused on identifying and reducing life stressors. By managing stressors better, depressed women in this condition may have reduced their emotional distress such that they were able to make changes in their risk behaviors. These studies' findings emphasize the importance of considering depression when choosing the delivery mode and optimal content of safer sex interventions for adolescents.

IMPLICATIONS FOR RESEARCH

Much work remains to be done to determine the nature of the relation between depression and sexual risk behavior in adolescents. Studies need to attend to potential gender, racial/ethnic, and developmental differences in the association, as well as to modifying and mediating associations with other factors such as socioeconomic status and social support. Longitudinal studies must be performed to enhance our understanding of the development of depression and sexual risk over time, with an eye on clarifying the probable bidirectionality of the link. It is likely that there is a cycle to the associations, such that sexual risk behavior during adolescence is related to subsequent depression, which is related to subsequent sexual risk behavior, as suggested by others (Ethier et al., 2006). Predisposition to depression, or the presence of factors contributing to both depression and sexual risk behavior, may predict this cycle.

Additional research is needed to delve into *how* depression leads to sexual risk behaviors, and vice versa. Several questions should be addressed. Is sexual behavior, or social interactions that may lead to sexual intercourse, used to regulate affect? In what way does depressed or irritable mood influence cognition, social interactions, risk perceptions, partner choice, and sexual decision making? And for the reverse relationship, how does initiating sexual intercourse, having multiple or high-risk partners, and not using condoms contribute to the development of depression? Especially for girls, do these behaviors decrease self-esteem and increase stigma, which leads to depression? Other research has suggested that exploring early life experiences may aid in understanding these relationships, for example, testing attachment theory as a means of explaining how the health of intimate relationships may predict depression status (Pielage, Luteijn, & Arrindell, 2005).

Most important, research must try to distinguish among the types of and motivations for sexual risk behavior among depressed adolescents. Not using a condom in a supportive, loving relationship that may be part of a functional response to depressive symptoms should be differentiated from sex with unfamiliar, high-risk, or multiple partners as part of a high-risk or unconventional lifestyle that may include other health risk behaviors such as substance use and violence (Jessor & Jessor, 1977). Although having sexual intercourse and not using a condom increases risk of adverse outcomes, not all sexual events are equal in terms of risk, and healthy sexual relationships are beneficial in achieving developmental milestones (Furman & Wehner, 1994; Weinstein & Rosen, 1991) and improving affective states (Shrier et al., 2007). For example, more frequent sexual behaviors are related to longer relationship duration in adolescent couples (Rostosky, Galliher, Welsh, & Kawaguchi, 2000). Attention to relationship and partner (for example, Shrier et al., 2008) characteristics will be imperative in future research.

Sexual risk intervention studies are needed that both target and assess the effects of depression, are conducted in large samples of diverse populations, and include cognitive, behavioral, and biological outcomes.

Studies of depression and sexual risk in adolescents should try to address the limitations in previous research, including lack of a theoretical framework, incongruent time frames for assessing depressive symptoms and sexual risk behaviors (for example, Hutton et al., 2004), exclusion of male adolescents (for example, Rink et al., 2007), and analyses that do not account for the possibility of a nonlinear relationship between depressive symptoms and sexual risk behaviors (Dawson et al., 2008; Kalichman & Weinhardt, 2001; Waller et al., 2006). Because there are racial and ethnic differences in rates of sexual risk behaviors and STIs (Eaton et al., 2006; Ellen, Aral, & Madger, 1998), depressive symptoms (Eaton et al., 2006) and disorders (Riolo et al., 2005), and in responses on mental health assessments (e.g., Azocar, Arean, Miranda, & Munoz, 2001), research is also needed to better understand sociodemographic differences in the link between depression and sexual risk. Studies should also focus on understudied populations at particularly high risk for both depression and sexual risk, such as youth who are engaging in same-sex sexual behaviors, abusing drugs, involved in the sex trade, incarcerated, homeless, runaway, or living in rural areas. Most important, sexual risk intervention studies are needed that both target and assess the effects of depression, are conducted in large samples of diverse populations, and include cognitive, behavioral, and biological outcomes.

IMPLICATIONS FOR HEALTH CARE

Regardless of what is known about directionality and causality, there is strong evidence to support clinical practice that is attentive to the link between depression and sexual risk. As suggested by health care guidelines such as Bright Futures (Hagan, Shaw, & Duncan, 2007), clinicians need to screen adolescents for both depressive symptoms and sexual risk behaviors. If a problem is detected in one domain, the clinician should promptly and thoroughly assess the other domain and continue to do so in an ongoing manner, recognizing that problems may develop over time. Once sexual risk behavior is identified, risk reduction counseling strategies may need to differ substantially depending on the presence of depression (Lightfoot et al., 2007).

When depression is diagnosed, affected adolescents should be assessed for sexual risk behaviors and history of STI. Mental health clinicians need to recognize the importance of assessing sexual risk in their depressed adolescent clients and may need to acquire the skills and comfort to do so. Mental health professional training programs must include education on adolescent sexual risk assessment, service needs, and referral options.

Screening, evaluation, and treatment for depression should be considered an essential part of sexual health care for adolescents.

Clinicians who diagnose and manage STIs and pregnancy in adolescents need to treat each encounter as an opportunity to screen for depressive symptoms. If mental health assessment and treatment are not available on site, affected adolescents need to be referred to appropriate resources. As Hutton et al. (2004) noted, "depression is a barrier to behavior change," which is the most effective strategy available to health care providers to decrease risk for STIs and unintended pregnancy in adolescents. Therefore, screening, evaluation, and treatment for depression should be considered an essential part of sexual health care for adolescents.

SUMMARY

Depressed adolescents are more likely to engage in sexual risk behavior, acquire STIs, and have unplanned pregnancies than their nondepressed peers. Further, adolescents who engage in sexual risk behaviors and those who acquire STIs are at increased risk for depression. Cognitive, affective, social, and behavioral processes may contribute to the link between depression and sexual risk, with different mechanisms likely at play for male and female adolescents; other characteristics may distinguish which adolescents are most vulnerable. Although it is critical that further research is designed specifically to examine the nature of depression–sexual risk associations, clinicians caring for sexually active adolescents and for those who are depressed need to recognize and intervene with those at increased risk. For adolescents in general, but especially for those who are depressed, safer sex interventions need to be developed that recognize and reduce depressive symptoms as they influence sexual behavior, emphasize self-worth and cultivate optimism and future orientation, teach self-assessment of maladaptive efforts at affect regulation, and promote healthier strategies to manage depressed mood.

KEY TERMS

Dysthymia   Social capital

DISCUSSION QUESTIONS

1. In the literature on depression and sexual risk outlined in this chapter, what behavioral associations have been found among adolescents with depressive symptomatology? Do these associations vary by age?

2. Explain the bidirectional relationship between depression and sexual risk. Be sure to include cognitive, behavioral, and relational processes that may exist in this relationship.

3. In addition to the author's recommendations for future research in this area, what else can be done from a clinician's or principal investigator's point of view to better address and possibly reduce sexual risk among adolescents?

REFERENCES

Azocar, F., Arean, P., Miranda, J., & Munoz, R. F. (2001). Differential item functioning in a Spanish translation of the Beck Depression Inventory. *Journal of Clinical Psychology, 57,* 355–365.

Bachanas, P. J., Morris, M. K., Lewis-Gess, J. K., Sarett-Cuasay, E. J., Sirl, K., Ries, J. K., & Sawyer, M. K. (2002). Predictors of risky sexual behavior in African American adolescent girls: Implications for prevention interventions. *Journal of Pediatric Psychology, 27,* 519–530.

Baker, J. G., Succop, P. A., Boehner, C. W., Biro, F. M., Stanberry, L. R., & Rosenthal, S. L. (2001). Adolescent girl's coping with an STD: Not enough problem solving and too much self-blame. *Journal of Pediatric and Adolescent Gynecology, 14,* 85–88.

Bancroft, J., Janssen, E., Strong, D., Carnes, L., Vukadinovic, Z., & Long, J. (2003). The relation between mood and sexuality in heterosexual men. *Archives of Sexual Behavior, 32*(3), 217–230.

Birmaher, B., Ryan, N. D., Williamson, D. E., Brent, D. A., & Kaufman, J. (1996). Childhood and adolescent depression: A review of the past 10 years. Part II. *Journal of the American Academy of Child and Adolescent Psychiatry, 35*(12), 1575–1583.

Biro, F. M., & Rosenthal, S. L. (1992). Psychological sequelae of sexually transmitted diseases in adolescents. *Obstetrics and Gynecology Clinics of North America, 19*(1), 209–218.

Brown, L., Danovsky, M., Lourie, K., & DiClemente, R. (1997). Adolescents with psychiatric disorders and the risk of HIV. *Journal of the American Academy of Child and Adolescent Psychiatry, 36,* 1609–1615.

Brown, L. K., Reynolds, L. A., & Lourie, K. J. (1997). A pilot HIV prevention program for adolescents in a psychiatric hospital. *Psychiatric Services, 48,* 531–533.

Brown, L. K., Tolou-Shams, M., Lescano, C., Houck, C., Zeidman, J., Pugatch, D., & Lourie, K. J. (2006). Depressive symptoms as a predictor of sexual risk among African American adolescents and young adults. *Journal of Adolescent Health, 39,* 444, e441–448.

Compton, W. M., Cottler, L. B., Ben-Abdallah, A., Cunningham-Williams, R., & Spitznagel, E. L. (2000). The effects of psychiatric comorbidity on response to an HIV prevention intervention. *Drug and Alcohol Dependence, 58,* 247–257.

Cooper, M., Shapiro, C., & Powers, A. (1998). Motivations for sex and risky sexual behavior among adolescents and young adults: A functional perspective. *Journal of Personality and Social Psychology, 75,* 1528–1558.

Dawson, L. H., Shih, M.-C., de Moor, C., & Shrier, L. A. (2008). Reasons why adolescents and young adults have sex: Associations with psychological characteristics and sexual behavior. *Journal of Sex Research, 45,* 225–232.

Diagnostic and statistical manual of mental disorders (4th ed.). (1994). Washington, DC: American Psychiatric Association.

DiClemente, R. J., & Ponton, L. E. (1993). HIV-related risk behaviors among psychiatrically hospitalized adolescents and school-based adolescents. *American Journal of Psychiatry, 150,* 324–325.

DiClemente, R. J., Wingood, G. M., Crosby, R. A., Sionean, C., Brown, L. K., & Rothbaum, B. (2001). A prospective study of psychological distress and sexual risk behavior among black adolescent females. *Pediatrics, 108,* e85.

Eaton, D. K., Kann, L., Kinchen, S., Ross, J., Hawkins, J., & Harris, W. A. (2006). Youth risk behavior surveillance: United States, 2005. *Morbidity and Mortality Weekly Reports Surveillance Summaries, 55*(SS05), 1–108.

Ellen, J. M., Aral, S. O., & Madger, L. S. (1998). Do differences in sexual behaviors account for the racial/ethnic differences in adolescents' self-reported history of a sexually transmitted disease? *Sexually Transmitted Disease, 25,* 125–129.

Erbelding, E. J., Hutton, H. E., Zenilman, J. M., Hunt, W. P., & Lyketsos, C. G. (2004). The prevalence of psychiatric disorders in sexually transmitted disease clinic patients and their association with sexually transmitted disease risk. *Sexually Transmitted Disease, 31,* 8–12.

Ethier, K. A., Kershaw, T. S., Lewis, J. B., Milan, S., Niccolai, L. M., & Ickovics, J. R. (2006). Self-esteem, emotional distress and sexual behavior among adolescent females: Inter-relationships and temporal effects. *Journal of Adolescent Health, 38,* 268–274.

Fitzpatrick, K. M., Piko, B. F., Wright, D. R., & LaGory, M. (2005). Depressive symptomatology, exposure to violence, and the role of social capital among African American adolescents. *American Journal of Orthopsychiatry, 75,* 262–274.

Fortenberry, J. D., Temkit, M., Tu, W., Graham, C. A., Katz, B. P., & Orr, D. P. (2005). Daily mood, partner support, sexual interest, and sexual activity among adolescent women. *Health Psychology, 24,* 252–257.

Furman, W., & Wehner, E. A. (1994). Romantic views: Toward a theory of adolescent romantic relationships. In R. Montemayor, G. R. Adams, & G. P. Gullota (Eds.), *Advances in adolescent development: Vol. 6. Relationships during adolescence* (pp. 168–175). Thousand Oaks, CA: Sage.

Guttmacher Institute. (2006). *U.S. teenage pregnancy statistics: National and state trends and trends by race and ethnicity.* New York: Author.

Hagan, J. F., Shaw, J. S., & Duncan, P. (Eds.). (2007). *Bright futures: Guidelines for health supervision of infants, children, and adolescents* (3rd ed.). Elk Grove, IL: American Academy of Pediatrics.

Hallfors, D. D., Waller, M. W., Bauer, D., Ford, C. A., & Halpern, C. T. (2005). Which comes first in adolescence: Sex and drugs or depression? *American Journal of Preventive Medicine, 29,* 163–170.

Hofferth, S. L., Reid, L., & Mott, F. L. (2001). The effects of early childbearing on schooling over time. *Family Planning Perspectives, 33,* 259–267.

Hutton, H. E., Lyketsos, C. G., Zenilman, J. M., Thompson, R. E., & Erbelding, E. J. (2004). Depression and HIV risk behaviors among patients in a sexually transmitted disease clinic. *American Journal of Psychiatry, 161,* 912–914.

Jessor, R., & Jessor, S. (1977). *Problem behavior and psychosocial development: A longitudinal study of youth.* New York: Academic.

Joiner, T. E., Alfano, M. S., & Metalsky, G. I. (1992). When depression breeds contempt: Reassurance seeking, self-esteem, and rejection of depressed college students by their roommates. *Journal of Abnormal Psychology, 101,* 165–173.

Kalichman, S. C., Kelly, J. A., Johnson, J. R., & Bulto, M. (1994). Factors associated with risk for HIV infection among chronic mentally ill adults. *American Journal of Psychiatry, 151,* 221–227.

Kalichman, S. C., & Weinhardt, L. (2001). Negative affect and sexual risk behavior: Comment on Crepaz and Marks. *Health Psychology, 20,* 300–301.

Katz, R. C., Mills, K., Singh, N. N., & Best, A. M. (1995). Knowledge and attitudes about AIDS: A comparison of public high school students, incarcerated delinquents, and emotionally disturbed adolescents. *Journal of Youth and Adolescence, 24,* 117–131.

Lehrer, J. A., Shrier, L. A., Gortmaker, S., & Buka, S. (2006). Depressive symptoms as a longitudinal predictor of sexual risk behaviors among US middle and high school students. *Pediatrics, 118,* 189–200.

Lewinsohn, P., Hoberman, H., Teri, L., & Hautzinger, M. (1985). An integrative theory of depression. In S. Reiss & R. Bootzin (Eds.), *Theoretical issues in behavior therapy* (pp. 331–359). San Diego, CA: Academic Press.

Lewinsohn, P. M., Hops, H., Roberts, R. E., Seeley, J. R., & Andrews, J. A. (1993). Adolescent psychopathology: I. Prevalence and incidence of depression and other DSM-III-R disorders in high school students. *Journal of Abnormal Psychology, 102,* 133–144.

Lewinsohn, P. M., Petit, J. W., Joiner, T. E., Jr., & Seeley, J. R. (2003). The symptomatic expression of major depressive disorder in adolescents and young adults. *Journal of Abnormal Psychology, 112,* 244–252.

Lightfoot, M., Tevendale, H., Comulada, W. S., & Rotheram-Borus, M. J. (2007). Who benefited from an efficacious intervention for youth living with HIV: A moderator analysis. *AIDS and Behavior, 11,* 61–70.

Locke, K. D., & Horowitz, L. M. (1990). Satisfaction in interpersonal interactions as a function of similarity in level of dysphoria. *Journal of Personality and Social Psychology, 58,* 823–831.

Lorant, V., Deliege, D., Eaton, W., Robert, A., Philippot, P., & Ansseau, M. (2003). Socioeconomic inequalities in depression: A meta-analysis. *American Journal of Epidemiology, 157,* 98–112.

Mazzaferro, K. E., Murray, P. J., Ness, R. B., Bass, D. C., Tyus, N., & Cook, R. L. (2006). Depression, stress, and social support as predictors of high-risk sexual behaviors and STIs in young women. *Journal of Adolescent Health, 39,* 601–603.

Morris, W. N., & Reilly, N. P. (1987). Toward the self-regulation of mood: Theory and research. *Motivation and Emotion, 11,* 215–249.

Office of National AIDS Policy. (1996). *Youth and HIV/AIDS: An American agenda.* Retrieved August 1, 2003, from http://clinton5.nara.gov/ONAP/youth/youth4.html.

Orr, S. T., Celentano, D. D., Santelli, J., & Burwell, L. (1994). Depressive symptoms and risk factors for HIV acquisition among black women attending urban health centers in Baltimore. *AIDS Education and Prevention, 6,* 230–236.

Orvaschel, H., Beeferman, D., & Kabacoff, R. (1997). Depression, self-esteem, sex, and age in a child and adolescent clinical sample. *Journal of Clinical Child Psychology, 26,* 285–289.

Pao, M., Lyon, M., D'Angelo, L. J., Schuman, W. B., Tipnis, T., & Mrazek, D. A. (2000). Psychiatric diagnoses in adolescents seropositive for the human immunodeficiency virus. *Archives of Pediatrics and Adolescent Medicine, 154,* 240–244.

Paxton, R. J., Valois, R. F., Watkins, K. W., Huebner, E. S., & Drane, J. W. (2007). Associations between depressed mood and clusters of health risk behaviors. *American Journal of Health Behavior, 31,* 272–283.

Pielage, S. B., Luteijn, F., & Arrindell, W. A. (2005). Adult attachment, intimacy and psychological distress in a clinical and community sample. *Clinical Psychology and Psychotherapy, 12,* 455–464.

Planalp, S. (2003). The unacknowledged role of emotion in theories of close relationships: How do theories feel? *Communication Theory, 13,* 78–99.

Pogarsky, G., Thornberry, T. P., & Lizotte, A. J. (2006). Developmental outcomes for children of young mothers. *Journal of Marriage and Family, 68,* 332–344.

Ponton, L., DiClemente, R., & McKenna, S. (1991). An AIDS education and prevention program for hospitalized adolescents. *Journal of the American Academy of Child and Adolescent Psychiatry, 30,* 729–734.

Ramrakha, S., Caspi, A., Dickson, N., Moffitt, T. E., & Paul, C. (2000). Psychiatric disorders and risky sexual behaviour in young adulthood: Cross-sectional study in birth cohort. *British Medical Journal, 321,* 263–266.

Rao, U., Daley, S. E., & Hammen, C. (2000). Relationship between depression and substance use disorders in adolescent women during the transition to adulthood. *Journal of the American Academy of Child and Adolescent Psychiatry, 39,* 215–222.

Resnick, M. D., Bearman, P. S., Blum, R. W., Bauman, K. E., Harris, K. M., Jones, J., Tabor, J., Beahring, T., Sieving, R. E., Shew, M., Ireland, M., Bearinger, L. H., & Udry, J. R. (1997). Protecting adolescents from harm: Findings from the National Longitudinal Study on Adolescent Health. *Journal of the American Medical Association, 278,* 823–832.

Rink, E., Tricker, R., & Harvey, S. M. (2007). Onset of sexual intercourse among female adolescents: The influence of perceptions, depression, and ecological factors. *Journal of Adolescent Health, 41,* 398–406.

Riolo, S. A., Nguyen, T. A., Greden, J. F., & King, C. A. (2005). Prevalence of depression by race/ethnicity: Findings from the National Health and Nutrition Examination Survey III. *American Journal of Public Health, 95,* 998–1000.

Roberts, J. E., Gotlib, I. H., & Kassel, J. D. (1996). Adult attachment security and symptoms of depression: The mediating roles of dysfunctional attitudes and low self-esteem. *Journal of Personality and Social Psychology, 70,* 310–320.

Rosenberg, P. S., Biggar, R. J., & Goedert, J. J. (1994). Declining age at HIV infection in the United States. *New England Journal of Medicine, 330,* 789–790.

Rosenthal, S. L., Biro, F. M., Cohen, S. S., Succop, P. A., & Stanberry, L. R. (1995). Strategies for coping with sexually transmitted diseases by adolescent females. *Adolescence, 30,* 655–666.

Rostosky, S. S., Galliher, R. V., Welsh, D. P., & Kawaguchi, M. C. (2000). Sexual behaviors and relationship qualities in late adolescent couples. *Journal of Adolescence, 23,* 583–597.

Rotheram-Borus, M. J., Swendeman, D., Comulada, W. S., Weiss, R. E., Lee, M., & Lightfoot, M. (2004). Prevention for substance-using HIV-positive young people: Telephone and in-person delivery. *Journal of Acquired Immune Deficiency Syndrome, 37,* S68–S77.

Saluja, G., Iachan, R., Scheidt, P. C., Overpeck, M. D., Sun, W., & Giedd, J. N. (2004). Prevalence of and risk factors for depressive symptoms among young adolescents. *Archives of Pediatrics and Adolescent Medicine, 158,* 760–765.

Santelli, J. S., Lowry, R., Brener, N. D., & Robin, L. (2000). The association of sexual behaviors with socioeconomic status, family structure, and race/ethnicity among US adolescents. *American Journal of Public Health, 90,* 1582–1588.

Shrier, L., Braslins, P., Christiansen, D., Markowitz, L. E., Fortenberry, J. D., & Orr, D. (2003, July 30). *Gender differences in the associations of mental health, sexual risk behavior, and sexually transmitted infection among adolescents and young adults.* Paper presented at the International Society for Sexually Transmitted Disease Research, Ottawa, Ontario.

Shrier, L., Harris, S., & Beardslee, W. (2002). Temporal associations between depressive symptoms and self-reported sexually transmitted disease among adolescents. *Archives of Pediatrics and Adolescent Medicine, 156,* 599–606.

Shrier, L., Shih, M.-C., Hacker, L., & de Moor, C. D. (2007). A momentary sampling study of the affective experience following coital events in adolescents. *Journal of Adolescent Health, 40,* 357. e1–e8.

Shrier, L. A., Shih, M. -C., Beardslee, W. R. (2005). "Affect and sexual behavior in adolescents: a review of the literature and comparison of momentary sampling with diary and retrospective self-report methods of measurement." *Pediatrics, 115:* e573–e581.

Shrier, L. A., Schillinger, J. A., Aneja, P., Rice, P. A., Batteiger, B. E. Braslins, P. G., Orr, D. P., Fortenberry, J. D. (In press). Depressive symptoms and sexual risk behavior in young, Chlamydia-infected, heterosexual dyads. *Journal of Adolescent Health.*

Shrier, L. A., Koren, S., Aneja, P., & de Moor, C. (2008). Affect regulation, social context, and sexual intercourse in adolescents. *Archives of Sexual Behavior.* DOI 10.1007/s10508-008-9394-1.

Shrier, L. A., Emans, S. J., Woods, E. R., & DuRant, R. H. (1997). The association of sexual risk behaviors and problem drug behaviors in high school students. *Journal of Adolescent Health, 20,* 377–383.

Shrier, L. A., Harris, S. K., Kurland, M., & Knight, J. R. (2003). Substance use problems and associated psychiatric symptoms among adolescents in primary care. *Pediatrics, 111,* e699–e705.

Shrier, L. A., Harris, S. K., Sternberg, M., & Beardslee, W. R. (2001). Associations of depression, self-esteem, and substance use with sexual risk among adolescents. *Preventive Medicine, 33,* 179–189.

Siegel, S. J., & Alloy, L. B. (1990). Interpersonal perceptions and consequences of depressive-significant other relationships: A naturalistic study of college roommates. *Journal of Abnormal Psychology, 99,* 361–373.

Slonim-Nevo, V., Ozawa, M. N., & Auslander, W. F. (1991). Knowledge, attitudes and behaviors related to AIDS among youth in residential centers: Results from an exploratory study. *Journal of Adolescence, 14,* 17–33.

Smith, M. D. (2001). HIV risk in adolescents with severe mental illness: Literature review. *Journal of Adolescent Health, 29,* 320–329.

Spencer, J. M., Zimet, G. D., Aalsma, M. C., & Orr, D. P. (2002). Self-esteem as a predictor of initiation of coitus in early adolescents. *Pediatrics, 109,* 581–584.

Sterk, C. E., Theall, K. P., & Elifson, K. W. (2006). The impact of emotional distress on HIV risk reduction among women. *Substance Use and Misuse, 41,* 157–173.

Stiffman, A. R., Dore, P., Earls, F., & Cunningham, R. (1992). The influence of mental health problems on AIDS-related risk behaviors in young adults. *Journal of Nervous and Mental Disease, 180,* 314–320.

Tapert, S. F., Aarons, G. A., Sedlar, G. R., & Brown, S. A. (2001). Adolescent substance use and sexual risk-taking behavior. *Journal of Adolescent Health, 28,* 181–189.

Thurstone, C., Riggs, P. D., Klein, C., & Mikulich-Gilbertson, S. K. (2007). A one-session human immunodeficiency virus risk-reduction intervention in adolescents with psychiatric and substance use disorders. *Journal of the American Academy of Child and Adolescent Psychiatry, 46,* 1179–1186.

Valois, R. F., Bryant, E. S., Rivard, J. C., & Hinkle, K. T. (1997). Sexual risk-taking behaviors among adolescents with severe emotional disturbance. *Journal of Child and Family Studies, 6,* 409–419.

Waller, M. W., Hallfors, D. D., Halpern, C. T., Iritani, B. J., Ford, C. A., & Guo, G. (2006). Gender differences in associations between depressive symptoms and patterns of substance use and risky sexual behavior among a nationally representative sample of U.S. adolescents. *Archives of Women's Mental Health, 9,* 139–150.

Weinstein, E., & Rosen, E. (1991). The development of adolescent sexual intimacy: Implications for counseling. *Adolescence, 26,* 331–339.

Weinstock, H., Berman, S., & Cates, W., Jr. (2004). Sexually transmitted diseases among American youth: Incidence and prevalence estimates, 2000. *Perspectives on Sexual and Reproductive Health, 36,* 6–10.

CHAPTER

19

CONNECTEDNESS IN THE LIVES OF ADOLESCENTS

DEBRA H. BERNAT ▪ MICHAEL D. RESNICK

LEARNING OBJECTIVES

After studying this chapter, you will be able to

- Define connectedness and explain its association with adolescent health risk behavior.
- Summarize key theoretical frameworks for understanding connectedness as a protective factor against adolescent risk behavior.
- Describe how adolescent connectedness in various contexts influences subsequent risk behavior.

Connections that young people have to adults, the schools they attend, and the communities in which they live are key determinants of the health and well-being of adolescents. Research during the past two decades shows that a sense of connectedness to others and key institutions in their lives is protective against an array of health risk behaviors and is associated with better mental health outcomes (Hawkins, Catalano, Kosterman, Abbott, & Hill, 1999; Resnick et al., 1997). The 2003 Commission on Children at Risk, a group of prominent physicians, research scientists, and youth service professionals, identified a lack of connectedness as a major contributor to deteriorating behavioral and mental health among youth in the United States (Commission on Children at Risk, 2003). Specifically, they concluded:

> In large measure, what's causing this crisis of American childhood is a lack of connectedness. We mean two kinds of connectedness—close connections to other people, and deep connections to moral and spiritual meaning. Where does this connectedness come from? It comes from groups of people organized around certain purposes—what scholars call social institutions. In recent decades, the U.S. social institutions that foster these two forms of connectedness for children have gotten significantly weaker. That weakening, this report argues, is a major cause of the current mental and behavioral health crisis among U.S. children [pp. 1–2].

Based on current research from neuroscience and biology, the commission concluded that children are biologically primed to connect from birth, and the more this need is met the less likely it is that problems will develop.

KEY CONCEPTS AND RESEARCH FINDINGS: WHAT IS MEANT BY "CONNECTEDNESS"?

Connectedness is increasingly being used to refer to protective relationships that exist between adolescents and their environment. These include relationships that adolescents have with individuals (inside and outside of the family), as well as within their broader social context, including schools and other institutions (Allen, McElhaney, Kuperminc, & Jodl, 2004; Resnick, 2008). These anchoring points in the lives of young people represent the opposite of social isolation and disconnection, which is now described as a threat equal to that of tobacco use in terms of contribution to mortality (Putnam, Feldstein, & Cohen, 2003).

Theoretical Models

Several theories and models—including attachment theory, Hirschi's theory of deviant behavior, and Hawkins' social development model—serve as the foundation for understanding why connectedness may serve as a protective factor in the lives of adolescents. Perhaps the most important theory suggesting the strength of connectedness is attachment theory (Bowlby, 1980). *Attachment theory* describes the process by which infants become attached to their parents and provides a basis for how children form connections to others. Thus, interactions between infants and their caregivers form the foundation for connecting with others.

Hirschi's theory of deviant behavior (Hirschi, 1969) states that bonding within a socialization unit, such as school or family, consists of four elements: (1) involvement in the unit, (2) attachment or affective relationships, (3) investment or commitment to the unit, and (4) belief in the values of the unit. According to the theory of deviant behavior, once a bond is established, it will likely affect future behavior.

Finally, the *social development model* incorporates ideas from numerous theories including social learning theory, social control theory, and differential association theory (Catalano & Hawkins, 1996). This model suggests that socialization occurs through (1) perceived opportunities to participate in activities with others, (2) development of skills for involvement, and (3) rewards for involvement. The model suggests that involvement that is skillful is more likely to be reinforced, and this reinforcement is more likely to lead to attachment and commitment. It is believed that individuals' behavior will conform to the norms and behaviors of the unit they are bonded to, whether prosocial or antisocial. In each of the above instances, interaction is the basis for the development of a sense of connection to others, and through that sense of connectedness come identity, meaning, and internalization of norms, beliefs, values, as well as behaviors that reflect those internalized standards and preferences.

As suggested by the theories just described, health risk behavior takes place in the contexts in which adolescents live. Comprehensive models of adolescent development emphasize the importance of considering factors at all levels of influence. Thus, this chapter reviews research related to adolescents' connectedness as it pertains to religion, parents, nonparental adults, school, and the community.

Religiosity and Spiritual Connectedness

Interest in the role that religiosity and spirituality can play in the lives of adolescents has grown significantly in recent years. Adolescence may be an important time to study religiosity and spirituality (R/S), because it is a time when youths are seeking a sense of belonging and meaning in their life. However, little attention has been given to religiosity and spirituality in the scientific literature. Several studies, for example, suggest that less than one percent of articles on children and adolescents address religiosity (Boyatzis, 2003) and spirituality (Benson, Roehlkepartain, & Rude, 2003).

Measurement. In the majority of studies, *religiosity* refers to behavior, such as religious service attendance, prayer, and meditation, while *spirituality* refers to an internal process, such as spiritual well-being, support, and coping. Spirituality has also been characterized as development and deepening of a sense of awe, wonder, and mystery about the world and the universe (Lerner, 2000). A recent review of forty-three studies assessing the relationship between R/S and adolescent health found that more than half of the studies measured R/S as participation in religious activities or services (Rew & Wong, 2006). Other common measures of R/S include importance of religion and religious affiliation.

A substantial limitation of current research on religiosity and spirituality is related to the measurement of these constructs. Although religiosity is widely accepted as a multidimensional construct, single-item measures are often used. A recent review, for example, showed that of forty-three R/S studies, only fifteen studies on religiosity and three studies on spirituality included multi-item measures (Rew & Wong, 2006). Multidimensional, reliable, and valid measures are needed to better understand the relationship between spiritual connectedness and adolescent health and indicators of well-being, particularly those including beliefs, knowledge, and behaviors.

Research Findings. Data from the Monitoring the Future survey indicate that 43 percent of eighth graders, 40 percent of tenth graders, and 33 percent of twelfth graders attend religious services at least once a week (Child Trends, n.d.). These data are consistent with several studies showing that church attendance declines during the high school years (Kerestes, Youniss, & Metz, 2004). Interestingly, the importance of religion appears to remain stable across adolescence. These findings have been reported across various samples of adolescents. It is possible that younger adolescents go to church with their parents, but this practice becomes less common as youth get older. It is also possible that adolescents explore different ways to express beliefs as they reach young adulthood.

Spiritual or religious connectedness has been described as a protective factor against health risk behaviors and negative health outcomes. Numerous literature reviews have recently been conducted showing that adolescents with higher levels of spirituality and religiosity are less likely to engage in risky sexual behavior (Rostosky, Wilcox, Wright, & Randall, 2004) and substance use (Michalak, Trocki, & Bond, 2007) and have better mental health outcomes (Wong, Rew, & Slaikeu, 2006). These findings appear to hold true, regardless of denominational affiliation. Interestingly, adolescents from different denominational affiliations appear to be similar on measures of religiosity, including attendance and importance (Kerestes et al., 2004).

Exposure to more conventional beliefs, opportunities, and connections with others through church attendance may be the mechanism by which religiosity serves as a protective factor.

Adolescents for whom religiosity is important may engage in fewer health risk behaviors for several reasons. Religion may expose youth to more conventional beliefs and values (Walker, Ainette, Wills, & Mendoza, 2007), provide opportunities for adolescents to engage in prosocial activities, and connect youth to the broader community (King, 2003). One study, for example, found that regular church attendance was associated with more positive outcomes, regardless of whether adolescents believed in a higher power (Good & Willoughby, 2006). This finding supports the view that exposure to more conventional beliefs, opportunities, and connections with others through church attendance may be the mechanism by which religiosity serves as a protective factor.

The social context of religious group membership and religious observance may also invite a predilection toward an array of affiliative behaviors above and beyond the underlying human need for meaning and belonging (Boyden, 1978). Particularly in religious groups where emphasis is placed on service, communality, and empathy, group norms and expectations might then reinforce the value placed on social bonding, close emotional communication, and responsiveness to the needs of others (Bakan, 1966).

Future Directions. Further research is needed to develop multidimensional measures of religiosity and to better operationalize the more complex and elusive concept of spirituality. In addition, research is needed that examines religiosity and spirituality as dynamic processes during the adolescent years and to examine how social influences (such as parents and peers) relate to religiosity and spiritual connectedness across this developmental period. Finally, more research is needed to better understand how both religiosity and spirituality relate to positive outcomes in the lives of adolescents.

Parent-Child and Family Connectedness

Parents have perhaps the most influential role on their children. Although adolescence is often a time of gaining independence from one's family, research suggests that adolescents want close relationships with their parents and rely on them for support and guidance (Ungar, 2004). Strong bonds between parents and adolescents protect youth from engaging in health risk behaviors, particularly when parents recognize, value, and reward prosocial behaviors (Resnick et al., 1997).

Measurement. Parent-child connectedness (PCC) generally refers to the quality of the bond between a parent and a child (Lezin, Rolleri, Bean, & Taylor, 2004). A recent review suggests that PCC measures generally assess characteristics such as attachment and bonding (parents and child share thoughts and feelings, for example), warmth and caring (parents help child), cohesion (family spends time together), support and involvement (parents attend school events), communication (frequency of discussions), monitoring and control (parental presence), autonomy (child has voice in family decisions), and maternal and paternal characteristics (depression, for example) (Lezin et al., 2004). A closely related construct is family connectedness, which refers to a sense of belonging and closeness to one's family more broadly.

Research Findings. It has been well established that PCC is associated with lower levels of health risk behaviors. Using a nationally representative data set, for example, Resnick et al. examined the relationship between family connectedness and eight areas including emotional distress, suicide, violence, substance use (tobacco, alcohol, and marijuana use), sexual debut, and pregnancy (Resnick et al., 1997). Family connectedness (defined as closeness to parents, perceived caring, satisfaction, and feeling loved and wanted) was protective against all outcomes examined, except history of pregnancy. They also found that parental presence, shared family activities, and high expectations were important predictors of adolescent health outcomes. In a review of connections in the lives of adolescents, Blum and Rinehart noted: "Time and time again, the home environment emerges as central in shaping health outcomes for American youth. Controlling for the number of parents in a household, controlling for whether families are rich or poor, controlling for race and ethnicity, children who report feeling connected to a parent are protected against many different kinds of health risk, including emotional distress, and suicidal thoughts and attempts; cigarette, alcohol, and marijuana use; violent behavior; and early sexual activity" (Blum & Rinehart, 1997, p. 16).

Family connectedness has been referred to as one of the most powerful protective factors in the lives of adolescents (Resnick, Harris, & Blum 1993). Questions used to assess family connectedness often do not specify the nature of family. Family connectedness in its most basic form refers to connectedness with at least one competent and caring adult. Thus, families of many different types may play a protective role in the lives of adolescents. Indeed, analyses have indicated the primacy of family dynamics over family structure in terms of buffering effects against self-destructive, risky behaviors in adolescents (Gil, Vega, & Biafora, 1998).

Research has begun to investigate how PCC may work to reduce negative outcomes and increases the likelihood of positive outcomes. Although extensive research exists on the importance of *parental monitoring* (parents knowing where their children are and who they are with), research indicates that parental monitoring is particularly effective when it increases communication between a parent and child and the child informs parents of his or her whereabouts (Stattin & Kerr, 2000). Thus, direct control of a child's behavior does not necessarily explain the protective effect of parental monitoring on health outcomes of adolescents. However, parents who are close to their children may be better able to monitor and control how their children spend their time, which may reduce the likelihood that they will become involved in health risk behaviors (Henrich, Brookmeyer, & Shahar, 2005). To date, it is unclear whether PCC is protective once adolescents have become engaged in risky behaviors. A recent study on weapon violence, for example, found that relationships with parents were not as protective once youth became engaged in these behaviors. This suggests that promoting parent-child connectedness may be particularly important for primary prevention programs that begin prior to adolescence or before the onset of particular health risk behaviors.

Another line of research has begun to examine the interplay of family characteristics and PCC in relationship to health risk behaviors. For example, it is known from previous research that parents' own behaviors play an important role in adolescent development, as parents are primary role models for their children. For example, a recent study examined the interplay between parental tobacco smoking and PCC on youth smoking (Tilson, McBride, Lipkus, & Catalano, 2004). This study found that high PCC was not protective against smoking among youth whose parents smoked. The findings showed that adolescents whose parents smoked were equally likely to become smokers, regardless of how connected they were to their parents.

Future Directions. Future research should continue to examine how and when PCC is protective for adolescents. It is also critical to continue to examine how PCC interacts with other parental influences and family characteristics. Also, examining differential effects of connections adolescents have to mothers and fathers is an important direction for future research.

Connections to Nonparental Adults

Although parents are among the most influential adults in the lives of young people, adolescents develop important relationships with adults besides their parents. These relationships may include teachers, coaches, friends' parents, neighbors, counselors, and religious leaders. The relationships may develop through existing social networks or as part of formal mentoring programs. Research shows that relationships with prosocial nonparental adults can have a strong positive effect on adolescent development.

The majority of adolescents report having at least one important relationship with a nonparental adult. In a recent study, nearly three quarters (73 percent) of adolescents from a nationally representative sample reported having a mentor (DuBois & Silverthorn, 2005). Extended family members (such as aunts, uncles, cousins, and grandparents) are among those most commonly reported as *mentors* (Rhodes, Ebert, & Fischer, 1992; Zimmerman, Bingenheimer, & Notaro, 2002). Other commonly reported mentors included those involved in the day-to-day lives of adolescents, including teachers, religious leaders, coaches, and friends' parents; some of this research has suggested the particular salience of the parent(s) of a best friend, in terms of willingness to communicate and confide (Benson, 2006).

Measurement. Researchers have used different terminology to study the role of nonparental adults in the lives of adolescents. The two terms most commonly used are "natural mentors" (DuBois & Silverthorn, 2005; Zimmerman et al., 2002) and "very important nonparental adults" (Beam, Chen, & Greenberger, 2002). There is general agreement, however, that mentors are nonparental adults who provide support and guidance to adolescents. *Natural mentors* are individuals within the adolescent's existing social network, as opposed to a relationship that develops through a formal mentoring program.

> *Mentors are nonparental adults who provide support and guidance to adolescents.*

Research Findings. Studies have been conducted to assess the overall effects of both natural mentors and formal mentoring programs (such as Big Brothers Big Sisters of America) on a range of outcomes including academic achievement, problem behaviors, physical health, and mental health. A recent study of the effects of natural mentors on adolescents using a nationally representative sample found that adolescents with natural mentors were more likely to complete high school and college, have higher self-esteem and life satisfaction, and engage in healthy lifestyle behaviors such as physical activity and birth control use (DuBois & Silverthorn, 2005). Adolescents with natural mentors were also less likely to engage in problem behaviors such as violence. Overall, these results show that natural mentors can have a broad effect on the health and well-being of adolescents. Further, findings did not vary by individual or environmental risk factors, suggesting that all adolescents can benefit from relationships with nonparental adults. It is worth noting, however, that the effects of natural mentors do not completely offset individual and environmental risk factors, suggesting that natural mentors alone are not enough to undo multiple risk factors that may exist in the lives of adolescents. An enduring research agenda with substantive implications for health and social service providers is the extent to which the protective effects of connectedness to natural mentors can offset the deleterious effects of neglectful or overtly damaging family environments. Many interventions are grounded in the assumption that when families cannot be a source of nurturance for adolescents, the protective effects of connectedness with caring, competent adults can be transplanted into the lives of adolescents who are bereft of such nourishment (Bernat & Resnick, 2006).

Although many adolescents have natural mentors, many also receive mentoring through formal mentoring programs. Although the benefits of having natural mentors have been well documented, it is unclear whether mentoring relationships through a formal program can produce similar results. A recent meta-analysis including fifty-five evaluations of formal mentoring programs found positive effects of formal mentoring programs on emotional, behavioral, and educational outcomes; however, the overall effect was small (DuBois, Holloway, Valentine, & Cooper, 2002). Mentoring programs in general had the largest effect on adolescents from disadvantaged backgrounds, which may be because formal mentoring programs are often designed specifically for those at higher risk for negative outcomes. A critical aspect of formal mentoring programs is the quality of program implementation. This meta-analysis revealed substantial heterogeneity in estimates of effect size for the programs included, which may account for the overall small effect found. Future evaluations of formal mentoring programs need to give careful consideration to quality of implementation.

Beyond understanding the overall effects that mentoring can have on the lives of adolescents, researchers have also been working to understand the role that nonparental adults play in the lives of adolescents and how they may benefit from these relationships. Research suggests that mentors may affect adolescent development both directly and indirectly. Because mentors are outside the family context, mentors provide a safe context for adolescents to talk about their lives and at the same time provide opportunities for mentors to instill adults' values and perspectives. Thus, mentors may directly reduce the likelihood of adolescents engaging in risky behaviors by conveying messages about the dangers associated with these behaviors. Mentors may indirectly affect health-compromising behaviors by affecting factors related to these behaviors, such as self-worth, future aspirations, and academic achievement. Positive effects of mentors may also be the result of improving relationships with parents and peers. Mentors have been shown to improve relationship skills, which may improve adolescents' ability to communicate with parents and build relationship with prosocial peers (Rhodes, Haight, & Briggs, 1999).

School Connectedness

Adolescents' relationship to school plays an important role in their development. Work by the Search Institute in Minneapolis, Minnesota, and results from the National Longitudinal Study of Adolescent Health (Add Health) have increased attention to school connectedness as an important protective factor in the lives of adolescents during the past decade. Greater school connectedness has been associated with (1) better academic outcomes, including higher academic performance (Anderman & Freeman, 2004) and school completion (Bond et al., 2007); and (2) lower levels of involvement in health-risk behaviors, including substance use (Catalano, Haggerty, Oesterle, Fleming, & Hawkins, 2004), violent behavior (Karcher, 2002), and risky sexual behavior (Catalano et al., 2004). The Institute of Medicine (1997) suggests that "in some situations, a healthful psychosocial environment (in school) may be as important—or even more important—than classroom health education in keeping students away from drugs, alcohol, violence, risky sexual behavior, and the rest of today's social morbidities."

Measurement. School connectedness generally refers to students' beliefs that adults in their school care about them as students and as individuals (Blum & Libbey, 2004). A variety of constructs have been used to evaluate a student's relationship to school, including school connectedness, school attachment, school bonding, orientation toward school, school engagement, school involvement, satisfaction with school, identification with school, and teacher support (Libbey, 2004). Many of these constructs measure similar aspects of a student's relationship to school, including academic engagement, belonging, fairness in discipline practices, participation in extracurricular activities, liking school, student voice, peer relationships, safety, and teacher support (Libbey, 2004).

Summary of Research Findings. Despite various measures of school connectedness, research consistently shows that students who feel connected to school report higher levels of academic performance and lower levels of involvement in health risk behaviors compared to those who feel less connected to school. In a nationally representative sample of adolescents across the United States, school connectedness was found to be protective against emotional distress, suicidal thoughts and behaviors, violence, substance use, and age of sexual debut (Resnick et al., 1997). As noted previously, in this study school connectedness was related to all health outcomes examined, except history of pregnancy. Some research suggests this relationship may be causal, because interventions designed to increase school bonding or school connectedness have resulted in decreases in health risk behavior (Hawkins, Guo, Hill, Battin-Pearson, & Abbott, 2001).

Because school connectedness measures tap different dimensions of a student's relationship to school, research has begun assessing which aspects of school connectedness relate to positive outcomes. A review of the most recent theoretical and empirical work on school connectedness suggests that the most important environmental factors associated with school connectedness include high expectations for academic success, perceived support from school staff, and a safe school environment (Blum & Libbey, 2004). These findings are consistent with research that has compared effects of teacher support versus social belonging on health outcomes. One study, for example, found that students who felt their teachers were fair and cared about them were less likely to initiate six health risk behaviors (smoking tobacco, drinking to the point of getting drunk, marijuana use, suicidal ideation or attempt, sexual intercourse, and weapon-related violence), whereas feeling a part of school and enjoying school were not protective against any of these behaviors (McNeely & Falci, 2004).

> *Research has begun assessing which aspects of school connectedness relate to positive outcomes.*

Understanding why some students feel connected to school but other students do not has also been a focus of numerous studies. Research consistently shows that school connectedness is higher in younger students, students from two-parent households, students who perform well in school, students who participate in extracurricular activities, and students with more friends (McNeely, Nonnemaker, & Blum, 2002; Thompson, Iachan, Overpeck, Ross, & Gross, 2006). Studies also suggest a relationship between connectedness and gender, race, and having educated parents, but current findings regarding these factors are equivocal. Some studies, for example, show that males are more connected to school than females, while other studies show higher connectedness among females. More recent studies have also examined how school and neighborhood characteristics may be associated with school connectedness. Connectedness appears to be higher in schools with wealthier students and lower in neighborhoods with more renters, which may be related to living in a more transient environment.

Future Directions. Future research on school connectedness should continue to identify individual, school, and community characteristics associated with connectedness that could be modified through interventions. In addition, identifying aspects of school connectedness that are most strongly related to health outcomes could clarify intervention targets. It is also important to assess school connectedness over time. Age clearly plays an important role in school connectedness, and understanding the needs of students at various ages is critical. In the context of eroding school budgets and the growing complexity of health and social issues presented at school by young people, educators and school administrators have a particular interest in research that informs the question of how to enhance and deepen school connectedness and positive school climate, particularly in a context of scarce resources and little discretionary funding for schools.

Community Connectedness

Research designed to better understand how the broader social context affects adolescent health is growing. Research to date suggests that connection to one's community is associated with lower levels of health risk behaviors and higher levels of prosocial behavior.

Measurement. Community connectedness often refers to adolescents' perceptions of caring by adults in the community (Rauner, 2000). Several terms are used in the scientific literature to refer to *community connectedness*, including collective efficacy, social capital, social cohesion, and community attachment. Measures of caring by adults in the community often ask about adolescents' perception of caring by adults, including neighbors, school staff, and church leaders (Borowsky, Resnick, Ireland, & Blum, 1999). *Sense of community* refers to emotional connection and belonging in the neighborhood (Chavis & Pretty, 1999; Chavis & Wandersman, 1990). This is often measured by items such as "I feel connected to this neighborhood," "I feel at home in this neighborhood," and "It is very important to me to live in this particular neighborhood." In addition, community connectedness measures often assess collective action, such as how much neighbors will work together to solve problems, how much neighbors are willing to share, and how much fun neighbors have with each other. To be clear, most measures of community connectedness could rightly be viewed as subsumed under the larger construct of social capital, of which community identification and collective efficacy are a part.

Research Findings. Research to date suggests that connection to community is associated with lower levels of health risk behaviors and higher levels of prosocial behavior among adolescents. A recent study, for example, found that communities with greater social capital (measured as resources for adolescents in the community) had lower rates of health risk behaviors, higher rates of health care utilization, and lower health care expenditures than communities with less social capital (Youngblade, Curry, Novak, Vogel, & Shenkman, 2006). Another study using a large sample of adolescents from the National Survey of Children's Health found that adolescents who lived in neighborhoods with greater connectedness (measured as how much neighbors help each other) had greater social competence and health-promoting behavior compared to adolescents living in less connected communities (Youngblade et al., 2007). This finding was consistent across sociodemographic groups.

Research to date suggests that connection to community is associated with lower levels of health risk behaviors and higher levels of prosocial behavior.

For community connectedness, the most influential factors are relations between adults and adolescents, voice in the community, attitudes toward adolescents, and opportunities for creative engagement.

Future Directions. The work of Putnam, Feldstein, and Cohen (2003) demonstrates that even in the context of poverty, health is better in communities characterized by strong social capital and interpersonal bonds. Little, however, is known about the potentially detrimental effects of feeling closely connected to a community where there is substantial role modeling of antisocial behavior—where negative, antisocial behaviors are perceived to be (or may actually be) the norm. In such instances, it might be expected that community connectedness would portend more, rather than fewer, risky behaviors, consistent with evidence, for example, that the social norms of groups that teens are connected to will influence their sexual behavior (Kirby, 2001).

SUMMARY

The research summarized in this chapter indicates the importance of adolescents' connections to others and institutions for their health and well-being. A sense of connectedness has been found to be protective against an array of health risk behaviors including substance use, risky sexual behavior, and violence (Catalano et al., 2004; Resnick et al., 1997; Resnick, Harris, & Blum, 1993). Research suggests that positive connections are beneficial for all adolescents—across gender and racial, ethnic, and social class groups (Bernat & Resnick, 2006; Resnick et al., 1997). This is important insofar as most interventions are designed to target specific groups of adolescents, but this also suggests the utility of broad, adolescent development–focused strategies that seek to promote universal, cross-cutting protective factors across social groups of youth (Resnick, 2005).

It is important to note, however, that connections to others may not always provide protection to adolescents. In particular, connections to peers (as well as adults) have been shown to relate to both positive and negative outcomes, depending on whether their peers are engaging in prosocial or antisocial behavior. Thus, it is critical that connections involve prosocial adults and prosocial peers to create a positive effect on adolescent development.

In this chapter, we have synthesized five areas of connectedness that have been related to better health outcomes among adolescents. These areas are not independent of one another. For example, schools and nonparental adults exist within communities and may represent an important aspect of community connectedness. Furthermore, the more connected adolescents feel in one area, the more likely they are to feel connected in another (analogous to a long-standing line of research that documents the clustering of health-jeopardizing behaviors). It is possible that when adolescents feel connected in one area, this builds skills and access to resources that are transferable to other settings. Thus, interventions designed to build connectedness in one aspect of adolescents' lives may have implications for other areas—as has been amply demonstrated by successful service-learning programs, where participation in community service in the second decade of life is predictive of future civic engagement (Zaff, Malanchuk, Michelsen, & Eccles, 2003).

Overall, connectedness is a dynamic process that varies throughout adolescence. Adolescents may need different relationships, opportunities, and experiences to maintain a sense of connectedness to prosocial individuals, groups, and institutions over time. The opportunities and experiences adolescents need may vary greatly from ninth to twelfth grade. Thus, it is critical to better understand the needs of adolescents over time and, in a corresponding fashion, how institutions and adults can support these needs as they change, particularly as young people grow in their need for differentiation, independence, and autonomy.

Despite tremendous growth in the area of connectedness research in the past two decades, research in this area is still limited. Given the various definitions that have been assigned to the concept of connectedness and the challenges in implementing and maintaining longitudinal studies that include both large and socially diverse groups of adolescents, we still need to explore the more encompassing question, What forms of connectedness have what kinds of impact and outcomes among what groups of adolescents? This question alone creates a substantive, long-term agenda for research, with potentially great implications for understanding both fundamental processes of healthy adolescent development, as well as the application of such knowledge to programs, policy, and practice among the wide array of adults working with and on behalf of adolescents.

KEY TERMS

Attachment theory
Community connectedness
Connectedness
Family connectedness

Hirschi's theory of deviant behavior
Mentors
Natural mentors
Parent-child connectedness (PCC)

Parental monitoring

Religiosity

School connectedness

Sense of community

Social development model

Spirituality

DISCUSSION QUESTIONS

1. Elaborate on some of the challenges faced by researchers when trying to measure connectedness in different contexts.

2. Does one level of connectedness have more influence over another in terms of reducing risk behavior among adolescents (such as school connectedness versus parent-child connectedness)? Explain.

3. How can health interventionists better incorporate the concept of connectedness when targeting adolescents? Is it possible to alter or strengthen connections that have already been formed to promote behavior change?

REFERENCES

Allen, J. P., McElhaney, K. B., Kuperminc, G. P., & Jodl, K. M. (2004). Stability and change in attachment security across adolescence. *Child Development, 75*(6), 1792–1805.

Anderman, L. H., & Freeman, T. M. (2004). Students' sense of belonging to school. In P. R. Pintrich & M. L. Maehr (Eds.), *Advances in motivation and achievement* (Vol. 13, pp. 27–63). Oxford, England: Elsevier.

Bakan, D. (1966). *The duality of human existence: Isolation and communion in Western man.* Boston: Beacon Press.

Beam, M. R., Chen, C., & Greenberger, E. (2002). The nature of adolescents' relationships with their "very important" nonparental adults. *American Journal of Community Psychology, 30*(2), 305–325.

Benson, P. (2006). *All kids are our kids: What communities must do to raise caring and responsible children and adolescents* (2nd ed.). New York: Wiley.

Benson, P. L., Roehlkepartain, E. C., & Rude, S. P. (2003). Spiritual development in childhood and adolescence: Toward a field of inquiry. *Applied Developmental Science, 7,* 204–212.

Bernat, D. H., & Resnick, M. D. (2006). Healthy youth development: science and strategies. *Journal of Public Health Management and Practice,* Suppl., S10–S16.

Blum, R. W., & Libbey, H. P. (2004). Executive summary. *Journal of School Health, 74*(7), 231.

Blum, R. W., & Rinehart, P. M. (1997). Reducing the risk: Connections that make a difference in the lives of youth (No. 40). Minneapolis: University of Minnesota, Division of Pediatrics and Adolescent Health.

Bond, L., Butler, H., Thomas, L., Carlin, J., Glover, S., Bowes, G., & Patton, G. (2007). Social and school connectedness in early secondary school as predictors of late teenage substance use, mental health, and academic outcomes. *Journal of Adolescent Health, 40*(4): 357. e9–18.

Borowsky, I. W., Resnick, M. D., Ireland, M., & Blum, R. W. (1999). Suicide attempts among American Indian and Alaska Native youth: Risk and protective factors. *Archives of Pediatric and Adolescent Medicine, 153*(6), 573–580.

Bowlby, J. (1980). *Attachment and loss: Sadness and depression.* London: Hogarth Press.

Boyatzis, C. J. (2003). Religious and spiritual development: An introduction. *Review of Religious Research, 44,* 213–219.

Boyden, S. (1978). *Western civilization in biological perspective.* Cambridge: Oxford University Press.

Catalano, R. F., Haggerty, K. P., Oesterle, S., Fleming, C. B., & Hawkins, J. D. (2004). The importance of bonding to school for healthy development: Findings from the Social Development Research Group. *Journal of School Health, 74*(7), 252–261.

Catalano, R. F., & Hawkins, J. D. (1996). The social development model: A theory of antisocial behavior. In J. D. Hawkins (Ed.), *Delinquency and crime: Current theories.* New York: Cambridge University Press.

Chavis, D., & Pretty, G. (1999). Sense of community: Advances in measurement and application. *Journal of Community Psychology, 27,* 635–642.

Chavis, D., & Wandersman, A. (1990). Sense of community in the urban environment: A catalyst for participation and community development. *American Journal of Community Psychology, 18,* 55–81.

Child Trends. (n.d.). Religious services attendance. Washington, DC: Author.

Commission on Children at Risk. (2003). Hardwired to connect: The new scientific case for authoritative communities. New York: Institute for American Values.

DuBois, D. L., Holloway, B. E., Valentine, J. C., & Cooper, H. (2002). Effectiveness of mentoring programs for youth: A meta-analytic review. *American Journal of Community Psychology, 30*(2), 157–197.

DuBois, D. L., & Silverthorn, N. (2005). Natural mentoring relationships and adolescent health: Evidence from a national study. *American Journal of Public Health, 95*(3), 518–524.

Gil, A. G., Vega, W. A., & Biafora, F. (1998). Temporal influences of family structure and family risk factors on drug use initiation in a multiethnic sample of adolescent boys. *Journal of Youth and Adolescence, 27*(3), 373–393.

Good, M., & Willoughby, T. (2006). The role of spirituality versus religiosity in adolescent psychosocial adjustment. *Journal of Youth and Adolescence, 35*(1), 41–55.

Hawkins, J. D., Catalano, R. F., Kosterman, R., Abbott, R., & Hill, K. G. (1999). Preventing adolescent health-risk behaviors by strengthening protection during childhood. *Archives of Pediatric Adolescent Medicine, 153*(3), 226–234.

Hawkins, J. D., Guo, J., Hill, K. G., Battin-Pearson, S., & Abbott, R. D. (2001). Long-Term Effects of the Seattle Social Development Intervention on School Bonding Trajectories. *Applied Developmental Science, 5*(4), 225–236.

Henrich, C. C., Brookmeyer, K. A., & Shahar, G. (2005). Weapon violence in adolescence: Parent and school connectedness as protective factors. *Journal of Adolescent Health, 37*(4), 306–312.

Hirschi, T. (1969). *Causes of delinquency.* Berkeley: University of California Press.

Institute of Medicine. (1997). *Schools and health: Our nation's investment.* Washington, DC: National Academy Press.

Karcher, M. J. (2002). Connectedness and school violence: A framework for developmental interventions. In E. Gerler (Ed.), *Handbook of school violence* (pp. 7–40). Binghamton, NY: Haworth.

Kerestes, M., Youniss, J., & Metz, E. (2004). Longitudinal patterns of religious perspective and civic integration. *Applied Developmental Science, 8*(1), 39–46.

King, P. E. (2003). Religion and identity: The role of ideological, social, and spiritual contexts. *Applied Developmental Science, 7,* 197–204.

Kirby, D. (2001). Understanding what works and what doesn't in reducing adolescent sexual risk-taking. *Family Planning Perspectives, 33*(6), 276–281.

Lerner, M. (2000). *Spirit matters.* Charlottesville, VA: Hampton Roads.

Lezin, N., Rolleri, L. A., Bean, S., & Taylor, J. (2004). Parent-child connectedness: Implications for research, interventions, and positive impacts on adolescent health. Scotts Valley, CA: ETR Associates.

Libbey, H. P. (2004). Measuring student relationships to school: Attachment, bonding, connectedness, and engagement. *Journal of School Health, 74*(7), 274–283.

McNeely, C., & Falci, C. (2004). School connectedness and the transition into and out of health-risk behavior among adolescents: A comparison of social belonging and teacher support. *Journal of School Health, 74*(7), 284–292.

McNeely, C. A., Nonnemaker, J. M., & Blum, R. W. (2002). Promoting school connectedness: Evidence from the National Longitudinal Study of Adolescent Health. *Journal of School Health, 72*(4), 138–146.

Michalak, L., Trocki, K., & Bond, J. (2007). Religion and alcohol in the U.S. National Alcohol Survey: How important is religion for abstention and drinking? *Drug and Alcohol Dependence, 87*(2–3), 268–280.

Putnam, R. D., Feldstein, L. M., & Cohen, D. J. (2003). *Better together: Restoring the American community.* New York: Simon & Schuster.

Rauner, J. (2000). *The role of caring in youth development and community life.* New York: Columbia University Press.

Resnick, M. D. (2005). Healthy youth development: Getting our priorities right. *Medical Journal of Australia, 183*(8), 398–400.

Resnick, M. D. (2008). Best bets for improving the odds for optimum youth development. In K. K. Kline (Ed.), *Authoritative communities: The scientific case for nurturing the whole child* (pp. 137–150). New York: Springer.

Resnick, M. D., Bearman, P. S., Blum, R. W., Bauman, K. E., Harris, K. M., Jones, J., Tabor, J., Beuhring, T., Sieving, R. E., Shew, M., Ireland, M., Bearinger, L. H., & Udry, J. R. (1997). Protecting adolescents from harm: Findings from the National Longitudinal Study on Adolescent Health. *Journal of the American Medical Association, 278*(10), 823–832.

Resnick, M. D., Harris, L. J., & Blum, R. W. (1993). The impact of caring and connectedness on adolescent health and well-being. *Journal of Paediatrics and Child Health, 29*(Suppl. 1), S3–S9.

Rew, L., & Wong, Y. J. (2006). A systematic review of associations among religiosity/spirituality and adolescent health attitudes and behaviors. *Journal of Adolescent Health, 38*(4), 433–442.

Rhodes, J. E., Ebert, L., & Fischer, K. (1992). Natural mentors: An overlooked resource in the social networks of young, African American mothers. *American Journal of Community Psychology, 20,* 445–461.

Rhodes, J. E., Haight, W. L., & Briggs, E. C. (1999). The influence of mentoring on the peer relationships of foster youth in relative and nonrelative care. *Journal of Research on Adolescence, 9*(2), 185–201.

Rostosky, S. S., Wilcox, B. L., Wright, M.L.C., & Randall, B. A. (2004). The impact of religiosity on adolescent sexual behavior: A review of the evidence. *Journal of Adolescent Research, 19*(6), 677–697.

Stattin, H., & Kerr, M. (2000). Parental monitoring: A reinterpretation. *Child Development, 71*(4), 1072–1085.

Thompson, D. R., Iachan, R., Overpeck, M., Ross, J. G., & Gross, L. A. (2006). School connectedness in the Health Behavior in School-Aged Children Study: The role of student, school, and school neighborhood characteristics. *Journal of School Health, 76*(7), 379–386.

Tilson, E. C., McBride, C. M., Lipkus, I. M., & Catalano, R. F. (2004). Testing the interaction between parent-child relationship factors and parent smoking to predict youth smoking. *Journal of Adolescent Health, 35*(3), 182–189.

Ungar, M. (2004). The importance of parents and other caregivers to the resilience of high-risk adolescents. *Family Process, 43*(1), 23–41.

Walker, C., Ainette, M. G., Wills, T. A., & Mendoza, D. (2007). Religiosity and substance use: Test of an indirect-effect model in early and middle adolescence. *Psychology of Addictive Behaviors, 21*(1), 84–96.

Wong, Y. J., Rew, L., & Slaikeu, K. D. (2006). A systematic review of recent research on adolescent religiosity/spirituality and mental health. *Issues in Mental Health Nursing, 27*(2), 161–183.

Youngblade, L. M., Curry, L. A., Novak, M., Vogel, B., & Shenkman, E. A. (2006). The impact of community risks and resources on adolescent risky behavior and health care expenditures. *Journal of Adolescent Health, 38*(5), 486–494.

Youngblade, L. M., Theokas, C., Schulenberg, J., Curry, L., Huang, I. C., & Novak, M. (2007). Risk and promotive factors in families, schools, and communities: A contextual model of positive youth development in adolescence. *Pediatrics, 119*(Suppl. 1), S47–S53.

Zaff, J. F., Malanchuk, O., Michelsen, E., & Eccles, J. (2003). Identity development and feelings of fulfillment: Mediators of future civic engagement (CIRCLE working paper No. 4). Medford, MA: Center for Information and Research on Civic Learning and Engagement.

Zimmerman, M. A., Bingenheimer, J. B., & Notaro, P. C. (2002). Natural mentors and adolescent resiliency: A study with urban youth. *American Journal of Community Psychology, 30*(2), 221–243.

CHAPTER

FAMILY INFLUENCES ON ADOLESCENT HEALTH

SUSAN L. DAVIES ▪ RICHARD A. CROSBY ▪ RALPH J. DICLEMENTE

LEARNING OBJECTIVES

After studying this chapter, you will be able to

- Classify the family unit as the primary source of transmission of basic socio-cultural factors that influence adolescent health behavior.

- Indicate how relationships within the family can positively and negatively influence adolescent risk.

- Explain how structural and socioeconomic factors can directly or indirectly shape adolescent behavior.

Adolescent development is a complex and interactive process involving individuals, families, groups, and communities. Families serve as adolescents' primary learning resource, preparing them to function successfully. In this chapter, we will explore the family unit as the primary source of transmission of basic social and cultural factors that influence adolescents' health behaviors.

KEY CONCEPTS AND RESEARCH FINDINGS

Primacy of the Family System in Adolescent Development

In the time since Freud first took interest in the family, its function has been studied in historical, economic, scientific, and cultural contexts. The family is considered to be an adolescent's most powerful influence, as its effect continues long after leaving home (Szapocznik & Coatsworth, 1999; Novak & Pelaez, 2004). In meeting the adolescent's psychological needs, the family engages in bonding and attachment, provides intimacy, and conveys mutual respect. In socializing children, the family conveys cultural, societal, and religious beliefs and traditions to the next generation.

Norms, values, and models of behavior introduced in the family serve as building blocks for the development of the adolescent's personality, beliefs, and attitudes. In nurturing family environments, interactions between members demonstrate and reinforce healthy, effective norms of behavior. Adolescents internalize the family's conception of health—and the beliefs and behaviors that support it.

The Capability of Families to Protect and Prepare Adolescents

Marked changes in the structure of families took place in the United States between 1970 and 2000. Census data show three notable trends: a decrease in families with children, a decrease in the number of traditional nuclear families, and an increase in the number of single-parent, mother-headed families (Fields & Casper, 2001). Although the structure of families has changed, society still expects the family system to be competent in performing its essential functions (McCubbin, McCubbin, Thompson, Han, & Allen, 1997). Individuals across the sociodemographic spectrum rarely possess the complex cadre of affirmative parenting skills when they first become parents, including tools to effectively address the negative behaviors that are a normal part of early childhood. At-risk families often face a number of additional challenges (such as poverty, substance abuse, or mental illness) that can thwart development. At greatest peril are those families experiencing a cluster of concurrent risks and living in resource-poor communities with few safety nets in the way of social services or access to training and education.

Theoretical Foundations

Family theories can increase our understanding of how factors from multiple systems of influence interact to shape adolescent risk and protective behaviors. According to White and Klein (2002), several dimensions of families make them unique to other social groups: families last longer than most social groups; they have intergenerational relationships unlike other social groups; and they are part of a kinship, a larger type of social organization. Coleman (1990) noted that attempts to explain family behavior with the same processes that govern other social groups would remove or ignore many critical aspects of family phenomena. Being a biological and a social unit, the family has a connection with history.

Some family theories are grounded in the fundamental notion of *dynamic interaction,* which states that the individual and his or her environment interact in ways that change both. Development is not seen as linear but spiral, where this constant interaction and reciprocal influence lead to future interactions that have been influenced by the perception of past interactions (Salt, 1991). Family systems research highlights how the family's relational environment shapes adolescent risk and protection. Family systems theories have also been used to understand adult behavior in later life, suggesting that the family continues to exert influence over an individual's daily experiences well into adulthood (Fingerman & Bermann, 2000).

Family continues to exert influence over an individual's daily experiences well into adulthood.

Bowen's (1978) Family Systems Theory is a comprehensive model of human behavior that represents a family's emotional and relational life. *Family Systems Theory* (FST) contends that adolescent risk behaviors are symptomatic of unresolved relationship difficulties in the family (Knauth, Skowron, & Escobar, 2006; Gilbert, 1999). FST also contends that engaging in risk behavior is one way in which adolescents respond to the difficulty they experience in differentiating themselves within the family. FST posits several constructs that together shape family functioning: differentiation, triangles, nuclear family emotional system, emotional cutoff, the family projection process, the multigenerational transmission process, sibling position, and societal regression. First, all families can be characterized on a continuum of *differentiation* that reflects each family member's tolerance for individuality and intimacy. A well-differentiated individual demonstrates intact personal boundaries and effective problem-solving skills, whereas an undifferentiated person may largely base his or her decisions on the attitudes and opinions of significant others.

Bowen's theory further asserts that the nuclear family is an *emotional system* that functions as one emotional unit, rather than many individuals with their own emotions. This view implies that (1) anything that affects one member affects each member in the system and (2) family members trade self in the family relationship togetherness for a family fusion of selves. Because the actions of one affect everyone else, anxiety is infectious and easily passed from one person to another in the group. The concept of emotional cutoff reflects how, in the presence of excessive emotional intensity, a family member separates from the rest of the family, or vice versa. This occurs when individuals behave in such a way that they are cut off emotionally from the rest of the family. Adolescent pregnancy, disapproval of partner choice, homosexuality, and addiction are common situations leading to emotional cutoff.

Fundamental Relationships Within Family Systems

The impact of familial interactions on adolescents' adoption and maintenance of health-compromising and protective behaviors has received increasing attention in the adolescent development literature. Within family systems, parenting is considered the most potent force in shaping adolescents' social, emotional, and cognitive development. Child and adolescent development literature first linked parenting practices to early childhood attachment and conduct problems and then to the development of aggressive, antisocial behavior (Jacob, Moser, Windle, Loeber, & Stouthamer-Loeber, 2000). This literature has continued to grow, expanding its scope to adolescent risk behaviors including substance use and abuse, violence, delinquency, and sexual risk behaviors that lead to pregnancy and sexually transmitted infections.

A healthy parent-adolescent relationship and positive communication are important protective factors against risk behaviors among adolescents (Ary, Duncan, Duncan, & Hops, 1999; DiClemente, Wingood, Crosby, Cobb, Harrington, & Davies, 2001). Parent-adolescent connectedness has been positively associated with delayed sexual debut (McBride, Paikoff, & Holmbeck, 2003) and increased resilience to negative risk behaviors including violence, delinquency, and substance use (Aronowitz & Morrison-Beedy, 2004). Conversely, poor parent-adolescent relationships and family disruption have been shown to be uniquely predictive of adolescent risk behavior (Conger & Ge, 1999). Shared parent-adolescent time during pre-, early, and midadolescence has also been linked to reduced family conflict in later years (Dubas & Gerris, 2002). Although closeness in adolescent-parent relationships generally declines during adolescence (Conger & Ge, 1999), more secure attachment to parents during adolescence is linked to greater social competence and better psychosocial adjustment (Allen, Moore, Kuperminc, & Bell, 1998).

Research suggests that the adolescent individuation process does not require detachment from parents and that close relationships with parents continue throughout adolescence.

Early research suggested that highly conflictual parent-adolescent relationships were not only normative but necessary for adolescent autonomy development. Some studies indicate that parent-adolescent conflict in early adolescence serves a positive function in transforming family relationships; in fact, moderate conflict with parents has been associated with better adjustment than either no conflict or frequent conflict (Smetana, Metzger, & Campione-Barr, 2004). Other research suggests that the adolescent individuation process does not require detachment from parents and that in most cases close relationships with parents continue throughout adolescence (Petersen, Leffert, & Graham, 1995). However, parents do perceive adolescence to be the most challenging and difficult stage of childrearing (Smetana, Campione-Barr, & Metzger, 2006). At the outset of adolescence, family relationships tend to be hierarchical but change into more egalitarian relationships by late adolescence, as parental supervision decreases to allow greater adolescent autonomy (Smetana et al., 2006).

Parenting Practices

Parenting practices are the proximal means through which adolescents develop and change. These practices serve as a critical interface between family contexts and child adjustment (Forgatch, DeGarmo, & Beldavs, 2005). Specific parenting behaviors that have been found to influence adolescent health risk and protective behaviors include type of discipline, level of parental involvement, level of parental monitoring, and quality and quantity of communication. The element most frequently examined and implicated in adolescent risk is parental monitoring. Across problem behaviors, parental monitoring appears highly predictive of negative peer group affiliation and early involvement in risk behaviors. Less perceived parental monitoring, especially adolescents' perceptions of low parental monitoring, has been associated with increases in violence (Botvin, Griffin, & Nichols, 2006), sexual risk taking (Sieverding, Adler, Witt, & Ellen, 2005), and substance use (Dishion et al., 1996). However, both authoritative and authoritarian parents monitor, making its protective ability less clear. Stattin and Kerr (2000) added clarity by exploring the various methods parents use to monitor their children and found that when parental monitoring is assessed using child disclosure as a source of parent knowledge, this aspect appears to be most predictive of risk.

Parenting practices that encourage high levels of autonomy and individualism should not be confused with failing to set limits or provide structure—common elements of indulgent and neglectful parenting styles, which are consistently associated with increased risk and decreased achievement. Trends toward increased authoritative parenting can be seen as a widespread societal movement encouraging parents to embrace autonomy, independence, and individualism in their children.

Mason, Cauce, Gonzales, and Hiraga (1994) created the term *precision parenting* to describe the difficulty African American parents face in finding the appropriate amount of control to exert in order to encourage both independence and respect for authority among adolescents experiencing structural racism. This delicate balance perhaps explains why a study of African American parents found them to score high on measures of both authoritative and authoritarian parenting (Dornbusch, Ritter, Liederman, & Fraleigh, 1987). For some families living in communities of low socioeconomic status, parents show higher levels of power assertion and lower levels of autonomy granting (McElhaney & Allen, 2001), and children's well-being is associated with firm parental control and heightened supervision, reflecting the need to enforce rules in dangerous environments (Gonzales, Cauce, Friedman, & Mason, 1996; McLoyd, 1998). Luthar (1999) asserted that the optimal amount of control used by African American parents can vary as a function of the negative influences in the community. The culminating literature on parenting practices and child outcomes within African American families shows significant variability (Mandara & Murray, 2002; McBride et al., 2003), with some risks and assets influenced predominantly by socioeconomic status (such as use of harsh discipline and heightened control) and others associated more with sociocultural contexts (such as academic involvement) (Chavous et al., 2003; Giles-Sims & Lockhart, 2005; Lansford, Dodge, Pettit, Bates, Crozier, & Kaplow, 2002). These and other studies highlight the need for culture-specific and ecologically grounded approaches to conceptualization, research, and intervention (Gorman-Smith, Tolan, Henry, & Florsheim, 2000).

In examining family and parenting variables, it is especially important to recognize the unique differences that exist among individuals within various racial, ethnic, and cultural groups (Broman, Reckase, & Freedman-Doan, 2006). Cohen and Rice (1997) reported that white students perceived parents as less authoritarian than Hispanic and Asian students, and Radziszewska and colleagues (1996) found that white parents were more likely to be rated as authoritative, and African American and Hispanic parents were more likely to be rated as autocratic (Radziszewska, Richardson, Dent, & Flay, 1996).

Studies conducted in both African American and white families indicate that children and adolescents raised by parents who exhibit both acceptance (warmth and support), and firm, consistent control (discipline and monitoring) exhibit better adjustment outcomes (Steinberg, 2001; Querido, Warner, & Eyberg, 2002). Unlike parental *psychological* control, which has been associated with increased adolescent sexual and other risk behavior, supportive and noncoercive parenting practices (or *behavioral* control) have been shown to facilitate positive identity formation (Arnett, 2001), develop effective self-regulatory skills and positive emotional adjustment, and buffer children from the negative effects of economic hardship (Mistry, Vandewater, Huston, & McLoyd, 2002). There is evidence that parent-adolescent relationship quality and parental attitudes and behaviors mediate the relation between financial strain and adolescents' academic achievement (Gutman & Eccles, 1999). Similar studies have shown the same protective capabilities for adverse sexual and other risk behaviors (Kilgore, Snyder, & Lentz, 2000). In sum, the research indicates that it is the combination of parenting style characteristics (such as high monitoring and high nurturance) that leads to positive outcomes in children (Baumrind, 2005; Mboya, 1995). These complex processes should not be examined only for their main effects, because nurturance has consistently been shown to moderate the relationships between risk practices in adolescents and their parents' use of monitoring and strong discipline. One common thread appears to be authoritative parenting with high levels of demand tempered by high levels of warmth.

Influence of Marital Instability

Another relational dynamic within family systems that influences adolescent health is the quality of the parents' relationship with one another. Marital instability or discordant marital environments (often characterized by stress, estrangement, detachment, or unhealthy boundaries) have been associated with various child adjustment and behavioral outcomes, including increased delinquency (Gorman-Smith, Tolan, Loweber, & Henry, 1998), substance abuse (Sanders, 2000), conduct disorder, and aggression (Snyder, 2000). How marital conflict is handled appears to be key: if handled well, the children learn positive conflict resolution, coping, and problem-solving skills that can serve them well in future interpersonal interactions; if managed poorly, conflict can affect exposed children behaviorally and emotionally (Kitzmann, 2000).

Growing up in a single-parent family has been associated with a series of correlated disadvantages, including lower maternal age, lower levels of parental education, poorer socioeconomic status, more family problems, exposure to childhood sexual and physical abuse, parental illicit drug use and criminal offending, and lower scores on standardized tests of intelligence (Stewart-Brown, Patterson, Mockford, Barlow, Klimes, & Pyper, 2004). However, when these disadvantages are accounted for, exposure to single parenthood is largely unrelated to adjustment in young adulthood.

If managed poorly, conflict can affect exposed children behaviorally and emotionally.

Influence of Siblings

Although the importance of familial relationships on child and adolescent development has long been recognized, sibling relationships have only recently become a focus of research. Sibling relationships are among the most enduring relational contexts, affecting individual development across the life span (Branje, Van Lieshout, Van Aken, & Haselager, 2004; Brody, 1998). Sibling relationships have been studied from various perspectives, though most commonly as a collection of demographic variables (such as birth order, gender considerations, and age differences), which in numerous studies have failed to demonstrate strong direct effects on adolescent development.

The contamination hypothesis suggests that sibling relationships are likely to be poorer in high-conflict homes, either as a result of competition for scarce parental resources or modeling of conflicted interpersonal relationships.

Siblings have a socializing effect on one another through their daily conflicts and negotiations, and they carry those skills with them into other social settings. Downey and Condron (2004) showed that kids who practiced the best conflict resolution skills at home carried those abilities into the classroom. Sibling relationship quality has been associated with levels of family harmony (Whiteman, McHale, & Crouter, 2007). Two competing hypotheses attempt to explain how family systems influence sibling relationships (Deater-Deckard, Dunn, & Lussier, 2002). The *contamination hypothesis* suggests that sibling relationships are likely to be poorer in high-conflict homes, either as a result of competition for scarce parental resources or modeling of conflicted interpersonal relationships. In this situation, it is likely that siblings in high-conflict families will have less influence on each other's behavior. In contrast, the *compensation hypothesis* suggests that family dysfunction, especially as it causes conflict between parents, often serves to bring siblings closer together in order to buffer themselves from unstable relationships with their parents. Accordingly, this hypothesis predicts that siblings in high-conflict families will exert stronger influences on each other's behavior.

The roles of parents and peers in modeling in the development of adolescent alcohol use have been well documented, whereas the potential influence of siblings has been understudied (van der Vorst, Engels,

Meeus, Dekovic, & Vermulst, 2006). Given the long-term nature of sibling relationships, it is likely that their influence is significant. Studies of sibling influence on alcohol use have indicated that older siblings' use predicts younger siblings' association with peers who use alcohol, which in turn predicts the younger siblings' alcohol use (Conger & Rueter, 1996; Windle, 2000). Other research has shown that older sibling alcohol use predicted younger sibling alcohol use only among sibling pairs who were of the same gender, closer in age, and from higher-conflict families (Trim, Leuthe, & Chassin, 2006). A review of studies assessing the association between adolescent smoking and parent and sibling smoking behaviors showed that across studies sibling smoking was a stronger and more consistent predictor of adolescent smoking than parent smoking (Avenevoli & Merikangas, 2003). Older siblings' risk behavior may predict younger siblings' risk behavior both directly and indirectly through peer selection. Although peer influences are often considered the strongest, most proximal correlates of adolescent risk, siblings often have overlapping peer networks.

The Role of Fathers

Societal expectations of fatherhood shifted dramatically in the later decades of the twentieth century. Increased father participation in families, particularly in sharing child care duties, has been the result of men's desire to be more involved with their children, the fact that both parents are more likely to be employed than in past years, and also the contribution of the feminist movement that helped to redistribute household responsibilities (Tiedje & Darling-Fisher, 1996). There is considerable research to indicate that fathers contribute to their children's healthy development in ways that are unique from mothers. This literature is not universally consistent, however, and methodologically rigorous research on father involvement has lagged behind that of family structure. Earlier research focused on structural factors of the father's role, including living in the home, provision of child support, and division of labor for child-rearing responsibilities. More recent studies reflect increased recognition of process-related variables between fathers and adolescent offspring. Benefits of father involvement reported in empirical studies include higher levels of cognitive development, greater expression of empathy, fewer behavior problems, greater social skills, and greater school performance (Mosley & Thompson, 1995).

Fathers contribute to their children's healthy development in ways that are unique from mothers.

An area of research that needs further exploration is postdivorce father involvement. Factors associated with positive child outcomes after divorce include father visitation, financial support, positive parental relationship, and a positive father-child relationship before and after the divorce (Tiedje & Darling-Fisher, 1996). Socioeconomic indicators are the strongest predictors of father involvement among fathers who do not live with their children. Fathers who are able to provide economic support for their children are more likely to be engaged with their children, even if not physically present. Conversely, unemployed or underemployed fathers are less likely to be involved in their children's lives. Fathers with more than one family (those who have fathered children with different mothers) find it especially difficult to fulfill financial and social responsibilities, with children from previous relationships more likely to be adversely affected (Logan, Manlove, Ikramullah, & Cottingham, 2006). Other factors that negatively affect paternal involvement include conflicts with the child's mother, lack of financial resources, new spouse or partner, and geographic mobility. Perhaps because of societal expectations of fathers as economic providers, economic hardship has been associated with increased father-initiated relationship strain even within married couples (Elder, Conger, Foster, & Ardelt, 1992). Research on fathers' provision of child support shows positive child outcomes, including increased cognitive development, academic achievement, and prosocial behavior (Graham, Beller, & Hernandez, 1994). The relationship between informal child support provision and adolescent outcomes has been understudied. However, father-child relationship quality has been suggested to be more predictive of child outcomes than the frequency of contact (Furstenberg & Harris, 1993). Father involvement that is nurturing and positive may benefit the father and the child's mother, in addition to the child. Moreover, fathers' use of harsh and inconsistent discipline or an aloof parenting style has been associated with poorer emotional adjustment and lower school achievement (Davidov & Grusec, 2006).

One overall conclusion that can be drawn from the substantial family, child, and adolescent development literature is that a stable emotional connection and a predictable caretaking relationship are two key variables that predict positive well-being among adolescents (Silverstein & Auerbach, 1999).

Influence of Family Socialization

A family systems perspective can also help to understand the family's role in children's gender development by recognizing the need to examine an adolescent's relationship with one parent in the context of his or her relationship with the other parent (Minuchin, 1985). Children learn about gender roles and norms largely by observing their mother's and father's gender-typed behavior during parental interactions. Research suggests that boys and girls may be exposed to different socialization settings, which contribute to gender-typed behavior and cognitive schemas. Gender socialization practices that encourage girls' self-regulation, sensitivity to others, and support seeking from parents and peers may place girls at higher risk for internalizing problems; similarly, boys' greater socialization for self-assertion and away from empathy may increase their vulnerability to externalizing problems (Leadbeater, Kuperminc, Blatt, & Hertzog, 1999). Evidence suggests that parents may engage in different behavior patterns with their sons than with their daughters, especially in the presence of the other spouse (Smetana et al., 2000). Research has found that boys are more likely than girls to be exposed to interparental conflict (Grych & Fincham, 1990). Boys in families with marital distress have also been shown to experience more competitive interaction between parents (McHale, 1995). Gender roles within families can be viewed as transactional patterns of the family as a whole. For example, adolescents of both genders are more likely to receive emotional support from their mothers and informational and instrumental support from their fathers (Steinberg & Silk, 2002).

Recent work on the effects of parenting behaviors on adolescent risk by gender suggests a need for gender-specific parenting practices. McBride et al. (2003) found that among African American families living in high-risk environments autonomy granting is protective for adolescent girls, but has the opposite effect on teen boys. Authors speculated that when adolescent daughters are given a significant amount of household responsibilities, they benefit from having some level of control over the decision making, whereas boys benefit most from strict parental control. A study by Fasula, Miller, and Wiener (2007) identified a "sexual double standard" in African American mothers' socialization patterns toward sexual risk reduction. This qualitative study of mothers' sexual communication messages to their children indicated gender-specific differences through messages that allowed more freedom and power in heterosexual interactions to adolescent males than females. Findings suggest that mothers are more likely to approach sexual risk reduction efforts proactively with their sons and neutrally or prohibitively with their daughters. A common saying among African Americans is that "Mothers raise their daughters and love their sons." The most consistent message African American girls report receiving from their mothers is to be self-reliant and resourceful (Cauce, Hiraga, Graves, Gonzales, Ryan-Finn, & Grove, 1996). Many daughters perceive their brothers as being given significantly fewer responsibilities than they have, leading to many African American daughters' perception that their mothers place a higher value on their sons than their daughters (Cauce et al., 1996).

Role of Socioeconomic Disadvantage

Many factors make it difficult for parents, especially those living in poverty, to provide the guidance needed by adolescents, including the challenges of daily living that must take precedence, the lack of adequate time or skills, and other priorities. A recent meta-analysis indicated that socioeconomic disadvantage is strongly and consistently related to harsh, unresponsive parenting (Grant, Compas, Stuhlmacher, Thurm, McMahon, & Halpert, 2003). Economic hardship has been shown to adversely impact parental nurturance and disciplinary practices, leading parents to value obedience over autonomy and independence (Taylor & Robert, 1995). Socioeconomic status is one of the most formidable and least changeable contextual factors. It is undoubtedly more difficult for parents to put forth effort to improve their parenting practices when they are struggling to meet the family's most primary needs. However, even in highly disadvantaged populations, parenting style has been shown to be protective. Parental discipline and monitoring has been shown in numerous models to mediate the association between family income and child conduct problems in youth of varying age, gender, and ethnicity (Kilgore et al., 2000). McLoyd (1998) showed that economic stressors affected adolescent social and emotional functioning not directly but indirectly through their impact on maternal psychological functioning and subsequent parenting and parent-child relations. Brody, Flor, and Gibson (1999) traced the links among family financial resources, maternal parenting efficacy, developmental goals, parenting practices, and children's academic and psychosocial competence among rural, single-parent African American families. Using a multimethod, multi-informant design, adequate financial resources were associated with mothers' child-rearing efficacy, which in turn was correlated to parenting practices indirectly through developmental goals. Competence-promoting parenting practices were indirectly linked with children's academic and psychosocial competence through their association with children's self-regulation. Brody and colleagues (2001) further found that community disadvantage had a significant positive effect on deviant peer affiliations. Nurturing or involved parenting and collective socialization processes were inversely associated, and harsh or inconsistent parenting was positively associated with deviant peer affiliations. The effects of nurturing or involved parenting and collective socialization were most pronounced for children residing in the most disadvantaged neighborhoods.

Poverty is the single most powerful risk for families and children and affects families in many ways.

Poverty is the single most powerful risk for families and children and affects families in many ways. Poverty exerts its greatest impact during children's preschool years, the age group in which children are most likely to live in poverty. Parents' economic status (education, occupation, and income) limits their ability to provide adequate housing, a safe environment, and responsible child care while working.

Family Influences on Adolescents' Substance Use Behaviors

An area where familial influences may be most pronounced is adolescent substance abuse. Authoritative parenting is consistently shown to be highly protective against tobacco (Chassin, Presson, Rose, Sherman, Davis, & Gonzalez, 2005; O'Byrne, Haddock, & Poston Walker, 2002) and other drug use (Adalbjarnardottir & Hafsteinsson, 2001; Patock-Peckham & Morgan-Lopez, 2006). The detrimental effects of neglectful or unengaged parenting and authoritarian parenting on increased risk for drinking, smoking, and other drug use is also well documented (Bronte-Tinkew, Moore, & Carrano, 2006). Permissive parenting practices have also been associated with increased adolescent alcohol and tobacco use (Cohen & Rice, 1997; Slicker, 1998). Studies of associations or relationships between parenting styles and adolescent alcohol and other drug use behaviors have indicated some incongruencies, depending on whether the parenting style was rated by adolescents or parents, suggesting the importance of considering both parent and adolescent reports (Chassin et al., 2005; Cohen & Rice, 1997). Cohen and Rice (1997) found that alcohol and tobacco use among a sample of eighth- and ninth-grade students was associated with a child perception of lower authoritativeness and higher permissiveness, but that there was no relationship between parental perceptions of their parenting style and child alcohol or tobacco use. These researchers concluded that parents may benefit from understanding how their children perceive them and suggested that even though the child's perception of parenting style may be biased, it was most useful in predicting substance use. Other research indicated that adolescents perceived their mothers' parenting style to differ from that of their fathers. Bronte-Tinkew, Moore, and Carrano (2006) found that adolescents were more likely to rate their mothers as authoritative and more likely to rate their fathers as uninvolved. Other researchers have reported significant gender differences in the strength of relationships between parenting styles and adolescent substance use, and findings suggest that the parenting style of the parent of the same sex has the strongest relationship with self-regulation and substance use (Patock-Peckham & Morgan-Lopez, 2006).

Family Influences on Adolescents' Sexual Behavior

The family is a primary part of adolescents' socialization to sexual values, sex roles, and expected sexual behaviors. Evidence suggests that adolescents' sexual health may be particularly influenced by their mothers (DiLorio, Kelley, & Hockenberry-Eaton, 1999; Dutra, Miller, & Forehand, 1999; Miller, Kotchick, Dorsey, Forehand, & Ham, 1998). Mothers are more likely than fathers to communicate with their adolescents about sex-related topics (such as STDs and AIDS, partner selection, and sexual development), and mothers are often a primary source of adolescents' information about sex. There is a dearth of literature on the role of fathers in communicating about sexuality, and what little there is frequently relies on mothers as proxies for fathers (Kirkman, Rosenthal, & Feldman, 2002). Even when fathers and mothers assume equal responsibility in communicating with their children about sexuality, in practice it is usually mothers who perform this role. Three factors have been posited to explain this: mothers spend more time with their children, women have greater communication skills, and they are often the family's primary nurturers. Kirkman, Rosenthal, and Feldman (2002) posit that the task of communicating with their children about sexuality puts fathers awkwardly between the contradictory issues of traditional masculinity and involved fatherhood.

A particularly important form of family influence on adolescents' sexual risk behavior pertains to parental monitoring. Indeed, parental monitoring may be the most robust of the influences that shape adolescents' sexual risk and protective behaviors. For example, infrequent monitoring has been associated with adolescents' lack of condom use for penile-vaginal sex (Crosby, Voisin, et al., 2006; Crosby, DiClemente, Wingood, et al., 2003; DiClemente, Wingood, Crosby, et al., 2001; Li, Stanton, & Feigelman, 2000; Li, Feigelman, & Stanton, 2000). Similarly, infrequent monitoring has also been associated with earlier initiation of sexual activity (Rosenthal et al., 2001; Romer et al., 1999). These two findings alone (early age of initiation and lack of condom use) set the stage for increased risk of STD acquisition and unintended conception. Other observed associations are between infrequent monitoring and adolescent females' reporting sex with nonmonogamous male partners, as well as sex with multiple male partners (DiClemente, Wingood, Crosby, et al., 2001).

Evidence also suggests that parents should not decrease their frequency of monitoring as adolescents move through their teen years. One study found that the number of females who had ever had sex increased with increasing age, particularly among adolescents who perceived that their peers were supportive of sexual activity and who perceived low parental monitoring (Romer, Stanton, Galbraith, et al., 1999). Other studies have also demonstrated the importance of frequent monitoring for older adolescents (Li, Stanton, & Feigelman, 2000; Li, Feigelman, & Stanton, 2000).

Consistent with the findings from these studies, which showed associations between infrequent parental monitoring and sexual risk behaviors, are other studies that have shown an association between parental monitoring and two outcomes of unprotected sexual intercourse: sexually transmitted diseases (STDs) and pregnancy. Two studies, for example, have demonstrated significant associations between infrequent parental monitoring and biologically confirmed incidence of STDs. In the first study, among a community sample of African American adolescent females, those who perceived infrequent parental monitoring at baseline assessment were 1.8 and 2.5 times more likely to acquire chlamydia or trichomoniasis, respectively, compared to adolescents who perceived more frequent monitoring. Adolescents who perceived infrequent parental monitoring were 2.1 times more likely to test positive for an STD (chlamydia, trichomoniasis, or gonorrhea) over an eighteen-month observation period (Crosby, DiClemente, Wingood, Lang, & Harrington, 2003). The second study assessed a racially diverse sample of male and female adolescents sentenced to short-term detention facilities in the state of Georgia (Crosby, Voisin, et al., 2006). This study found that infrequently monitored adolescents were 1.8 times more likely to be diagnosed with chlamydia or gonorrhea compared to those who perceived frequent monitoring. However, the association was modified by age, gender, and race, and the effect was present for older adolescents, females, and minority adolescents.

A recent study also demonstrated that infrequent parental monitoring predicted subsequent pregnancy among minority teens (Crosby, DiClemente, Wingood, et al., 2002). More than four hundred adolescent females who initially tested negative for pregnancy were followed for a six-month period. Those reporting infrequent monitoring at baseline were 2.5 times more likely to test positive for pregnancy at the conclusion of this observation period.

Family Influences on Adolescents' Depression and Suicide

Several studies have examined relationships between adolescent depression and parenting behaviors. Pineda, Cole, and Bruce (2007) assessed maternal critical and positive interaction behaviors among mothers of moderately depressed fourteen- to eighteen-year-old, predominantly Caucasian adolescents, compared with mothers of adolescents who did not have symptoms of depression. Adolescents with depressive symptoms responded to maternal criticism with depressive behavior, and adolescent depressed affect was followed by less positive and supportive responses from mothers, compared to mothers of nondepressed adolescents. Similarly, Gonzales, Deardorff, Formoso, Barr, and Barrera (2006), in studying 175 Mexican-origin families of eleven- to fifteen-year old adolescents from low-income inner-city areas in the Southwest United States, found that maternal support—defined as acceptance and attachment—was negatively related to adolescent depression. Barber, Stolz, and Olsen (2005) conducted a cross-national study of the interrelationships of parenting and adolescent outcomes in the United States and eleven other countries. A complex dominance analysis of three parenting aspects (parental support, psychological control, and behavioral control) was conducted based on adolescent reports regarding both mothers and fathers. Parental

Several studies have examined relationships between adolescent depression and parenting behaviors.

support was consistently linked to lower levels of depressive feeling in adolescents across groups both cross-sectionally and longitudinally, demonstrating causal linkages. Hill, Bush, and Roosa (2003) studied the different influences of parenting style on adolescent mental health that were due to acculturative status by examining low-income Mexican American and Euro American families of children eight to thirteen years of age. Both Mexican American and Euro American families with low levels of conflict and hostile control, and who were accepting and used consistent discipline, were more likely to have children with fewer depressive symptoms and conduct disorder.

Finkelstein, Donenberg, and Martinovich (2001) examined the relationship of controlling parenting style with adolescent depression in a multiethnic balanced sample of Caucasian, Latina, and African American girls. There was no significant relationship between firm maternal control and depression in Caucasian and Latino girls, but a negative relationship of firm control with depression was found in the African American group.

Radziszewska and Hafsteinsson (2001) examined relationships between parenting styles and depression among 3,993 fifteen-year-olds in California and found that adolescents who reported that their parents had an authoritative style were least likely to have depressive symptoms, followed by adolescents who had permissive, autocratic, and unengaged parenting. These authors identified three subgroups at particular risk for depression: African American boys with unengaged parents and Asian American girls with either autocratic or unengaged parents.

Parental caring, warmth, control, conflict, and authoritarianism have been examined in relation to adolescent suicidal ideation or self-harm. Pearce, Martin, and Wood (1995) found that more negative touch from family and friends and less positive touch was related to greater suicidal ideation and deliberate self-harm among thirteen- to fifteen-year-old middle-class Caucasian adolescents.

FUTURE DIRECTIONS FOR FAMILY-FOCUSED RESEARCH

The magnitude of influence that family interactions and behaviors exert on adolescent risk and protective behaviors indicates an urgent need for more research-based, family-centered interventions to improve adolescent health outcomes. Rigorously designed family intervention research will play an increasingly important role in addressing the needs of families. Heightened recognition of the diversity of the adolescent population, the families in which they live, and community contexts that they operate under will also be essential. Particularly needed are family etiological models that fit unique cultural and socioeconomic needs of specific populations (such as minority, rural, or low income). Because family-focused research is so complex, it requires equally complex methods for examining family phenomena. Beyond recognizing a significant association, the contribution of parenting style to their adolescent's health behaviors is not well understood. Hypotheses regarding the multiple, recursive, and sequential influences of parents on children (and vice versa) has often exceeded the capacity of research designs and analytic tools to test them (Snyder & Kazak, 2005). An example of this difficulty is the inability to parcel out various confounders and contextual factors that carry great weight in shaping adolescents' behavior.

A richer understanding of multiple family process variables will require prospective, multi-informant, multilevel research designs that account for an ecological context. Indications of such methodological advancements are starting to emerge. For example, Brickner, Peterson, Andersen, Sarason, Rajan, and Leroux (2007) developed a social transmission probability model in a prospective study to clarify conflicting findings of previous, less methodologically rigorous studies with regard to whether siblings, peers, or parents exert the strongest influence on adolescent smoking behaviors. This model predicts the probability that an individual will make a behavioral transition in terms of the number of persons engaging in the behavior in their social environment, context-specific probabilities of influencing that individual regarding the behavior in question, and the relative predictive influences of specific persons in different social contexts. Similar social transmission probability models could be created based on Brickner's (2007) model.

Rigorously designed family intervention research will play an increasingly important role in addressing the needs of families.

It is quite likely that the best time to intervene to protect adolescents is to engage their parents well before adolescence begins, during the middle childhood years (Hawkins, Catalano, Kosterman, Abbot, & Hill, 1999). Family research to change parenting behaviors can be challenging, because parents are less accessible than their children, who can be reached through school and various community venues. Compounding this challenge, interventions targeted at changing parenting styles may be more difficult than interventions to change specific behaviors related to risky health behaviors (Chassin et al., 2005). For example, it may be easier to engage in parental monitoring and communicate about substance use than it will be to adopt a nurturing, autonomy-granting parenting style. This provides further justification for starting family interventions earlier. There are numerous examples of effective family interventions (see Biglan & Taylor, 2000; Kumpfer & Alder, 2003; Webster-Statton & Taylor, 2001, for reviews).

SUMMARY

The tremendous advantages to be gained from effective family interventions argue for continued efforts to develop them. Lessons learned in the family continue to guide individuals throughout their lives. However, few parents or family members receive training before they impart these powerful lessons. Although economic resources are a critical determinant of child health and well being, there are countless examples of families with abundant resources who lack essential competencies for effective child rearing. The substantial influence of parenting practices on adolescent developmental trajectories is increasingly clear: adolescents raised in authoritative households consistently demonstrate higher protective and fewer risk behaviors than adolescents from nonauthoritative families. Parenting practices that have consistently led to greater physical, mental, and social outcomes in their children include developmentally appropriate supervision, control, and monitoring; consistent positive discipline; clear, supportive communication; and demonstration of warmth, affection, encouragement, and approval (Stewart-Brown et al., 2004).

Concerted, multilevel efforts to support the development of positive parenting and healthy family functioning are needed. Family-centered interventions that integrally involve parents and adolescents together have the potential to be ongoing, forming more adaptive interaction and communication patterns that will continue to insulate youth throughout their lives, particularly at times when risk opportunities occur. Judging by data from a number of studies supporting the intergenerational transmission of parenting behaviors, such interventions could even have implications for future generations.

KEY TERMS

Compensation hypothesis
Contamination hypothesis
Differentiation
Dynamic interaction

Emotional system
Family Systems Theory (FST)
Parenting practices
Precision parenting

DISCUSSION QUESTIONS

1. What are the differences between parenting styles and parenting practices? How do these concepts interact to influence adolescent risk and protective behaviors?

2. Imagine that you are brought into a civil court custody hearing between a divorced couple as an expert in the field of family health. The mother of a five-year-old girl is trying to get full custody of her daughter. Conversely, the father of the same five-year-old girl is also fighting for full custody. Both parents are fully capable and financially able to care for their daughter. Given your knowledge on family influence and subsequent adolescent health risk, discuss your opinions (pros and cons) for your decision on who should be granted full custody.

3. Because the family unit plays such a vital role in the behavioral development of adolescents transitioning into adulthood, how can health promotion interventions engage families to become more involved, especially those of lower socioeconomic status or in unstable households, where adolescents are at highest risk?

REFERENCES

Adalbjarnardottir, S., & Hafsteinsson, L. G. (2001). Adolescents' perceived parenting styles and their substance use: Concurrent and longitudinal analyses. *Journal of Research on Adolescence, 11*(4), 401–423.

Allen, J. P., Moore, C. M., Kuperminc, G. P., & Bell, K. L. (1998). Attachment and adolescent psychosocial functioning. *Child Development, 69,* 1406–1419.

Arnett, J. (2001). *Adolescence and emerging adulthood*. Englewood Cliffs, NJ: Prentice Hall.

Aronowitz, T. & Morrison-Beedy, D. (2004). Resilience to risk-taking behaviors in impoverished African American girls: The role of mother-daughter connectedness. *Research in Nursing and Health, 27*(1), 29–39.

Ary, D. V., Duncan, T. E., Duncan, S. C., & Hops, H. (1999). Adolescent problem behavior: The influence of parents and peers. *Behaviour Research and Therapy, 37*(3), 217–230.

Avenevoli, S., & Merikangas, K. R. (2003). Familial influences on adolescent smoking. *Addiction, 98*(Suppl. 1), 1–20.

Barber, B. K., Stolz, H. E., & Olsen, J. A. (2005). Trajectories of physical aggression from toddlerhood to middle childhood. *Monographs of the Society for Research in Child Development, 70,* 1–137.

Baumrind, D. (2005). Patterns of parental authority and adolescent autonomy. In J. Smetana (Ed.), *New Directions for Child and Adolescent Development* (pp. 61–69), No. 108. San Francisco: Jossey-Bass.

Bowen, M. (1978). *Family therapy in clinical practice*. New York: Jason Aronson.

Branje, S.J.T., Van Lieshout, C.F.M., Van Aken, M.A.G., & Haselager, G.J.T. (2004). Perceived support in sibling relationships and adolescent adjustment. *Journal of Child Psychology and Psychiatry, 45*(8), 1385–1396.

Brody, G. H. (1998). Sibling relationship quality: Its causes and consequences. *Annual Review of Psychology, 49,* 1–24.

Brody, G. H., Flor, D. L., & Gibson, N. M. (1999). Linking maternal efficacy beliefs, developmental goals, parenting practices, and child competence in rural single-parent African American families. *Child Development, 70*(5), 1197–1208.

Brody, G. H., Ge, X., Conger, R., Gibbons, F. X., Murry, V. M., Gerrard, M., & Simons, R. L. (2001). The influence of neighborhood disadvantage, collective socialization, and parenting on African American children's affiliation with deviant peers. *Child Development, 72*(4), 1231–1246.

Broman, C. L., Reckase, M. D., & Freedman-Doan, C. R. (2006). The role of parenting in drug use among black, Latino and white Adolescents. *Journal of Ethnicity in Substance Abuse, 5*(1), 39–50.

Bronte-Tinkew, J., Moore, K. A., & Carrano, J. (2006). The father-child relationship, parenting styles, and adolescent risk behaviors in intact families. *Journal of Family Issues, 27*(6), 850–881.

Cauce, A. M., Hiraga, Y., Graves, D., Gonzales, N., Ryan-Finn, K., & Grove, K. (1996). African American mothers and their adolescent daughters: Intimacy, autonomy, and conflict. In B. J. Leadbeater & N. Way (Eds.), *Urban girls: Resisting stereotypes, creating identities*. New York: New York University Press.

Chassin, L., Presson, C. C., Rose, J., Sherman, S. J., Davis, M. J., & Gonzalez, J. L. (2005). Parenting style and smoking-specific parenting practices as predictors of adolescent smoking onset. *Journal of Pediatric Psychology, 30*(4), 334–344.

Chavous, T. M., Bernat, D. H., Schmeelk-Cone, K., Caldwell, C. H., Kohn-Wood, L., & Zimmerman, M. A. (2003). Racial identity and academic attainment among African American adolescents. *Child Development, 74*(4), 1076–1090.

Cohen, D. A., & Rice, J. (1997). Parenting styles, adolescent substance use, and academic achievement. *Journal of Drug Education, 27*(2), 199–211.

Coleman, J. S. (1990). *Foundations of social theory*. Cambridge, MA: Belknap.

Conger, R. D., & Ge, X. (1999). Conflict and cohesion in parent-adolescent relations: Changes in emotional expression from early to mid-adolescence. In M. J. Cox & J. Brooks-Gunn (Eds.), *Conflict and cohesion in families: Causes and consequences* (pp. 185–206). Mahwah, NJ: Erlbaum.

Crosby, R. A., DiClemente, R. J., Wingood, G. M., Harrington, K., Davies, S. L., Hook, E. W., III, & Oh, M. K. (2002). Low parental monitoring predicts subsequent pregnancy among African American adolescent females. *Journal of Pediatric and Adolescent Gynecology, 15*: 43–46.

Crosby, R. A., DiClemente, R. J., Wingood, G. M., Lang, D., & Harrington, K. F. (2003). Infrequent parental monitoring predicts sexually transmitted infections among low-income African American adolescent females. *Archives of Pediatric and Adolescent Medicine, 157,* 169–173.

Crosby, R. A., Voisin, D., Salazar, L. F., DiClemente, R., Yarber, W., & Caliendo, A. (2006). Family influences and biologically confirmed sexually transmitted infections among detained adolescents: An exploratory study. *American Journal of Orthopsychiatry, 76,* 389–394.

Davidov, M., & Grusec, J. E. (2006). Untangling the links of parental responsiveness to distress and warmth to child outcomes. *Child Development, 77*(1), 44–58.

DiClemente, R. J., Wingood, G. M., Crosby, R., Sionean, C., Cobb, B. K., Harrington, K., Davies S., Hook, E. W., III, & Oh, M. K. (2001). Parental monitoring: Association with adolescents' risk behaviors. *Pediatrics, 107,* 1363–1368.

Dornbusch, S. M., Ritter, P. L., Leiderman, P. H., Roberts, D. F., & Fraleigh, M. J. (1987). The relation of parenting style to adolescent school performance. *Child Development, 58,* 1244–1257.

Downey, D. B., & Condron, D. J. (2004). Playing well with others in kindergarten: The benefit of siblings at home. *Journal of Marriage and Family, 66,* 333–350.

Dubas, J. S., & Gerris, J. R. (2002). Longitudinal changes in the time parents spend in activities with their adolescent children as a function of child age, pubertal status, and gender. *Journal of Family Psychology, 16*(4), 415–427.

Fasula, A. M., Miller, K. S., & Wiener, J. (2007). The sexual double standard in African American adolescent women's sexual risk reduction socialization. *Women and Health, 46,* 3–21.

Fields, J., & Casper, L. M. (2001). *America's families living arrangements: March 2000* (Current population reports, series P20–537). Washington, DC: U.S. Bureau of the Census.

Fingerman, K. L., & Bermann, E. (2000). Applications of family systems theory to the study of adulthood. *International Journal of Aging and Human Development, 51*(1), 5–29.

Finkelstein, J. S., Donenberg, G. R., & Martinovich, Z. (2001). Maternal control and adolescent depression: Ethnic differences among clinically referred girls. *Journal of Youth and Adolescence, 30,* 155–172.

Gilbert, R. (1999). *Connecting with our children: Guiding principles for parents in a troubled world.* New York: Wiley.

Giles-Sims, J., & Lockhart, C. (2005). Culturally shaped patterns of disciplining children. *Journal of Family Issues, 26*(2), 196–218.

Gonzales, N. A., Deardorff, J., Formoso, D., Barr, A., & Barrera, M. (2006). Family mediators of the relation between acculturation and adolescent mental health. *Family Relations, 55,* 318–330.

Gonzales, N. A., Cauce, A. M., Friedman, R. J., & Mason, C. A. (1996). Family, peer, and neighborhood influences on academic achievement among African-American adolescents: One-year prospective effects. *American Journal of Community Psychology, 24*(3), 365–387.

Gorman-Smith, D., Tolan, P. H., Henry, D. B., & Florsheim, P. (2000). Patterns of family functioning and adolescent outcomes among urban African American and Mexican American families. *Journal of Family Psychology, 14*(3), 436–457.

Gorman-Smith, D., Tolan, P. H., Loweber, R., & Henry, D. B. (1998). Relation of family problems to patterns of delinquent involvement among urban youth. *Journal of Abnormal Child Psychology, 26,* 5.

Grant, K. E., Compas, B. E., Stuhlmacher, A., Thurm, A., McMahon, S., & Halpert, J. (2003). Stressors and child and adolescent psychopathology: Moving from markers to mechanisms of risk. *Psychological Bulletin, 129,* 447–466.

Gutman, L. M., & Eccles, J. S. (1999). Financial strain, parenting behaviors, and adolescents' achievement: Testing model equivalence between African American and European American single- and two-parent families. *Child Development, 70*(6), 1464–1476.

Hawkins, J. D., Catalano, R. F., Kosterman, R., Abbot, R., & Hill, K. G. (1999). Preventing adolescent health-risk behaviors by strengthening protection during childhood. *Archives of Pediatrics and Adolescent Medicine, 153*(3), 226–234.

Hill, N. E., Bush, K. R., & Roosa, M. W. (2003). Parenting and family socialization strategies and children's mental health: Low-income Mexican-American and Euro-American mothers and children. *Child Development, 74,* 189–204.

Jacob, T., Moser, R. P., Windle, M., Loeber, R., & Stouthamer-Loeber, M. (2000). A new measure of parenting practices involving preadolescent- and adolescent-aged children. *Behavior Modification, 24*(5), 611–634.

Kilgore K., Snyder, J., & Lentz, C. (2000). The contribution of parental discipline, parental monitoring, and school risk to early-onset conduct problems in African American boys and girls. *Developmental Psychology, 36*(6), 835–845.

Kirkman, M., Rosenthal, D. A., & Feldman, S. S. (2002). Talking to a tiger: Fathers reveal their difficulties in communicating about sexuality with adolescents. In S. S. Feldman & D. A. Rosenthal (Eds.), *New Directions for Child and Adolescent Development* (pp. 57–74), No. 97. San Francisco: Jossey-Bass.

Kitzmann, K. M. (2000). Effects of marital conflict on subsequent triadic family interactions and parenting. *Developmental Psychology, 36*(1), 3–13.

Knauth, D. G., Skowron, E. A., & Escobar, M. (2006). Effect of differentiation of self on adolescent risk behavior: Test of the theoretical model. *Nursing Research, 55*(5), 336–345.

Lansford, J. E., Dodge, K. A., Pettit, G. S., Bates, J. E., Crozier, J., & Kaplow, J. (2002). A 12-year prospective study of the long-term effects of early child physical maltreatment on psychological, behavioral, and academic problems in adolescence. *Archives of Pediatrics and Adolescent Medicine, 156*(8), 824–830.

Leadbeater, B. J., Kuperminc, G. P., Blatt, S. J., & Hertzog, C. (1999). A multivariate model of gender differences in adolescents' internalizing and externalizing problems. *Developmental Psychology, 35*(5), 1268–1282.

Li, X., Feigelman, S., & Stanton, B. (2000). Perceived parental monitoring and health risk behaviors among urban low-income African-American children and adolescents. *Journal of Adolescent Health, 27,* 43–48.

Logan, C., Manlove, J., Ikramullah, E., & Cottingham, S. (2006). Men who father children with more than one woman: A contemporary portrait of multiple-partner fertility (Child Trends Research Brief, Publication No. 2006–10). Washington, DC: Child Trends.

Luthar, S. (1999). *Poverty and children's adjustment.* Thousand Oaks, CA: Sage.

Mandara, J., & Murray, C. B. (2002). Development of an empirical typology of African American family functioning. *Journal of Family Psychology, 16*(3), 318–337.

Mboya, M. M. (1995). Variations in parenting practices: gender- and age-related differences in African adolescents. *Adolescence, 30*(120), 955–962.

McBride, C. K., Paikoff, R. L., & Holmbeck, G. N. (2003). Individual and familial influences on the onset of sexual intercourse among urban African American adolescents. *Journal of Consulting and Clinical Psychology, 71*(1), 159–167.

McCubbin, H. I., McCubbin, M. A., Thompson, A. I., Han, S., & Allen, C. T. (1997). Families under stress: What makes them resilient. *Journal of Family and Consumer Sciences, 89*(3), 2–11.

McElhaney, K. B., & Allen, J. P. (2001). Autonomy and adolescent social functioning: The moderating effect of risk. *Child Development, 72*(1), 220–235.

McLoyd, V. C. (1998). Socioeconomic disadvantage and child development. *American Psychologist, 53*(2), 185–204.

Miller, K. S., Kotchick, B. A., Dorsey, S., Forehand, R., & Ham, A. Y. (1998). Family communication about sex: What are parents saying and are their adolescents listening? *Family Planning Perspectives, 30*(5), 218–222, 235.

Mistry, R. S., Vandewater, E. A., Huston, A. C., & McLoyd, V. C. (2002). Economic well-being and children's social adjustment: The role of family process in an ethnically diverse low-income sample. *Child Development, 73*(3), 935–951.

Minuchin, P. (1985). Families and individual development: Provocations from the field of family therapy. *Child Development, 56,* 289–302.

Novak, G., & Pelaez, M. (2004). *Child and adolescent development: A behavioral systems approach.* Thousand Oaks, CA: Sage.

O'Byrne, K. K., Haddock, C. K., & Poston Walker, S. C. (2002). Parenting style and adolescent smoking. *Journal of Adolescent Health, 30*(6), 418–425.

Patock-Peckham, J. A., & Morgan-Lopez, A. A. (2006). College drinking behaviors: Mediational links between parenting styles, impulse control, and alcohol-related outcomes. *Psychology of Addictive Behaviors, 20*(2), 117–125.

Pearce, C. M., Martin, G., & Wood, K. (1995). Significance of touch for perceptions of parenting and psychological adjustment among adolescents. *Journal of the American Academy of Child and Adolescent Psychiatry, 34,* 160–167.

Pineda, A. Q., Cole, D. A., & Bruce, A. E. (2007). Mother-adolescent interactions and adolescent depressive symptoms: A sequential analysis. *Journal of Social and Personal Relationships, 24,* 5–19.

Querido, J. G., Warner, T. D., & Eyberg, S. M. (2002). Parenting styles and child behavior in African American families of preschool children. *Journal of Clinical Child Psychology, 31*(2), 272–277.

Radziszewska, B., Richardson, J. L., Dent, C. W., & Flay, B. R. (1996). Parenting style and adolescent depressive symptoms, smoking, and academic achievement: Ethnic, gender, and SES differences. *Journal of Behavioral Medicine, 19*(3), 289–305.

Romer, D., Stanton, B., Galbraith, J., Feigelman, S., Black, M. M, & Li, X. (1999). Parental influence on adolescent sexual behavior in high-poverty settings. *Archives of Pediatric Adolescent Medicine, 153,* 1055–1062.

Rosenthal, S. L., von Ranson, K. M., Cotton, S., Biro, F. M., Mills, L., & Succop, P. A. (2001). Sexual initiation: Predictors and developmental trends. *Sexually Transmitted Diseases, 28,* 527–532.

Salt, R. E. (1991). Affectionate touch between fathers and preadolescent sons. *Journal of Marriage and the Family, 53,* 545–554.

Sanders, M. R. (2000). Community-based parenting and family support interventions and the prevention of drug abuse. *Addictive Behaviors, 25*(6), 929–942.

Sieverding, J. A., Adler, N., Witt, S., & Ellen, J. (2005). The influence of parental monitoring on adolescent sexual initiation. *Archives of Pediatric and Adolescent Medicine, 159*(8), 724–729.

Silverstein, L. B., & Auerbach, C. F. (1999). Deconstructing the essential father. *American Psychologist, 54*(6), 397–407.

Slicker, E. K. (1998). Relationship of parenting style to behavioral adjustment in graduating high school seniors. *Journal of Youth and Adolescence, 27*(3), 345–372.

Stattin, H., & Kerr, M. (2000). Parental monitoring: A reinterpretation. *Child Development, 71*(4), 1072–1085.

Steinberg, L. (2001). We know some things: Parent-adolescent relationships in retrospect and prospect. *Journal of Research on Adolescence, 11*(1), 1–19.

Stewart-Brown, S., Patterson, J., Mockford, C., Barlow, J., Klimes, I., & Pyper, C. (2004). Impact of a general practice based group parenting programme: Quantitative and qualitative results from a controlled trial at 12 months. *Archives of Disease in Childhood, 89,* 519–525.

Szapocznik, J., & Coatsworth, J. D. (1999). An ecodevelopmental framework for organizing the influences on drug abuse: A developmental model of risk and protection. In M. Glantz & C. R. Hartel (Eds.), *Drug abuse: Origins and interventions.* Washington, DC: American Psychological Association.

Taylor, R. D., & Robert, D. (1995). Kinship support and maternal and adolescent well-being in economically disadvantaged African American families. *Child Development, 66,* 1585–1597.

Trim, R. S., Leuthe, E., & Chassin, L. (2006). Sibling influence on alcohol use in a young adult, high-risk sample. *Journal of Studies on Alcohol, 67*(3), 391–398.

van der Vorst, H., Engels, R.C.M.E., Meeus, W., Dekovic, M., & Vermulst, A. (2006). Family factors and adolescents' alcohol use: A reply to Chassin and Handley (2006) and Fromme (2006). *Psychology of Addictive Behaviors, 20*(2), 140–142.

White, J. M., & Klein, D. M. (2002). *Family theories.* Thousand Oaks, CA: Sage.

Whiteman, S. D., McHale, S. M., & Crouter, A. C. (2007). Explaining sibling similarities: Perceptions of sibling influences. *Journal of Youth and Adolescence, 36*(7), 963–972.

Windle, M. (2000). Parental, sibling, and peer influences on adolescent substance use and alcohol problems. *Applied Developmental Science, 4*(2), 98–110.

CHAPTER

21

MEDIA EXPOSURE AND ADOLESCENTS' HEALTH BEHAVIOR

VICTOR C. STRASBURGER ▪ MARJORIE J. HOGAN

LEARNING OBJECTIVES

After studying this chapter, you will be able to

- Recognize the vast influence media has on adolescent development and health behavior.

- Identify how different forms of media affect adolescents' perceptions of violence, sex, body image, and drugs.

- Summarize possible solutions for altering messages that are portrayed within the media to promote healthier behaviors among adolescents.

True, media violence is not likely to turn an otherwise fine child into a violent criminal. But, just as every cigarette one smokes increases a little bit the likelihood of a lung tumor someday, every violent show one watches increases just a little bit the likelihood of behaving more aggressively in some situation.

—BRAD J. BUSHMAN AND L. ROWELL HUESMANN, IN *HANDBOOK OF CHILDREN AND THE MEDIA*

By baring a single breast in a slam-dunk publicity stunt of two seconds' duration, [Janet Jackson] also exposed just how many boobs we have in this country. We owe her thanks for a genuine public service.

—FRANK RICH, *NEW YORK TIMES*

A cigarette in the hands of a Hollywood star onscreen is a gun aimed at a twelve- or fourteen-year-old.

—JOE ESZTERHAS, *HOLLYWOOD ANIMAL*

My six-year-old daughter turned to me and said, "What's a four-hour erection?" said Kelly Simmons, executive vice president at Tierney Communications in Philadelphia. "How do you explain it?"

—STUART ELLIOTT, *NEW YORK TIMES*

Those most concerned about adolescent health—parents, teachers, adolescent health care providers and researchers, and public policy analysts and advocates—are discovering that virtually every health or behavioral concern relates in some significant way to media influence during the child and teen years. Teens spend more time with media than any other activity except sleeping; no wonder media messages and images influence teen knowledge, attitudes, and behavior about violence and aggression, sex, eating disorders and obesity, substance use, and school performance (Strasburger, 2006).

Failure to appreciate the teen cultural milieu may result in an adolescent health care provider's inability to recognize and address key health issues with a patient. An obese adolescent presenting to his doctor's office should be asked about hours spent with media. Heavy media use may displace the teen's other pursuits, including physical activity. Unhealthy ads for food and drink may be a contributing factor as well. A middle school student struggling at home or in school should be asked about her "media diet" and the media environment in her home. Key questions to address during routine health care visits are simply: How much time do you spend with electronic media daily? Is there a TV set or Internet connection in your bedroom? (Strasburger, 2005a). Asking these two key media use questions in the office or clinic will consume little time, but will yield salient clues about significant adolescent health problems and potential solutions.

Practitioners also need to be aware of the fact that young children are uniquely susceptible to media influence, but that their behavior may not show that influence until they are older (Strasburger, Wilson, & Jordan, 2009). Therefore, when thinking about the effect of media messages and images, we must consider the entire range of childhood through the teen years. Research shows that media can be a powerful teacher for all ages (Strasburger, 2006; Stranger, 2002). By sheer time standards alone, media represent a major influence on adolescents—one that must be acknowledged properly by all adults who care about teens and their well-being.

Media represent a major influence on adolescents—one that must be acknowledged properly by all adults who care about teens and their well-being.

TEENS AND MEDIA USE

By the time they reach the age of seventy, teenagers will have spent seven to ten years of their lives in front of a television screen (Strasburger et al., 2009). Although television remains the predominant medium for children and adolescents, there is now an astounding range of media for teens to choose, use, and abuse—TV, movies, video games, the Internet, cell phones, iPods, and magazines. A 2005 sample of more than two thousand children in elementary through high school found that young people spend an average of 6.5 hours daily with a variety of media (Rideout, Roberts, & Foehr, 2005). Although television remains popular for all ages, adolescents tend to branch out into computer and video games, music, music videos, and film (see Figure 21.1A; Rideout et al., 2005).

American teens have unprecedented access to media: two-thirds of American children and teens have a television set in their bedrooms, one-half have a VCR or DVD player, one-half have a video game console, and almost 33 percent have Internet access or a computer (see Figure 21.1B; Rideout et al., 2005).

The context is critical as well, in that the average American household has 3.6 CD or tape players, 3.5 TV sets, 3.3 radios, 2.9 VCR or DVD players, 2.1 video game consoles, and 1.5 computers (Rideout et al., 2005).

Teenagers live in a media-saturated world, and many studies show that children and teens with a TV set in their own bedroom are at increased risk for adverse health outcomes (see Figure 21.1C; Strasburger, 2006).

THE INFLUENCE OF MEDIA ON ADOLESCENTS

For teens seeking answers to crucial questions—"Who am I?" "What should I be when I grow up?" "When should I start having sex with my boy- or girlfriend?" "When should I begin drinking alcohol?"—media provide plenty of answers, unlike parents, schools, and sex education or drug education programs. Media portrayals of casual

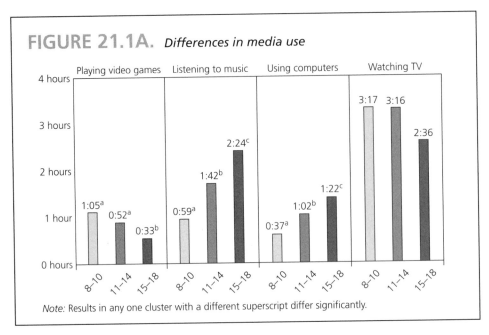

FIGURE 21.1A. *Differences in media use*

Note: Results in any one cluster with a different superscript differ significantly.

Source: From Rideout, Roberts, and Foehr (2005). Used with permission.

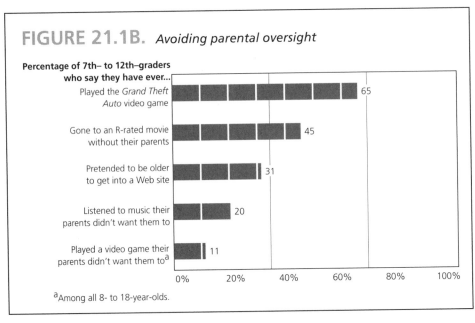

FIGURE 21.1B. *Avoiding parental oversight*

[a]Among all 8- to 18-year-olds.

Source: From Rideout, Roberts, and Foehr (2005). Used with permission.

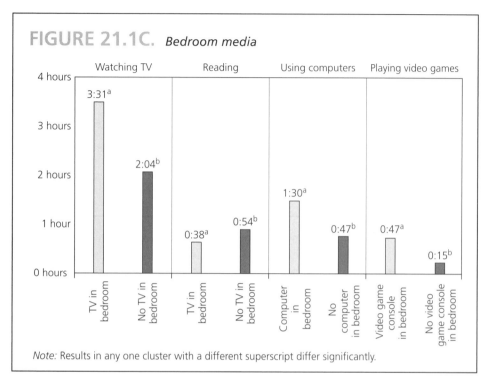

FIGURE 21.1C. *Bedroom media*

Note: Results in any one cluster with a different superscript differ significantly.

Source: From Rideout, Roberts, and Foehr (2005). Used with permission.

sex, violence as a solution to problems, and drug use give susceptible teens the impression that these behaviors are normal and acceptable. This is media as *super-peer*, (Strasburger et al., 2009) giving teens a glimpse into the adult world of sex, drugs, and relationships, as well as "scripts" to use as they navigate the adolescent years. Scripts offered by attractive people on popular television shows, movies, and even video games may provide teens with approaches to a host of adolescent issues: gender identity, conflict resolution, sexual gratification, stress, and parent relationships, to name but a few (Strasburger, 2006). For example, studies show that teens routinely overestimate the number of their peers who are sexually active (Strasburger, 2005a) and that television "encourages" them to have sex (Brown, Childers, & Waszak, 1990). Girls who mature early are likely to seek out sexual media and interpret these portrayals as approving teen sexual activity (Brown, Halpern, & L'Engle, 2005).

Children and teens tend to blur the media world and the real world, believing that the media portray real people behaving like real adults.

In addition to the super-peer theory, media influence on teens is also explained by the *cultivation hypothesis* (Gerbner, Gross, Morgan, & Signorelli,

1994). Children and teens tend to blur the media world and the real world, believing that the media portray real people behaving like real adults (violently, sexually, with drug use thrown in). In addition, Bandura's social cognitive theory posits that children and teens learn by observing others, both directly in real life and vicariously on the media screen (Bandura, 1986). Ironically, although adolescents acknowledge the power of media to teach and influence behavior, the *third-person effect* applies—like adults, teens believe that media images and messages influence everyone except them (Kaiser Family Foundation, 2002).

Media Violence

Because more than a thousand studies and another 2,500 reviews in various scholarly fields employing different methodologies (classic laboratory experiments, cross-sectional correlational studies, longitudinal studies, and meta-analyses) have demonstrated that media violence affects children and adolescents, the controversy should be over (Wartella, Olivarez, & Ennings, 1998). Only thirty studies observed no impact. Undeniably, social science research presents challenges, but the effect size of media violence exposure on young viewers is significant. The societal scourge of smoking allows a ready comparison. Not all smokers develop cancer, but the connection

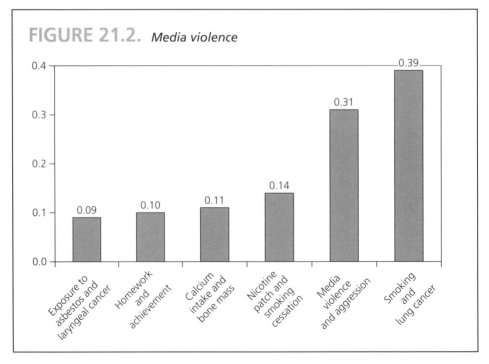

FIGURE 21.2. *Media violence*

Source: From Strasburger, Wilson, and Jordan (2009). Used with permission.

between smoking cigarettes and developing lung cancer later in life is clear and readily acknowledged by most segments of society (see Figure 21.2).

Similarly, although not every young consumer of media violence will become aggressive or violent, the epidemiological connection is strong. Approximately 10 to 30 percent of violent incidents in society can be attributed to media violence (Strasburger et al., 2008; Comstock & Strasburger, 1993). Clearly, media violence is not the sole or most important factor leading to societal violence, but an effect of this magnitude demands attention.

Media violence is particularly pernicious for children and teens; the lesson learned and reinforced at young ages is that violence is an acceptable solution to conflict (Strasburger et al., 2008; Hogan, 2005; Bushman & Huesmann, 2006). Violent means are used not only by the "bad guys," but also by the heroes. Media violence is often sanitized—without consequences or repercussions for those who are violent—and humor is commonly juxtaposed with gunplay. Justified violence ("she asked for it") is a powerful and strongly reinforcing message for young viewers. Particularly confusing and harmful for young viewers of TV and film—and even more, in popular video games—is the combination of violence and sex.

Several longitudinal studies provide scholarly support for the power of violent media to lead to aggressive and antisocial behavior. A study begun in 1960 with third graders found exposure to violent television predictive of aggressive behavior eleven and twenty-two years later (Eron, Huesmann, Lefkowitz, & Walder, 1972; Huesmann, Eron, Lefkowitz, & Walder, 1984). A similar study followed children ages one through ten for seventeen years in New York: time spent watching television was a risk factor for interpersonal aggression, especially for boys (Johnson, Cohen, Smailes, Kasen, & Brook, 2002). Finally, a study from 1977 through 2003 found violent media exposure at ages six through nine years predicted adolescent aggression, criminal behavior, and spousal abuse (Huesmann, Moise-Titus, Podolski, & Eron, 2003). Researchers conclude that children and teens learn attitudes about violence when very young, and these attitudes and beliefs may become entrenched, carried to adulthood, and difficult to modify. In the longitudinal studies, the three most important variables were how much violence was viewed, identification of the child with violent characters, and the perception that TV violence was actually real (Huesmann et al., 2003). A recent review of the longitudinal data concluded that media violence produces aggression both in the short- and long-term (Bushman & Huesmann, 2006). Adding its voice to the debate, a recent Federal Communications Commission (FCC) report agrees with the research that media violence is one cause of aggressive behaviors, especially in the short term (FCC, 2007).

Studies show effects of media violence on young viewers beyond aggressive and antisocial behavior (Strasburger et al., 2009; Hogan, 2005; Anderson, Carnagey, & Eubanks, 2003). Exposure to violent images and messages leads to desensitization; hence the increasing "body count" in violent movie sequels. People tend to become a bit more callous about death and crime in their lives when they see countless

Studies show effects of media violence on young viewers beyond aggressive and antisocial behavior.

violent events on their screens. Finally, heavy viewers of media violence develop the notion that the world is a "mean and scary place"—a blurring of the real and the media world. Perhaps this fear plays a role in the apparently increasing hostile interactions between people. A combination of fear of the world around us, justifiable violence in the media, and acceptance of violence for conflict resolution may help to explain some of the recent shootings in schools and on the streets (Strasburger, 2006; Strasburger et al., 2009; Anderson, Berkowitz, et al., 2003).

Concerns have also been raised about violence in sports, especially professional wrestling. A recent survey of 2,228 students found significant correlations between watching wrestling on TV and date fighting, fighting in general, and weapon carrying for both males and females (DuRant, Champion, & Wolfson, 2006).

Guns, Media, and Teens

Media—whether television, film, or violent video games—normalize and glamorize guns. It should be no surprise to pediatricians that guns, especially handguns, represent a real threat to young people in the United States; American youth are twelve times more likely to die from gun violence than a child in the other top twenty-five industrialized nations, and 75 percent of all youth homicides in the world occur in this country (see Figure 21.3; National Institutes of Health and Prevention, 1997).

Japan outlaws the individual ownership of guns, whereas in the United States there are more guns than households. In Japan there were twenty-eight gun-related

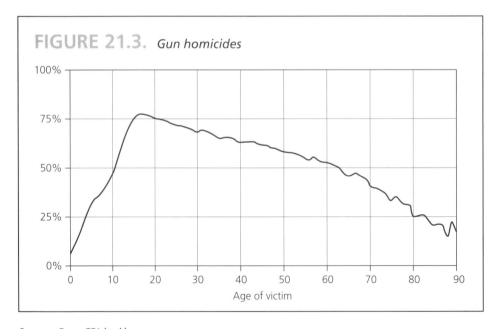

FIGURE 21.3. *Gun homicides*

Source: From FBI (n.d.).

deaths in 1990; in the United States there were 30,694 gun-related deaths in the year 2005 (Centers for Disease Control, 2005; Davidson, 1993).

Guns are prevalent in media portrayals: on television 25 percent of violent scenes involve the use of a gun (Federman, 1998), 40 percent of the top-grossing G- and PG-rated films featured at least one major character carrying a gun (Ramsey & Pelletier, 2004), and a meta-analysis of fifty-six studies found that the mere presence of a gun in a movie or TV show increases the likelihood of aggressive behavior (Carlson, Marcus-Newhall, & Miller, 1990). A 2007 analysis of seventy-seven recent PG-13-rated films found a total 2,251 violent occurrences, nearly half of which were "lethal" (Webb, Jenkins, Browne, Abdelmonen, & Kraus, 2007).

Video games, an increasingly popular form of media for children and youth, seem to be even more problematic, because many are so-called "first-person shooter games" (Strasburger, 2006). Although some can be entertaining and even educational, many video games are exceedingly violent. One study found even E-rated (for everyone) games to have violent content (Thompson & Haninger, 2001). A meta-analysis of fifty-four studies involving nearly five thousand children and youth found that playing violent video games increased aggressive thoughts, feelings, and behavior (Anderson & Bushman, 2001). A survey of six hundred early adolescents found that frequent players not only got into more arguments with teachers and physical fights with peers, but also viewed the world as a more aggressive place (Gentile, Lynch, Linder, & Walsh, 2004).

Ironically, the U.S. Army uses adaptations of commonly played video games to teach new recruits how to kill (Strasburger & Grossman, 2001). Law enforcement agencies use a firearm training simulator similar to arcade video games. In some instances, the shooters in recent school shootings were frequent players of violent video games. The adolescent shooter in Paducah, Kentucky, had never used an actual gun, but learning to fire from playing first-person video games, his eight shots had eight hits in the upper torso or head—three victims were dead and one paralyzed. It is likely that the skill reinforced by violent video games—firing once at popups on the screen—trains those inclined to kill with a firearm (Strasburger & Grossman, 2001).

According to the most recent data from the 2005 Youth Risk Behavior Surveillance System, 22 percent of female teens and 12 percent of male teens have seriously considered suicide, the third leading cause of death in the adolescent years (Centers for Disease Prevention and Control, 2006). The prevalence of firearm use in media and the glamorization of gun violence are alarming and unwise trends. Additionally, several studies demonstrate a link between media coverage of a prominent suicide (even sensitively produced movies) and a subsequent increase in adolescent suicide (Gould, Jamieson, & Romer, 2003; Phillips & Paight, 1987). This is known as *suicide contagion,* and it seems stronger in youth than adults (Gould, Wallerstein, Kleinman, O'Carroll, & Mercy, 1990); the CDC recently issued guidelines for media reports of suicide and urged that sensationalizing or glorifying the event be avoided (Strasburger, 2006).

Sex and the Media

For two principal reasons, the mass media now provide sex education for a growing number of children and adolescents in America (Strasburger, 2005b). Traditional sex education—formerly offered in schools—is often absent, inadequate, or constrained and ineffective because of a "just-say-no," abstinence-only approach (Kaiser Family Foundation, 2004). In addition, parents and physicians may be ill equipped or lack opportunities to educate youth about healthy sexuality. Curious adolescents turn to sexual images and messages in the media, or increasingly to the Internet, to learn about sex and birth control—and there is no shortage of material available. A 2004 national survey of teens found that media far outranked parents or schools as a source of contraceptive information (National Public Radio, 2004). The Internet does offer valuable information, but viewers must be appropriately savvy and mature to avoid dangerous misinformation and easily accessed, explicit pornography (Rideout, 2001).

The mass media now provide sex education for a growing number of children and adolescents in America.

Secondly, American media have become effective sex educators because they are extremely titillating to young, curious teens. American media are among the most sexually suggestive in the world (see Figure 21.4; Strasburger, 2005).

Television and movie portrayals offer attractive scripts for sexual behaviors, notably without acknowledgement of the dangers and emptiness of casual sex. Only 14 percent of television programs with sexual content mention risks or responsibilities that accompany sex; the figure drops to 10 percent for shows aimed at adolescent viewers (see Figures 21.5A and 21.5B; Kunkel, Eyal, Finnerty, Biely, & Donnerstein, 2005).

The sheer amount of sex in the media is astounding: more than 75 percent of primetime shows feature sexual content (see Figure 21.5B); popular teen shows have more sex than shows aimed at adults; and one in ten programs portrays actual or implied sexual intercourse (Kunkel et al., 2005).

Sex draws viewers' eyes to the program, but doesn't stop there: sex is also used to sell everything from shampoo to cars, from beer to vacations (Strasburger, 2006). These portrayals normalize sex (everyone is doing it!) and sanitize sex (there are no risks!)—powerful messages for young teens.

Research on the effect of sexual media on young viewers is sparse, especially compared to the robust media violence data. However, three very recent longitudinal studies do shed light on the impact of sexual media on adolescent behavior, allowing examination of cause and effect. A 2004 RAND study of about 1,800 teens found that those most exposed to sex in the media were two times more likely to initiate intercourse or other sexual activities at a younger age (Collins et al., 2004). A 2006 study of North Carolina young adolescents concluded that exposure to sexual content in a variety of media accelerated the sexual activity of white teens and doubled the risk of early sexual intercourse (Brown et al., 2006). This unique study was based on an analysis of the "media diet" of the participating teens—a useful concept for interested adults. Finally, using data from

FIGURE 21.4. *Are you hot?*

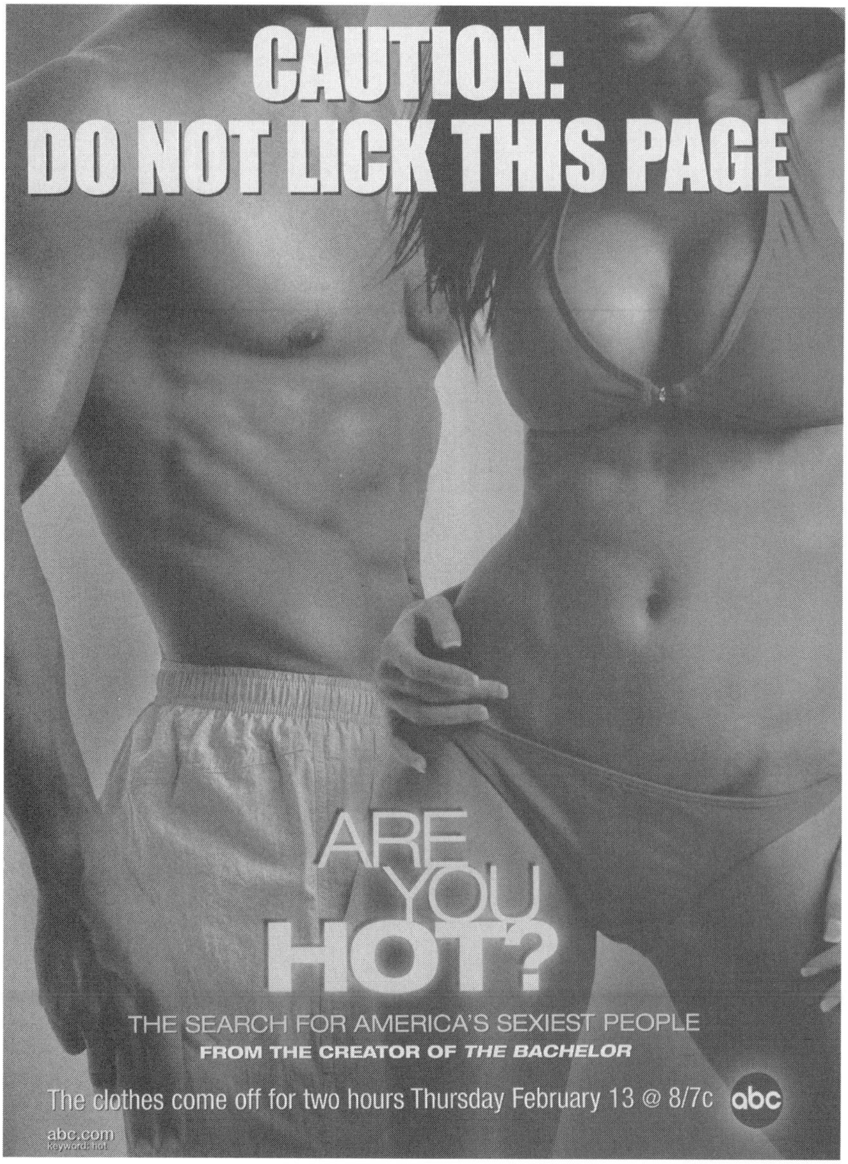

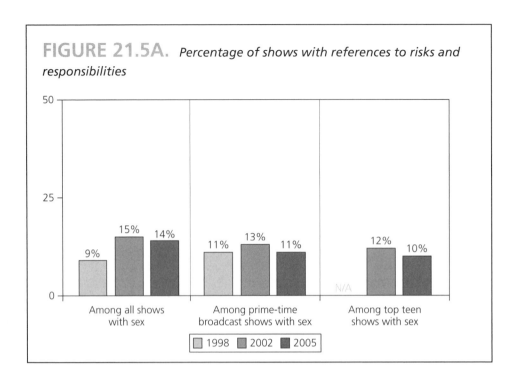

FIGURE 21.5A. *Percentage of shows with references to risks and responsibilities*

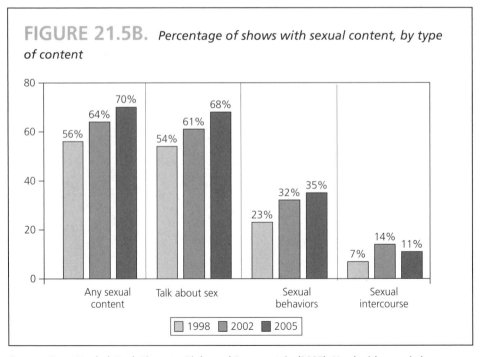

FIGURE 21.5B. *Percentage of shows with sexual content, by type of content*

Source: From Kunkel, Eyal, Finnerty, Biely, and Donnerstein (2005). Used with permission.

the National Longitudinal Study of Adolescent Health, University of Wisconsin researchers scrutinized the media diet of 5,000 teens less than sixteen years old. After one year, those watching two or more hours of television daily or reporting lack of parental regulation of media use had a significantly higher rate of initiating sexual intercourse (Ashby, Arcari, & Edmonson, 2006). Several correlational studies also exist. Although they do not allow cause-and-effect conclusions, they do support a relationship between frequent use of sexualized media and sexual behavior (Strasburger, 2005b).

Clearly, media serve as an access point for adolescents seeking information and validation about sexuality. Ironically, young viewers do not see advertisements for safe birth control methods, condoms, or emergency contraception (Strasburger, 2006). The United States continues to have unacceptably high rates of teen pregnancy and sexually transmitted infections, yet providing potentially life-saving information to young people is considered immoral (Abma, Martinez, Mosher, & Dawson, 2002). Several clinical trials demonstrate that enabling access to condoms increases condom use only for those already sexually active; it is a myth that access to birth control entices youth to have sex at younger ages (Strasburger, 2006). At the same time, the networks who refuse to air ads for condoms flood the air waves with suggestive ads for Viagra, Cialis, and Levitra—warning about four-hour erections and viewed by people of all ages—and drug companies spent nearly half a billion per year for erectile dysfunction drug advertising (see Figures 21.6A and 21.6B; Strasburger, 2006; Snobeck, 2005) The media are decidedly *not* abstinence-only.

> *Ironically, young viewers do not see advertisements for safe birth control methods, condoms, or emergency contraception.*

In a positive step, the American Academy of Pediatrics has called on TV networks to advertise safe, effective birth control options and to delay airing of erectile dysfunction ads until after 10 PM (American Academy of Pediatrics, 2006). Ironically, a recently produced condom commercial was rejected by FOX and CBS because it dared to mention condoms preventing pregnancy instead of HIV; the ad will run on several more enlightened networks this year (Newman, 2007).

Unique Internet Risk

Youth are Internet-savvy in increasing numbers. Recent surveys show that 75 percent of all U.S. children and teens are online (Wolnak, 2007). Most often young users are far more knowledgeable than parents about surfing the Net, and whether or not a computer is in a youth's bedroom, many parents are clueless about the power of the medium. Especially for young teens, social networking sites, chat rooms, and instant messaging offer connection and affirmation during these difficult years. More than half of youth ages twelve through seventeen have profiles on social networking sites such as MySpace and FaceBook (Wolnak, 2007). Concerns arise when time spent in online relationships exceeds time and energy in real face-to-face interactions with friends and family.

FIGURE 21.6A. *Viagra ad*

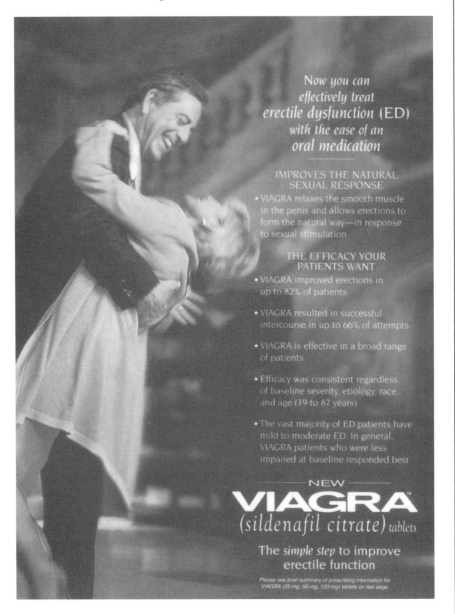

FIGURE 21.6B. *Trojan condom ad*

"I didn't use one because I didn't have one with me."

GET REAL

If you don't have a parachute, don't jump, genius.

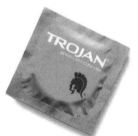

Helps reduce the risk

One in five youngsters may be solicited for sex on the Internet (Nelson, 2007). Those at greatest risk are lonely young teens or those who are aggressively seeking relationships on interactive sites, specifically chat rooms. Internet contacts between young adolescents and older opportunists may culminate in sexual abuse, as reported in the media (Wolnak, 2007). The Internet Crimes Against Children (ICAC) task force recommends talking to kids about online sexual activities, including visiting X-rated chat rooms, talking about sex with people they meet online, "cybersex," and viewing pornography (Wolnak, 2007). Parents and practitioners must be aware of how easily pornography is accessed on the Internet, conservatively estimated to account for millions of sites and to be very lucrative (Nelson, 2007). Research is needed on the impact of sexually explicit material on adolescents and how adults can best intervene to protect youth.

Media and Body Image, Eating Disorders, and Obesity

Adolescence is a period of life dominated by challenging tasks, including comfort with self-identity and establishing future orientation. Teens are asking themselves, Who am I? Where am I going? What is success? What is beauty? They look to family, peers, but also to the ubiquitous media for guidance and answers. Young adolescent females may be especially vulnerable to media portrayals, whether on TV, in movies, or in popular magazines. The ideal mature woman's body has gone through many evolutions over years and centuries: consider the voluptuous figures in classical painting to the size 14 Marilyn Monroe in the 1950s to the ever-thinning Miss America candidates (now 13 to 19 percent thinner than expected for age) to Twiggy to today's often gaunt models or large-breasted yet skinny teen idols (see Figures 21.7A and 21.7B; Strasburger, 2006; Kilbourne, 1999).

It must be extremely confusing for a twelve-year-old girl bombarded by thousands of images on a daily basis. No wonder nearly one-third of third-grade girls have dieted; by sixth grade, an astounding 60 percent have dieted (Maloney, McGuire, Daniels, & Specker, 1989). In addition, as many as one-half of normal-weight teen girls consider themselves overweight (Krowchuk, Dreiter, Woods, Sinal, & DuRant, 1998).

A large study showed that young female teens hoping to look like their favorite teen idols are more likely to be concerned about their weight, to be constantly on a diet, or to use purging behavior (Field, Cheung, et al., 1999). In another study, more than two-thirds of fifth- through twelfth-grade girls reported that their ideal body shape was influenced by portrayals in fashion magazines (Field, Camargo, Taylor, Berkey, & Colditz, 1999). The connection between body image and eating disorders certainly exists, but a cause-and-effect link is as yet unproven (Strasburger et al., 2006). Two recent studies have shed more light on the possibility that media may actually help to *cause* eating disorders. A study of Spanish adolescents ages twelve to twenty-one found that those reading popular girls' magazines had twice the risk of developing an eating disorder (Martinez-Gonzalez et al., 2003). And a naturalistic study after introduction of American TV to Fiji found 15 percent of teen girls in Fiji reported vomiting to control weight, compared with 3 percent before. Furthermore, 75 percent of the girls reported feeling "too big or fat" after being introduced to American programming (Becker, 2002).

The link between media and obesity is complex (Jordan, 2007). The epidemic of obesity in America is a well-documented public health nightmare. Could there be a connection between accelerating body mass indexes (BMIs) and the fact that 50 percent of the 40,000 TV ads viewed yearly by children and teens are for unhealthy foods, particularly sugary cereal and high-calorie snacks (Reece, Rifon, & Rodriguez, 1999; Taras & Gage, 1995; Institute of Medicine, 2006)? There are also 4,500 Pizza Huts and 3,000 Taco Bells in school cafeterias around the United States (Oleck, 1994), and many schools negotiate exclusive contracts with soft drink companies to peddle their unhealthy drinks (Hays, 2000). New research shows that soft drink consumption contributes to obesity (Ludwig, Peterson, & Gortmaker, 2001; Giammattei, Blix, Marshak, Wollitzer, & Pettitt, 2003). The literature on media and obesity doesn't solve the cause-and-effect conundrum. Five large cross-sectional studies find a correlation between television viewing and obesity, but it is unclear what comes first (Strasburger, 2006; Robinson, 1998). Do

FIGURE 21.7A. *Style.com ad*

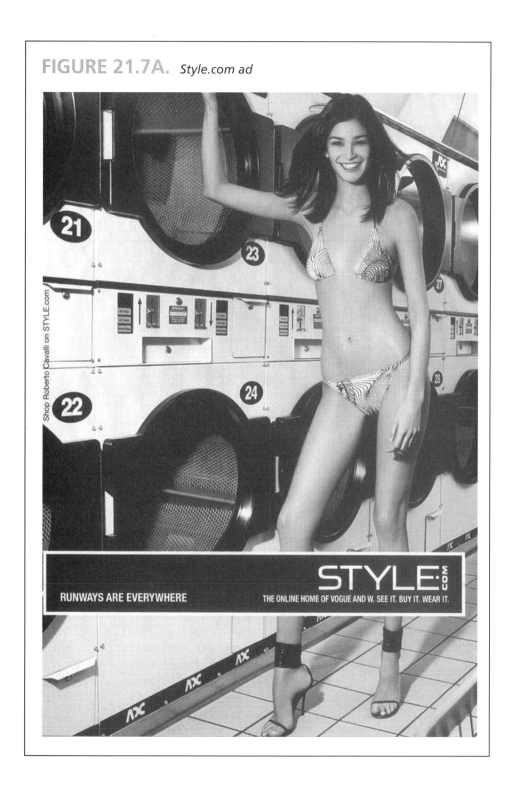

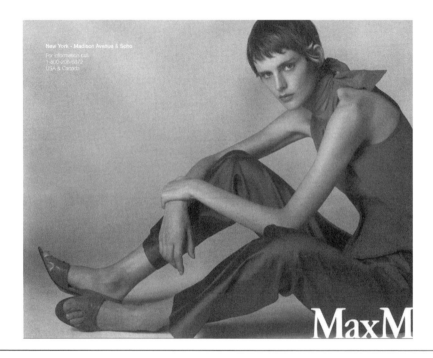

FIGURE 21.7B. *Max Mara ad*

fat, sedentary children watch more TV, does TV viewing lead to obesity, or is it a combination of the two? Children with a TV set in the bedroom watch more TV and have a 30 percent increased risk of a BMI higher than the eighty-fifth percentile (Dennison, Erb, & Jenkins, 2002). An innovative study showed that a simple six-month classroom curriculum in elementary school emphasizing less media use led to decreased BMI, skin-fold thickness, and waist measurement (Robinson, 1999).

The question still remains: Does media use cause obesity? An excess of merely fifty kilocalories daily leads to a five-pound weight gain in one year (Dietz, 1993). Consequently, if TV and other media cause even a small imbalance in the intake-output energy equation, their role could be significant. Media use displaces other pursuits, including physical activity, among children and teens (Robinson et al., 1993); they spend more time with media than any other activity except sleeping (Strasburger et al., 2008). However, sedentary teenagers who do not watch TV sometimes choose other sedentary activities instead (Strasburger et al., 2009). TV watching also increases snacking behavior and poor nutritional choices (Dietz, 1993) and may result in actually burning fewer calories than resting quietly or reading a good book (Klesges, Shelton, & Klesges, 1993).

Drugs and the Media

Ironically, American society expects youth to "just say no" to drug use at the same time that phenomenal amounts of money are spent each year to advertise cigarettes, alcohol, and prescription drugs in every possible venue—in excess of $20 billion annually (Strasburger, 2006). The vast majority of adult smokers picked up the habit as young teenagers. Does any health professional still honestly believe that tobacco companies do not target youth? Tobacco companies spend $11.2 billion dollars yearly on ads, and two large studies found that one-third of teen smoking behavior is attributable to the influence of tobacco advertising and promotions (see Figure 21.8A; Federal Trade Commission, 2003; Pierce, Choi, Gilpin, Farkas, & Beryy, 1998; Biener & Siegel, 2000). Young people exposed to cigarette ads or promotions are more likely to be smokers (Sargent, Dalton, & Beach, 2000).

American society expects youth to "just say no" to drug use at the same time that phenomenal amounts of money are spent each year to advertise cigarettes, alcohol, and prescription drugs in every possible venue.

The alcohol industry spends $5 billion yearly on advertising (Center on Alcohol Marketing and Youth, 2003), and teens see an average of two thousand alcohol ads yearly on TV alone (Strasburger, 2006). Ads for alcohol products have been shown to influence adolescents' intention to drink (Grube, 1995; Wyllie, Zhang, & Casswell, 1998; Grube, 1999). The overwhelming number of alcohol ads generally depict appealing, sexy people having fun and give the clear message that drinking is normative and glamorous (see Figure 21.8B). Two surveys of nearly two thousand preteens and young teens in North Dakota found a 50 percent increased risk of drinking with exposure to alcohol ads (Collins, Ellickson, McCaffrey, & Hambarsoomians, 2007).

Prescription drugs are increasingly advertised directly to a public eager for a cure for all ills. Drug companies spend about $4 billion yearly, more than twice the amount spent on research and development (Rubin, 2004). The message is clear: there is a drug available to fix all problems, heal all pain . . . a drug for every occasion, even sexual intercourse (Strasburger, 2006; Thomaselli, 2003).

In addition to advertising, young viewers are frequently exposed to drug use in the media (see Figures 21.9A and 21.9B; Strasburger, 2006).

Increasingly, smoking is portrayed in the media, both television and film: 85 percent of the top grossing movies since 1988 feature smoking cigarettes (Sargent, Beach, et al., 2001) far outstripping the actual rate of smoking in society (Charlesworth & Glantz, 2005). A 2007 study estimates that thirty recent popular movies collectively delivered more than one million smoking images to young people worldwide (Sargent, Tanski, & Gibson, 2007). In a 2006 survey of youth, 95 percent of all youth twelve to seventeen years of age saw at least one movie trailer during the year on TV depicting tobacco use, and 89 percent saw at least one trailer three or more times

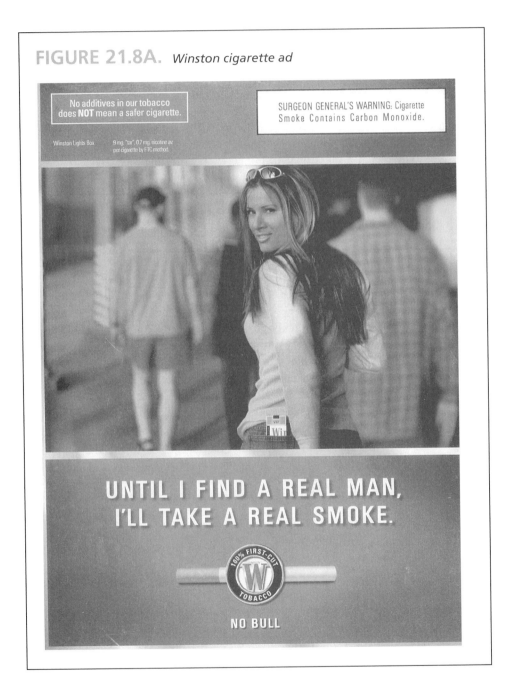

FIGURE 21.8A. *Winston cigarette ad*

FIGURE 21.8B. *Sauza tequila ad*

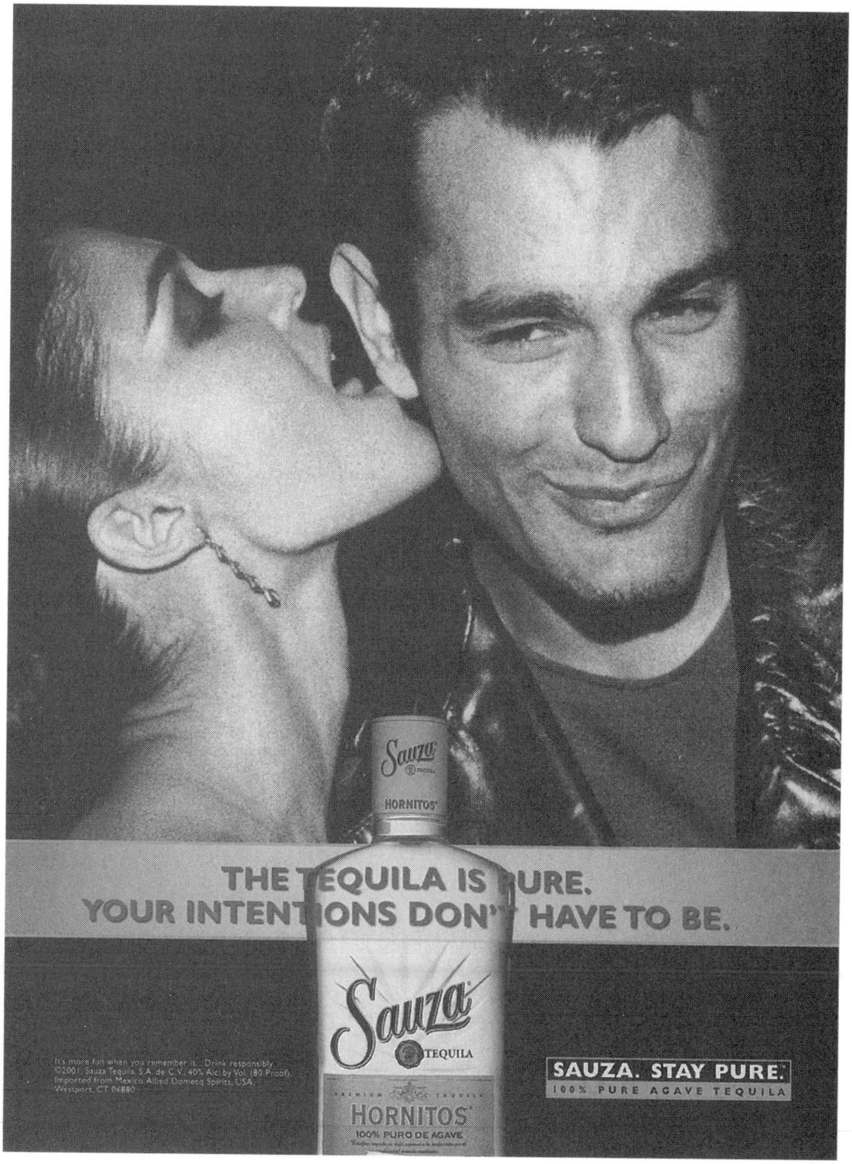

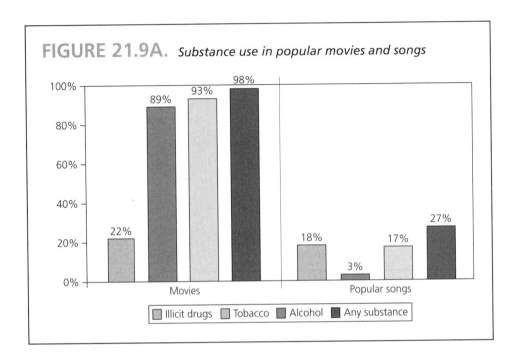

FIGURE 21.9A. *Substance use in popular movies and songs*

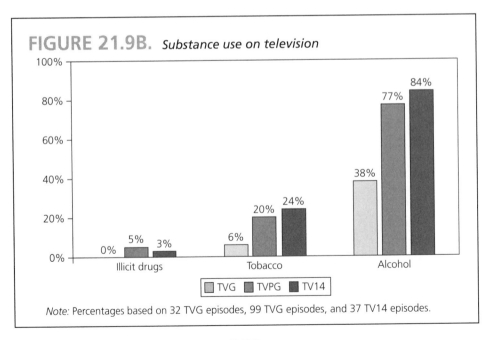

FIGURE 21.9B. *Substance use on television*

Note: Percentages based on 32 TVG episodes, 99 TVG episodes, and 37 TV14 episodes.

Source: Roberts, Henrikson, and Christenson (2000).

(Healton et al., 2006). These depictions flagrantly undermine the ban on tobacco advertising on television. On prime-time TV, alcohol use is seen in 71 percent of shows, while in the movies drinking is portrayed in a remarkable 93 percent of films (Christenson, Henrikson, & Roberts, 2000; Roberts, Henrikson, & Christenson, 2000). Teens are heavy viewers of MTV, and this medium depicts alcohol use every fourteen minutes for the average viewer (Gerbner & Ozyegin, 1997). On MTV, VH1, and BET, alcohol use is commonly juxtaposed with sexual activity or eroticism (Roberts, Christenson, Henrikson, & Bandy, 2002).

The government has declared a war on drugs focused on illegal drugs such as marijuana, cocaine, and ecstasy, and these substances are rarely depicted in the media. However, there seems to be little outrage about the legal but highly dangerous use of tobacco and alcohol, even though alcohol is implicated in many adolescent deaths from injury (Strasburger, 2006). Children who watch more than four hours of television daily are five times more likely to start smoking than those who view less than two hours each day (Gidwani, Sobol, DeJohng, Perrin, & Gortmaker, 2002). Similarly, studies indicate that viewing smoking in movies increases the risk of adolescent smoking initiation and teens' perception that most adults smoke (a salient example of the cultivation hypothesis discussed earlier; Sargent et al., 2002). A survey of 735 young teens found an association between exposure to R-rated movies, a TV in the bedroom, and an increased risk of smoking for white, but not black, youth (Jackson, Brown, & L'Engle, 2007).

Most school systems provide some degree of drug and sex education, using primarily abstinence-only approaches. These programs are ineffective, according to recent Congressionally mandated studies (Trenholm et al., 2007; Botvin & Griffin, 2005). In a May 2007 press release, the MPAA added smoking as film rating factor, but how this factor will be used remains unclear (Germain, 2007).

Other Concerns About Media Effects on Youth

Research is ongoing and sorely needed about the following other potential effects of media exposure on adolescent well-being.

- *School and Learning.* In a novel study, researchers showed that the hours of TV viewed during early childhood was associated with attentional problems at age seven (Christakis, Zimmerman, DiGiuseppe, & McCarty, 2004). New Zealand researchers followed one thousand children until the age of twenty-six, finding an adverse association between childhood and adolescent TV viewing and later educational achievement. Heavy viewing strongly predicted dropping out of high school (Hancox, Milne, & Poulton, 2005). Two recent U.S. studies found cognitive effects and poorer academic performance associated with television viewing, especially when the TV was in the child's bedroom (Borzekowski & Robinson, 2005; Zimmerman & Christakis, 2005). In 2007, a study found that teens watching more than one hour of TV daily are at much higher risk for academic difficulty.

Those watching more than three hours every day were at particular risk, and they had more attentional problems (Johnson et al., 2007).

■ *Bullying.* One study using data from the National Longitudinal Study of Youth found that each hour of TV viewed daily at age four was associated with an increased risk of bullying behavior in later years (Zimmerman, Glew, Christakis, & Katon, 2005). A cross-sectional study of more than 31,000 adolescents from eight different countries, including the U.S., found an association between TV viewing and physical forms of bullying (Kuntsche et al., 2006).

■ *Music.* Most studies have not found a clear association between popular music and music videos and negative behavior in adolescents, despite depictions of violence, sex, and drug use. Older studies show that most listeners don't know or understand the lyrics to their favorite tunes (Greenfield et al., 1987) or that comprehension is age-dependent (Strasburger & Hendren, 1996). A new study finds that songs with violent lyrics can have an impact on listener thoughts and feelings of hostility (Anderson, Carnagey, & Eubanks, 2003). A 2006 survey of almost 1500 teens found that those listening to "degrading" music lyrics were more likely to initiate intercourse at an earlier age or have more advanced sexual activity (Martino et al., 2006). Rap music videos have also been linked recently with binge drinking, marijuana use, and multiple sexual partners among African American female teens (Peterson, Wingood, DiClemente, Harrington, & Davies, 2007).

■ *Television News.* Given the magnitude and impact of current events, including terrorism, war, Hurricane Katrina, and 9/11, many children and adolescents see frightening images on television; researchers are examining the possible effects, including fear and posttraumatic stress (Cantor, 1998; Van der Molen, 2004).

SOLUTIONS: IMPROVING MEDIA FOR ADOLESCENTS

No one doubts that we live in a media world; complexities and interconnection will progress in tandem with media trends. Within a few years, the TV screen and the computer screen will be inextricably linked. Teenagers will be able to point and click on a pizza commercial and order a pizza from their local pizzeria. In addition, more of the phones we use will be minicomputers with Internet linkages. Adults concerned about the well-being of teens must seek solutions to the risks posed by media, so that the benefits of media may be recognized and enjoyed. The basic solution to media concerns is media literacy: in today's world, literacy extends far beyond comprehending the printed word to understanding all the complexities in the mediated world (Committee on Public Education, 1999). A media-educated consumer of any medium comprehends the following concepts (Strasburger & Hogan, 2005; Hogan, 2001; British Medical Association, 2000):

- Media have a political, social, and economic basis

- Media are created, not real

- Every user imbues media images and messages with his or her unique interpretation

- Media can be deconstructed

No doubt Hollywood—dubbed Notmyfaultywood in one cartoon (Strasburger, 2006)—has a role to play, but writers, directors, and producers are notoriously resistant to change, citing First Amendment protection and creative license to "push the envelope." Madison Avenue, as well, bears responsibility to scrutinize advertising, especially for unhealthy foods, cigarettes, and alcohol, to children and teens. In Britain, advertisers, representatives from the media industry, and public health advocates have decided on voluntary restrictions on the use of anorectic models in media (Gentile, Oberg, et al., 2004). Other countries ban advertising aimed at children (American Academy of Pediatrics, 2006).

Adults concerned about the well-being of teens must seek solutions to the risks posed by media, so that the benefits of media may be recognized and enjoyed.

Although advocates for improving media for youth are against censorship (with some exceptions), the federal government could ban cigarette advertising in all media and restrict alcohol to "tombstone" ads (boxed, text-only print ads; see Figure 21.10)—no cute frogs or sexy beach babes. The government could also pass laws mandating media education in all schools for all ages and include a media component in every sex or drug education program in schools. Media research must be funded and encouraged (Strasburger, 2006).

Despite shouldering countless unfunded mandates, schools must recognize the importance of media in the lives of their students. Solutions include teaching media literacy in an age-appropriate way to all grades, incorporating media education into existing sex and drug education programs, and encouraging students to use media more creatively.

Parents could and should be the primary media educators in their children's lives (Strasburger & Hogan, 2005; British Medical Association, 2000). For young children, parents should control the media choices and media habits in the home. Children and teens should not have a television set, video game console, or Internet access in the bedroom. Establishing media use as a family event encourages an intelligent approach to choices of programs and makes parent involvement more likely. Parents asking questions like the following about media images and messages is the cornerstone of media literacy:

- Why does this alcohol company use appealing little dogs to sell a brand of beer?

- How do you feel about the way adolescent girls are behaving in this TV show?

- Is using a gun to solve this conflict the best solution?

FIGURE 21.10. *Bombay Sapphire tombstone ad*

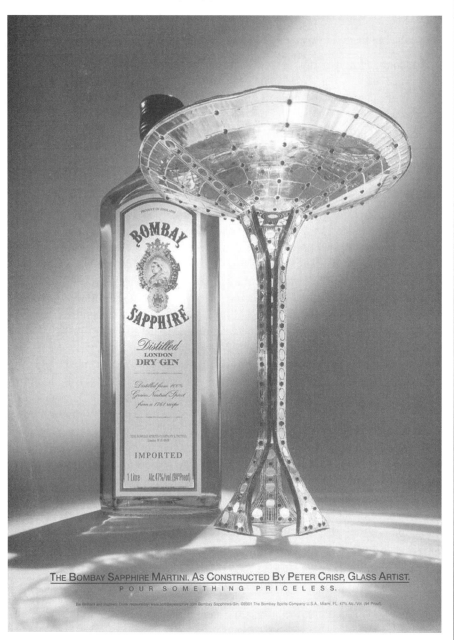

- What do you think about the words in that song?

- Who sponsored the Internet site you are using for your research?

- What does being "part of a nutritional breakfast" mean?

Parents should also be positive media role models. Kids see and learn from adult media habits in the home. If parents choose quality media and spend most of their time on other activities, including reading and active pursuits, a healthy message is being taught in the home. Despite the confusing nature of existing systems, parents should be aware of the ratings of various media products and monitor the content of media offerings (British Medical Association, 2000).

Pediatricians and other health care providers have unique access to youth and families, but many are not cognizant of the huge and growing role media play in the lives and health of young people. A recent survey of 365 pediatricians found that only half recommend limiting media use to one to two hours per day (which is American Academy of Pediatrics policy), and half were not interested in learning more about media effects on their patients through media education. Pediatricians admitting to watching more TV themselves were more pessimistic about being able to effect any changes (Media Matters, 1997).

Adolescent health care providers are already asked to provide anticipatory guidance on myriad topics, from car seats to nutrition to gun safety—how can one more topic, arguably extremely important, be squeezed into a tight schedule? Parents or teens themselves can fill out a simple questionnaire about media use, for example, the American Academy of Pediatrics Media History Form (Committee on Public Education, 2001). Practitioners may amplify this information by asking focused questions about hours spent with media daily and the home media environment, specifically: Does your teen have a TV or Internet access in his or her bedroom? If a teen has problems with aggressive behavior, substance abuse, suicidal thoughts, obesity, or school problems, among other red flags, a more intense interview about media is encouraged.

Adolescent health care providers can also work within their own professional organizations to improve the current media climate. The American Academy of Pediatrics (AAP), a national leader in the area of media education and recognizing the burgeoning role of media in the lives of children and teens, offers a variety of materials and policy statements relevant to media. Major recommendations for pediatricians and other adolescent health care providers, researchers, and public policy analysts and advocates include the following (Strasburger & Hogan, 2005; Hogan & Strasburger, 2008):

- Total daily media time should be no more than one to two quality hours

- Avoid a TV set, video game console, or Internet access in the bedroom

- Severely restrict media time for children less than two years old

- Incorporate media education into daily life

The AAP, the American Psychological Association, the American Medical Association, and a variety of advocacy groups for children, youth, and media health have provided leadership and recommendations for professionals, parents, and the general public about media. Some ideas include the following (Strasburger, 2006; Strasburger & Hogan, 2005; Hogan & Strasburger, 2008):

- Mandate appropriate media education for students in all grades

- Mandate a media education component in sex and drug education curricula (see Figure 21.11A)

- Increase funding for violence prevention programs that include a media component

- Educate writers, directors, and producers about health effects related to the media by increasing interaction between the public health community and the media industry

- Target cigarette smoking in the media, possibly urging ratings to reflect smoking or designating movie sets as "nonsmoking zones"

- Create counteradvertising campaigns against the mainstream drugs tobacco and alcohol (see Figures 21.11B and 21.11C)

- Pressure Congress to ban cigarette ads in all media and limit alcohol advertising to tombstone ads

- Support and encourage the media industry to air ads for contraceptives during prime-time programming

- Create voluntary standards for the advertising industry in the use and depiction of anorectic or severely underweight models

- Create a voluntary universal ratings system for all media (the current use of a different system for each medium is impractical, confusing, inaccurate, and non-user-friendly for parents; a unified system should use content-based, not arbitrary age-based, categories)

- Eliminate or severely restrict school advertising and in-school snack foods and fast foods

- Increase pressure on Congress to place restrictions on fast food advertising and tie-ins between children's movies and fast food restaurants

- Provide adequate funding for media research (more information is sorely needed on the effect of the Internet on child and adolescent behavior, the individual variations in how youth process different media, and ongoing content analyses of violence, sex, and drugs in current media)

FIGURE 21.11A. *The high failure rate of abstinence*

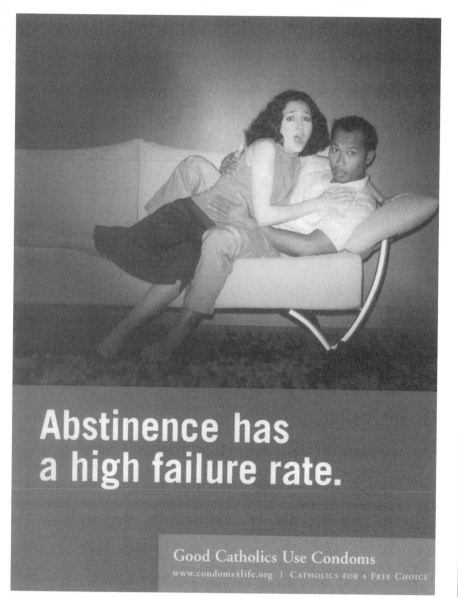

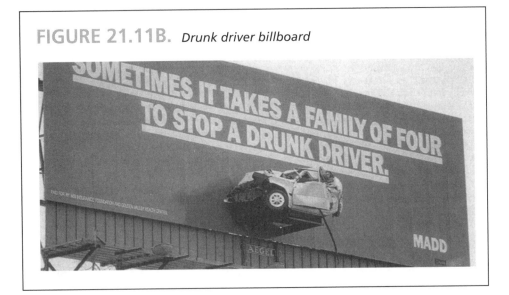

FIGURE 21.11B. *Drunk driver billboard*

SUMMARY

In an ever more complicated media world, we must continue to monitor the impact of media on our young patients. Decades ago, no one could have anticipated that there would be limitations on cigarette advertising, smoke-free restaurants and work places, a multi-billion dollar settlement against Big Tobacco, or that public opinion would be solidly mobilized against the unhealthy practice of smoking. All these changes came about because of public health activism. Media, unlike tobacco, can be prosocial, educational, and entertaining (Hogan & Strasburger, 2008). But media are also associated with serious, well-documented negative outcomes. Despite the power of multinational media conglomerates and the intransigence of the media industry, we can make a difference in the future.

KEY TERMS

Cultivation hypothesis

Suicide contagion

Super-peer

Third-person effect

DISCUSSION QUESTIONS

1. With approximately 75 percent of prime-time shows including sexual content, how, if at all, can the media alter messages being sent to adolescents to promote healthier behaviors?

FIGURE 21.11C. *Getting plastered counterad*

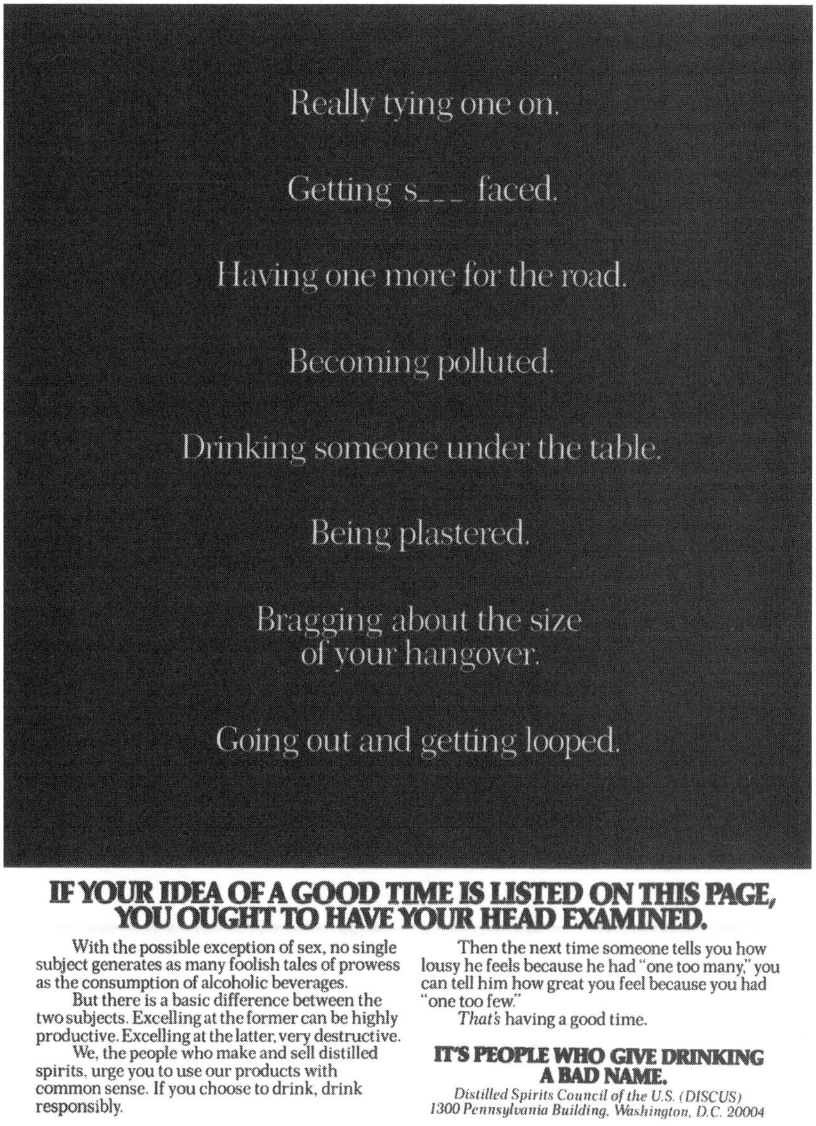

Really tying one on.

Getting s___ faced.

Having one more for the road.

Becoming polluted.

Drinking someone under the table.

Being plastered.

Bragging about the size
of your hangover.

Going out and getting looped.

IF YOUR IDEA OF A GOOD TIME IS LISTED ON THIS PAGE, YOU OUGHT TO HAVE YOUR HEAD EXAMINED.

With the possible exception of sex, no single subject generates as many foolish tales of prowess as the consumption of alcoholic beverages.

But there is a basic difference between the two subjects. Excelling at the former can be highly productive. Excelling at the latter, very destructive.

We, the people who make and sell distilled spirits, urge you to use our products with common sense. If you choose to drink, drink responsibly.

Then the next time someone tells you how lousy he feels because he had "one too many," you can tell him how great you feel because you had "one too few."

That's having a good time.

IT'S PEOPLE WHO GIVE DRINKING A BAD NAME.

Distilled Spirits Council of the U.S. (DISCUS)
1300 Pennsylvania Building, Washington, D.C. 20004

2. Discuss your views on the following statement: adolescents seek the media as a source of guidance and information (about guns, sex, body image, and so forth) because their parents are not around or are unapproachable.

3. How will media exposure change over the next ten years? What preventive measures can be taken to protect youth? Think about prevention in different contexts.

REFERENCES

Abma, J. C., Martinez, G. M., Mosher, W. D., & Dawson, B. S. (2002). Teenagers in the U.S.: Sexual activity, contraceptive use, and childbearing. *Vital Health Statistics, 23,* 1–48.

American Academy of Pediatrics. (2006). Children, adolescents and advertising. *Pediatrics, 118,* 2563–2569.

Anderson, C. A., Berkowitz, L., Donnerstein, E., Huesmann, L. R., Johnson, J. D., Linz, D., Malamuth, N. M., & Wartella, E. (2003). The influence of media on youth. *Psychological Science in the Public Interest, 4,* 81–110.

Anderson, C. A., & Bushman, B. J. (2001). Effects of video games on aggressive behavior, aggressive cognition, aggressive affect, physiological arousal, and prosocial behavior: A meta-analytic review of the scientific literature. *Psychological Science, 12,* 353–359.

Anderson, C. A., Carnagey, N. L., & Eubanks, J. (2003). The effects of songs with violent lyrics on aggressive thoughts and feelings. *Journal of Personality and Social Psychology, 84,* 960–971.

Ashby, S. L., Arcari, C. M., & Edmonson, M. B. (2006). Television viewing and risk of sexual initiation by young adolescents. *Archives of Pediatric and Adolescent Medicine, 160,* 375–380.

Bandura, A. (1986). *Social foundations of thought and action: A social cognitive theory.* Englewood Cliffs, NJ: Prentice Hall.

Becker, A. E. (2002). Eating behaviours and attitudes following prolonged exposure to television among ethnic Fijian adolescent girls. *British Journal of Psychiatry, 180,* 509–514.

Biener, L., & Siegel, M. (2000). Tobacco marketing and adolescent smoking: More support for a causal inference. *American Journal of Public Health, 90,* 407–411.

Borzekowski, D.L.G., & Robinson, T. N. (2005). The remote, the mouse, and the no. 2 pencil: The household media environment and academic achievement among third grade students. *Archives of Pediatric and Adolescent Medicine, 159,* 607–613.

Botvin, G. J., & Griffin, K. W. (2005). Models of prevention: School-based programs. In J. H. Lowinson, P. Ruiz, R. B. Millman, & J. G. Langrod (Eds.), *Substance abuse: A comprehensive textbook* (4th ed., pp. 1211–1229). Philadelphia: Lippincott, Williams & Wilkins.

British Medical Association. (2000). Eating disorders, body image and the media. London: Author.

Brown, J. D., Childers, K. W., & Waszak, C. S. (1990). Television and adolescent sexuality. *Journal of Adolescent Health, 11,* 62–70.

Brown, J. D., Halpern, C. T., & L'Engle, K. L. (2005). Mass media as a sexual super peer for early maturing girls. *Journal of Adolescent Health, 36,* 420–427.

Brown, J. D., L'Engle, K. L., Pardun, C. J., Guo, G., Kenneavy, K., & Jackson, C. (2006). Exposure to sexual content in music, movies, television and magazines predicts black and white adolescents' sexual behavior. *Pediatrics, 117,* 1018–1027.

Bushman, B. J., & Huesmann, L. R. (2001). Effects of televised violence on aggression. In D. Singer & J. Singer (Eds.), *Handbook of children and the media* (pp. 223–254). Thousand Oaks, CA: Sage.

Bushman, B. J., & Huesmann, L. R. (2006). Short-term and long-term effects of violent media on aggression in children and adults. *Archives of Pediatric and Adolescent Medicine, 160,* 348–352.

Cantor, J. (1998). *"Mommy, I'm scared": How TV and movies frighten children and what we can do to protect them.* San Diego, CA: Harcourt Brace.

Carlson, M., Marcus-Newhall, A., & Miller, N. (1990). Effects of situational aggression cues: A quantitative review. *Journal of Personality and Social Psychology, 58,* 622–633.

Center on Alcohol Marketing and Youth. (2003). Alcohol advertising and youth. Washington, DC: Author.

Centers for Disease Prevention and Control. United States, 2005. *Firearm Healths and Rates per 100,000.* Available at www.cdc.gov. Accessed 1/29/2009.

Centers for Disease Prevention and Control. (2006). Youth Risk Behavior Surveillance: United States, 2005. *Morbidity and Mortality Weekly Reports, 55*(SS-5), 1–108.

Charlesworth, A., & Glantz, S. A. (2005). Smoking in the movies increases adolescent smoking: A review. *Pediatrics, 116,* 1516–1528.

Christakis, D. A., Zimmerman, F. J., DiGiuseppe, D. L., & McCarty, C. A. (2004). Early television exposure and subsequent attentional problems in children. *Pediatrics, 113,* 708–713.

Christenson, P. G., Henrikson, L., & Roberts, D. F. (2000). Substance use in popular prime-time television. Washington, DC: Office of National Drug Control Policy.

Collins, R. L., Ellickson, P. L., McCaffrey, D., & Hambarsoomians, K. (2007). Early adolescent exposure to alcohol advertising and its relationship to underage drinking. *Journal of Adolescent Health, 40,* 527–534.

Collins, R.L., Elliot, M. N., Berry, S. H., Kanouse, D. E., Kunkel, D., Hunter, S. B., & Miu, A. (2004). Watching sex on television predicts adolescent initiation of sexual behavior. *Pediatrics, 114,* e280–e289.

Committee on Public Education, American Academy of Pediatrics. (1999). Media education. *Pediatrics, 104,* 341–343.

Committee on Public Education, American Academy of Pediatrics. (2001). Children, adolescents, and television. *Pediatrics, 107,* 423–426.

Comstock, G. A., & Strasburger, V. C. (1993). Media violence. *Adolescent Medicine Clinics, 4,* 495–509.

Davidson, O. G. (1993). Under fire: The NRA and the battle ground for gun control. New York: Holt, Rinehart, and Winston.

Dennison, B. A., Erb, T. A., & Jenkins, P. L. (2002). Television viewing and television in bedroom associated with overweight risk among low-income preschool children. *Pediatrics, 109,* 1028–1035.

Dietz, W. H. (1993). Television, obesity, and eating disorders. *Adolescent Medicine: State of the Art Reviews, 4,* 543–549.

DuRant, R. H., Champion, H., & Wolfson, M. (2006). The relationship between watching professional wrestling on television and engaging in date fighting among high school students. *Pediatrics, 118,* e265–e272.

Elliott, S. (2004). Viagra and the battle of the awkward ads. *New York Times*, April 25, 2004. Available at http://www.nytimes.com. Accessed 1/29/2009.

Eron, L., Huesmann, L. R., Lefkowitz, M. M., & Walder, L. O. (1972). Does television violence cause aggression? *American Psychologist, 27,* 253–263.

Eszterhas, J. (2004). *Hollywood animal.* New York: Knopf.

Federal Bureau of Investigation. (n.d.). Supplementary homicide reports, 1976–2004. Washington, DC: Bureau of Justice Statistics, U.S. Department of Justice. Retrieved October 22, 2007, from www.ojp.usdoj.gov/bjs.

Federal Communications Commission. (2007, April 25). *In the matter of violent television programming and its impact on children* (MB Docket No. 04–261). Washington DC: Author.

Federal Trade Commission. (2003). *Cigarette report for 2003.* Washington DC: Author.

Federman, J. (Ed). (1998). *National Television Violence Study: Vol. 3.* Thousand Oaks, CA: Sage.

Field, A. E., Camargo, C. A., Taylor, C. B., Berkey, C. S., & Colditz, G. A. (1999). Relation of peers and media influences to the development of purging behaviors among preadolescent and adolescent girls. *Archives of Pediatric and Adolescent Medicine, 153,* 1184–1189.

Field, A. E., Cheung, L., Wolf, A. M., Herzog, D. B., Gortmaker, S. L., & Colditz, G. A. (1999). Exposure to the mass media and weight concerns among girls. *Pediatrics, 103,* e236.

Gentile, D. A., Lynch, P. J., Linder, J. R., & Walsh, D. A. (2004). The effects of violent video game habits on adolescent hostility, aggressive behaviors and school performance. *Journal of Adolescence, 27,* 5–22.

Gentile, D. A., Oberg, C., Sherwood, N. E., Story, M., Walsh, D. A., & Hogan, M. J. (2004). Well-child visits in the video age: Pediatricians and the American Academy of Pediatrics' guidelines for children's media use. *Pediatrics, 114,* 1235–1241.

Gerbner, G., Gross, L., Morgan, M., & Signorelli, N. (1994). Growing up with television: The cultivation perspective. In J. Bryant & D. Zimmerman (Eds.), *Media effects: Advances in theory and research.* Hillsdale, NJ: Lawrence Erlbaum.

Gerbner, G., & Ozyegin, N. (1997). Alcohol, tobacco, and illicit drugs in entertainment television, commercials, news, "reality shows," movies, and movie channels. New York: Robert Wood Johnson Foundation.

Germain, D. (2007, May 13). MPAA adds smoking as a film-rating factor. *ABC News.* Retrieved April 14, 2008, from http://abcnews.go.com/print?id=3162588.

Giammattei, J., Blix, G., Marshak, H. H., Wollitzer, A. O., & Pettitt, D. J. (2003). Television watching and soft drink consumption: Associations with obesity in 11–13-year-old schoolchildren. *Archives of Pediatric and Adolescent Medicine, 157,* 882–886.

Gidwani, P. P., Sobol, A., DeJohng, W., Perrin, J. M., & Gortmaker, S. L. (2002). Television viewing and initiation of smoking among youth. *Pediatrics, 110,* 505–508.

Gould, M., Jamieson, P., & Romer, D. (2003). Media contagion and suicide among the young. *American Behavioral Scientist, 46,* 1269–1284.

Gould, M. S., Wallerstein, S., Kleinman, M. H., O'Carroll, P., & Mercy, J. (1990). Suicide cluster: An examination of age-specific effects. *American Journal of Public Health, 80,* 211–212.

Greenfield, P. M., Bruzzone, L., Koyamatsu, K., Satuloff, W., Nixon, K., Brodie, M., & Kingsdale, D. (1987). What is rock music doing to the minds of our youth? A first experimental look at the effect of rock music lyrics and music videos. *Journal of Early Adolescence, 7,* 315–329.

Grube, J. W. (1995). Television alcohol portrayals, alcohol advertising, and alcohol expectancies among children and adolescents. In S. E. Martin (Ed.), *The effects of the mass media on use and abuse of alcohol.* Bethesda, MD: National Institute on Alcohol Abuse and Alcoholism.

Grube, J. W. (1999). Alcohol advertising and alcohol consumption: A review of recent research. National Institute on Alcohol Abuse and Alcoholism, 10th Special Report to Congress on alcohol and health. Bethesda, MD: National Institute on Alcohol Abuse and Alcoholism.

Hancox, R. J., Milne, B. J., & Poulton, R. (2005). Association of television viewing during childhood with poor educational achievement. *Archives of Pediatric and Adolescent Medicine, 159,* 614–618.

Hays, C. (2000, September 14). New report examines consumerism in U.S. schools. *New York Times.*

Healton, C. G., Watson-Stryker, E. S., Allen, J. A., Vallone, D. M., Messeri, P. A., Graham, P. R., Stewart, A. M., Dobbins, M. D., & Glantz, S. A. (2006). Televised movie trailers: Undermining restrictions on advertising tobacco to youth. *Archives of Pediatric and Adolescent Medicine, 160,* 885–888.

Hogan, M. J. (2001). Parents and other adults: Models and monitors of healthy media habits. In D. Singer & J. Singer (Eds.), *Handbook of children and the media.* Thousand Oaks, CA: Sage.

Hogan, M. J. (2005). Adolescents and media violence: Six crucial issues for practitioners. *Adolescent Medicine Clinics, 16,* 249–268.

Hogan, M. J., & Strasburger, V. C. (2008). Media and prosocial behavior in children and adolescents. In L. Nucci & D. Narvaez (Eds.), *Handbook of moral and character education* 537–553. Mahwah, NJ: Lawrence Erlbaum.

Huesmann, L. R., Eron, L. D., Lefkowitz, M. M., & Walder, L. O. (1984). Stability of aggression over time and, generations. *Developmental Psychology, 20,* 1120–1134.

Huesmann, L. R., Moise-Titus, J., Podolski, C., & Eron, L. D. (2003). Longitudinal relations between children's exposure to TV violence and their aggressive and violent behavior in young adulthood. *Developmental Psychology, 39,* 201–221.

Institute of Medicine. (2006). *Food marketing to children and youth: Threat or opportunity?* Washington, DC: National Academies Press.

Jackson, B., Brown, J. D., & L'Engle, K. L. (2007). R-rated movies, bedroom televisions, and initiation of smoking by white and black adolescents. *Archives of Pediatric and Adolescent Medicine, 161,* 260–268.

Johnson, J. G., Cohen, P., Kasen, S., & Brook, J. S. (2007). Extensive television viewing and the development of attention and learning difficulties during adolescence. *Archives of Pediatric and Adolescent Medicine, 161,* 480–486.

Johnson, J. G., Cohen, P., Smailes, E. M., Kasen, S., & Brook, J. S. (2002). Television viewing and aggressive behavior during adolescence and adulthood. *Science, 295,* 2468–2472.

Jordan, A. B. (2007). Heavy television viewing and childhood obesity. *Journal of Children and Media, 1,* 45–54.

Kaiser Family Foundation. (2002). *Teens, sex, and TV.* Menlo Park, CA: Author.

Kaiser Family Foundation, Seventeen Magazine. (2004). *Sex smarts: Birth control and protection.* Menlo Park, CA: Author.

Kilbourne, J. (1999). *Deadly persuasion: Why women and girls must fight the addictive power of advertising.* New York: Free Press.

Klesges, R. C., Shelton, M. L., & Klesges, L. M. (1993). Effects of television on metabolic rate: Potential implications for childhood obesity. *Pediatrics, 91,* 281–286.

Krowchuk, D. P., Dreiter, S. R., Woods, C. R., Sinal, S. H., & DuRant, R. H. (1998). Problem dieting behaviors among young adolescents. *Archives of Pediatric and Adolescent Medicine, 152,* 884–888.

Kunkel, D., Eyal, K., Finnerty, K., Biely, E., & Donnerstein, E. (2005). *Sex on TV 4*. Menlo Park, CA: Kaiser Family Foundation.

Kuntsche, E., Pickett, W., Overpeck, M., Craig, W., Boyce, W., & Gaspar de Matos, M. (2006). Television viewing and forms of bullying among adolescents from eight countries. *Journal of Adolescent Health, 39,* 908–915.

Ludwig, D. S., Peterson, K. E., & Gortmaker, S. L. (2001). Relation between the consumption of sugar-sweetened drinks and childhood obesity: A prospective, observational analysis. *Lancet, 357,* 505–508.

Maloney, M. J., McGuire, J., Daniels, S. R., & Specker, B. (1989). Dieting behavior and eating attitudes in children. *Pediatrics, 84,* 482–489.

Martinez-Gonzalez, M. A., Gual, P., Lahortiga, F., Alonso, Y., Irala-Esevez, J., & Cervera, S. (2003). Parental factors, mass media influences, and the onset of eating disorders in a prospective population-based cohort. *Pediatrics, 111,* 315–320.

Martino, S. C., Collins, R. L., Elliot, M. N., Strachman, A., Kanouse, D. E., & Berry, S. H. (2006). Exposure to degrading versus nondegrading music lyrics and sexual behavior among youth. *Pediatrics, 118,* e430–e441.

Media Matters. (1997). *Media history form*. Elk Grove Village, IL: American Academy of Pediatrics.

National Institutes of Health and Prevention. (1997). Rates of homicide, suicide, and firearm-related death among children: 26 industrialized nations. *Morbidity and Mortality Weekly Reports, 46,* 101–105.

National Public Radio, Kaiser Family Foundation, Kennedy School of Government. (2004). *Sex education in America: Principals survey*. Menlo Park, CA: Kaiser Family Foundation.

Nelson, N. (2007). Internet crimes against children. Speech at Hennepin County Medical Center SCANT Conference, ICAC Task Force, St. Paul, MN.

Newman, A. A. (2007). Pigs with cell phones, but no condoms. *New York Times*. Retrieved April 14, 2008, from www.nytimes.com/2007/06/18/business/media.

Oleck, J. (1994, July 20). Go ahead, make my lunch: Restaurant chains vying for school media market. *Restaurant Business*.

Peterson, S. H., Wingood, G. M., DiClemente, R. J., Harrington, K., & Davies, S. (2007). Images of sexual stereotypes in rap videos and the health of African American female adolescents. *Journal of Women's Health, 16,* 1157–1164.

Phillips, D. P., & Paight, D. J. (1987). The impact of televised movies about suicide: A replicative study. *New England Journal of Medicine, 317,* 809–811.

Pierce, J. P., Choi, W. S., Gilpin, E. A., Farkas, A. J., & Berry, C. C. (1998). Industry promotion of cigarettes and adolescent smoking. *Journal of the American Medical Association, 279,* 511–515.

Ramsey, L. T., & Pelletier, A. R. (2004). Update on firearms use in G- and PG-rated movies. *Journal of the American Medical Association, 292,* 2836–2837.

Reece, B. B., Rifon, N. J., & Rodriguez, K. (1999). Selling food to children: Is fun part of a balanced breakfast? In M. C. Macklin & L. Carlson (Eds.), *Advertising to children: Concepts and controversies*. Thousand Oaks, CA: Sage.

Rich, F. (2004, February 15). *New York Times*, section 2, p. 1.

Rideout, V. (2001). *Generation Rx.com: How young people use the Internet for health information*. Menlo Park, CA: Kaiser Family Foundation.

Rideout, V., Roberts, D. F., & Foehr, U. G. (2005). *Generation M: Media in the lives of 8–18-year-olds*. Menlo Park, CA: Kaiser Family Foundation.

Roberts, D. F., Christenson, P. G., Henrikson, L., & Bandy E. (2002). *Substance use in popular music videos*. Washington, DC: Office of National Drug Control Policy.

Roberts, D. F., Henrikson, L., & Christenson, P. G. (2000). *Substance use in popular movies and music*. Washington, DC: Office of National Drug Control Policy.

Robinson, T. N. (1998). Does television cause childhood obesity? *Journal of the American Medical Association, 279,* 959–960.

Robinson, T. N. (1999). Reducing children's television viewing to prevent obesity: A randomized controlled trial. *Journal of the American Medical Association, 282,* 1561–1567.

Robinson, T. N., Hammer, L. D., Killen, J. D., Kraemer, H. C., Wilson, D. M., Hayward, C., & Taylor, C. B. (1993). Does television viewing increase obesity and reduce physical activity? Cross-sectional and longitudinal analysis among adolescent girls. *Pediatrics, 91,* 273–280.

Rubin, A. (2004, November 6). Prescription drugs and the cost of advertising them. *The Rubins.com*. Retrieved April 14, 2008, from www.therubins.com/geninfo/advertise.

Sargent, J. D., Beach, M. L., Dalton, M. A., Mott, L. A., Tickle, J. J., Ahrens, M. B., & Heatherton, T. F. (2001). Effect of seeing tobacco use in films on trying smoking among adolescents. *British Medical Journal, 323,* 1394–1397.

Sargent, J. D., Dalton, M., & Beach, M. (2000). Exposure to cigarette promotions and smoking uptake in adolescents: Evidence of a dose-response relation. *Tobacco Control, 9,* 163–168.

Sargent, J. D., Dalton, M. A., Beach, M. L., Mott, L. A., Tickle, J. J., Ahrens, M. B., & Heatherton, T. F. (2002). Viewing tobacco use in the movies: Does it shape attitudes that mediate adolescent smoking? *American Journal of Preventive Medicine, 22,* 137–145.

Sargent, J. D., Tanski, S. E., & Gibson, J. (2007). Exposure to movie smoking among U.S. adolescents aged 10 to 14 years: A population estimate. *Pediatrics, 119,* e1167–e1176.

Snobeck, C. (2005). FDA tells Levitra to cool it with ad. *Business News.* Retrieved April 14, 2008, from www .post-gazette.com.

Stranger, J. D. (2002). Television in the home 1998: The third annual national survey of parents and children. Philadelphia, PA: Annenberg Public Policy Center.

Strasburger, V. C. (2005a). Adolescents and the media: Why don't pediatricians and parents "get it"? *Medical Journal of Australia, 183,* 425–426.

Strasburger, V. C. (2005b). Adolescents, sex, and the media: Oooo, baby, baby—a Q&A. *Adolescent Medicine Clinics, 16,* 269–288.

Strasburger, V. C. (2006). Risky business: What primary care practitioners need to know about the influence of media on adolescents. *Primary Care Clinics in Office Practice, 33,* 317–348.

Strasburger, V. C., Brown, R. T., Braverman, P. K., Rogers, P. D., Holland-Hall, C., & Coupey, S. (2006). *Adolescent medicine: A handbook for primary care.* Philadelphia, PA: Lippincott Williams & Wilkins.

Strasburger, V. C., & Grossman, D. (2001). How many more Columbines? What can pediatricians do about school and media violence? *Pediatric Annals, 30,* 87–94.

Strasburger, V. C., & Hendren, R. O. (1995). Rock music and music videos. *Pediatric Annals, 24,* 97–103.

Strasburger, V. C., & Hogan, M. J. (Eds.). (2005). Adolescents and the media. *Adolescent Medicine Clinics, 16,* 249–284.

Strasburger, V. C., Wilson, B. J., & Jordan, A. (2009). *Children, adolescents, and the media* (2nd ed.). Thousand Oaks, CA: Sage.

Taras, H. L., & Gage, M. (1995). Advertised foods on children's television. *Archives of Pediatric and Adolescent Medicine, 149,* 649–652.

Thomaselli, R. (2003, January 23). 47% of doctors feel pressured by DTC drug advertising. *Advertising Age.* Retrieved April 14, 2008, from www.adage.com/news.cms?newsID=36897.

Thompson, K. M., & Haninger, K. (2001). Violence in E-rated video games. *Journal of the American Medical Association, 286,* 591–598.

Trenholm, C., Devaney, B., Fortson, K., Quay, L., Wheeler, J., & Clark, M. (2007). *Impacts of four Title V, Section 510, abstinence education programs: Final report.* Princeton, NJ: Mathematica Policy Research.

Van der Molen, J.H.W. (2004). Violence and suffering in the televisions news: Toward a broader conception of harmful television content for children. *Pediatrics, 113,* 1771–1775.

Wartella, E., Olivarez, A., & Ennings, N. (1998). Children and television violence in the United States. In U. Carlsson & C. von Feilitzen (Eds.), *UNESCO international clearinghouse on children and violence on the screen.* Paris: United Nations Educational, Scientific and Cultural Organization.

Webb, T., Jenkins, L., Browne, N., Abdelmonen, A., & Kraus, J. (2007). Violent entertainment pitched to adolescents: An analysis of PG-13 films. *Pediatrics, 119,* e1219–e1229.

Wolnak, J. (2007). Internet crimes: Myths and realities. Speech at Hennepin County Medical Center SCANT Conference, Crimes Against Children Research Center, University of New Hampshire, Durham, NH.

Wyllie, A., Zhang, J. F., & Casswell, S. (1998). Positive responses to televised beer advertisements associated with drinking and problems reported by 18–29-year-olds. *Addiction, 93,* 749–760.

Zimmerman, F. J., & Christakis, D. A. (2005). Children's television viewing and cognitive outcomes. *Archives of Pediatric and Adolescent Medicine, 159,* 619–625.

Zimmerman, F. J., Glew, G. M., Christakis, D. A., & Katon, W. (2005). Early cognitive stimulation, emotional support, and television watching as predictors of subsequent bullying among grade-school children. *Archives of Pediatric and Adolescent Medicine, 159,* 384–388.

CHAPTER

22

TECHNOLOGICAL ADVANCES IN MODIFYING ADOLESCENT HEALTH RISK BEHAVIORS

NATALIE C. KAISER ▪ JASON E. OWEN ▪ ANDREW J. WINZELBERG

LEARNING OBJECTIVES

After studying this chapter, you will be able to

▪ Interpret the effectiveness of randomly controlled technological interventions that address adolescent health risk behaviors.

▪ Recall the application of different technologies as a mode of intervention for targeting risk behaviors among adolescents.

▪ Formulate conclusions regarding the benefits and drawbacks to developing a technological intervention as opposed to more traditional methods.

Developing efficacious interventions for improving adolescent health behaviors has proved to be a significant challenge, as evidenced by the abundance of inconsistent findings in the literature (Clemmens & Hayman, 2004; Muller, Danielzik, & Pust, 2005; Timperio, Salmon, & Ball, 2005). Engaging adolescents in efforts to make long-term behavioral changes at the expense of behaviors that provide more immediate gratification is quite difficult (Reynolds, 2004). Thus, the potential application of emerging technologies to entrenched problems such as overweight, tobacco use, risky sexual behaviors, and eating disorders in adolescents is appealing for a number of reasons. Adolescents are early adopters of new technologies and use new technologies at much higher rates than their older counterparts. By way of example, 87 percent of twelve- to seventeen-year olds reported using the Internet regularly (31 percent to access health information), compared with only 66 percent of U.S. adults (Lenhart, Madden, & Hitlin, 2005).

In part, adolescents may be adopting newer technologies because of the advantages these technologies bring to the process of disseminating information and connecting with highly valued peer communities (Houston & Ehrenberger, 2001). New technologies are interactive, more likely to contain up-to-date information, peer-based and peer-led, convey a greater sense of privacy to users, present information dynamically, and have greater accessibility with respect to time and place of use (Marcus, Nigg, Riebe, & Forsyth, 2000). Technological interventions may also be particularly compelling for health care professionals: cost is relatively low, dissemination to large numbers of individuals is possible, information can be easily updated and individually tailored, interventions can be readily incorporated into more traditional interventions (as supplements in primary care settings, for example) or provided remotely, and there is potential for greater adherence, engagement, and candor with respect to sensitive topics such as substance abuse and sexual behavior (Houston et al., 2001; Robinson, Patrick, Eng, & Gustafson, 1998; Simoes, Bastos, Moreira, Lynch, & Metzger, 2006; Webb, Zimet, Fortenberry, & Blythe, 1999).

The purpose of this chapter is to review systematically identified, randomized studies that have evaluated technological interventions for health behaviors associated with adolescents' obesity and physical activity; substance, alcohol, and tobacco use; sexual risk behaviors; and eating disorders and to characterize the state of the literature with respect to these kinds of interventions. We focus on these specific health behaviors because they are the most prevalent, pressing, and widely researched health behaviors pertaining to adolescents. We chose to focus our review on innovative recent technological media, including interactive compact discs (CD-ROMs), DVDs, computers, internet applications, telephones and cell phones, online chat rooms, instant messaging services, and pagers that have been used to address these health behaviors. Systematic literature searches were performed using PubMed and PsychInfo to identify all studies employing a randomized, controlled design that allowed for the specific evaluation of the effects of one of the technological media listed above on each of the four broad categories of health behaviors. Studies that evaluated the use of technology as a component of a broader intervention methodology were not included, but have been described when results have suggested a particularly promising application of that technology.

KEY CONCEPTS AND RESEARCH FINDINGS

Results are presented separately here for each category of adolescent health behavior: obesity and physical activity; substance, alcohol, and tobacco use; sexual risk behaviors; and eating disorders.

Overweight and Physical Activity

More than one out of seven adolescents are currently overweight or obese, and the majority of these adolescents are expected to experience compromised mental and physical health over their lifetimes (Cielo, 2005). Technological interventions have been applied for purposes of preventing overweight and to target adolescents who are at risk or already overweight. Identified and reviewed studies primarily employed CD-ROM, internet, and video-game technologies to address the significant problem of adolescent overweight (see Table 22.1).

Randomized Trials To evaluate possible advantages of innovative and interactive forms of behavioral and psychosocial interventions over more static approaches, several studies have compared computer-based approaches to print media for the promotion of physical activity. Results from these studies are mixed. Casazza and Ciccazzo (2007) found interactive CD-ROM to be more effective than printed pamphlets for reducing BMI and increasing physical activity, but no differences between the two types of media were observed for changes in nutrition knowledge, dietary habits (such as total caloric intake), perceived social support, and self-efficacy for diet and exercise-related behaviors. In a similar study comparing the effectiveness of Web versus print media for physical activity promotion among youth, Marks et al. (2006) found print materials to be superior for promoting changes in physical activity. Kypri et al. (2005) assessed health behaviors in older adolescents and young adults and evaluated the effects of tailored, Web-based feedback on these health behaviors. The investigators reported that Web-based feedback was associated with significant improvements in fruit and vegetable consumption and physical activity, but had no effect on alcohol use.

Video games may play a role in contributing to the childhood obesity epidemic. The popularity of video games has coincided with the jump in obese and overweight children over the past two decades (Brown, 2006). Some researchers have attempted to harness interest in video games to provide behavior change interventions. For example, Baronowski et al. (2003) described the development of a game called *Squire's Quest* in which players accumulate points by having their character consume fruit, 100 percent juice, and vegetables. The game character also prepares healthy food recipes in a virtual kitchen to provide energy for the king and court to fight the invaders. Results indicated that children who played the game increased their fruit, 100 percent juice, and vegetable consumption by one serving per day (Baronowski et al., 2003). Game

TABLE 22.1. Randomized, controlled trials of technological interventions for obesity and physical inactivity in adolescents

Reference	Intervention	Sample	Target Behavior	Posttest Results
Goldfield et al. (2006)	Accelerometers to reinforce counts of physical activity with one hour of sedentary TV time; control = open loop feedback only	30 overweight or obese 8- to 12-year-olds	Increased physical activity, reduced sedentary behavior	Intervention improved physical activity counts and time spent in moderate to vigorous physical activity; reduced time spent engaged in sedentary behavior, BMI, weight
Saelens et al. (2002)	Computer-guided assessment of eating and activity behaviors, tailored physician counseling session, telephone consultations, and self-monitoring booklet; control = single-session weight counseling	44 overweight 12- to 16-year-olds	Increased physical activity, reduced BMI	Intervention group: significant improvements in BMI, but did not alter physical activity, sedentary behavior, total energy intake, or dietary fat intake
Casazza & Ciccazzo (2007)	Guided CD-ROM providing dietary information and recommendations; control = traditional education or nothing at all	275 13- to 18-year-olds	BMI, improved dietary habits, physical activity, knowledge, self-efficacy, perceived support	CD-ROM group resulted in significantly reduced BMI and increased physical activity; no differences on changes in nutrition knowledge, total dietary intake, dietary and exercise social support, and self-efficacy
Resnicow, Taylor, Baskin, & McCarty (2005)	Physical activity, group retreat, two-way pagers for reminders, telephone-administered motivational interviewing	147 overweight adolescent African American females	BMI, percentage body fat, waist or hip circumference, blood pressure, lipids, insulin, glucose, cardiovascular fitness	No between-group differences at six-month or one-year follow-up

Study	Intervention	Sample	Measure	Results
White et al. (2004)	Internet-based information regarding nutrition, physical activity, and healthy food choices; control = educational information on nutrition and physical activity	57 overweight African American adolescent girls (ages 11 to 15) with one obese parent	BMI	Significant body fat and weight changes in experimental versus control group
Marks et al. (2006)	Web-based physical activity intervention with identical content delivered in a printed workbook; control = print intervention	319 girls in grades 6 to 8	Improvements in physical activity, self-efficacy, and intention	Both Web and print group had significant changes in physical activity and self-efficacy; print group demonstrated significantly greater increases in intentions
Jago et al. (2006)	Boy scout troop and internet program tracking physical activity with accelerometers; control = mirror image fruit and veggie intervention	472 10- to 14-year-old Houston-based Boy Scouts	Physical activity skills, self-efficacy, and goal setting	Small decrease in sedentary behavior and increased light-intensity physical activity among spring participants only
Kypri & McAnally (2005)	Web-based assessment and personalized feedback for experimental group; control = assessment only or minimal contact	218 17- to 24-year-olds who attended a New Zealand university	Fruit, juice, vegetable consumption, smoking behaviors, and alcohol consumption	Significant differences in meeting recommendations for fruit and vegetable consumption and physical activity
Baronowski et al. (2003)	Psychoeducational multimedia intervention to facilitate fruit and vegetable consumption; control = no program	1,578 fourth-grade students	Healthy food choices for snacks measured by Food Intake Recording Software System	Increased fruit, vegetable, and juice consumption by one serving more than the children not receiving the program

maker Konami has had success with the popular game *Dance Dance Revolution,* which requires players to engage in a series of increasingly rapid dance moves involving substantial aerobic activity. Other video games, including Sony's interactive Eye Toy, QMotion's PC virtual reality games, and *Escape from Obeez City* have been developed, but no randomized trials have been conducted on these games to date.

Innovative, Untested Applications of Technology   Although technology as a mode of intervention for targeting obese youth has been tested in a handful of randomized clinical trials in recent years, the latest technologies—particularly those delivered via the Web, such as streaming video, Flash content, and video chats—suggest great promise but have not yet been evaluated with controlled trials. For example, Long et al. (2006) described the development of an "edutainment" interactive Web site that included an engaging portal designed to have a "space station look" from which participants could choose to enter a kitchen to access links to nutrition-related Web sites or a gym to access links to exercise-related Web sites. Frenn et al. (2005) have also reported the use of a Web site for delivery of stage-matched videos and tailored feedback based on responses to stage or motivation questions. Finally, accelerometers have been used in conjunction with a Web-based health promotion intervention, allowing individuals to upload objectively measured physical activity data to a Web site and to then receive personally tailored activity goals (Slootmaker, Chin A Paw, Schuit, Seidell, & van Mechelen, 2005).

Alcohol and Substance Use Behaviors

Alcohol and substance use among adolescents is alarmingly prevalent. Nearly 44 percent of college students report having had one or more heavy drinking periods in the past two weeks, and over 37 percent meet criteria for alcohol abuse or dependence (Knight et al., 2002). Alcohol use is also common among younger adolescents, with about 25 percent reporting drinking before age thirteen (Swahn & Bossarte, 2007). Technology may have a role to play in reducing the severity of this public health problem. Roughly 25 percent of adolescent and young adult internet users have searched for information related to drug or alcohol problems (Kaiser Family Foundation, 2001). Relative to other health behaviors, technology-based interventions for improving alcohol and drug-related behaviors have received considerable attention in the literature (see Table 22.2).

Randomized Trials Addressing Alcohol Use, Abuse, and Dependence   Recent use of technology to improve alcohol-related behaviors in particular has focused on CD-ROM, internet, and stand-alone computer-based methods. While these technologies show promise, tested technologies have not so far been shown to be superior to more traditional intervention methodologies. Moore et al. (2005), for example, found comparable effects of Web and print-delivered health risk information interventions on binge drinking behaviors. To take advantage of "teachable moments," Malo et al. (2005) compared an emergency department–based laptop computer intervention with standard of care to reduce alcohol misuse. No significant decreases in alcohol misuse or binge drinking episodes were observed between control and intervention groups. Schinke et al. (2005) evaluated the effects of a ten-week skills-based interactive intervention using CD-ROM information to teach assertiveness skills, goal setting, coping, peer pressure, and decision making to adolescents. Although the intervention resulted in significant increases in perceived harm of alcohol use and increased assertiveness skills, there was no effect of the intervention on actual alcohol use.

Randomized Trials Addressing Substance Use, Abuse, and Dependence Studies targeting substance use behaviors in adolescents have employed interactive CD-ROM materials disproportionately more than other technologies. Duncan et al. (2000) have succinctly described the advantages of CD-ROM for these purposes: providing practice opportunities for decision-making and refusal skills, giving users the ability to dynamically select content areas of interest, focusing users' attention on the topic, and establishing an easily disseminated and standardized model of intervention. Schinke and Schwinn (2005) compared the effects of twenty- to thirty-minute exposure to a CD-ROM providing peer-delivered information on stress reduction and the relationship between drugs and stress management strategies to a more traditional teacher-delivered drug prevention program among seventh-grade females. Results suggested that the CD-ROM intervention resulted in significant reductions in attitudes associated with substance use relative to the control group. Williams et al. (2005) reported a similar set of positive outcomes on attitudes toward substance use and skills for stress or anxiety for a CD-ROM intervention provided to a mixed-gender group of sixth and seventh graders. Duncan et al. (2000) also employed a CD-ROM intervention to provide socially acceptable refusal skills needed to effectively deal with substance use situations, particularly marijuana. Results indicated that the CD-ROM significantly improved self-efficacy for refusing drug offers, intention to refuse drug offers, and perceived social norms associated with substance use. CD-ROMs do appear to be effective in improving attitudes about substance abuse among early adolescents, but little is known about how they might affect attitudes or behavior among older adolescents and those at greatest risk for substance use, abuse, and dependence.

Randomized Trials Addressing Tobacco Use Several studies have evaluated Internet-based methods for delivering smoking cessation treatments to adolescent smokers. Patten et al. (2006) evaluated the hypothesis that an Internet-based smoking cessation program for adolescents would result in significantly greater abstinence rates and declines in smoking compared with four brief office visits over a twenty-four-week period. Contrary to expectations, however, results of the study revealed that: (1) use of the internet service was quite low, with steep drop-off rates over time, (2) internet treatment did not outperform brief office visits with respect to smoking abstinence or reduction in cigarettes smoked per day, and (3) confirmed abstinence rates appeared to be substantially higher in the brief office visit group (Patten et al., 2006). Using a novel virtual reality chat room intervention, Woodruff et al. (2007) reported that compared

TABLE 22.2. Randomized, controlled trials of technological interventions for substance and alcohol use in adolescents

Reference	Intervention	Sample	Target Behavior	Posttest Results
Moore, Soderquist, & Werch (2005)	Drinking prevention delivered via Internet; control = print-based intervention	116 college students	Binge drinking (four to five drinks on one occasion)	Intervention effective for those who already had engaged in binge drinking behaviors, regardless of intervention method
Malo et al. (2005)	Emergency department–based laptop computer alcohol intervention; control = standard of care method	329 adolescents aged 14 to 18	Reduce normative age-related increase in alcohol misuse to prevent alcohol-related injury	No significant decrease in alcohol misuse among intervention versus standard of care
Saitz et al. (2007)	Minimal (control) versus more extensive online alcohol brief interventions	4,008 freshman university students	Alcohol consumption and related attitudes	More extensive interventions associated with intention to seek help in men and greater increase in readiness for change in women; no significant drinking differences versus intervention group
Schinke, Schwinn, & Ozanian (2005)	Skills-based interactive CD-ROM to prevent alcohol abuse; CD-ROM-only arm, CD 1 parent involvement, no intervention control	489 youths from after-school agencies for underprivileged	Assertion skills; ability to perceive harm; self-efficacy, problem solving, peer interactions	Intervention arm had positive increase in perceived harm of alcohol use and increased assertiveness skills; posttest drinking unchanged from pretest
Kypri et al. (2004)	Web-based brief intervention to reduce hazardous drinking; control = leaflet information only	167 college students	Hazardous drinking behaviors	Six-week follow-up: lower total alcohol consumption, heavy episode frequency, personal problems; six-month follow-up: lower personal problems and academic problems, but no lower alcohol consumption

Study	Intervention	Sample	Outcome measures	Results
Bersamin, Paschall, Fearnow-Kenney, & Wyrick (2007)	Online alcohol misuse prevention program (College Alc); control = no intervention	622 incoming college freshmen	Reducing alcohol use and related consequences among drinkers and non-drinkers	Three-month follow up: among those who already drank, heavy drinking, drunkenness, and negative related outcomes decreased; no effects for those who did not drink before intervention
Duncan, Duncan, Beauchamp, Wells, & Ary (2000)	Interactive CD-ROM program to reduce adolescent substance use; control = classroom with no intervention	74 public school students; multicultural sample	Reduce marijuana use and increase refusal techniques	Increased self-efficacy to refuse, intention to refuse, and perceptions of social norms associated with substance use in treatment group; higher recall in treatment group of information
Fishbein, Von Haeften, Hall-Jamieson, Johnson, & Kirkland Ahern (2000)	Antidrug PSAs delivered via TV versus laptop computer; control = political PSAs	154 adolescents from Boys and Girls Clubs	Effectiveness, realism, positive or negative emotional response, and amount learned	Minimal differences between use of computer versus TV or pencil-and-paper methodology; computer more effective for Caucasians
Schinke & Schwinn (2005)	Substance abuse gender-specific intervention; control = conventional intervention in group setting	Seventh-grade middle school girls	Responses to stress, attitude toward self, substance use items	Treatment group: more stress reduction methods; lower approval of cigarettes, alcohol, drugs; lower likelihood of substance abuse if asked by best friend; stronger plans to avoid substance use in next year
Williams et al. (2005)	Life Skills Training interactive CD-ROM, interactive audiovisual content to reduce substance use; control = delayed intervention	123 sixth- and seventh-grade students (ages 12 to 13)	Rates of substance use behavior, attitudes, knowledge, normative expectations	Significant intervention effects on prodrug attitudes, normative expectations for peer and adult substance abuse, anxiety, reduction skills, and relaxation skills knowledge

(Continued)

TABLE 22.2. *(Continued)*

Reference	Intervention	Sample	Target Behavior	Posttest Results
Patten et al. (2006)	Stomp Out Smokers: Internet-based smoking intervention; control = clinic-based, brief office intervention with counseling sessions	Adolescent smokers aged 11 to 18	Severity of nicotine dependence, current smoking status, smoking reduction, treatment compliance	Greater smoking abstinence rates for control than internet group at thirty days and six months; among those who continued to smoke, internet group associated with significant reduction in average number of days smoked versus control
Woodruff, Conway, Edwards, Elliott, & Crittendon (2007)	Internet-based, virtual reality world combined with motivational interviewing; control = measurement only	136 adolescent smokers recruited from high schools	Smoking status, smoking behavior, quitting history, readiness to quit	Intervention group significantly more likely to quit smoking within one week of treatment, smoke fewer days in past week, fewer cigarettes in past week, and consider themselves former smokers; at one-year follow-up, only number of times quit significant

with a no-intervention control the chat room was associated with short-term (seven-week) improvements in abstinence and smoking behavior. However, no differences between the virtual reality chat and no-treatment controls were observed at three- and twelve-month follow-ups. Similar to results reported by Patten et al. (2006), adherence to the treatment protocol was low for virtual chat participants, with fewer than 10 percent of those randomized to the chat group participating in all sessions and nearly 20 percent not completing a single chat session.

Innovative Approaches and Promising Technologies Many of the studies that use technological interventions to address adolescent alcohol and substance use have used nonrandomized study designs or designs that did not explicitly evaluate the role of the technology itself, but these studies may shed some light on how these technologies may be used to maximize effects in future applications. In an uncommon use of CD-ROMs, Schinke, Di Noia, Schwinn, and Cole (2006) used interactive CDs to facilitate communication between urban African American mothers and their adolescent daughters. While study personnel watched passively, mother-daughter dyads used the interactive CD to perform a series of communication-building exercises with one another. Although the study did not specifically evaluate substance abuse outcomes, results revealed significantly increased feelings of closeness and improved communication outcomes that could reduce likelihood of acquiring adverse health behaviors. In a departure from adolescent-focused interventions, Di Noia, Schwinn, Dastur, and Schinke (2003) evaluated the relative accessibility of drug prevention education materials disseminated via CD-ROM, pamphlet, and Internet among professionals involved in planning and recommending these materials to adolescents and others in their communities. Results from this study suggest that community professionals at the front line implementing substance abuse prevention strategies find Internet-based materials to be more accessible and more likely to be used than either CD-ROM or pamphlet materials. Speaking to the validity of this finding, Saitz et al. (2007) have reported that adolescents are substantially more willing to receive information about alcohol use via the Web than via telephone.

The lack of robust effects for Internet-based technologies is somewhat surprising, but some promising studies have reported findings that may help with the development of more effective internet interventions. For example, Chen and Yeh (2006) described a face-to-face plus Internet-based intervention for adolescent smoking that was compared with a no-treatment control group. The combined face-to-face and Internet group resulted in significant improvements in smoking-related behaviors and attitudes. Combining face-to-face and Internet modalities may be important for maximizing outcomes, because some degree of personal contact may be necessary to enhance the amount of time and attention spent interacting with a Web site. At a population level, Klein, Havens, and Carlson (2005) have reported evidence that a public media campaign to promote an adolescent-themed smoking

Some promising studies have reported findings that may help with the development of more effective internet interventions.

cessation Web site was particularly effective in reaching its target population. At the end of the campaign, nearly all adolescent smokers in the study had heard of the Web site (GottaQuit.com, which is no longer operational), and over 25 percent of these had actually visited the Web site. The success of massive social networking sites suggests that Web sites that promote a sense of community and are "sticky" enough to keep users interested and engaged in the content and community provided by the Web site have the potential to reach a large number of adolescents.

Sexual Risk Behaviors

HIV and other sexually transmitted diseases, in conjunction with high sexual activity rates, pose a serious risk to the health of adolescents (Centers for Disease Control and Prevention [CDC], 2000). In 2000, among young people aged thirteen to nineteen, 61 percent of infections of HIV occurred in females (CDC, 2002). These rates are similar across infections of other sexually transmitted diseases. Technologically based interventions for reducing sexual risk behaviors have appropriately targeted groups at greatest risk for sexually transmitted infections (STIs; Di Noia, Schinke, Pena, & Schwinn, 2004; Downs et al., 2004; Roye, Silverman, & Krauss, 2007; see Table 22.3).

Randomized Trials Using Computer-Based Approaches A number of research teams have evaluated whether technological interventions are superior to more conventional health behavior change methodologies, including educational lectures, pamphlets, or face-to-face interactions. For example, Evans, Edmundsen-Drane, and Harris (2006) compared the effectiveness of a computer-assisted instruction intervention to a traditional lecture-based intervention for influencing psychosocial correlates of HIV preventive behaviors. The computer-based system, AIDS Interactive, targeted self-efficacy by allowing students opportunities to rehearse communication skills related to HIV risk behaviors by responding to comments made by an imaginary partner in a sexual situation. Di Noia et al. (2004) also evaluated a computer-based intervention designed to increase self-efficacy for engaging in sexual risk reduction behaviors among adolescent females. Outcomes from both studies suggested that computer-based technologies may be more effective than traditional methods. Similarly, Lightfoot, Comulada, and Sotver (2007) tested the hypothesis that a computerized intervention would be as efficacious as an in-person small-group intervention for reducing sexual risk behaviors, and results from the study generally confirmed this hypothesis. Kiene and Barta (2006) evaluated the effectiveness of a custom computerized HIV/AIDS risk intervention at increasing HIV/AIDS preventive behaviors. Results indicated that participants interacting with the computer-delivered risk reduction intervention exhibited a significant increase in frequency of keeping condoms readily available and displayed greater condom-related knowledge at a four-week follow-up session.

Randomized Trials Using Video-Based Approaches Video-based interventions have the potential to deliver health messages while providing entertainment and social modeling. Video also makes it possible to tailor demographic characteristics of the narrator or characters to specifically increase personal relevance and strengthen social modeling. Furthermore, video as a health education tool reaches those who are illiterate or unwilling to read text-based health messages (such as brochures and pamphlets). Downs et al. (2004) compared the effects of a video targeting adolescent females to two types of written control material. The video attempted to create opportunities for personal decision making in hypothetical sexual situations while providing crucial information on the subject. In a like manner, Roye et al. (2007) evaluated the effects of video to provide information about risky sexual behaviors and HIV transmission, counseling, and video plus counseling on condom use in black and Latina adolescent females. The video also directly addressed perceived barriers to condom use that had previously been identified in focus groups. Results suggested that neither video nor counseling alone significantly affected condom use, but the combined intervention improved condom use.

Innovative, Untested Applications of Technology   The future of video and computer for providing health-based messages is particularly promising given the availability and popularity of Web-based video sharing services (such as YouTube.com) and the capability of social networking sites popular among adolescents to share video. Such technologies have made it possible for individuals to engage in a limited degree of dialogue related to an original video by posting video responses, and the rapid increase in availability of Web cams has made this type of dialogue popular among adolescents. However, researchers and health educators have yet to evaluate the potential of these types of video networks to disseminate health messages to adolescents.

Eating Disorders

Eating disorders are most commonly found in female adolescents (Striegel-Moore et al., 2003). Between 2 and 4 percent of female adolescents and young adults develop full syndrome eating disorders (anorexia nervosa, bulimia, or binge-eating disorder) and subclinical eating concerns are estimated to affect up to a quarter of adolescent women (Fairburn & Beglin, 1990; Striegel-Moore et al., 2003; Hart & Kenny, 1997). The typical age of onset occurs in late adolescence, between sixteen and twenty. Risk factors for the development of eating disorders include dietary restraint and excessive weight and shape concerns (Stice, 2002; Jacobi, Hayward, de Zwaan, Kraemer & Agras, 2004). Eating disorders are known to be chronic, persistent, and difficult to treat (Fairburn & Harrison, 2003).

A number of technological interventions have been developed by patients and health professionals to prevent and treat eating disorders in adolescents. These interventions take the form of peer-led and professionally led support or discussion groups, psychoeducation, and combined psychoeducation and support or therapy group interventions. These interventions have addressed both *universal prevention*—interventions that seek to reduce the incidence of a disease by eliminating or reducing risk factors that are prevalent in a population—and *targeted prevention,* which focuses on reducing risk factors in populations at high risk of developing subclinical or full syndrome disorders.

TABLE 22.3. Randomized, controlled trials of technological interventions for sexual risk behaviors in adolescents

Reference	Intervention	Sample	Target Behavior	Posttest Results
Kiene & Barta (2006)	Computer-delivered interactive software targeting information, motivation, and behavioral skills; control = nutrition education	157 college students	Changes in predictors of safer sex behavior and in preventive behavior	Significant reduction in risk behaviors in computer group
Evans et al. (2000)	Computer-assisted to increase HIV preventive behaviors; control = lecture or no intervention	152 university students in human sexuality class	HIV preventive behaviors such as consistent, correct condom use	Significantly higher AIDS knowledge, self-evaluative motivation, and intention to practice HIV preventive behaviors in computer intervention
Di Noia et al. (2004)	Keeping It Safe computer software: HIV/AIDS knowledge, protective attitudes, self-efficacy; control = different site, no intervention	Early adolescent females ages 11 to 14	HIV/ AIDS-related knowledge, protective attitudes, and self-efficacy for HIV risk reduction	Experimental arm youths evidenced greater improvements from pretest to posttest than control arm youths

Lightfoot et al. (2007)	Experimental group = computer-based; control = no intervention or small-group face-to-face	133 at-risk 14- to 18-year-old students	Sexual intercourse in past three months (0 = no; 1 = yes); type of sexual activity in past three months	Computerized intervention group significantly less likely to engage in sexual activity and reported significantly fewer partners
Downs et al. (2004)	Video intervention; two controls: brochure or book form	300 sexually active 14- to 18-year-olds	Knowledge about STD risk behavior, STD acquisition, and risky sexual behavior	No group differences in knowledge or use of condoms; video condition had significantly lower likelihood of self-reporting a new STD at follow-up
Roye et al. (2007)	Video with ethnic diversity targeting barriers to condom use; control = counseling or care as usual	400 sexually active black and Latina 15- to 21-year-olds	Self-reported condom use at last intercourse	Video alone and counseling alone not significantly different from usual care; combined video and counseling intervention improved condom use at last intercourse

TABLE 22.4. Randomized, controlled trials of technological interventions for eating disorders in adolescents

Reference	Intervention	Sample	Target Behavior	Posttest Results
Taylor et al. (2006)	Student Bodies eating disorder prevention; self-help psycho-education with moderated asynchronous discussion group; control group = no intervention	480 college-aged women	Weight and shape concerns, eating pathology, and eating disorders	Improved weight and shape concerns, reduction of eating disorders in subgroups
Zabinski et al. (2004)	Chat room eating disorder prevention, newsgroup, psychoeducation, and weekly homework; control = wait list or no intervention	60 college-aged women	Weight and shape concerns, eating pathology, and eating disorders	Significantly reduced eating pathology and improved self-esteem
Heinicke, Paxton, McLean, & Wertheim (2007)	Eating disorder prevention chat room facilitated by a therapist and manual; control = delayed treatment control	73 young female adolescents	Body image and eating pathology	Treatment group participants significantly reduced their body image dissatisfaction and eating pathology

Gollings & Paxton (2006)	Set Your Body Free Group Body Image Program: manualized group treatment program with chat rooms; control = face-to-face group	40 college-aged women with body image dissatisfaction and disordered eating	Disordered eating behaviors and attitudes, body image dissatisfaction	Significant improvement on all outcome measures pre-post intervention
Franko et al. (2005)	Food, Mood, and Attitude Interactive CD-ROM; control = video and attention	240 college women prescreened for intensity of eating disorder	Knowledge, internalization of sociocultural idea, weight concerns, shape concerns, and restraint	Significant gain of knowledge in intervention versus control; significantly less internalization of sociocultural ideal, weight concerns, and restraint
Bergh et al. (2002)	Computer feedback on eating rate and satiety; control = no treatment	19 patients with bulimia, 13 with anorexia (inpatient and outpatient)	Eating rate, satiety level, remission rate, BMI, psychopathology, medical status, and social adjustment	Greater remission rates in experimental group; significantly improved eating rates among both anorexics and bulimics

Of note, most of the interventions discussed in this chapter have been designed for late adolescent and early adult females. In addition, for unknown reasons most of the interventions developed have been limited to delivery by computer. However, this delivery method has been employed in various adaptations. See Table 22.4.

Internet Interventions Emphasizing Prevention of Eating Disorders The earliest and most extensively developed intervention, Student Bodies, has been evaluated as both a universal and targeted intervention. Since the creation of the Student Bodies program, a number of iterations have been developed and evaluated with adolescent high school– and college-aged students (Winzelberg et al., 1998; Winzelberg et al., 2000; Celio et al., 2000; Zabinski et al., 2001; Jacobi et al., 2007; Abascal, Bruning, Winzelberg, Dev, & Taylor, 2004; Bruning-Brown, Winzelberg, Abascal, & Taylor, 2004; Low et al., 2006; Luce et al., 2005; Jacobi et al., 2005; Taylor et al., 2006). Each new version of the program has been revised to incorporate research findings and feedback from participants. Overall, participants completing Student Bodies reported significant improvements in weight and shape concerns and healthier eating attitudes and behaviors, as well as reducing the onset of eating disorders (Taylor et al., 2006).

Three other eating disorder interventions have been shown to reduce eating pathology in adolescents. The first intervention, created by Zabinski, Wilfley, Calfas, Winzelberg, and Taylor (2004), used a synchronous (chat room) format for delivering the intervention. The program, loosely based on the Student Bodies intervention described earlier, provided an eight-week professionally moderated discussion group focused on improving body image and eating behaviors for college-aged women. Participants in the intervention were found to significantly reduce their eating pathology. The second intervention, developed by Heinicke, Paxton, McLean, and Wertheim (2007), offered six ninety-minute group sessions in synchronous format to young adolescents. Compared to the control group, participants significantly reduced their body image dissatisfaction and eating pathology.

The last chat-based intervention, developed by Gollings and Paxton (2006), evaluated an adaptation of their Set Your Body Free Group Body Image Program. In this pilot study, forty young women with disordered eating patterns and high levels of body dissatisfaction were assigned to either a synchronous chat-based or face-to-face group intervention. The manualized group intervention was facilitated by a psychotherapist and based on cognitive behavioral therapy and motivational interviewing. Women in both groups were found to improve their eating patterns and body image.

Internet Interventions Emphasizing Treatment of Eating Disorders The most widely evaluated treatment program for bulimia has been the SALUT intervention. Project SALUT (Intelligent Environment for the Diagnostics, Treatment, and Prevention of Eating Disorders) is a self-help eating disorder prevention and treatment program that is available in seven European languages. Like the Student Bodies program described above, studies evaluating the SALUT intervention have varied slightly in design (length of treatment and type of control group, for example), but the core features of the program include a self-help guide, the ability to self-monitor behaviors and track them over time, and weekly e-mails from an online therapist. Overall, studies found that the SALUT intervention reduces the eating disorder symptoms of bingeing and purging (Liwowsky, Cebulla, & Fichter, 2006; Carrard, Rouget, Volkart, Carola, & Lam, 2005; Fernandez-Aranda, Nunez, Martinez, & Granero Perez, 2005; Rouget et al., 2005). Furthermore, in 2007 Ljottsson and colleagues reported on the results of their twelve-week-long program for women with bulimia nervosa. Their intervention combined a self-help program based on cognitive-behavioral therapy with a moderated support group. At the end of treatment, participants had reduced their eating pathology, with 37 percent reporting the cessation of binge eating or purging.

CD-ROM Intervention Franko et al. (2005) introduced an interactive CD-ROM program called Food, Mood, and Attitude. This approach incorporated aspects of interpersonal and rational theory as well as cognitive-behavioral theory, which have both been widely used by eating disorder researchers and clinicians (Stein et al., 2001). The user navigates as a peer counselor in a virtual university addressing the problem of eating disorders. Results indicated that such interventions could benefit both at-risk college women who have not yet pursued treatment and low-risk women who simply want to know more about eating disorder risk.

Computer Feedback Intervention Bergh, Brodin, Lindberg, and Sodersten (2002) used computer feedback to focus on disordered eating behavior and altered perceptions of satiety (which are thought to characterize anorexia and bulimia). Researchers hooked up a computer to a scale holding a plate of food and gave feedback to participants about the reduced weight of the food plate, while they were simultaneously able to record corresponding satiety levels and the eating rate. Eventually, participants were asked to follow a set eating rate, training to eat a certain amount of food within a given time. Results indicated significantly greater remission rates for those in the intervention condition and the eating rate and amount were significantly improved for both anorexics and bulimics.

Innovative, Untested Applications of Technology Today, the number of consumer-created eating disorder support and discussion groups and Web sites far exceeds the number of interventions developed by health professions. For example, dozens of profiles and forums created by adolescents that address eating disorders are available on MySpace, Facebook, Yahoo, and Google groups. Almost all of these discussion and support groups are unstructured, peer-led, open-ended, and open to all participants. Despite their wide acceptance on the Internet, no studies have examined the participation rates and effectiveness of these Web sites.

The number of consumer-created eating disorder support and discussion groups and Web sites far exceeds the number of interventions developed by health professions.

SUMMARY

Technological interventions appear to be at least as effective as more traditional methods, but results vary considerably across health behaviors. Additionally, technology has been used in quite different ways in each category of health behavior. We found that few studies evaluated similar technologies in comparable samples, making it quite difficult to draw generalizable conclusions about each technology, particularly with respect to identifying which individuals are most likely to benefit from which treatment.

Technology may in some cases provide more cost-effective solutions for providing some level of intervention at a population level, but the strength of these interventions may ultimately be attenuated by low levels of adherence. Where the norm would be professional or peer-based counseling, technology is likely to be a less efficacious alternative, but where a standard intervention might be written psychoeducational materials, technological interventions may offer greater efficacy by providing tailored messages, interactive presentation of information, and feedback or reinforcement. Technological alternatives to paper- and pamphlet-based and lecture-based psychoeducational interventions allow for greater degrees of interaction between the content material and the user, thereby improving the "match" between an individual and the nature of the information being presented, promoting depth of processing of the content material, and enhancing opportunities for practicing responses to a wide variety of situations.

Extant studies have begun to provide some insights into boundary conditions that establish for whom and under what circumstances technology-based interventions may be most effective. For example, across all health behaviors discussed in this chapter, technological interventions that were found to be most effective tended to be interactive and composed of multiple sessions. More extensive evaluations, however, are warranted. Thus, it is essential that technologically focused interventions be evaluated in trials that choose appropriate control groups. It is equally essential that technologically driven interventions be evaluated in programs of research that allow for systematic, empirically based improvements. Unfortunately, the pace of technological innovation makes such programs of research quite difficult to establish. Given the time-intensive nature of designing, developing, implementing, evaluating, and reporting scientific studies, it is not surprising that the research literature can accurately be characterized as outdated with respect to existing technologies.

As might be expected, interventions across all the health behaviors reviewed appear to show stronger effects for adolescents who have already engaged in high-risk behaviors than those who have yet to undertake these behaviors. For example, college-aged women were often targeted in eating disorder interventions, because this is the population considered to be at greatest risk (Franko et al., 2005; Mintz, O'Halloran, Mulholland, & Schneider, 1997; Drewnowski, Yee, Kurth, & Krahn, 1994). These findings suggest that tailoring interventions more specifically to the severity of the problem behavior could further enhance outcomes, because Marks et al. (2006) demonstrated that Web-based and print-based interventions were most effective for study participants who entered the study with the lowest levels of physical activity.

We identified a number of limitations of this literature as a whole. Across all the reviewed studies, we did not find studies that evaluated differential effects of technological intervention by age. In adolescent populations, it is particularly important to account for developmental stages of the participants and to clearly articulate how the effects of a specific technology might differ with respect to these developmental stages. Second, the number of studies identified was surprisingly small, and inconsistent results are magnified by the lack of overlapping studies for specific technologies applied to similar populations within a given health behavior. Third, many of the studies included the use of a specific technology as a single component in a larger, multi-component intervention (such as Internet plus face-to-face counseling), precluding our ability to isolate the effects of the technology on the health behavior. Finally, those studies reporting significant effects of a technological intervention frequently failed to identify effects that were sustained over multiple follow-up observations.

In light of these shortcomings, we offer several recommendations for future research. Most important, we believe it is important for editors, reviewers, and funding agencies to recognize the complexity of the research designs required to adequately evaluate technological interventions (such as the process of obtaining consent for a minor's participation in an Internet-based study). Rapidly changing technology makes it difficult to evaluate these interventions using controlled research designs, and systematic research can take years to complete. Often, by the time a research team publishes its results, the technology has advanced, and we believe there is potential for bias against programs of research involving now outdated technologies. However, without those systematic programs of research, we are unlikely to learn important lessons about how and under what circumstances technological interventions can be used to successfully promote adolescent behavior change. Moreover, researchers may be able to achieve stronger effect sizes by attempting to improve adherence to the intervention and paying attention to sustainability of effects over longer periods of time. Also, evaluating users' qualitative experiences with the technology is likely to drive innovation toward greater usability, adherence, and efficacy. Future studies need to evaluate existing, real-world technologies used by the general public—such as popular peer-based Web sites—rather than focusing exclusively on interventions that have been developed and facilitated by health care professionals. Additionally, investigations need to determine how to integrate self-help and professionally moderated Internet-delivered interventions within a stepped-care approach for treatment, and educators need to determine how to best deliver universal and targeted psychoeducational interventions to adolescents.

In summary, *technology* is a broad term that encompasses a variety of applications and changes on a seemingly daily basis, with new and more sophisticated technological innovations emerging all the time. What these technologies have in common is that they each attempt, in some way, to improve the level and quality of feedback, personalized information, and interactivity that influence the way in which adolescents process health-related information. The state of the literature suggests that there is a substantial role for technological interventions in improving adolescent health behaviors, at the very least as a supplement to more traditional methods. Additional research is needed to identify for whom these types of technological interventions are most efficacious and to characterize mechanisms of action that could further enhance effect sizes. Further, because the use of technology is often accompanied by the absence of, or only minimal exposure to, person-to-person contact, more work is needed to understand how and under what circumstances limited human contact can enhance or detract from treatment efficacy.

KEY TERMS

Targeted prevention intervention

Universal prevention intervention

DISCUSSION QUESTIONS

1. Out of the different innovative technological media discussed in this chapter, which is most accessible by adolescents on a daily basis (not necessarily just those participating in an intervention)? Does the level of use vary according to gender or age?

2. How do you think traditional intervention methodologies compare to technological interventions in terms of sustainable intervention effects and cost?

3. Briefly outline an innovative technological intervention. Think about your research design, type of technology, risk behavior to modify, target population, length of study, and your evaluation plan.

REFERENCES

Abascal, L., Bruning, J., Winzelberg, A. J., Dev, P., & Taylor, C. B. (2004). Combining universal and targeted prevention for school based eating disorder programs. *International Journal of Eating Disorders, 35*(1), 1–9.

Baronowski, T., Baronowski, J., Cullen, K. W., Marsh, T., Islam, N., & Zakeri, I. (2003). Squire's quest! Dietary outcome evaluation of a multimedia game. *American Journal of Preventive Medicine, 24*(1), 52–61.

Bergh, C., Brodin, U., Lindberg, G., & Sodersten, P. (2002). Randomized controlled trial of treatment for anorexia and bulimia nervosa. *Proceedings of the National Academy of Sciences, 99*(14), 9486–9491.

Bersamin, M., Paschall, M. J., Fearnow-Kenney, M., & Wyrick, D. (2007). Effectiveness of a Web-based alcohol-misuse and harm-prevention course among high- and low-risk students. *Journal of American College Health, 55*(4), 247–255.

Brown, D. (2006). Playing to win: Video games and the fight against obesity. *Journal of the American Dietetic Association, 106*(2), 188–189.

Bruning-Brown, J., Winzelberg, A., Abascal, L., & Taylor, C. B. (2004). An evaluation of an Internet-delivered eating disorder prevention program for adolescents and their parents. *Journal of Adolescent Health, 35*(4), 290–296.

Carrard, I., Rouget, P., Volkart, A., Carola, M., & Lam, T. (2005, September 9). Efficacy evaluation of the French version of the Web-based self-help guide for bulimia nervosa in Switzerland. Paper presented at the European Council on Eating Disorders 9th General Meeting, Innsbruck, Austria.

Casazza, K., & Ciccazzo, M. (2007). The method of delivery of nutrition and physical activity information may play a role in eliciting behavior changes in adolescents. *Eating Behaviors, 8,* 73–82.

Celio, A. A., Winzelberg, A. J., Wilfley, D. E., Eppstein-Harald, D., Springer, E. A., Dev, P., & Taylor, C. B. (2000). Reducing risk factors for eating disorders: Comparison of an Internet- and a classroom-delivered psychoeducation program. *Journal of Consulting and Clinical Psychology, 68,* 650–657.

Centers for Disease Control and Prevention. (2000). *Tracking the hidden epidemics 2000: Trends in STDs in the United States.* Atlanta, GA: Author.

Centers for Disease Control and Prevention. (2002). *Young people at risk: HIV/AIDS among America's youth.* Atlanta, GA: Author.

Chen, H., & Yeh, M. (2006). Developing and evaluating a smoking cessation program combined with an Internet-assisted instruction program for adolescents with smoking. *Patient Education and Counseling, 61,* 411–418.

Cielo, A. (2005). Early intervention of eating and weight-related problems via the Internet in overweight adolescents: A randomized controlled trial. *Dissertation Abstracts International: Section B—the Sciences and Engineering, 66*(4-B), 2299.

Clemmens, D., & Hayman, L. L. (2004). Increasing activity to reduce obesity in adolescent girls: A research review. *Journal of Obstetric and Gynecological Neonatal Nursing, 33,* 801–808.

Di Noia, J., Schinke, S. P., Pena, J. B., & Schwinn, T. M. (2004). Evaluation of a brief computer-mediated intervention to reduce HIV risk among early adolescent females. *Journal of Adolescent Health, 35,* 62–64.

Di Noia, J., Schwinn, T. M., Dastur, Z. A., & Schinke, S. P. (2003). The relative efficacy of pamphlets, CD-ROM, and the Internet for disseminating adolescent drug abuse prevention programs: An exploratory study. *Preventive Medicine, 37,* 646–653.

Downs, J. S., Murray, P. J., Bruine de Bruine, W., Penrose, J., Palgren, C., & Fischhoff, B. (2004). Interactive video behavioral intervention to reduce adolescent females' STD risk: A randomized controlled trial. *Social Science and Medicine, 59*(8), 1561–1572.

Duncan, T. E., Duncan. S. C, Beauchamp, N., Wells, J., & Ary, D. V. (2000). Development and evaluation of an interactive CD-ROM refusal skills program to prevent youth substance use: "Refuse to use." *Journal of Behavioral Medicine, 23*(1), 59–72.

Drewnowski, A., Yee, D. K., Kurth, C. L., & Krahn, D. D. (1994). Eating pathology and DSM-III-R: A continuum of bulimic behaviors. *American Journal of Psychiatry, 151,* 1217–1219.

Evans, A. E., Edmundsen-Drane, E. W., & Harris, K. K. (2006). Computer-assisted instruction: An effective instructional method for HIV prevention education? *Journal of Adolescent Health, 26,* 244–51.

Fairburn, C. G., & Beglin, S. J. (1990). Studies of the epidemiology of bulimia nervosa. *American Journal of Psychiatry, 147*(4), 401–408.

Fairburn, C. G., & Harrison, P. J. (2003). Eating disorders. *Lancet, 361,* 407–416.

Fernandez-Aranda, F., Nunez, A., Martinez, C., & Granero Perez, R. (2005, September 9). Efficacy evaluation of the Spanish version of the Web-based self-help guide for bulimia nervosa: A controlled study. Paper presented at the European Council on Eating Disorders 9th General Meeting, Innsbruck, Austria.

Fishbein, M., Von Haeften, I., Hall-Jamieson, K., Johnson, B., & Kirkland Ahern, R. (2000). Evaluation of anti-drug public service announcements (PSAs): Comparison of computer-assisted and paper and pencil methodologies in a sample of adolescents from the Boys and Girls Clubs of Metropolitan Philadelphia. *Psychology, Health, and Medicine, 5,* 259–270.

Franko, D. L., Mintz, L. B., Villapiano, M., Green, T. C., Mainelli, D., & Folensbee, L. (2005). Food, mood, and attitude: Reducing risk for eating disorders in college women. *Health Psychology, 24*(6), 567–578.

Frenn, M., Malin, S., Brown, R. L., Greer, Y., Fox, J., Greer, J., & Smyczek, S. (2005). Changing the tide: An Internet/video exercise and low-fat diet intervention with middle-school students. *Applied Nursing Research, 18,* 13–21.

Goldfield, G. S., Malloy, R., Parker, T., Cunningham, T., Legg, C., Lumb, A., Prud'homme, D., Gaboury, I., & Adamo, K. B. (2006). Effects of open-loop feedback on physical activity and television viewing in overweight and obese children: A randomized, controlled trial. *Pediatrics, 118*(1), 157–166.

Gollings, E. K., & Paxton, S. J. (2006). Comparison of Internet and face-to-face delivery of a group body image and disordered eating intervention for women: A pilot study. *Eating Disorders, 14*(1), 1–15.

Hart, K., & Kenny, M. (1997). Adherence to the super woman ideal and eating disorder symptoms among college women. *Sex Roles, 36,* 461–478.

Heinicke, B. E., Paxton, S. J., McLean, S. A., & Wertheim, E. H. (2007). Internet-delivered targeted group intervention for body dissatisfaction and disordered eating in adolescent girls: A randomized controlled trial. *Journal of Abnormal Child Psychology, 35*(3), 379–391.

Houston, T. K., Cooper, L. A., Vu, H. T., Kahn, J., Toser, J., & Ford, D. E. (2001). Screening the public for depression through the internet. *Psychiatric Services, 52,* 362–367.

Houston, T. K., & Ehrenberger, H. E. (2001). The potential of consumer health informatics. *Seminars in Oncology Nursing, 17,* 41–47.

Jacobi, C., Hayward, C., de Zwaan, M., Kraemer, H. C., & Agras, W. S. (2004). Coming to terms with risk factors for eating disorders: Application of risk terminology and suggestions for a general taxonomy. *Psychological Bulletin, 130*(1), 19–65.

Jacobi, C., Morris, L., Beckers, C., Bronisch-Holtze, J., Winter, J., Winzelberg, A. J., & Taylor, C. B. (2007). Maintenance of Internet-based prevention: A randomized controlled trial. *International Journal of Eating Disorders, 40*(2), 114–119.

Jacobi, C., Morris, L., Bronisch-Holtze, J., Winter, J., Winzelberg, A., & Taylor, C. B. (2005). Reduktion von Risikofaktoren für gestörtes Essverhalten: Adaptation und erste Ergebnisse eines Internet-gestützten Präventionsprogramms. *Zeitschrift für Gesundheitspsychologie, 13,* 92–101.

Jago, R., Baranowski, T., Baronowski, J. C., Thompson, D., Cullen, K. W., Watson, K., et al. (2006). Fit for life boy scout badge: Outcome evaluation of a troop and Internet intervention. *Preventive Medicine, 42,* 181–187.

Kaiser Family Foundation. (2001). GenerationRx.com: How young people use the Internet for health information. Retrieved August 6, 2007, from www.kff.org/entmedia/20011211a-index.cfm.

Kiene, S. M., & Barta, W. (2006). A brief individualized computer-delivered sexual risk reduction intervention increases HIV/AIDS preventive behavior. *Journal of Adolescent Health, 39,* 404–410.

Klein, J. D., Havens, C. F., & Carlson, E. J. (2005). Evaluation of an adolescent smoking-cessation media campaign: GottaQuit.com. *Pediatrics, 116,* 950–956.

Knight, J. R., Wechsler, H., Kuo, M., Seibring, M., Weitzman, E. R., & Schuckit, M. A. (2002). Alcohol abuse and dependence among U.S. college students. *Journal of Studies on Alcohol, 63,* 263–270.

Kypri, K., & McAnally, H. M. (2005). Randomized controlled trial of a Web-based primary care intervention for multiple health risk behaviors. *Preventive Medicine, 41,* 76–6.

Kypri, K., Saunders, J. B., Williams, S. M., McGee, R. O., Langley, J. D., Casheel-Smith, M. L., & Gallagher, S. J. (2004). Web-based screening and brief intervention for hazardous drinking: A double-blind randomized controlled trial. *Addiction, 99,* 1410–1417.

Lenhart, A., Madden, M., & Hitlin, P. (2005). Teens and technology: Youth are leading the transition to a fully wired and mobile nation. *Pew Internet and American Life Project.* Retrieved August 28, 2007, from www.pewinternet.org/pdfs/PIP_Teens_Tech_Julsy2005web.pdf.

Lightfoot, M., Comulada, W. S., & Sotver, G. (2007). Computerized HIV preventive intervention for adolescents: Indications of efficacy. *American Journal of Public Health, 97*(6), 1027–1030.

Liwowsky, I., Cebulla, M., & Fichter, M. (2006). New ways to combat eating disorders: Evaluation of an Internet-based self-help program in bulimia nervosa. *MMW Fortschritte der Medizin, 148*(31–32), 31–33.

Long, J. D., Armstrong, M. L., Amos, E., Shriver, B., Roman-Shriver, C., Feng, D., Harrison, L., Luker, S., Nash, A., & Blevins, M. W. (2006). Pilot using World Wide Web to prevent diabetes in adolescents. *Clinical Nursing Research, 15*(1), 67–79.

Low, K. G., Charanasomboon, S., Lesser, J., Reinhalter, K., Martin, R., Jones, H., Winzelberg, A., Abascal, L., & Taylor, C. B. (2006). Effectiveness of a computer-based interactive eating disorder prevention program at long-term follow-up. *Eating Disorders, 14*(1), 17–30.

Luce, K. H., Osborne, M., Winzelberg, A., Abascal, A., Celio, A., Wilfley, D., Stevenson, D., Dev, P., & Taylor, C. B. (2005). Application of an algorithm-driven protocol to simultaneously provide universal and targeted prevention programs. *International Journal of Eating Disorders, 37*(3), 220–226.

Malo, R. F. Shope, J. T., Blow, F. C., Gregor, M. A., Zakrajsek, J. S, Weber, J. E., & Nypaver, M. M. (2005). A randomized controlled trial of an emergency department-based interactive computer program to prevent alcohol misuse among injured adolescents. *Annals of Emergency Medicine, 45*(4), 420–429.

Marcus, B. H., Nigg, C. R., Riebe, D., & Forsyth, L. H. (2000). Interactive communication strategies: Implications for population-based physical-activity promotion. *American Journal of Preventive Medicine, 19,* 121–126.

Marks, J. T., Campbell, M. K., Ward, D. S., Ribisl, K. M., Wildemuth, B. M., & Symons, M. J. (2006). A comparison of Web and print media for physical activity promotion among adolescent girls. *Journal of Adolescent Health, 39,* 96–104.

Mintz, L. B., O-Halloran, S. M., Mulholland, A. M., & Schneider, P. A. (1997). Questionnaire for eating disorder diagnoses: Reliability and validity of operationalizing DSM-IV criteria into a self-report format. *Journal of Counseling Psychology, 44,* 63–79.

Moore, M. J., Soderquist, J., & Werch, C. (2005). Feasibility and efficacy of a binge drinking prevention intervention for college students delivered via the Internet versus postal mail. *Journal of American College Health, 54*(1), 38–44.

Muller, M. J., Danielzik, S., & Pust, S. (2005). School- and family-based interventions to prevent overweight in children. *Proceedings of the Nutrition Society, 64,* 249–254.

Patten, C. A., Croghan, I. T., Meis, T. M., Decker, P. A., Pingree, S., Colligan, R. C., Dornelas, E. A., Offord, K. P., Boberg, E. W., Baumberger, R. K., Hurt, R. D., & Gustafson, D. H. (2006). Randomized clinical trial of an Internet-based versus brief office intervention for adolescent smoking cessation. *Patient Education and Counseling, 64,* 249–258.

Resnicow, K., Taylor, R., Baskin, M., & McCarty, F. (2005). Results of go girls: A weight control program for overweight African American adolescent females. *Obesity Research, 13*(10), 1739–1748.

Reynolds, B. (2004). Do high rates of cigarette consumption increase delay discounting? A cross-sectional comparison of adolescent smokers and young-adult smokers and nonsmokers. *Behavioral Processes, 67,* 545–549.

Robinson, T. N., Patrick, K., Eng, T. R., & Gustafson, D. (1998). An evidence-based approach to interactive health communication: A challenge to medicine in the information age. *Journal of the American Medical Association, 280,* 1264–1269.

Rouget, P., Carrard, I., Nevonen, L., Fernandex-Aranda, F., Norring, C., Cebulla, M., Fichter, M., Liwowsky, I., Crola, J., Volkart, A. C., & Lam, T. (2005, September 9). Results from the European multi-centre study on the efficacy of a Web-based self-help guide for the treatment of bulimia. Paper presented at the European Council on Eating Disorders 9th General Meeting, Innsbruck, Austria.

Roye, C., Silverman, P. P., & Krauss, B. (2007). A brief, low-cost, theory-based intervention to promote dual method use by Black and Latina female adolescents: A randomized clinical trial. *Health Education Behavior, 34,* 608–621.

Saelens, B. E., Sallis, J. F., Wilfley, D. E., Patrick, K., Cella, J. A., & Buchta, R. (2002). Behavioral weight control for overweight adolescents initiated in primary care. *Obesity Research, 10*(1), 22–32.

Saitz, R., Palfai, T. P., Freedner, N., Winter, M. R., MacDonald, A., Lu, J., Ozonoff, A., Rosenbloom, D. L., & Dejong, W. (2007). Screening and brief intervention online for college students: The iHealth study. *Alcohol and Alcoholism, 42,* 28–36.

Schinke, S., Di Noia, J., Schwinn, T., & Cole, K. (2006). Drug abuse risk and protective factors among Black, urban adolescent girls: A group randomized trial of computer-delivered, mother-daughter intervention. *Psychology of Addictive Behaviors, 20,* 496–500.

Schinke, S., & Schwinn, T. (2005). Gender-specific computer-based intervention for preventing drug abuse among girls. *American Journal of Drug and Alcohol Abuse, 31,* 609–616.

Schinke, S. P., Schwinn, T. M., & Ozanian, A. J. (2005). Alcohol abuse prevention among high-risk youth: computer-based intervention. *Journal of Prevention and Intervention in the Community, 29*(1/2), 117–130.

Simoes, A. A., Bastos, F. I., Moreira, R. I., Lynch, K. G., & Metzger, D. S. (2006). A randomized trial of audio computer and in-person interview to assess HIV risk among drug and alcohol users in Rio De Janeiro, Brazil. *Journal of Substance Abuse Treatment, 30,* 237–243.

Slootmaker, S. M., Chin A Paw, M. J., Schuit, A. J., Seidell, J. C., & van Mechelen, W. (2005). Promoting physical activity using an activity monitor and tailored Web-based advice: design of a randomized controlled trial. *BMC Public Health, 5*(143), 1–9.

Stein, R. I., Saelens, B. E., Zoler-Dounchis, J., Lewczyk, C. M., Swenson, A. K., & Wilfley, D. E. (2001). Treatment of eating disorders in women. *The Counseling Psychologist, 29,* 695–732.

Stice, E. (2002). Risk and maintenance factors for eating pathology: a meta-analytic review. *Psychological Bulletin, 128*(5), 825–848.

Striegel-Moore, R. H., Dohm, F. A., Kraemer, H. C., Taylor, C. B., Daniels, S., Crawford, P. B., & Schreiber, G. B. (2003). Eating disorders in white and black women. *American Journal of Psychiatry, 160*(7), 1326–1331.

Swahn, M. H., & Bossarte, R. M. (2007). Gender, early alcohol use, and suicide ideation and attempts: Findings from the 2005 Youth Risk Behavior Survey. *Journal of Adolescent Health, 41*(2), 175–181.

Taylor, C. B., Bryson, S. W., Luce, K. H., Cunning, D., Celio, A., Abascal, M. A., Roxwell, R., Pavarti, D., Winzelberg, A. J., & Wilfley, D. E. (2006). Prevention of eating disorders in at-risk college-age women. *Archives of General Psychiatry, 63,* 881–888.

Timperio, A., Salmon, J., & Ball, K. (2004). Evidence-based strategies to promote physical activity among children, adolescents, and young adults: Review and update. *Journal of the Science of Medicine in Sport, 7,* 20–29.

Webb, P. M., Zimet, G. D., Fortenberry, J. D., & Blythe, M. J. (1999). Comparability of a computer-assisted versus written method for collecting health behavior information from adolescent patients. *Journal of Adolescent Health, 24,* 383–388.

White, M. A., Martin, P. D., Newton, R. L., Walden, H. M., York-Crowe, E. E., Gordon, S. T., Ryan, D. H., & Williamson, D. A. (2004). Mediators of weight loss in a family-based intervention presented over the internet. *Obesity Research, 12*(7), 1050–1059.

Williams, C., Griffin, K. W., Macaulay, A. P., West, T. L., & Gronewold, E. (2005). Efficacy of a drug prevention CD-ROM intervention for adolescents. *Substance Use and Misuse, 40,* 869–877.

Winzelberg, A., Epstein, D., Eldredge, K., Wilfley, D., Dasmahapatra, R., Dev, P., & Taylor, C. B. (2000). Effectiveness of an Internet-based program for reducing risk factors for eating disorders. *Journal of Consulting and Clinical Psychology, 68*(2), 346–350.

Winzelberg, A., Taylor, C. B., Altman, T., Eldredge, K., Dev, P., & Constantinou, P. (1998). Evaluation of a computer-mediated eating disorder prevention program. *International Journal of Eating Disorders, 24,* 339–350.

Woodruff, S. I., Conway, T. L., Edwards, C. C., Elliott, S. P., & Crittenden, J. (2007). Evaluation of an Internet virtual world chat room for adolescent smoking cessation. *Addictive Behaviors, 32,* 1769–1786.

Woodruff, S. I., Edwards, C. C., Conway, T. L., & Elliott, S. P. (2001). Pilot test of an Internet virtual world chat room for rural teen smokers. *Journal of Adolescent Health, 29,* 239–243.

Zabinski, M., Wilfley, D., Calfas, K., Winzelberg, A., & Taylor, C. B. (2004). An interactive psychological intervention for women at risk of developing an eating disorder. *Journal of Clinical and Consulting Psychology, 72*(5), 914–919.

Zabinski, M. F., Pung, M. P., Wilfley, D. E., Eppstein, D. L., Winzelberg, A. J., Celio, A., & Taylor, C. B. (2001). Reducing risk factors for eating disorders: Targeting at-risk women with a computerized psychoeducational program. *International Journal of Eating Disorders, 29*(4), 401–408.

Ziemlis, A., Bucknam, R. B., & Elfessi, A. M. (2002). Prevention efforts underlying decreases in binge drinking at institutions of higher education. *Journal of American College Health, 50,* 238–252.

CHAPTER

MEASURING ADOLESCENT HEALTH BEHAVIORS

RENEE E. SIEVING ▪ LYDIA A. SHRIER

LEARNING OBJECTIVES

After studying this chapter, you will be able to

- Illustrate the importance of using accurate measures when evaluating adolescent health behavior

- Classify different types of measurement available for assessing adolescent health behaviors

- Categorize strengths and weaknesses of different measurement modes: self-report, observational, and biological

- Compare factors that threaten the validity of adolescents' self-reported behavior

Graduate students are often surprised to learn that the measurement of adolescent health behaviors requires special focus. Yet a close examination of the work of adolescent health professionals reveals the pervasiveness of measurement issues. Consider, for example, Gwen, employed by a state health department as the state's adolescent health coordinator. Every year, Gwen makes recommendations to the state health commissioner about allocating state-level funds for preventing alcohol, tobacco, and other drug use among adolescents. To make these recommendations, Gwen uses information on the current prevalence of alcohol and other drug use among adolescents from every region of the state, obtained from a statewide survey of adolescents conducted every three years. Self-report measures from this statewide survey help Gwen determine which groups of adolescents are at risk for negative health outcomes related to alcohol, tobacco, and other drug use.

Other adolescent health professionals have similar experiences. For example, Luis works as a project director of a recently funded prevention program. The purpose of this program is to reduce sexually transmitted infections among adolescent males involved in a local Job Corps training program. Luis's responsibilities include locating measures of sexual risk behaviors appropriate to use with adolescent males, using these measures to create a screening instrument to be given to all local Job Corps trainees, and utilizing findings from the screening instrument to determine specific behaviors for the program to target.

Jane is director of clinical services for a school-based clinic system. Over the past two school years, primary care providers and mental health professionals in the clinics have noted substantial increases in levels of emotional distress and depression among students. Responding to this trend, Jane wrote a foundation grant to provide additional school-based mental health services. To meet funding requirements, the clinics must document alterations in the prevalence of depression among the student population as a result of these added services, as well changes in risk and protective factors for depression that are targeted for change by these services.

These examples illustrate the importance of accurate measures of adolescent health behaviors for developing and evaluating health programs and services for young people. Minimizing error related to the measurement of health behaviors is of critical importance to adolescent health service providers, program planners, policy makers, and researchers.

Two fundamental measurement concepts are reliability and validity. *Reliability* refers to consistency: Does a measure produce the same results with repeated trials? A scale that indicates that a person weighs 150 pounds at one moment and 170 pounds half an hour later is not considered reliable. *Validity* refers to accuracy: Does a given instrument measure what it purports to measure? To be valid, a measure must be reliable; however, reliability does not guarantee validity. Later in this chapter, we will consider key factors—including cognitive and situational factors—that can affect the reliability and validity of measures of adolescent health behavior.

TYPES OF MEASURES

In this section, we discuss the types of measures available for assessing adolescent health behaviors. *Measurement modes* are broadly classified as self-reported, observational, and biological. We highlight strengths and limitations of each mode and discuss special considerations for use with adolescents.

Self-Report

The most common mode for collecting data about adolescent health behaviors are methods in which young people provide a direct report of their behaviors. *Self-report methods* include interviews, surveys, diaries, and momentary sampling methods. Key considerations with self-report methods are the sensitivity of specific information and the level of privacy associated with a given method, because adolescents' perceptions of privacy can dramatically affect their reporting of sensitive, stigmatized, and illicit behaviors (Supple, Aquilio, & Wright, 1999; Turner et al., 1998).

Interviews Broadly defined, an *interview* is a situation in which a respondent is asked questions about a phenomenon by an individual trained in interviewing techniques. Interviews can range from relatively unstructured events to highly structured ones. In an *unstructured interview,* an interviewer asks broad, open-ended questions about a phenomenon, and the respondent is expected to reply. Researchers use unstructured formats in exploratory and qualitative research. In contrast, in a *structured interview,* an interviewer reads items verbatim from a script and records the respondent's answers. Structured interviews are commonly used in adolescent health behavior research. A *semistructured interview* combines elements of unstructured and structured interviews. An interviewer uses both closed-ended and open-ended questions; for example, closed-ended questions may be followed by open-ended questions to clarify selected responses. Semistructured interviews are used to explore opinions, perceptions, or attitudes about specific topics. A focus group is an excellent example of a semistructured interview with a group of people.

> *The most common mode for collecting data about adolescent health behaviors are methods in which young people provide a direct report of their behaviors.*

Although face-to-face interviews allow an interviewer to clarify ambiguous responses, they may pose a privacy threat to respondents who may underestimate or deny certain sensitive behaviors because of fear of embarrassment or disclosure. Respondents may be reluctant to disclose sensitive behaviors if they are not assured that their responses will be held in confidence by the interviewer (Durant & Carey, 2000). Compared to other self-report methods, face-to-face interviews are relatively labor-intensive and expensive (Durant & Carey, 2000). Evidence suggests that telephone interviews may be more effective than face-to-face interviews as a means for collecting unbiased reports of sensitive behaviors. However, telephone interviewing often cannot access very high-risk populations such as street youth or young people from families living in extreme poverty (Gribble et al., 1999).

In addition to utility in assessing behaviors, telephone interviews are an effective method for surveillance of content and quality of health services received by adolescents. Klein and colleagues (1999) reached 95 percent of fourteen- to twenty-one-year-olds ($n = 354$) who took part in a study of content covered during preventive care clinic visits. Comparing self-reports to audiotaped records of preventive visits, adolescents recalled discussing topics including confidentiality, cigarette and alcohol use, exercise, family, school, steroid use, sex, and condom use with high levels of sensitivity and specificity. Self-reports were least sensitive for blood pressure and cholesterol screening and for discussions of dental care, over-the-counter drug use, fighting, and violence.

Surveys Self-reported assessments of behavior over some retrospective time period (such as the past three months) are a mainstay of research on adolescent health behavior. In group situations, surveys are perhaps the most economical self-report method. Compared to interviews, *self-report surveys* provide a more private and less threatening means of reporting sensitive behaviors such as sexual activity, violence, and drug use (Gribble et al., 1999; Turner et al., 1998).

The most common form of self-report surveys is the paper-and-pencil questionnaire with forced-choice response items. Adolescents' ability to read and comprehend questions is critical to the effectiveness of *self-administered paper-and-pencil questionnaires* (SAQs). SAQs are problematic with groups who have limited literacy, including those for whom English may be a second language. SAQs collecting information on complex behaviors (such as sexual behaviors or school performance) often include branching or skip patterns that can be difficult to follow (Gribble et al., 1999). In addition to problems related to correct administration, problems with data quality can arise with SAQs. Certain types of questions (such as questions about sexual orientation or sexual abuse) are often associated with high rates of refusing to answer (Gribble et al., 1999). In addition, youth may answer every question, but their answers may be logically inconsistent (Upchurch et al., 2002).

Studies examining the validity of self-reported anthropometric measures have shown that young people tend to underreport their weight; differences between self-reported and measured weight are greatest among youth who are overweight and adolescent girls (Brener, McManus, et al., 2003; Lee, Valeria, Kochman, & Lenders, 2006; Strauss, 1999). Adolescents' self-perception of overweight may be particularly inaccurate; the sensitivity of self-reports of being "very overweight" was only 24 percent in a national sample of youth (Goodman, Hinden, & Khandewal, 2000). Although findings are less consistent for height (Strauss, 1999), adolescents' self-reported height tends to be taller than their measured height; this discrepancy is most common among older and Caucasian youth (Brener, McManus, et al., 2003). Overweight adolescents, however, tend to underestimate their height (Lee et al., 2006).

As a result of inaccurate self-reports, body mass index calculated using self-reported height and weight may underestimate the prevalence of overweight among adolescents (Brener, McManus, et al., 2003). Studies suggest that effects of misclassification of overweight status are relatively small (Strauss, 1999) especially for those at greatest risk (such as persistently overweight adolescents). In a national sample of youth, only 3.8 percent were misclassified as obese (Goodman et al., 2000).

Some research with adolescents requires evaluation of pubertal stage, which is most practically achieved via self-report. Studies comparing pubertal self-report (using standardized pictures and text) with clinician exam have found that adolescents self-report pubertal stages with only fair accuracy (Desmangles, Lappe, Lipaczewski, & Haynatzki, 2006). Adolescents may overreport pubertal stage early in development (Bonat, Pathomvanich, Keil, Field, & Yanovski, 2002; Lee et al., 2006) and underreport their stage as development progresses (Lee et al., 2006; Schlossberger, Turner, & Irwin, 1992). Of note, obese young teens may overestimate breast development (females) and underestimate pubic hair and genital development (females and males; Bonat et al., 2002; Lee et al., 2006). Girls with anorexia nervosa may underestimate breast development (Hick & Katzman, 1999).

In the 1990s, adolescent health behavior studies began using computer-driven technologies to administer survey questions in an audio format. This approach, known as *audio computer-assisted self-interviewing* (A-CASI), allows respondents to listen with headphones to questions that have been digitally recorded. Questions are also displayed on the computer's screen, allowing respondents to respond to a visual presentation of the question rather than wait until an audio reading has been completed. *Telephone computer-assisted self-interviewing* (T-CASI), a recent variation on A-CASI, allows respondents to listen to prerecorded survey questions via phone. A-CASI and T-CASI offer several advantages over SAQs that are particularly relevant for adolescents. With these methods, respondents can answer survey questions in complete privacy, even if their reading ability is limited. Second, computer-assisted methods reduce the likelihood of missing and inconsistent data through computer-controlled branching of complex question sets and automated question consistency checks. Finally, many adolescents enjoy interactive computer-assisted formats more than paper-and-pencil formats (Rew et al., 2004; Turner et al., 1998).

Computer-assisted methods reduce the likelihood of missing and in-consistent data through computer-controlled branch-ing of complex question sets and automated ques-tion consistency checks.

Several researchers have tested the hypothesis that adolescents are more willing to self-report sensitive and stigmatized behaviors via A-CASI as compared to alternative methods. For example, Turner and colleagues (1998) found that adolescent males' reports of particularly sensitive, stigmatized, or illegal behaviors—including injecting drug use, male-male sexual contacts, and sexual contacts with intravenous drug users—were substantially higher with A-CASI than with SAQ format. A study using qualitative data found that the majority of respondents indicated that A-CASI elicited more honest responses than face-to-face interviews (Metzger et al., 2000). Early studies with T-CASI suggest that the prevalence of self-reported health behaviors derived from this mode may be comparable to A-CASI (Ellen et al., 2002).

Survey methods, which rely on retrospective self-reports, have certain limitations related to accurate measurement of adolescent health behaviors. The accuracy of self-reports may be compromised in part, because some health-related behaviors are difficult to recall. Asking adolescents to recall behaviors over longer versus shorter periods of time and asking them to recall the frequency of commonly occurring behaviors increases the inaccuracy of their reports. Questions about age of initiation of health risk behaviors (such as alcohol and tobacco use or sex) tend to elicit inaccurate responses, which is partly a function of forgetting over time (Brener, Billy, & Grady, 2003). With some behaviors, the accuracy of adolescents' self-reports may also be compromised by situational factors. Certain health-related behaviors are so sensitive that respondents may elect not to report them on a survey. In addition, adolescents may purposely underreport or overreport certain behaviors on surveys because they believe engaging in these behaviors is either socially undesirable or desirable (Brener, Billy, & Grady, 2003).

Diaries *Daily diaries* are an unobtrusive method for obtaining data on behaviors for which more distal recall may prove problematic. Specific behaviors or mood states that occur frequently may be difficult to recollect at a later date when numerous occasions of similar events have occurred in the interval between the event of interest and the assessment. It may also be challenging to remember specifics of an infrequent behavior if much time has elapsed since the behavior occurred. With interviews or surveys, cognitive errors such as forgetting, minimizing, exaggerating, or averaging behaviors introduce recall bias into reporting. These errors are reduced with daily diaries because no more than twenty-four hours will have passed since the most recent behavior event. Because the time interval between reports is short, daily diaries are better able to assess event-specific details than interviews or surveys, which require recall over longer time periods and collect aggregate information on behaviors (Fortenberry, Cecil, & Zimet, 1997).

Daily diaries have several other advantages. The format gives the impression of privacy and is therefore well suited for reporting on sensitive behaviors. Because diaries are completed in a respondent's natural environment, there may be fewer problems with reactivity bias than with data collected in research settings. Some adolescents prefer diaries to interviews or surveys (McLaws et al., 1990; Shrier, Shih, & Beardslee, 2005). Repeated assessments of behaviors through daily diary reports permit within-person analyses of associations with behaviors. For example, an eight-week daily diary study examining drinking and sexual intercourse among 112 youth found no within-person differences in the proportion of times condoms were used when drinking occurred before sex compared to when it did not (Morrison et al., 2003).

Despite these advantages, features of diaries can compromise data quality. As with other self-report methods, youth may exaggerate or minimize certain behaviors. Other shortcomings are specific to diaries. Keeping daily diaries requires effort and may involve recording sensitive information. As a result, diary study participants may self-select and not represent a population of interest. Further, respondents may fatigue from daily reporting, making inaccurate entries (Ramjee, Weber, & Morar, 1999). Respondents may habituate to completing the same daily form, reducing response accuracy. Some may alter behaviors as a result of diary self-monitoring. Despite the illusion of privacy, respondents may wish to conceal diaries from partners (Ramjee et al., 1999) or others due to confidentiality concerns. Behaviors may be reported with greater (Ramjee et al., 1999) or lesser (Coxon, 1999) frequency on diaries versus surveys.

Diaries may be kept with paper-and-pencil formats, scannable forms (Fortenberry et al., 2005), via telephone (Wiener et al., 2004; Bailey, Gao, & Clark, 2006), electronically (Shrier et al., 2005), or using video recordings (Rich & Patashnick, 2002). Electronic diaries minimize errors associated with incomplete reporting and data transfer. Although self-created video diaries can be costly and present analytic challenges (Rich & Patashnick, 2002), the resultant data are rich, detailed, and based in life context (Davies & Wilson, 2006; Holliday, 2004; Rich et al., 2000; Rich & Patashnick, 2002). A simple diary layout is preferred (Hays et al., 2001), but detailed formats (e.g., time-use diaries) are appropriate for certain research, such as studies on media use (Cummings & Vandewater, 2007; Rich et al., 2007) and other frequent daily activities. Diary completion, when reported, can be over 90 percent (Lex et al., 1989; Shrier et al., 2005; Wormald, 2003).

Momentary Sampling Methods In the 1970s, Csikszentmihalyi and colleagues (Csikszentmihalyi & Larson, 1984; Larson & Csikszentmihalyi, 1983) developed the *experience sampling method* (ESM) to gather psychological, behavioral, and social data on individuals' daily lives through momentary reports of experiences as they occur in the natural environment. One of the first applications of ESM was with the study of daily experiences of adolescents (Csikszentmihalyi & Larson, 1987; Csikszentmihalyi, Larson, & Prescott, 1977). Adolescents were given electronic pagers and pads of self-report forms and asked to respond to a signal emitted once every two hours over a one-week period. The detailed information that resulted provided eye-opening insights into adolescents' daily lives—who they were with, where they were, what they were doing and thinking—through sampling their waking moments. Since the original ESM studies, *momentary sampling* (MS) methods have evolved to use electronic devices for both signaling participants and collecting data. In addition, data may now be transferred electronically from the data collection device to a research database.

A variant of ESM, *ecological momentary assessment* (EMA), includes self-initiated reports of target behaviors to gather more detailed information on these behaviors than is assessed in random reports (Hufford et al., 2002; Shiffman, 2000). For example, an EMA study of thirty-seven heavy drinkers evaluated historical, treatment-related, and episode-specific mood correlates of excessive drinking in a drinking episode (Coxon, 1999). Positive mood before a drinking episode predicted excessive drinking, suggesting that drinking was used to maintain or enhance good mood (celebratory drinking). However, drinkers with positive mood after the episode were less likely to drink to excess, perhaps indicating that drinkers who feel good once they have started drinking do not continue to drink to experience positive mood. By acquiring both participant-level data (such as drinking history) and event-level data (such as mood before a drinking episode), MS methods permit examination of complex models of behavior.

Research has used MS methods to relate adolescents' moods to sensitive behaviors including sexual activity and substance use (Henker et al., 2002; Shrier et al., 2005; Shrier et al., 2007; Whalen et al., 2001; Whalen et al., 2002). One MS methods study found that over a day, positive affect was highest when adolescents were thinking about sex (Shrier et al., 2005). In another MS methods study, data from sixty-seven sexually active adolescents showed that a sexual intercourse event predicted improved affect (Shrier et al., 2007). These findings have important implications for safer sex interventions with adolescents, which typically target negative consequences of sexual behaviors and may not acknowledge potential affective benefits.

Unlike other self-report methods, MS data has minimal bias from recall, as the time period over which measures are assessed ranges from "that moment" to a few hours. Because links between event-level factors (such as affective states) and target behaviors are made analytically, errors related to an individual's cognitive processing are minimized. Random sampling of momentary states provides data that are more representative of daily experience than data collected by recall. Data are collected in vivo, enhancing ecological validity. Contextual factors such as location and companionship may be assessed and studied as predictors or modifiers of behavior. Studies have established the feasibility of using MS methods to assess a range of adolescent psychological states and health behaviors (Axelson, Bertocci, & Lewin, 2003; Henker et al., 2002; Rich et al., 2007; Shrier et al., 2005; Shrier et al., 2007; Whalen et al., 2001; Whalen et al., 2002).

Because links between event-level factors and target behaviors are made analytically, errors related to an individual's cognitive processing are minimized.

Despite clear advantages of MS methods, there are several notable disadvantages. Frequent data collection is burdensome to respondents and may adversely affect recruitment, retention, and adherence. The signal response rate varies greatly; adolescents participating in momentary sampling studies have responded to 52 to 90 percent of random signals (Larson & Lampman-Petraitis, 1989; Lex et al., 1989; Shrier et al., 2005; Shrier et al., 2007; Whalen et al., 2001; Whalen et al., 2002). Sample sizes tend to be small, limiting power to analyze individual-level factors. Ample resources are required to purchase and maintain electronic data collection devices. Because MS methods can be intrusive, the process of collecting data may influence the phenomena being measured (reactivity bias; Csikszentmihalyi & Larson, 1987; Hufford et al., 2002; Shrier et al., 2007). Finally, validity of MS data is often assumed based on in vivo collection, and reliability may be difficult to assess for highly changeable constructs such as affect. Therefore, formal psychometric testing of measures obtained via MS methods has not been developed.

Observation

Whereas self-report measures are the most common method of collecting data on adolescent health behaviors, observation is among the least used methods. While observations can provide extensive information that may be more accurate than self-report, they may be time-consuming, expensive, and inappropriate for certain behaviors such as drug use or sexual behavior. Researchers must establish procedures to assess reliability of each observation, increasing time and expense of data collection. Despite these drawbacks, researchers still use observational methods to collect interesting data, particularly in areas of health behavior where self-report is limited. Intervention studies focused on changing health behaviors often employ observations to assess fidelity to interventions (DiIorio, 2005).

The observation process is more rigorous than simply viewing an event. When properly performed, a systematic observation includes careful identification of the behaviors to be observed, definitions of behaviors to evaluate, including examples of what constitutes each behavior and what does not, development of an observation protocol, and training of observers to identify and classify behaviors of interest.

Various types of behaviors have been observed systematically, including conversations and interactions (Fredman, Chambless, & Steketee, 2004; Underwood, 2005), body movement and physical activity (Sirard & Pate, 2001), and facial expressions and responses. Observation can be used to document emotions such as aggression and empathy; quality and tone of verbal statements; and personal space between respondents. For the selected behavior, observers identify and code the presence or absence of the behavior, its frequency and/or its intensity.

Biological Methods

Biological measures include a variety of physical measures used to assess health behaviors and related outcomes and are often deemed the gold standard in validation studies of self-report measures because they are considered more objective and less susceptible to bias than other types of measures. For example, a teen may deny tobacco use on a survey, but a serum cotinine test may show evidence of recent use. Blood tests have been used to assess diabetes and other chronic disease management behaviors; blood, urine, and saliva biomarkers have been used to assess alcohol, tobacco, and other substance use; doubly labeled water techniques have been used to validate self-reports of food intake and physical activity; mechanical and electronic devices including accelerometers and heart rate monitors have been used to validate reports of physical activity; heart rate monitors and salivary cortisol levels have been used to assess adolescents' response to stress; biomarkers for pregnancy and sexually transmitted diseases including HIV have been used to corroborate self-reports of sexual behavior and contraceptive use. Reviews by Brener, Billy, and Grady (2003), Cone (1997), Kohl, Fulton, and Casperson (2000), and McPherson and colleagues (2000) provide detailed descriptions of strengths and limitations of using biomarkers to assess various adolescent health behaviors.

TABLE 23.1. **Common measurement approaches across domains of adolescent health behavior**

Domain of Adolescent Health Behavior	Self-Report Methods				Observation	Biological Methods
	Interview	Survey	Diary	Momentary Sampling		
Disease management behaviors	✓	✓	✓	✓	✓	✓
Contraceptive use	✓	✓	✓			✓
Depression, mood, affect	✓	✓	✓	✓	✓	✓
Dietary behaviors	✓	✓	✓			✓
Physical activity	✓	✓	✓		✓	✓
Sexual behaviors	✓	✓	✓	✓		✓
School involvement and performance	✓	✓	✓			
Substance use	✓	✓	✓	✓		✓
Violent and aggressive behaviors	✓	✓			✓	

As can be seen in the previous discussion, program evaluators and health behavior researchers have a variety of approaches at their disposal for measuring adolescent health behaviors; Table 23.1 shows which approaches are commonly used in measuring specific behaviors. Each approach has its strengths and weaknesses, and each must be evaluated individually to determine usefulness for a particular project with a specific group of adolescents. Because no perfect measure of behavior exists, optimal measurement may involve a combination of approaches to address the weaknesses of a single approach. For example, using a combination of self-report and accelerometry to measure physical activity allows an investigator to understand both specific types of activities performed and total energy expenditure. Self-report measures are the most efficient, feasible, and commonly used mode for collecting data about adolescents' health behaviors. Because of the importance of self-report measures, we will focus on them in the remaining sections of this chapter.

MEASUREMENT ERROR

No measure produces perfectly reliable or valid estimates of a behavior. The extent to which a measure deviates from perfect reliability and validity is known as *measurement error*. In this section, we describe two basic types of measurement error. We then discuss cognitive and situational factors that influence measurement of adolescent health behaviors.

Classification of Measurement Error

Measurement error can be thought of as random or systematic. *Random error* is due to chance factors that influence the measurement of behaviors or other attributes. Random error is unsystematic; it does not affect the behavior being measured in the same way each time a measurement is taken. Random error often decreases the reliability of a measure. *Systematic error* or bias is due to factors that systematically increase or decrease accurate measurement of behaviors or other attributes. Systematic error reduces the validity of measures. Random error does not influence the estimated mean value of a behavior within the group being measured, simply because the error is evenly distributed on both sides of the mean. Conversely, systematic error occurs only on one side of the mean, and thus it influences the mean in one direction—either upward or downward, depending on the nature of the bias.

The most serious type of systematic measurement error is differential error, which affects one or more groups of respondents but not others.

The most serious type of systematic measurement error is *differential error,* which affects one or more groups of respondents but not others. One or more groups may be more prone, or biased, to answer items in a certain way because of age, gender, education, or economic or cultural background. For example, a question on a standardized math test asking students to calculate costs of public transportation may favor youth who are familiar with metropolitan transit systems over those who live in rural areas. Bias in measuring health behaviors can lead to inaccurate prevalence estimates of those behaviors and misclassification of persons at risk, thereby hampering prevention efforts. Important intervention components may be overlooked or overemphasized in situations where systematic measurement error leads to biased estimates of relationships between variables (Catania et al., 1990). Thus, minimizing error related to the measurement of health behaviors is important to researchers, policy makers, program planners, and providers of adolescent health services.

Factors Influencing Measurement Error

The validity of adolescents' self-reported behaviors may be affected by cognitive factors and by factors related to the situation and setting in which measurement takes place.

Cognitive Factors The truthfulness and accuracy of self-reported health behaviors may be compromised because some aspects of behavior are relatively difficult to recall. Valid self-report of personal information and experiences requires that young people (1) understand the question to which they are responding, (2) retrieve the information from their autobiographical memory, (3) determine the accuracy of the information, and (4) develop a response (Jobe, 2000). The method of obtaining self-report data, the time period over which the information is being recalled, the behavior being assessed, and the type of information being solicited all influence the likelihood of error in the cognitive processes involved. Further, a respondent's emotional and physical state (such as fear of reprisal or pain) will influence each of the cognitive processes that lead to accurate responding.

Both written and spoken methods (such as A-CASI and interview) require comprehension of self-report questions; written methods require ability of respondents to read the words as well. Further, adolescents' varying ability to reason abstractly can affect comprehension of self-report questions. Reading questions aloud, either through A-CASI or standardized in-person approaches, can assist young people with limited reading abilities in comprehending questions (Overstreet et al., 1999). Being explicit, defining terms, and using straightforward, developmentally appropriate language also aid in comprehension. In general, use of adolescent idioms should be avoided.

The duration of time between acquisition of the information and its reporting affects respondents' ability to recall information; this time period may be days, weeks, months, or even years in interviews and written surveys, but is only twenty-four hours in a daily diary and can be immediate with momentary sampling techniques. For solitary, infrequent, severe, or salient experiences, such as first sexual intercourse, recall over a long period of time may be feasible, but accurate recall of recurring, relatively frequent, mild, or personally unimportant experiences, such as the specifics of drinking occasions over the past month, may be more difficult. In a national sample of high school seniors, Bachman and O'Malley (1981) found frequencies of self-reported past-month use of alcohol and other drugs were approximately three times greater than frequencies estimated from reports of past-year use. Adolescents also tend to be inconsistent and/or inaccurate in recalling health behaviors such as smoking patterns beyond a one-year period (Stanton et al., 1996), frequency of smoking on specific recent days (Means et al., 1992) "usual" intake of many types of foods (Brener et al., 2003), daily physical activity patterns for more than four days (Sallis, Buono, Roby et al., 1993), and frequency of vaginal intercourse over three- and six-month periods (Sieving et al., 2005). Conversely, adolescents are able to provide reliable estimates of interpersonal aggression over time periods ranging from the past month to the past twelve months (Hilton, Harris, & Rice, 1998). Even with salient information, asking adolescents to recall behavior over long periods of time may result in inaccurate information. For example, in a longitudinal study youths' estimates of lifetime suicidality underestimated its prevalence compared to estimates of suicidal thoughts or behaviors that were recalled every three years (Klimes-Dougan, 1998). The frequency of the behavior of interest must be considered in choosing the duration of the recall period. In a study assessing different durations of recall of adolescent sexual behaviors, behaviors that occurred less frequently were reported more consistently across recall periods than were more frequently occurring behaviors (McFarlane & St. Lawrence, 1999). The complexity of the behaviors being assessed may also influence adolescents' ability to recall them. For example, sexually active adolescents in monogamous relationships may give more reliable and accurate global estimates of condom use than adolescents who have multiple partners with condom use patterns that vary between partners. Finally, the circumstances in which the behavior occurred can influence the encoding of information about the experience and subsequent retrieval of that information. For example, the number and type of drinks an adolescent consumed may be difficult to recall the more intoxicated the respondent was at the time of drinking.

Information about specific occasions of recurrent behaviors may be difficult to retrieve individually; data are more likely to be blended, average, or otherwise presented in aggregate form. For example, adolescents may have difficulty recalling "usual" smoking patterns if they smoke infrequently or episodically (Brener et al., 2003). Adolescents may have difficulty recalling a specific physical activity over a year's time if they participate in that activity only seasonally (Rifas-Shiman et al., 2001). Retrieval cues, such as those used with timeline follow-back calendars (Weinhardt et al., 1998), may be useful in recalling distant or frequent events. However, without knowing details about the events specific to the respondent, the investigator can only provide general cues (such as reminding the respondent that he or she was on school vacation during the time period that an event of interest occurred).

Situational Factors Other threats to obtaining valid measures of health behaviors relate primarily to characteristics of the external environment. Young peoples' tendencies to distort self-disclosure in measurement situations may be influenced by two key variables: level of threat to self-esteem and level of emotional discomfort or distress posed by the questions (Catania, 1999). In turn, threat to self-esteem and emotional distress may be influenced by the interviewer, the respondent, the measurement instrument and related contextual factors. Interviewers may influence honest self-disclosure and accurate self-presentation in several key ways. Interviewers who exhibit comfort with interview topic(s) and term(s) and who convey nonjudgmental cues can enhance the likelihood of honest self-disclosure by respondents. Interviewers who know how to manage respondents' emotional reactions in ways that do not bias their answers can also enhance the likelihood of honest self-presentation. Interviewers' demographic characteristics are thought to be most relevant with research topics that have a large interpersonal component, such as sexuality. For example, Catania and colleagues (1996) found that same-gender interviewers significantly increased respondents' reports of some sexuality-related topics, including condom nonuse, sexual problems, and sexual violence.

Respondents exist in a broad social structure stratified by age, gender, class, race, and ethnicity; these factors may be important mediators of self-presentation bias. Gender is most likely to affect self-presentation of behaviors in which social norms and values differ for females and males. Similarly, ethnic and social class differences in self-presentation are most likely in situations where socially normative behaviors differ by race, ethnicity, and social class. In a national sample of sexually experienced youth, girls were less inconsistent than boys in reports of sexual behaviors; however, response inconsistencies did not differ between teens from different racial or ethnic groups (Upchurch et al., 2002). In this situation, respondent gender appeared to be more important than ethnicity in explaining self-presentation bias.

With regard to the interview itself, perceived lack of privacy, confidentiality, or anonymity can pose a substantial threat to honest self-disclosure. Adolescents' level of honesty in self-disclosure can be affected by interview mode, setting, and question content. In particular, behaviors that are illegal, stigmatized, or laden with moral implications may be underreported because of concerns about social desirability and fear of reprisal (Brener et al., 2003). Evidence suggests that self-presentation bias can be minimized using an interview mode that allows for more privacy than face-to-face interviewing typically permits, such as self-administered questionnaires and computer-assisted surveys. Mode effects have been found for adolescents' self-reported substance use, suicide and violence behaviors, weight control practices such as purging and binge eating, and sensitive sexual behaviors such as same-gender sex and anal intercourse (Catania et al., 1990; French et al., 1998; Klimes-Dougan, 1998; Turner et al., 1998).

Adolescents' level of honesty in self-disclosure can be affected by interview mode, setting, and question content.

The interview setting may also affect adolescents' perceptions of privacy and consequentially their level of honest self-disclosure. Research demonstrating higher prevalence of substance use, weapon carrying, and sexual risk behaviors in school-based surveys than in household-based surveys, with no differences in prevalence of physical activity between settings (Kann et al., 2002), suggests that privacy of the interview setting may be particularly important in assessing behaviors that are illegal or socially stigmatized. Although Santelli, Lindberg, Abma, McNeely, and Resnick (2000) found comparable trends over time for a range of sexual behaviors in four national surveys of youth, significant differences between surveys in prevalence estimates suggested important mode and setting effects.

Regardless of mode or setting, questions about sensitive, stigmatized, or illegal behaviors pose particular challenges to honest self-disclosure and accurate self-presentation. It is commonly assumed that more sensitive questions should be asked later in an interview, allowing respondents to gradually become desensitized to more intimate items. Instruments that provide explanations of terms and frame questions using nonjudgmental, supportive, and developmentally appropriate language may also help minimize self-disclosure bias (Catania, 1999; Romer et al., 1997; Sieving et al., 2005).

In summary, error is an inevitable and undesirable component of measurement. Error affects the reliability and validity of measures and, if severe, can lead to flawed interpretation of data. For example, errors in self-report can bias prevalence estimates of risky health behaviors and thus lead to misclassification of at-risk individuals, thereby hampering prevention efforts. Factors that create errors in measurement can be broadly thought of as those due to adolescents' cognitive processes and those due to the measurement situation and setting. Self-reports across domains of health behavior are affected to varying degrees by cognitive and situational factors.

SUMMARY

Health risk behaviors including substance use, violence involvement, unprotected sexual intercourse, physical inactivity, unhealthy eating, and school failure contribute to the leading causes of morbidity and mortality, as well as social problems among adolescents. Consequently, data are collected on these and other health behaviors of adolescents for many reasons. For example, policy makers and program planners use data on prevalence of these behaviors to monitor trends, set program goals, identify target populations, seek funding, and advocate for support. Researchers use data on health behaviors to examine associations between risk and protective factors, behaviors and health outcomes, build theories of behavior change, develop policies and programs designed to prevent risky behaviors, and evaluate these policies and programs. Thus, reliable and valid measurement of health behaviors is of real interest to program planners, policy makers, researchers, and adolescent health service providers.

A recent review of research on measurement of adolescent health risk behaviors by Brener and colleagues (2003) concludes that adolescents' self-reports related to various domains of health behaviors are affected by both cognitive and situational factors. However, these factors do not threaten the validity of self-reports within each behavior domain equally. Furthermore, domains of behavior differ in the extent to which they can be validated by biological measures. Researchers and program evaluators should familiarize themselves with particular threats to obtaining reliable and accurate measures of adolescent behaviors of particular interest and design measurement approaches that minimize these threats as much as possible.

Although measurement within some domains of adolescent health behavior as well as some modes of measurement are widely researched, relatively few studies have assessed the validity of other behavioral indicators and measurement modes. A recent review of self-report measures across domains of adolescent health risk behaviors highlighted a particular need for further research to validate self-report indicators of violence-related behaviors and suicidality (Brener et al., 2003). Further psychometric testing is needed to understand the reliability and validity of innovative measurement modes, including momentary sampling methods.

A final area for future measurement research is in refining behavioral indicators of positive development among young people. As noted in Chapters Four and Seven of this text, the field of adolescent health has a dual focus, considering both risk and protective factors that affect youth health outcomes. A growing body of research suggests that protective factors and prosocial behaviors may offset substantial risks and can enable young people to overcome stressful life circumstances (Klein et al., 2006). Considerable work remains in refining indicators of prosocial behaviors among young people (Moore & Lippman, 2005). The content and construct validity of multi-item measures of constructs such as civic engagement, prosocial school functioning, positive family functioning, and caring and empathy behaviors remains to be confirmed.

Bill O'Hare of the Annie E. Casey Foundation notes, "As a society, we measure what we value, and we value what we measure" (Forum for Youth Investment, 2004). In the realm of adolescent health behaviors, what we measure plays a central role in determining what and for whom we advocate, as well the effectiveness of our advocacy efforts. What we measure helps us understand important indicators and trends in adolescent health, as well as risk and protective factors for healthy and unhealthy behaviors and developmental trajectories. What we measure informs the development of programs and policies designed to promote adolescent health and well-being, as well as the evaluation of those programs and policies. Effective responses to fundamental threats to the health and well-being of young people require current, accurate, and inclusive assessment of their health and risk behaviors.

KEY TERMS

Audio computer-assisted
   self-interviewing (A-CASI)
Biological measures
Daily diaries
Differential error
Ecological momentary assessment
   (EMA)
Experience sampling method (ESM)
Interview
Measurement error
Measurement modes
Momentary sampling (MS) methods
Random error

Reliability
Self-administered paper-and-pencil
   questionnaires (SAQs)
Self-report methods
Self-report surveys
Semistructured interview
Structured interview
Systematic error
Telephone computer-assisted
   self-interviewing (T-CASI)
Unstructured interview
Validity

DISCUSSION QUESTIONS

1. *Reliability* and *validity* are two terms that often get confused. Briefly explain what each mean. Can a measure be reliable and not valid, or valid and not reliable?

2. Discuss the benefits and drawbacks in terms of privacy and cost when using the following self-report measurement methods: individual face-to-face interview, focus group, self-administered survey (paper and pencil), A-CASI, and daily diary.

3. Justify why a researcher would use momentary sampling methods over self-report methods as a means of data collection.

4. Why hasn't direct observation been used more often when collecting data on adolescent health behavior? When is it appropriate to use observation?

5. To ensure accurate measurement when collecting data, what measurement features should you incorporate in your study? Think about measurement mode, using dual modes, and ways to eliminate measurement error and bias.

REFERENCES

Axelson, D., Bertocci, M., Lewin, D., Trubnick, L., Birmaher, B., Williamson, D., Ryan, D., & Dahl, R. (2003). Measuring mood and complex behavior in natural environments: Use of ecological momentary assessment in pediatric affective disorders. *Journal of Child and Adolescent Psychopharmacology, 13*(3), 253–266.

Bachman J., & O'Malley, P. (1981). When four months equals a year: Inconsistencies in student reports of drug use. *Public Opinion Quarterly, 45,* 536–548.

Bailey, S., Gao, W., & Clark, D. (2006). Diary study of substance use and unsafe sex among adolescents with substance use disorders. *Journal of Adolescent Health, 38*(3), 297, e13–e20.

Bonat, S., Pathomvanich, A., Keil, M., Field, A., & Yanovski, J. (2002). Self-assessment of pubertal stage in overweight children. *Pediatrics, 110*(4), 743–747.

Brener, N., Billy, J., & Grady, W. (2003). Assessment of factors affecting the validity of self-reported health-risk behavior among adolescents: Evidence from the scientific literature. *Journal of Adolescent Health, 33*(6), 436–457.

Brener, N., McManus, T., Galuska, D., Lowry, R., & Wechsler H. (2003). Reliability and validity of self-reported height and weight among high school students. *Journal of Adolescent Health, 32*(4), 281–287.

Catania, J. (1999). A framework for conceptualizing reporting bias and its antecedents in interviews assessing human sexuality. *Journal of Sex Research, 36*(1), 25–38.

Catania, J., Binson, D., Canchola, J., Pollack, L., Hauck, W., & Coates, T. (1996). Effects of interviewer gender, interviewer choice, and item context on responses to questions concerning sexual behavior. *Public Opinion Quarterly, 60,* 345–375.

Catania, J., Chitwood, D., Gibson, D., & Coates, T. (1990). Methodologic problems in AIDS research: Influences on measurement error and participation bias in studies of sexual behavior. *Psychological Bulletin, 108*(3), 339–362.

Cone, E. (1997). New developments in biologic measures of drug use. In *The validity of self-reported drug use: Improving accuracy of survey estimates. NIDA Research Monograph Series, 167,* 108–129.

Coxon, A. (1999). Parallel accounts? Discrepancies between self-report (diary) and recall (questionnaire) measures of the same sexual behaviour. *AIDS Care, 11*(2), 221–234.

Csikszentmihalyi, M., & Larson, R. (1984). *Being adolescent: Conflict and growth in the teenage years.* New York: Basic Books.

Csikszentmihalyi, M., & Larson, R. (1987). Validity and reliability of the Experience-Sampling Method. *Journal of Nervous and Mental Disease, 175*(9), 526–536.

Csikszentmihalyi, M., Larson, R., & Prescott, S. (1977). The ecology of adolescent activity and experience. *Journal of Youth and Adolescence, 6,* 281–294.

Cummings, H., & Vandewater, E. (2007). Relation of adolescent video game play to time spent in other activities. *Archives of Pediatrics and Adolescent Medicine, 161*(7), 684–689.

Davies, J., & Wilson, A. (2006). "What's happening?" Examining the mental health needs of young people with learning disabilities. *Learning Disability Practice, 9*(5), 36–37.

Desmangles, J., Lappe, J., Lipaczewski, G., & Haynatzki, G. (2006). Accuracy of pubertal Tanner staging self-reporting. *Journal of Pediatric Endocrinology and Metabolism, 19*(3), 213–221.

DiIorio, C. (2005). *Measurement in health behavior: Methods for research and education.* San Francisco: Jossey-Bass.

Durant, L., & Carey, M. (2000). Self-administered questionnaires versus face-to-face interviews in assessing sexual behavior in young women. *Archives of Sexual Behavior, 29*(4), 309–322.

Ellen, J., Gurvey, J., Pasch, L., Tschann, J., Nanda, J., & Catania, J. (2002). A randomized comparison of A-CASI and phone interviews to assess STD/HIV-related risk behaviors in teens. *Journal of Adolescent Health, 31*(1), 26–30.

Fortenberry, J. D., Cecil, H., & Zimet, G. (1997). Concordance between self-report questionnaires and coital diaries for sexual behaviors of adolescent women with sexually transmitted infections. In J. Bancroft (Ed.), *Research sexual behavior: Methodological issues.* Bloomington: Indiana University Press.

Fortenberry, J. D., Temkit, M., Tu, W., Graham, C., Katz, B., & Orr, D. (2005). Daily mood, partner support, sexual interest, and sexual activity among adolescent women. *Health Psychology, 24*(3), 252–257.

Forum for Youth Investment. (2004). *What gets measured, gets done.* Retrieved September 17, 2005, from www .forumforyouthinvestment.org.

Fredman, S., Chambless, D., & Steketee, G. (2004). Development and validation of an observational coding system for emotional over involvement. *Journal of Family Psychology, 18*(2), 339–347.

French, S., Peterson, C., Story, M., Anderson, N., Mussell, M., & Mitchell, J. (1998). Agreement between survey and interview measures of weight control practices in adolescents. *International Journal of Eating Disorders, 23*(1), 45–56.

Goodman, E., Hinden, B., & Khandewal, S. (2000). Accuracy of teen and parental reports of obesity and body mass index. *Pediatrics, 106*(1 Pt 1), 52–58.

Gribble, J., Miller, H., Rogers, S., & Turner, C. (1999). Interview mode and measurement of sexual behaviors: Methodologic issues. *Journal of Sex Research, 36*(1), 16–24.

Hays, M., Irsula, B., McMullen, S., & Feldblum, P. (2001). A comparison of three daily coital diary designs and a phone-in regimen. *Contraception, 63*(3), 159–166.

Henker, B., Whalen, C., Jamner, L., & Delfino, R. (2002). Anxiety, affect, and activity in teenagers: Monitoring daily life with electronic diaries. *Journal of the American Academy of Child and Adolescent Psychiatry, 41,* 660–670.

Hick, K., & Katzman, D. (1999). Self-assessment of sexual maturation in adolescent females with anorexia nervosa. *Journal of Adolescent Health, 24*(3), 206–211.

Hilton, N., Harris, G., & Rice, M. (1998). On the validity of self-reported rates of interpersonal violence. *Journal of Interpersonal Violence, 13,* 58–72.

Holliday, R. (2004). Filming "The Closet": The role of video diaries in researching sexualities. *American Behavioral Scientist, 47*(12), 1597–1616.

Hufford, M., Shields, A., Shiffman, S., Paty, J., & Balabanis, M. (2002). Reactivity to ecological momentary assessment: An example using undergraduate problem drinkers. *Psychology of Addictive Behaviors, 16*(3), 205–211.

Jobe, J. (2000). Cognitive processes in self-report. In A. Stone, J. Turkkan, C. Bachrach, J. Jobe, H. Kurtzman, & V. Cain (Eds.), *The science of self-report: Implications for research and practice* (pp. 25–28). Mahwah, NJ: Erlbaum.

Kann, L., Brener, N., Warren, C., Collins, J., & Giovino, G. (2002). An assessment of the effect of data collection setting on the prevalence of health risk behaviors among adolescents. *Journal of Adolescent Health, 31*(4), 327–335.

Klein, J., Graff, C., Santelli, J., Hedberg, V., Allan, M., & Elster, A. (1999). Developing quality measures for adolescent care: validity of adolescents' self-reported receipt of preventive services. *Health Services Research, 34,* 391–404.

Klein, J., Sabaratnam, P., Auerbach, M., Smith, S., Kodjo, C., Lewis, K., Ryan, S., & Dandino, C. (2006). Development and factor structure of a brief instrument to assess the impact of community programs on positive youth development: The Rochester Evaluation of Asset Development for Youth tool. *Journal of Adolescent Health, 39*(2), 252–260.

Klimes-Dougan, B. (1998). Screening for suicidal ideation in children and adolescents: Methodological considerations. *Journal of Adolescence, 21*(4), 435–444.

Kohl, H., Fulton, J., & Caspersen, C. (2000). Assessment of physical activity by self-report: Status, limitations, and future directions. *Preventive Medicine, 31,* S54–S76.

Larson, R., & Csikszentmihalyi, M. (1983). The experience sampling method. In H. Reis (Ed.), *Naturalistic approaches to studying social interactions: Vol. 15.* San Francisco: Jossey-Bass.

Larson, R., & Lampman-Petraitis, C. (1989). Daily emotional states as reported by children and adolescents. *Child Development, 60*(5), 1250–1260.

Lee, K., Valeria, B., Kochman, C., & Lenders, C. (2006). Self-assessment of height, weight and sexual maturation: Validity in overweight children and adolescents. *Journal of Adolescent Health, 39*(3), 346–352.

Lex, B., Griffin, M., Mello, N., & Mendelson, J. (1989). Alcohol, marijuana, and mood states in young women. *International Journal of the Addictions, 24*(5), 405–424.

McFarlane, M., & St. Lawrence, J. S. (1999). Adolescents' recall of sexual behavior: Consistency of self-report and effect of variations in recall duration. *Journal of Adolescent Health, 25*(3), 199–206.

McLaws, M., Oldenburg, B., Ross, M., & Cooper, D. (1990). Sexual behaviour in AIDS-related research: Reliability and validity of recall and diary measures. *Journal of Sex Research, 27,* 265–281.

McPherson, S., Hoelscher, D., Alexander, M., Scanlon, K., & Serdula, M. (2000). Dietary assessment methods among school-aged children: Validity and reliability. *Preventive Medicine, 31,* S11–S33.

Means, B., Habina, K., Swan, G., & Jack, L. (1992). Cognitive research on response error in survey questions on smoking. *Vital and Health Statistics, 6*(5).

Metzger, D., Koblin, B., Turner, C., Navaline, H., Valenti, F., Holte, S., Gross, M., Sheon, A., Miller, H., Cooley, P., & Seage, G. (2000). Randomized controlled trial of audio computer-assisted self-interviewing: Utility and acceptability in longitudinal studies. HIVNET Vaccine Preparedness Study Protocol Team. *American Journal of Epidemiology, 152*(2), 99–106.

Moore, K., & Lippman, L. (2005). What do children need to flourish? Conceptualizing and measuring indicators of positive development. In *The Search Institute Series on Developmentally Attentive Community and Society: Vol. 3.* New York: Springer.

Morrison, D., Gillmore, M., Hoppe, M., Gaylord, J., Leigh, B., & Rainery, D. (2003). Adolescent drinking and sex: Findings from a daily diary study. *Perspectives on Sexual and Reproductive Health, 35*(4), 162–168.

Overstreet, S., Dempsey, M., Graham, D., & Moely, B. (1999). Availability of family support as a moderator of exposure to community violence. *Journal of Clinical Child Psychology, 28*(2), 151–159.

Ramjee, G., Weber, A., & Morar, N. (1999). Recording sexual behavior: comparison of recall questionnaires with a coital diary. *Sexually Transmitted Diseases, 26*(7), 374–380.

Rew, L., Horner, S., Riesch, L., & Cauvin, R. (2004). Computer-assisted survey interviewing of school-age children. *ANS: Advances in Nursing Science, 27*(2), 129–137.

Rich, M., Bickman, D., Koren, S., Aneja, P., de Moor, C., & Shrier, L. (2007). Measuring youth media exposure (MYME): A pilot study. *Journal of Adolescent Health, 40*(2, Suppl. 1), S5–S6.

Rich, M., Lamola, S., Amory, C., & Schneider, L. (2000). Asthma in life context: Video Intervention/Prevention Assessment (VIA). *Pediatrics, 105*(3 Pt. 1), 469–477.

Rich, M., & Patashnick, J. (2002). Narrative research with audiovisual data: Video Intervention/Prevention Assessment (VIA) and NVivo. *International Journal of Social Research Methodology: Theory and Practice, 5*(3), 245–261.

Rifas-Shiman, S., Gillman, M., Field, A., Frazier, A., Berkey, C., Tomeo, C., & Colditz, G. (2001). Comparing physical activity questionnaires for youth: seasonal vs. annual format. *American Journal of Preventive Medicine, 20*(4), 282–285.

Romer, D., Hornik, R., Stanton, B., Black, M., Xiannian, L., Ricardo, I., & Feigelman, S. (1997). "Talking" computers: A reliable and private method to conduct interviews on sensitive topics with children. *Journal of Sex Research, 34*(1), 3–9.

Sallis, J., Buono, M., Roby, J., Micale, F., & Nelson, J. (1993). Seven-day recall and other physical activity self-reports in children and adolescents. *Medicine and Science in Sports and Exercise, 25*(1), 99–108.

Santelli, J., Lindberg, L., Abma, J., McNeely, C., Resnick, M. (2000). Adolescent sexual behavior: Estimates and trends from four nationally representative surveys. *Family Planning Perspectives, 32*(4), 156–165, 194.

Schlossberger, N., Turner, R., & Irwin, C. (1992). Validity of self-report of pubertal maturation in early adolescents. *Journal of Adolescent Health, 13*(2), 109–113.

Shiffman, S. (2000). *Real-time self-report of momentary states in the natural environment: Computerized ecological momentary assessment.* Mahwah, NJ: Erlbaum.

Shrier, L., Shih, M., & Beardslee, W. (2005). Affect and sexual behavior in adolescents: A review of the literature and comparison of momentary sampling with diary and retrospective self-report methods of measurement. *Pediatrics, 115*(5), e573–e581.

Shrier, L., Shih, M., Hacker, L., & de Moor, C. (2007). A momentary sampling study of the affective experience following coital events in adolescents. *Journal of Adolescent Health, 40*(4), e351–e358.

Sieving, R., Hellerstedt, W., McNeely, C., Snyder, J., & Resnick, M. (2005). Reliability of self-reported contraceptive use and sexual behaviors among adolescent girls. *Journal of Sex Research, 42*(2), 159–166.

Sirard, J., & Pate, R. (2001). Physical activity assessment in children and adolescents. *Sports Medicine, 31*(6), 439–454.

Stanton, W., McClelland, M., Elwood, C., Ferry, D., & Silva, P. (1996). Prevalence, reliability and bias of adolescents' reports of smoking and quitting. *Addiction, 91*(11), 1705–1714.

Strauss, R. (1999). Self-reported weight status and dieting in a cross-sectional sample of young adolescents: National Health and Nutrition Examination Survey III. *Archives of Pediatrics and Adolescent Medicine, 153*(7), 741–747.

Supple, A., Aquilio, W., & Wright, D. (1999). Collecting sensitive self-report data with laptop computers: Impact on response tendencies of adolescents in a home interview. *Journal of Research on Adolescence, 9,* 467–488.

Turner, C., Ku, L., Rogers, S., Lindberg, L., Pleck, J., & Sonenstein, F. (1998). Adolescent sexual behavior, drug use, and violence: Increased reporting with computer survey technology. *Science, 280*(5365), 867–873.

Underwood, M. (2005). Observing anger and aggression among preadolescent girls and boys: Ethical dilemmas and practical solutions. *Ethics and Behavior, 15*(3), 235–245.

Upchurch, D., Lillard, L., Aneshensel, C., & Fang, L. (2002). Inconsistencies in reporting the occurrence and timing of first intercourse among adolescents. *Journal of Sex Research, 39*(3), 197–206.

Weinhardt, L., Carey, M., Maisto, S., Carey, K., Cohen, M., & Wickramasinghe, S. (1998). Reliability of the timeline follow-back sexual behavior interview. *Annals of Behavioral Medicine, 20*(1), 25–30.

Whalen, C., Jamner, L., Henker, B., & Delfino, R. (2001). Smoking and moods in adolescents with depressive and aggressive dispositions: Evidence from surveys and electronic diaries. *Health Psychology, 20*(2), 99–111.

Whalen, C., Jamner, L., Henker, B., Delfino, R., & Lozano, J. (2002). The ADHD spectrum and everyday life: Experience sampling of adolescent moods, activities, smoking, and drinking. *Child Development, 73*(1), 209–227.

Wiener, L., Riekert, K., Ryder, C., & Wood, L. (2004). Assessing medication adherence in adolescents with HIV when electronic monitoring is not feasible. *AIDS Patient Care and STDs, 18*(9), 527–538.

Wormald, H. (2003). Methodological issues in piloting a physical activity diary with young people. *Journal of Health Education, 62*(3), 220–233.

CHAPTER

24

BRIEF MOTIVATIONAL INTERVENTIONS FOR ADOLESCENT HEALTH PROMOTION IN CLINICAL SETTINGS

MARY ROJAS ▪ DEBRA BRAUN-COURVILLE ▪ ANNE NUCCI-SACK ▪ ANGELA DIAZ

LEARNING OBJECTIVES

After studying this chapter, you will be able to

- Understand that health promotion goes beyond presenting health education materials to assess readiness to change unhealthy behaviors.

- Differentiate between a brief intervention and motivational interview.

- Critique how brief interventions and motivational interviewing have used elements of behavioral change models.

- Assess the health promotion efficacy of brief interventions and motivational interviewing within the clinical setting.

"*Health promotion* is the process of enabling people to increase control over, and to improve, their health" (World Health Organization (WHO), 1986). Adolescence is a time filled with exploration and risk taking, with the potential for negative health consequences. During this stage, health behaviors are formed and often solidified, making the need for health promotion essential.

According to the 2006 National Health Interview Survey, more than 90 percent of adolescents aged twelve to seventeen report a usual place of health care, and more than 80 percent have seen a health care professional in the past year (Centers for Disease Control and Prevention, 2007). Data for older adolescents (aged eighteen to twenty-four years) is less promising, with 71 percent reporting a usual place of health care. Nevertheless, the health care visit is an ideal setting for health promotion because clinicians are well suited to educate patients about their health and guide them to healthy behaviors. The American Academy of Family Physicians (AAFP), American Academy of Pediatrics (AAP), American Medical Association (AMA), Maternal and Child Health Bureau, and the U.S. Preventive Services Task Force recommend adolescent clinical preventive services that include guidelines for health guidance, screening, physical assessment, tests, and immunizations. Perhaps the most significant contributions to risk assessment and health promotion of the adolescent patient in the primary care setting have been the development of the AMA's Guidelines for Adolescent Preventive Services (GAPS; Elster & Kuznets, 1994) and the Bright Futures Guidelines for Health Supervision (Hagan, Shaw, & Duncan, 2008). Both provide a comprehensive approach to risk assessment of the adolescent patient across the major biopsychosocial domains of risk. These tools provide clinicians with developmentally appropriate questions and recommendations for education and guidance, depending on the response of the adolescent. Parental assessments and anticipatory guidance are also built into the formats. Both guidelines are structured, designed for maximum efficiency, easy to implement, inexpensive, and can uncover areas of risky behaviors that would otherwise have gone unnoticed in the traditional biomedical model primary care visit. The GAPS and Bright Futures guidelines were developed by expert panel consensus. They standardize risk assessment of the adolescent patient and provide best-practice models for guidance and risk reduction in the primary care settings.

The medical visit offers several effective biomedical interventions to prevent or treat the outcomes of risky behaviors. Immunizations—particularly against human papillomavirus (HPV), hepatitis A, and hepatitis B—coupled with a comprehensive sex education program, screening and treatment, and guidance on sexual decision-making skills can reduce sexually transmitted infections (STIs). Early detection and treatment of chlamydia and gonorrhea infections has the potential to prevent adverse consequences such as pelvic inflammatory disease and infertility (Scholes et al., 1996). The CDC clinical guidelines recommend cervical swab testing for chlamydia every six months in all sexually active females less than twenty-six years (Centers for Disease Control and Prevention, 2006). The guidelines also suggest serologic testing for syphilis in high-risk populations and annual HIV testing in all sexually active adolescents. The American College of Obstetricians and Gynecology, in conjunction with the American Cancer Society, promote routine cervical cancer screening with annual Pap and HPV testing in women beginning at the age of twenty-one, or three years after sexual debut.

Primary care clinicians provide medication supplemented with education to help patients manage chronic diseases such as asthma, hypertension, and elevated cholesterol. They encourage patients to avoid cigarette smoking, eat a healthy diet, and engage in regular physical activity. They teach patients to recognize asthma symptoms and intervene early, which can help prevent exacerbations. And where necessary, primary care clinicians can step up disease management and treatment by referring adolescents for heightened subspecialty services.

The medical visit presents a natural setting for health promotion. It is focused on health issues, tailored to the patient's needs, and delivered by a highly knowledgeable expert. However, the actualization of health promotion in a primary care setting is complex. Issues of time restraints, limited resources, provider self-efficacy, cultural expectations, and lack of an evidence base have restricted the possibilities that primary care visits can offer.

As experts on health, clinicians caring for teenagers have the unique opportunity to engage adolescents in screening, anticipatory guidance, reducing risky behaviors, and promoting health lifestyles. Discussing health behaviors with adolescents in a private, confidential setting offers the potential for individualized attention, confidential disease screening, health education, counseling, and intervention. Providing adolescents with health education is a critical element to preventive health maintenance. Clinicians who feel uncomfortable providing health guidance due to lack of time, experience, or both may choose to promote healthy behaviors through pamphlets or displaying a video. However, health education alone, particularly without engagement and practical skills application, is limited. Presenting information without considering an adolescent's reasons for engaging in health risk behaviors and willingness to change those behaviors may also significantly limit its acceptance. Understanding why an adolescent engages in behaviors despite knowing its negative consequences may provide a clinician with more targeted methods to assess risk and promote healthy behaviors.

Bandura theorized that human psychosocial functioning could be altered fundamentally by empowering people with the coping competencies needed to gain mastery over their problems (Bandura, 1977). In *social cognitive theory,* human behavior is approached as a continuous reciprocal interaction among cognitive, behavioral, and environmental determinants (Baranowski, Perry, & Parcel, 1997). The *transtheoretical model of change* promoted by Prochaska and DiClemente attempts to explain and predict an individual's future success or failure in implementing and effecting a behavior change (DiClemente & Prochaska, 1982; Prochaska, 1979; Prochaska & DiClemente, 1982). They describe the stages of change as precontemplation, contemplation, action, maintenance, and relapse. Their model, developed as a consequence of studying smoking behaviors, recognizes that change unfolds over months and

Health education alone, particularly without engagement and practical skills application, is limited.

even years. Each change corresponds to an individual's readiness to change, which will vary over time. By matching an intervention to the appropriate stage (or readiness), program designers and clinicians can help improve the individual chances of success. Success is defined not just by altering the behavior, but also by any movement toward change, such as a shift from one stage of readiness to a more advanced stage. The stages of change model emphasizes maintaining change and understands that relapses are common and part of the process.

Behavioral change models provide an invaluable framework for understanding why adolescents engage in certain behaviors. However, implementation of these models into clinical settings is a formidable challenge. Two complementary techniques that integrate elements of behavioral change models and show promise for clinic-based health promotion are brief interventions and motivational interviewing. Many studies have examined the efficacy of brief interventions and motivational interviewing for changing negative health behaviors. However, most research has centered on adults, with only a few studies focusing on adolescents. For the purposes of this chapter, we have included those brief intervention and motivational interviewing studies that focus on adolescents in a clinic setting.

BRIEF INTERVENTION

Brief interventions are counseling strategies that primary care physicians can deliver during routine office visits to help patients change health risk behaviors and increase compliance with therapy. They are generally delivered over three to four visits and can last from five to fifteen minutes. The number of visits required to ensure treatment success can vary, but studies suggest that three to four visits or a combination of clinic visits with follow-up telephone counseling can increase the effectiveness of the brief intervention (Anderson & Scott, 1992; Fleming, Barry, Manwell, Johnson, & London, 1997; Kristenson, Ohlin, Hulten-Nosslin, Treli, & Hood, 1983; Wallace, Cutler, & Haines, 1988).

Brief interventions have been demonstrated to be effective in reducing unhealthy behaviors in adult populations in smoking cessation and reduction of alcohol consumption (Fleming, Barry, Manwell, Johnson, & London, 1997; Ockene et al., 1991; Soderstrom et al., 2007). Often the goals of these brief interventions are to reduce or minimize risky behaviors, but not necessarily completely resolve or abstain from them. This technique is used with adolescents often in the form of education, anticipatory guidance, and in some circumstances as pregnancy options counseling. However, its effectiveness on reducing risky behaviors has not been adequately examined.

Motivational Interviewing

Often paired with brief interventions is *motivational interviewing,* a client-centered, directive method for enhancing intrinsic motivation to change by exploring and resolving ambivalence.

Broadly based on Carl Rogers' client-centered therapy, motivational interviewing uses active cognitive and behavioral strategies targeted to the client's readiness to change (Miller & Rollnick, 2002; Rollnick, Miller, & Butler, 2007). It allows the client to build his or her own motivation and resolve toward changing a negative behavior. The four basic principles for motivational interviewing are expressing empathy, developing discrepancy, rolling with resistance, and supporting self-efficacy (Miller & Rollnick, 2002; Rollnick, Miller, & Butler, 2007). Motivational interviewing assumes that behavior change is affected more by motivation than information. The core interviewing skills are asking, informing, and listening (Rollnick et al., 2005). Because motivational interviewing attempts to increase patient awareness, it can be very effective at promoting healthy behaviors, changing unhealthy behaviors, and sustaining desirable behaviors. This may be especially true if the motivational interviewing is provided in combination with expert clinical advice (as in brief interventions).

The four basic principles for motivational interviewing are expressing empathy, developing discrepancy, rolling with resistance, and supporting self-efficacy.

Efficacy

In our search for evidence-based health promotion in clinical settings, we found several randomized controlled studies of brief interventions (BI) and motivational interviewing (MI). Most studies compared the efficacy of BI or MI against another intervention. However, the literature provides limited evidence of effectiveness for either approach. How well do BI and MI perform in real-world primary care settings? How much of a clinical impact do they have? The answers are not yet clear. Despite these shortcomings, the available data provide compelling evidence and reasons to suggest that they may be beneficial for health promotion in clinical settings.

Few comparative studies of BI and MI in primary care settings have examined their impact on key adolescent health problem areas: risky or problem behaviors, tobacco use, alcohol use, pregnancy and sexually transmitted infections, obesity, sun protection, and interpersonal violence (Borowsky, Mozayeny, Stuenkel, & Ireland, 2004; Hollis et al., 2005; Jemmott, Jemmott, Braverman, & Fong, 2005; Kamb et al., 1998; McCallum et al., 2007; McCambridge & Strang, 2004; Norman et al., 2007; Patten et al., 2006; Petersen, Albright, Garrett, & Curtis, 2007; Schwartz et al., 2007; Shrier, Ancheta, Goodman, Chiou, Lyden, & Emans, 2001; Walker et al., 2002). See Table 24.1. We were unable to identify randomized studies in a clinic setting related to substance use. There were also no clinical trials for adolescent obesity in the primary care clinical setting. As an alternative, we have included relevant studies in other pediatric populations or in the school setting. We report on twelve studies that evaluated the efficacy of BI or MI with adolescents or children. Study sample sizes ranged from 91 to 4,328 adolescents, with postintervention follow-up periods that ranged from three months (3) to six months (1), nine months (2), twelve months (6), or twenty-four months (1). All used some face-to-face intervention delivery administered by a practice nurse (1), clinician (6), or health educator, counselor, or study counselor (7). Three studies used computerized intervention delivery methods, and two included videotapes.

TABLE 24.1. Efficacy of face-to-face and computer-administered brief interventions in a clinic setting

Study	Population	Problem Area and Outcome	Intervention	Comparison Group	Results
Walker, Townsend, Oakley, Donovan, Smith, Hurst, Bell, & Marshall (2002)	970 teenagers ages 14–15 from eight general practices in Hertfordshire, UK	Risky behaviors: Health-related behaviors (diet, exercise, smoking, and drinking) and stages of change	RCT: twenty-minute consultation provided by a practice nurse reviewing general health-related behaviors, then focusing on a single area of risk as chosen by the adolescent	Usual care	Intervention group showed a greater change in health risk behaviors at three-month follow-up, though not statistically different. Positive momentum along the stages of change continuum for diet, exercise, and the combined health behavior measures. No twelve-month differences existed; however, at twelve months more of the intervention group knew where to go for confidential advice and family planning services.
Hollis, Polen, Hitlock, Lichtenstein, Mullooly, Velicer, & Redding (2005)	2,526 adolescents ages 14–17 being seen for routine care in seven large pediatric and family care practices (HMOs)	Tobacco use: abstinence and cessation and stages of change	RCT: individually tailored on the basis of smoking status and stage of change. Included a thirty-second clinician advice message, a ten-minute interaction with a computer program, a five-minute motivational interview, and up to two ten-minute telephone or in-person booster sessions.	Five-minute motivational intervention to promote increased consumption of fruits and vegetables	Abstinence rates after two years were significantly higher for the intervention arm relative to the control group, in the combined sample of baseline smokers and nonsmokers. Treatment effects were particularly strong among baseline self-described smokers, but were not significant for baseline nonsmokers or for those who had "experimented" in the past month at baseline.
Patten, Croghan, Meis, Decker, Pingree, Colligan, Dornelas, Offord, Boberg, Baumberger, Hurt, & Gustafson (2006)	139 adolescent smokers ages 11–18	Tobacco use: smoking abstinence rates	RCT: clinic-based, brief office intervention (BOI) consisting of four individual counseling sessions provided by a research counselor	Stomp Out Smokes (SOS), an Internet-based intervention. Adolescents in SOS had access to the SOS site for twenty-four weeks.	The thirty-day, twenty-four-week, and thirty-six-week smoking abstinence rates were greater for BOI than SOS; however, effects were not statistically different from one another. Among participants who continued to smoke, SOS was associated with a significantly greater reduction in average number of days smoked than BOI.

Study	Sample	Outcome measure	Intervention	Comparison	Results
McCambridge and Strang (2004)[a]	200 adolescents ages 16–20 years currently using drugs, recruited through school peers trained for the project	Drug use: self-reported use and perceptions of alcohol, tobacco, and illicit drugs and related risk and harm	CR: a single session of a sixty-minute MI (discussing alcohol, tobacco, and illicit drug use) delivered by one of the investigators. Initial discussion focused on the range of drugs used, which was then directed to particular areas of risk, problems, and concerns	Education as usual, which involved inquiry about sources of drug information and advice given	Statistically significant reduction in cigarette, alcohol, and drug use found at three-month follow-up among those in the intervention group compared to controls. Moderation of drug use among ongoing users was more pronounced and beneficial, as opposed to actual cessation.
Petersen, Albright, Garrett, & Curtis (2007)	764 women ages 16–44 at risk for unintended pregnancies attending one of three primary care facilities (41% between the ages of 16 and 25)	Pregnancy and STI: contraceptive use, consistency of use in the last thirty days, and intended use in next thirty days	RCT: Women's Reproductive Assessment Program (WRAP): pregnancy and STI prevention counseling delivered by experienced health educators associated with and trained for this study, provided through motivational interviewing at enrollment and two months later in a booster session	Brief general counseling with a health educator at enrollment (smoking, diet, and exercise) that excluded pregnancy and STI prevention	Significant increases in reported contraceptive use at two months, but no differences from intervention and control at eight or twelve months.
Shrier, Ancheta, Goodman, Chiou, Lyden, & Emans (2001)	123 adolescent females treated for cervicitis at an adolescent clinic or admitted to the hospital for pelvic inflammatory disease (all less than 24 years old; median age 17.2 years)	STI: condom use and recurrent STI	RCT: Safe sex education: seventeen-minute videotape adapted from *Time Out: The Truth About AIDS, HIV, and You*, where entertainers and sports figures discuss condoms. In addition, participants received one individualized intervention session delivered by a health educator. Opportunist intervention was implemented at the time of the STI treatment.	Safe sex education: standard education was provided at the discretion of clinician and included a discussion of STI transmission and the importance of consistent condom use. Participants were offered free condoms.	Compared with control participants, intervention participants tended to use condoms more with a nonmain partner at one month. At six months, fewer intervention participants than controls had sex with a nonmain sexual partner in the previous six months. At twelve months, intervention participants were less likely to have a current main partner (implying abstinence) and had a lower rate of recurrent STIs than controls, but these differences were not significant.

(Continued)

TABLE 24.1. (*Continued*)

Study	Population	Problem Area and Outcome	Intervention	Comparison Group	Results
Jemmott, Jemmott, Braverman, & Fong (2005)	682 sexually experienced African American and Latino girls, ages 12–19, recruited from an inner city adolescent medicine clinic	STI and HIV: unprotected sexual activity, STIs, and number of partners	RCT: Skills-based HIV/STI interventions, condom demonstrations with practicums, and negotiation strategies based on cognitive-behavioral theories. Interventions were delivered by African American adult facilitators. All three types of interventions included 250 minutes of group discussion, videotapes, games, and experiential exercises implemented in a single session with two to ten participants. The skills-based intervention addressed beliefs relevant to HIV/STI risk reduction, illustrated correct condom use, and depicted condom-use negotiation. Participants were allowed to practice the skills covered.	*Control 1:* Information-based intervention: discussions about risk reduction, HIV transmission, sexual responsibility, and importance of using condoms. Also included video demonstrations of correct condom use and negotiation of use. However, they were *not given the opportunity to practice skills.* *Control 2:* General health promotion: beliefs and skills relevant to other health behaviors (food selection, physical activity, breast self-examination, cigarette smoking, and alcohol use).	Efficacy analysis revealed differences twelve months postintervention: Skills-based participants reported less unprotected sex and fewer sexual partners, compared to information control (Control 1) or health promotion (Control 2). Skills-based participants were less likely to test positive for an STI compared to the health promotion control (Control 2). No differences were found at three- or six-month follow-up.

| Kamb, Fishbein, Douglas, Rhodes, Rogers, Bolan, Zenilman, Hoxworth, Malotte, Latesta, Kent, Lentz, Graziano, Byers, & Peterman (1998) | 4,328 HIV-negative men and women age 14 and older who came to one of five public inner city STI clinics | STI and HIV: condom use and STI incidence | RCT: all interventions encouraged consistent condom use for vaginal and anal sex with all partners; however, interventions were individualized to risk level and delivered by counselors.

Arm 1: enhanced counseling (four sessions)—based on reasoned action and social-cognitive theory. It sought to change self-efficacy, attitude, and perceived norms underlying condom use.

Arm 2: brief counseling (two sessions)—modeled after CDC's recommended HIV counseling. | Arm 3: didactic messages (two sessions)—brief messages about STI prevention, but did not engage the participant in interactive counseling.

Arm 4: didactic messages (two sessions)—same as Arm 3, except participants were not explicitly asked to return for follow-up visits. (Arms 1 through 3 included two-, six-, nine-, and twelve-month follow-up visits.) | At three and six months, condom use was higher in both the enhanced counseling and the brief counseling, compared to the didactic message arms. Across the five sites, new STIs were lower in the counseling arms than in the didactic arms. |

(Continued)

TABLE 24.1. *(Continued)*

Study	Population	Problem Area and Outcome	Intervention	Comparison Group	Results
Borowsky, Mozayeny, Stuenkel, & Ireland (2004)	224 children ages 7–15 who presented at eight pediatric practices and scored positive on a screen for violent or destructive behavior	Violent behavior	RCT: the intervention focused on two strategies to reduce violence involvement among youth: (1) identify, prevent, and treat mental health problems through psychosocial screening and appropriate referral and follow-up; and (2) promote healthy child-parent relationships through positive parenting. Clinicians saw the screening test results during the visit. The positive parenting intervention included one parent-educator contact via phone and a series of fifteen- to thirty-minute weekly telephone sessions. Parents also received two videotapes and a manual for the parenting course.	Clinicians did not see the screening test results.	Compared with control at nine months, children in the intervention group exhibited decreases in aggressive behavior, delinquent behavior, and attention problems. Children in the intervention group had lower rates of parent-reported bullying, physical fighting, and fight-related injuries requiring medical care and of child-reported victimization by bullying.

| McCallum et al. (2007) | 2,112 children ages 5–9 recruited in Australia; 160 were age- and weight-eligible (overweight or mildly obese) and randomized to the intervention or control groups | Obesity: BMI *Parent-reported:* child nutrition, physical activity, and health status *Child-reported:* health status, body satisfaction and appearance, self-worth | RCT: Live, Eat, and Play (LEAP) trial—four standard general practitioner (GP) consultations over twelve weeks, targeting change in nutrition, physical activity and sedentary behavior, supported by purpose-designed family materials. This was a family-based intervention. GPs were trained in three evening group sessions to provide didactic and reflective teaching regarding childhood obesity. The core component was a brief, solution-focused approach. The intervention focused on behavioral change, rather than weight change. | Control families were notified of their status; however, their status was not identified to the GP so they did not receive consultations. | *BMI:* at nine and twelve months, there were no statistical differences. *Nutrition scores:* intervention group had significantly better scores at nine and twelve months. *Physical activity:* no statistical difference at either follow-up. *Parent- and child-reported health status:* no difference. *Self-worth:* no difference. |

(Continued)

TABLE 24.1. (Continued)

Study	Population	Problem Area and Outcome	Intervention	Comparison Group	Results
Schwartz, Hamre, Dietz, Wasserman, Slora, Myers, Sullivan, Rockett, Thoma, Dumitru, & Resnicow (2007)	91 children ages 3–7 with BMIs between 85th and 95th percentile seen at a pediatric practice for a well-child care visit.	Obesity: BMI Behavioral patterns: consumption of sweetened drinks, snacks, and desserts; dining out; servings of fruits and vegetables; TV viewing	NRCT: pediatrician and registered dietitians provided motivational interviewing. Minimal intervention group received one MI session from the doctor for ten to fifteen minutes. Intensive intervention group received two MI sessions, each from the pediatrician (ten to fifteen minutes) and the dietitian (forty-five to fifty minutes). Pediatricians and dieticians in the intervention groups completed a two-day MI training session.	Standard care: pediatricians in this arm received instructions in the protocol, including BMI measurement technique, through a telephone conference.	*BMI* At six months there was no statistically significant decrease in BMI. 94% (15) of the parents reported that the intervention helped them think about changing their family's eating habits. *Behavioral outcomes* The minimal intervention group showed significant reductions in consumption of snacks and desserts (from baseline) compared to the control group. Dining out was reduced in the intervention group compared to the other two groups. No differences in consumption of sweetened drinks, fruits and vegetables intake, or TV viewing.

| Norman, Adams, Calfas, Covin, Sallis, Rossi, Redding, Cella, & Patrick (2007) | 819 adolescents ages 11–15 | Sun protection: self-reported composite measure of sun protection behavior | RCT: Sun Smart: at the study onset and the twelve-month follow-up, the adolescents engaged in an office-based expert system assessment of sun protection behaviors, followed by brief stage-based counseling from the primary care provider. Participants also received up to six system-generated personalized feedback reports, a brief printed manual, sunscreen samples, and periodic mailed tip sheets over a two-year period. Participants randomized to the comparison condition received a physical activity and nutrition intervention. | Greater adoption of sun protection behaviors over time was found in the intervention group compared with the control group. The intervention effect corresponded to between-group differences at twenty-four months in avoiding the sun and limiting exposure during midday hours and using sunscreen with a sun protection factor of at least 15. At twenty-four months, significantly more adolescents in the intervention group moved positively along the stages of change continuum to the action or maintenance stage of sun protective behaviors. |

Note: RCT = randomized controlled trial; NRCT = nonrandomized controlled trial; CR = cluster randomized; BI = brief intervention; MI = motivational interviewing.
[a]This study was done in a school setting, not a clinical setting, but it was included because of its relevance to RCT interventions in changing substance abuse behavior with adolescents.

Results of the comparative efficacy were mixed. Overall, findings leaned toward positive changes in the outcome in the short term, but were not sustained in the long term. Five studies found no statistically significant differences between the intervention group and the comparison group at the longest follow-up period (usually twelve months). Five studies found statistically significant effects in favor of the study intervention. Two found some differences in favor of some of the outcome measures. We caution the reader to resist drawing conclusions about the absence of statistically significant differences between the intervention and the control intervention. Failure to find a statistical difference is not necessarily indicative of lack of clinical effect. Some of these studies had small sample sizes at follow-up, not allowing for adequate statistical power to detect differences. Additionally, comparison groups were not the absence of intervention in most cases, but another intervention. Therefore, "no differences" does not mean that the techniques do not work, just that they are equally effective (or not effective) compared to the control intervention.

To demonstrate the potential beneficial effect of MI and BI for obesity-related outcomes, we included two randomized controlled studies targeting obesity-related outcomes in the pediatric population (McCallum et al., 2007; Schwartz et al., 2007). Although they failed to demonstrate sustained BMI reductions, there were positive changes in nutritional outcomes. The interventions targeted primarily parents, not children. Interventions with adolescents should be targeted to the adolescent at minimum and preferably to the whole family. Obesity is a multidimensional health problem involving a complex configuration of behaviors and people. Aside from the reduction in body size or weight, there are other outcomes that should be monitored. Environmental factors (eating habits, nutritional habits, food accessibility and costs, and exercise or activity), psychosocial factors (self-confidence, self-worth, and self-esteem), and biological factors (genetic and hormonal) may directly or indirectly play a role in weight reduction. Brief interventions and motivational interviewing should address all these factors, as well as take into account the amount of control an adolescent has over his or her time and diet.

Clearly, more research into the efficacy and effectiveness of motivational interviewing and brief interventions as a health promotion tool in a primary care setting is needed. Still, the current research provides several interesting learning points, as follows.

1. Providing adolescents with the opportunity to discuss general health risk behaviors with a health professional in a confidential setting may improve their ability to access needed health services in the future and ensure individual health promotion (Walker et al., 2002).

2. Individually tailored brief physician messages can substantially improve adolescent negative health behaviors such as smoking (Hollis et al., 2005) and drug use (McCambridge & Strang, 2004).

3. Motivational interviewing techniques need not be applied to multiple sessions. A single session can have a profound impact on reducing adolescent substance use (McCambridge & Strang, 2004).

4. Understanding why an adolescent participates in certain behaviors, and changing health attitudes and self-efficacy associated with those behaviors can also improve the health status of adolescents (Kamb et al., 1998). Risky sexual behaviors such as incorrect condom usage (Shrier et al., 2001) and inconsistent contraceptive use can also be improved with the use of short, personalized counseling sessions.

5. Skills training is a critical component of sexual health promotion, in addition to behavioral counseling and motivational interventions. Early and middle adolescents are concrete thinkers and need practical skills application of health information to solidify their education (Jemmott et al., 2005).

6. Health promotion messages given in a primary care setting do not necessarily need to be delivered by a physician, especially since a wide variety of health professionals participate in the care of adolescents. A session with a practice nurse can move patients forward in the stages of change continuum related to health risk behaviors (Walker et al., 2002). Health educators and counselors can also help reduce adolescent risk behaviors (Jemmott et al., 2005; Kamb et al., 1998; Petersen et al., 2007).

7. Brief physician counseling interventions can also be paired with other techniques and modalities, such as the Internet and computer models (Hollis et al., 2005; Norman et al., 2007; Patten et al., 2006). Even though some results of Internet-based smoking cessation programs (Patten et al., 2006) did not provide statistically significant results as compared to brief office interventions, the universal acceptance and availability of the Internet as a method of health education and promotion may appeal to certain audiences where face-to-face interventions do not work. Future research efforts may thus find the Internet to be a highly feasible and acceptable avenue of health promotion.

Health promotion messages given in a primary care setting do not necessarily need to be delivered by a physician.

SUMMARY

Brief interventions and motivational interviewing are techniques that lend themselves well to the adolescent clinic visit. The data suggest that BI and MI can be valuable tools in a clinician's arsenal to help adolescents change negative health behaviors and promote healthy behaviors. More research is needed on the efficacy of these techniques for other health topics such as drug use, pregnancy and STI prevention, diet, and exercise. We also need to evaluate and research the effectiveness of these techniques in a real-world clinic setting, and how to translate findings into clinically meaningful outcomes. Instead of limiting results and conclusions to statistically significant differences between intervention and control groups, it may be more advantageous to discuss degrees of risk reduction—was alcohol consumption reduced from four drinks a week to one? Was "rare" use of condoms changed to "sometimes" or "often" during sexual intercourse? Translation of scientific findings may increase their integration into adolescent health promotion and health behavioral change in the clinical care setting.

KEY TERMS

Brief interventions (BI)
Health promotion
Motivational interviewing (MI)

Social cognitive theory
Transtheoretical model of change

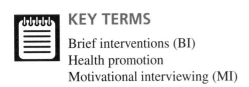

DISCUSSION QUESTIONS

1. If you were an adolescent health clinician and had to employ either the BI or MI health promotion technique to help change risk behavior, which would you choose? Why?

2. Are certain adolescent health risk behaviors (drug use, early sexual initiation, aggressive behavior, and overeating) better suited for BI as opposed to MI, or vice versa? Does it make a difference which health promotion technique is used to address a particular risk behavior?

3. Are BI and MI feasible health promotion techniques in today's society? Think about your last visit to the doctor, the time you spent with your provider, and your level of comfort. What are the pros and cons when utilizing these techniques with adolescents?

REFERENCES

Anderson, P., & Scott, E. (1992). The effect of general practitioners' advice to heavy drinking men. *British Journal of Addiction, 87,* 891–900.

Bandura, A. (1977). Self-efficacy: Toward a unifying theory of behavioral change. *Psychological Review, 84,* 191–215.

Baranowski, T., Perry, C., & Parcel, G. (1997). *How individuals, environments, and health behavior interact: Social cognitive theory.* San Francisco: Jossey-Bass.

Borowsky, I. W., Mozayeny, S., Stuenkel, K., & Ireland, M. (2004). Effects of a primary care-based intervention on violent behavior and injury in children. *Pediatrics, 114*(4), e392–399.

Centers for Disease Control and Prevention. (2006). Sexually transmitted diseases treatment guidelines, 2006. *Morbidity and Mortality Weekly Reports, 55*(RR-11).

Centers for Disease Control and Prevention. (2007). Early release of selected estimates based on data from the 2006 National Health Interview Survey. Retrieved from www.cdc.gov/nchs/data/nhis/earlyrelease/200706_02.pdf

DiClemente, C. C., & Prochaska, J. O. (1982). Self-change and therapy change of smoking behavior: A comparison of processes of change in cessation and maintenance. *Addictive Behaviors 7,* 133–142.

Elster, A. B., & Kuznets, N. (Eds.). (1994). *AMA Guidelines for Adolescent Preventative Services (GAPS): Recommendations and rationale.* Baltimore, MD: Williams and Wilkins.

Fleming, M., Barry, K. L., Manwell, L. B., Johnson, K., & London, R. (1997). Brief physician advice for problem alcohol drinkers: A randomized control trial in community-based primary care practices. *Journal of the American Medical Association, 277,* 1039–1045.

Hagan, J. F., Jr., Shaw, J. S., & Duncan, P. (Eds.). (2008). *Bright Futures: Guidelines for health supervision of infants, children and adolescents* (3rd ed.). Elk Grove Village, IL: American Academy of Pediatrics.

Hollis, J. F., Polen, M. R., Hitlock, E. P., Lichtenstein, E., Mullooly, J. P., Velicer, W. F., & Redding, C. A. (2005). Teen reach: Outcomes from a randomized, controlled trial of a tobacco reduction program for teens seen in primary medical care. *Pediatrics, 115*(4), 981–989.

Jemmott, J. B., Jemmott, L. S., Braverman, P. K., & Fong, G. T. (2005). HIV/STD risk reduction interventions for African American and Latino adolescent girls at an adolescent medicine clinic: A randomized controlled trial. *Archives of Pediatric Adolescent Medicine, 159*(5), 440–449.

Kamb, M. L., Fishbein, M., Douglas, J. M., Rhodes, F., Rogers, J., Bolan, G., Zenilman, J., Hoxworth, T., Malotte, C. K., Iatesta, M., Kent, C., Lentz, A., Graziano, S., Byers, R. H., & Peterman, T. A. (1998). Efficacy of risk-reduction counseling to prevent human immunodeficiency virus and sexually transmitted diseases: A randomized controlled trial—Project RESPECT Study Group. *Journal of the American Medical Association, 280*(13), 1161–1167.

Kristenson, H., Ohlin, H., Hulten-Nosslin, M., Treli, E., & Hood, B. (1983). Identification and intervention of heavy drinking in middle-aged men: Results and followup of 24–60 months of long-term study with randomized controls. *Alcoholism: Clinical and Experimental Research, 7,* 203–209.

McCallum, Z., Wake, M., Gerner, B., Baur, L., Gibbons, K., Gold, L., Gunn, J., Harris, C., Naughton, G., Riess, C., Sanci, L., Sheehan, J., Ukoumunne, O., & Waters, E. (2007). Outcome data from the LEAP (Live, Eat, and Play) trial: A randomized controlled trial of a primary care intervention for childhood overweight/mild obesity. *International Journal of Obesity, 31,* 630–636.

McCambridge, J., & Strang, J. (2004). The efficacy of single-session motivational interviewing in reducing drug consumption and perceptions of drug-related risk and harm among young people: Results from a multi-site cluster randomized trial. *Addiction, 99,* 39–52.

Miller, W. R., & Rollnick, S. (2002). *Motivational interviewing: Preparing people for change* (2nd ed.). New York: Guilford Press.

Norman, G., Adams, M., Calfas, K., Covin, J., Sallis, J., Rossi, J., Redding, C., Cella, J., & Patrick, K. (2007). A randomized trial of a multi-component intervention for adolescent sun protection behaviors *Archives of Pediatric and Adolescent Medicine, 161,* 146–152.

Ockene, J. K., Kristeller, J., Goldberg, R., Amick, T. L., Pekow, P. S., Hosmer, D., Quirk, M., & Kalan, K. (1991). Increasing the efficacy of physician-delivered smoking interventions: A randomized clinical trial. *Journal of General Internal Medicine, 6,* 1–8.

Patten, C. A., Croghan, I. T., Meis, T. M., Decker, P. A., Pingree, S., Colligan, R. C., Dornelas, E. A., Offord, K. P., Boberg, E. W., Baumberger, R. K., Hurt, R. D., & Gustafson, D. H. (2006). Randomized clinical trial of an Internet-based versus brief office intervention for adolescent smoking cessation. *Patient Education Counseling, 64*(1–3), 249–258.

Petersen, R., Albright, J., Garrett, J. M., & Curtis, K. M. (2007). Pregnancy and STD prevention counseling using an adaptation of motivational interviewing: A randomized controlled trial. *Perspectives on Sexual and Reproductive Health, 39*(1), 21–28.

Prochaska, J. O. (1979). *Systems of psychotherapy: A transtheoretical analysis.* Homewood, IL: Dorsey Press.

Prochaska, J. O., & DiClemente, C. (1982). Transtheoretical therapy: Toward a comprehensive model of change. *Psychotherapy Theory, Research, Practice, 19,* 267–288.

Rollnick, S., Butler, C. C., McCambridge, J., Kinnersley, P., Elwyn, G., & Resnicow, K. (2005). Consultations about changing behaviour. *British Medical Journal, 331*(7522), 961–963.

Rollnick, S., Miller, W. R., & Butler, C. C. (2007). *Motivational interviewing in health care: Helping patients change behavior.* New York: Guilford Press.

Scholes, D., Stergachis, A., Heidrich, F. E., Andrilla, H., Holmes, K. K., & Stamm, W. E. (1996). Prevention of pelvic inflammatory disease by screening for cervical chlamydial infection. *New England Journal of Medicine, 34*(21), 1362–1366.

Schwartz, R. P., Hamre, R., Dietz, W., Wasserman, R., Slora, E., Myers, E., Sullivan, S., Rockett, H., Thoma, K., Dumitru, G., & Resnicow, K. (2007). Office-based motivational interviewing to prevent childhood obesity. *Archives of Pediatric Adolescent Medicine, 161,* 495–501.

Shrier, L. A., Ancheta, R., Goodman, E., Chiou, V. M., Lyden, M. R., & Emans, S. J. (2001). Randomized controlled trial of a safer sex intervention for high-risk adolescent girls. *Archives of Pediatric Adolescent Medicine, 155*(1), 73–79.

Soderstrom, C. A., DiClemente, C. C., Dischinger, P. C., Hebel, R., McDuff, D. R., Auman, K. M., & Kufera, J. A. (2007). A controlled trial of brief intervention versus brief advice for at-risk drinking trauma center patients. *Journal of Trauma, Injury, Infection, and Critical Care, 62,* 1102.

Walker, Z., Townsend, J., Oakley, L., Donovan, C., Smith, H., Hurst, Z., Bell, J., & Marshall, S. (2002). Health promotion for adolescents in primary care: Randomised controlled trial. *British Medical Journal, 325*(7), 1–6.

Wallace, A. I., Cutler, S., & Haines, A. (1988). A randomised control trial of general practitioner intervention in patients with excessive alcohol consumption. *British Medical Journal, 297,* 663–668.

World Health Organization. (1986). *Ottawa charter for health promotion* (WHO/HPR/HEP/95.1). Geneva, Switzerland: Author.

CHAPTER

HEALTH POLICY APPROACHES TO REDUCE ADOLESCENT RISK BEHAVIOR AND ADVERSE HEALTH CONSEQUENCES

DAVID G. ALTMAN ▪ HEATHER CHAMPION ▪ ERIN L. SUTFIN

LEARNING OBJECTIVES

After studying this chapter, you will be able to

▪ Conclude that adolescent health is influenced by external social factors independent of the individual.

▪ Name policies designed to reduce adolescent health risk.

▪ Describe how the ecological model can be utilized to discern both adolescent behavior and policy approaches.

An influential report on the future of public health defined public health as what can be done collectively to create the conditions in which health is achieved (Institute of Medicine, 1988). Others have argued that effective health promotion is composed of educational and environmental supports that promote individual and collective action as well as the context that impedes or promotes health (Green & Kreuter, 1999). These perspectives point to the interdependent relationship between individuals and the context in which they live (compare Shinn & Toohey, 2003; Yancey et al., 2007). In a review of seventeen policy and environmental interventions for the prevention of chronic diseases associated with tobacco use, physical inactivity, and poor diet, Brownson, Haire-Joshu, and Luke (2006) found strong, sufficient, or promising evidence for all but four categories of intervention. These effects, however, were not just a function of adolescents' actions. Thus, health policy, formal and informal, plays an important role in creating the conditions in which adolescents thrive or not. Moreover, whether one evaluates adolescent health or adult health, disparities can be seen across socioeconomic strata, racial groups, and geography (Braveman, 2006). A key theme of this chapter is that adolescent health is influenced by factors in the social context that often reside outside of the direct, autonomous control of an individual (Brownson, Haire-Joshu, & Luke, 2006). Because of the health risks faced by adolescents, it is appropriate to enact policies that reduce risk and to pursue secondary or tertiary prevention policies (Robinson & Sirard, 2005).

Health policy, formal and informal, plays an important role in creating the conditions in which adolescents thrive or not.

THE ECOLOGICAL MODEL

One widely utilized framework for understanding policy is the *ecological model.* This model views behavior as a function of interdependent, nested, dynamic, and mutually influencing factors, such as biological, social, environmental, historical, and cultural factors (Schmid, Pratt, & Witmer, 2006; Smetana, Campione-Barr, & Metzger, 2006). This model is consistent with recent calls for transdisciplinary science (Stokols, 2006). At the policy or distal level of analysis, an intervention such as increasing the excise tax on alcohol or mandating air bags in automobiles will influence the actions that individuals take (such as not purchasing alcohol because it's too expensive) or provide protection of individuals regardless of their behavior (as with automatic deployment of an air bag). The reverse is also true. Some interventions at more proximal or lower levels of analysis (such as a school-based curriculum that motivates adolescents to exercise) can influence actions taken at higher levels of analysis (such as teens advocating for bike paths). Thus, the interdependent influences between policy-level and microlevel interventions illustrate the importance of multipronged, comprehensive interventions. Lerner and Galambos (1998) note that "policies indicate a society's investment in and care for its members" (p. 438); policies also reflect societal priorities for funding.

PRINCIPLES OF POLICY APPROACHES

There are a number of excellent papers on policy and environmental approaches (compare Brownson, Newschaffer, & Ali-Abarghoui, 1997; Sallis, Bauman, & Pratt, 1998; Schmid et al., 2006; Warner et al., 1990). Although these researchers approach policy from different perspectives, they share the following commonalities: (1) they communicate expectations and boundaries about behavior; (2) they are formal (such as laws, legislation, and regulations) and informal (such as rules, norms, and expectations); (3) they typically target the physical, social, economic, or legal context; (4) they can have direct effects or moderate the effects of other interventions; and (5) they can operate at multiple levels (such as worksite, community, local, state, national, or international) and across sectors (such as health, education, and transportation). Here, we examine these commonalities with respect to tobacco, alcohol, driving, physical activity and obesity, violence, and sexual health.

The interdependent influences between policy-level and micro-level interventions illustrate the importance of multipronged, comprehensive interventions.

TOBACCO

Adolescent tobacco use is a major public health problem. Although smoking rates among U.S. high school students have declined significantly since the early 1990s, studies show that tobacco use remained stable from 2003 to 2006, with 22 percent of twelfth graders being current smokers (Johnston, O'Malley, Bachman, & Schulenberg, 2007). Early tobacco use is troubling, because the earlier people start to smoke, the less likely they are to quit and the more likely they are to become heavy smokers (U.S. Department of Health and Human Services, 1994).

Marketing, Advertising, and Promotion

There is compelling evidence that adolescents are influenced by tobacco marketing. The National Cancer Institute (NCI) found that marketing was causally related to smoking initiation (NCI, 2002). A meta-analysis revealed that exposure to tobacco marketing more than doubles the odds of initiation among youth (under eighteen) and that marketing and pro-tobacco media depictions increased adolescent smokers' progression to heavier smoking by 42 percent (Wellman, Sugarman, DiFranza, & Winickoff, 2006). The *Master Settlement Agreement* (MSA), signed in 1998 by the Attorneys General of forty-six states and seven tobacco companies, identified several provisions aimed at reducing the exposure of youth to tobacco marketing. These included eliminating tobacco billboards and transit ads, prohibiting the use of cartoon characters to promote tobacco products, prohibiting tobacco brand-name sponsorship for most concerts or events in which contestants are under eighteen, limiting free tobacco-product distributions to locations where children are not permitted, and reaffirming the prohibition on tobacco product placement in movies and on TV (Campaign for Tobacco-Free Kids,

2003). Although the MSA was a constructive step, it failed to fundamentally change the marketing practices of the tobacco industry. Just one year after the MSA was signed, tobacco companies increased marketing expenditures by 22 percent (U.S. Federal Trade Commission, 2001). In response to the MSA, advertising in magazines with a significant youth readership increased for the brands most popular with adolescents—Marlboro, Camel, and Newport (King & Siegel, 2001). The MSA failed to address advertising in magazines and newspapers, thus leaving the industry free to use these media as ways to reach adolescents. Additionally, tobacco companies effectively use point-of-purchase marketing as a way to reach youth. In one study, 80 percent of all retail outlets had interior tobacco ads, and 60 percent had exterior ads (Wakefield et al., 2002). Point-of-purchase advertising, which is not restricted under the MSA, is linked to both initiation and escalation to regular smoking. Limiting or removing advertising at point-of-purchase locations was associated with reductions in youth smoking (Slater, Chaloupka, Wakefield, Johnston, & O'Malley, 2007). The MSA also failed to address marketing and sale of cigarettes on the Internet and direct-mail marketing (Campaign for Tobacco-Free Kids, 2003). Although the MSA altered some industry practices, it has not accomplished the intent of the agreement—to eliminate advertising and marketing of tobacco products to youth. Instead, tobacco companies have reached youth in new ways. Additional policies are needed to limit or restrict advertising at point-of-purchase, in newspapers and magazines, on the Internet, and through direct-mail advertising.

Youth Access to Tobacco

Most adolescents report easy access to tobacco (Johnston et al., 2007). Although it is illegal in most states for those under eighteen to purchase cigarettes, more than half of all youth report usually buying their own cigarettes from retailers or vending machines, from other kids, or by shoulder tapping (Substance Abuse and Mental Health Services Administration, 2004). Measures to reduce commercial access among youth have been incorporated into national and international tobacco control efforts (Etter, 2006). As part of the 1996 federal Synar amendment, the United States has required all states to have and enforce youth-access laws and document a specific level of compliance or risk loss of federal block grant funds (U.S. Department of Health and Human Services, 1996). The World Health Organization's (WHO's) Framework Convention on Tobacco Control requires ratifying nations to adopt and implement laws that prohibit the sale of tobacco to minors (WHO, 2007). Evidence on the efficacy of youth-access restrictions, however, remains mixed (Brownson et al., 2006; Thompson, Hamilton, Siegel, Biener, & Rigotti, 2007). Several policies can be implemented to reduce youth access to tobacco, including (1) minimum age-of-sale laws; (2) vendor compliance with age-of-sale laws; (3) laws directed at youth possession, purchase, or use of tobacco; (4) enforcement of laws; and (5) community mobilization. Combining multiple interventions in a coordinated manner with community mobilization is more effective than more narrowly focused interventions (Task Force on Community Preventive Services, 2005).

Tobacco Price

Although cigarette prices are largely determined by tobacco companies, state and federal excise taxes contribute to the cost. Econometric studies illustrate that increased taxes are an effective tool in reducing smoking among youth, with the median decrease in smoking approximately 3.7 percent for every 10 percent increase in the real price of cigarettes (Hopkins et al., 2001).

Clean Indoor Air Policies

Secondhand smoke (SHS) is a harmful combination of exhaled smoke and sidestream smoke. SHS contains at least 250 chemicals that are either toxic or carcinogenic (National Toxicology Program, 2000). Among U.S. nonsmokers, exposure to SHS is responsible for an estimated 3,000 annual deaths from lung cancer and 35,000 deaths from coronary heart disease, respiratory infections, asthma, and sudden infant death syndrome (NCI, 1999). Other SHS-related illnesses are experienced by children (CDC, 2002). A growing number of government agencies have implemented clean indoor air laws to limit exposure to SHS and encourage smoking cessation. Among adolescents, strict workplace restrictions have been found to be related to decreases in the number of cigarettes smoked per day, increases in attempts to stop smoking, and increases in smoking cessation rates (U.S. Department of Health and Human Services, 2006). Two large population-based surveys found that workplace bans were associated with a lower likelihood of an adolescent being a smoker, even though only about a quarter of adolescents work outside the home (Farkas, Gilpin, White, & Pierce, 2000). Moreover, household smoking bans are strongly related to lower levels of smoking among adolescents; full bans were more effective than partial bans and showed increased likelihood of cessation and lower rates of smoking (Farkas et al., 2000). By increasing public and household bans, the likelihood of adolescents' use of tobacco will decrease.

Cessation Policies

Cessation policies attempt to increase the number of smokers who make successful cessation attempts (Task Force on Community Preventive Services, 2005). Relative to other tobacco control interventions, less research has focused on adolescent cessation policies. In 2000, the U.S. Public Health Service Treatment Guidelines identified several effective strategies for cessation, many of which have policy implications for providers. These guidelines recommend the use of pharmacotherapy (where clinically appropriate) in conjunction with counseling, to increase the likelihood of successful cessation. Data from research with adults reveal that the reduction of out-of-pocket expenses for cessation treatments increases use of cessation therapies and successful quit attempts (Hopkins et al., 2001). Few studies have focused on adolescents, and those that study clinician interventions have shown mixed results (Mermelstein, 2003).

By increasing public and household bans, the likelihood of adolescents' use of tobacco will decrease.

ALCOHOL

An estimated five thousand adolescents under age twenty-one die annually from alcohol-related motor vehicle crashes (1,900), homicides (1,600), suicides (300), and other unintentional injuries (National Highway Traffic Safety Administration, 2003; Hingson & Kenkel, 2004). An estimated 20 percent of eighth graders, 65 percent of tenth graders, and 75 percent of twelfth graders have consumed alcohol (Johnston et al., 2005). Over 10 percent of eighth graders, 22 percent of tenth graders, and 29 percent of twelfth graders engaged in heavy episodic drinking (binge drinking) in the past two weeks. A substantial body of research has linked early age of initiation of alcohol use (less than fourteen years old) with subsequent increased rates of alcohol use, likelihood of engaging in other risky behaviors, and alcohol dependence (Grant & Dawson, 1998). A wide range of environmental approaches to reducing alcohol have been shown to be effective.

Alcohol Availability

Various state and federal policies to limit youth access to alcohol have been enacted. One of the most effective, the National Minimum Drinking Age Act, was passed by Congress in 1984. This law prohibited persons under twenty-one from purchasing or publicly possessing alcohol. If states did not comply, a portion of their federal highway funds were withheld. By 1988, all fifty states had passed legislation meeting the requirements for federal funding. The minimum legal drinking age has been attributed with saving twenty thousand lives between 1975 and 2000 (Wagenaar & Toomey, 2002). In addition, states have adopted policies to address underage drinking that apply to youth and to alcohol sellers, servers, and providers. These include underage possession of alcohol, consumption of alcohol, purchase of alcohol, and furnishing alcohol to minors or hosting underage drinking parties. Other policies, while not addressing underage youth directly, are nonetheless important. These include laws on minimum age for on-premises servers and bartenders, minimum age for off-premises sellers, false identification for obtaining alcohol, and keg registration. The effectiveness of these policies has been less extensively studied, and they report mixed findings (Wagenaar, Toomey, & Lenk, 2004/2005). Reducing the density of alcohol outlets limits access and availability, as well as reducing exposure to alcohol messages that contribute to social norms around drinking. Higher alcohol outlet density is associated with greater prevalence of driving after drinking among fifteen- to twenty-year-olds (Treno, Grube, & Martin, 2003).

Harm Minimization

Harm minimization policies include zero tolerance laws that limit blood alcohol concentration levels for drivers under twenty-one and loss of driving privileges for alcohol violations by minors. Data suggest that these policies can be effective in reducing crashes among drivers younger than twenty-one and have been attributed to a 24.4 percent reduction in fatal motor vehicle crashes (Voas, Tippetts, & Fell, 2003).

Alcohol Price

As with tobacco, the price of alcohol is inversely associated with consumption; as cost increases, alcohol use, heavy alcohol use, and consequences decrease (Chaloupka, Grossman, & Saffer, 2002).

Alcohol Marketing

Policies aimed at limiting exposure to alcohol marketing target social norms, including attitudes about the acceptability of alcohol use and the positive images associated with use. Specific *alcohol marketing* policies include limiting location and content of outdoor advertising, prohibiting the distribution or sale of promotional items to underage youth, and restricting or limiting alcohol industry sponsorship of local community events. The National Research Council (NRC) made several key recommendations related to advertising and underage drinking (NRC, 2003). These included recommendations to Congress to appropriate funding for the U.S. Department of Health and Human Services to monitor underage exposure to alcohol advertising on a consistent basis, media campaigns to reduce underage drinking, and intensive research and development for a youth-focused national media campaign to reduce underage drinking.

Enforcement

Limiting access to alcohol by youth is a key lever in reducing underage drinking. However, the effectiveness of these policies is diminished unless there is commensurate enforcement. Directing enforcement efforts at adults (such as retailers, servers, and parents) is more effective than efforts aimed at youth (Mosher, 1995). One area in which enforcement is challenging is the social provision of alcohol to underage youth. Social sources include parents, other relatives, and older friends and acquaintances. Stricter penalties for providing alcohol to minors need to be imposed. Instead of buying from commercial sources that are licensed to sell alcohol (such as bars, restaurants, and grocery stores), most underage drinkers obtain their alcohol from social sources, such as friends or parents (Jones-Webb et al., 1997; Hearst, Fulkerson, Maldonado-Molina, Perry, & Komro, 2007). In one study, 80 percent of underage drinkers obtained alcohol exclusively from social sources (Harrison, Fulkerson, & Park, 2000). To reduce access to alcohol, stricter penalties for providing alcohol to minors need to be imposed. Increasing and expanding social host liability is one way to provide a disincentive to parents and other adults who supply alcohol to underage youth.

Increasing and expanding social host liability is one way to provide a disincentive to parents and other adults who supply alcohol to underage youth.

Comprehensive Environmental Approaches

Several community-level interventions using comprehensive environmental approaches have been shown to be effective in reducing underage drinking. Communities Mobilizing for Change on Alcohol is an example of a communitywide program that focuses on policy changes to reduce youth access to commercial and social sources of alcohol. Youth ages eighteen to twenty in intervention communities that adopted the program had significantly fewer arrests for drinking and driving than did youth in the control communities (Wagenaar, Murray, Gehan, et al., 2000; Wagenaar, Murray, & Toomey, 2000). Likewise, Project Northland is an example of a comprehensive intervention that incorporated family, school, and community components to prevent or reduce alcohol use among adolescents. After three years, the prevalence of alcohol use by eighth-grade students was lower in the intervention communities than in the control communities. After intervention efforts were reduced, the impact was diminished; however, after intervention efforts were reintroduced, a positive impact on eleventh- and twelfth-grade students' alcohol use and binge drinking was reported (Perry et al., 2002). These interventions demonstrate the importance of policies aimed at reducing access to alcohol and increasing enforcement to reduce underage drinking.

DRIVING

Motor vehicle crashes (MVCs) are the leading cause of death for youth ages fifteen to twenty-four in the United States (Miniño, Heron, & Smith, 2006). The risk of death by MVC is highest among sixteen- to nineteen-year-olds compared to other age groups. The primary risk factors that increase the likelihood of youth being involved in a MVC are limited driving experience and skills. Additionally, factors that place adult drivers at greater risk for a MVC are more pronounced for young drivers and include carrying teenage passengers, driving late at night, driving under the influence of alcohol and other activities that create distractions (such as talking or text messaging on cell phones or listening to music). One of the primary policies targeted at reducing the risks associated with young drivers is *graduated drivers licensing* (GDL; National Highway Traffic Safety Administration [NHTSA], 1994). Most GDL policies involve delaying the onset of full driving privileges and minimizing riskier driving situations for newer drivers. GDL laws usually use a three-phase licensing process: learner's permit, provisional license, and full license. General recommendations for GDL programs include (1) specifying the number of hours of adult-supervised driving time (usually fifty hours over a six-month time period); (2) restricting night driving, especially between 10:00 PM and 5:00 AM; (3) excluding teen passengers unless a licensed adult over age twenty-one is present; (4) enforcing zero alcohol tolerance for those under age twenty-one; (5) revoking or suspending a license or permit if a teen drives in violation of the law—whether an at-fault accident, conviction, or an alcohol violation.

GDL programs have been associated with declines in MVCs, fatal crashes, and traffic convictions (NHTSA, 2007). A national evaluation of GDL at Johns Hopkins University attributed the most comprehensive GDL programs to an estimated 20 percent reduction in the rate of fatal crashes among sixteen-year-old drivers (Baker, Chen, & Li, 2006). Strengthening compliance with GDL laws is important for reducing motor vehicle crashes. Only states with at least five of the key GDL components had significantly lower fatal motor vehicle crashes (18 to 21 percent) among sixteen- to twenty-year-old drivers when compared to states without any of the seven GDL components. Programs demonstrating the greatest impact included age requirements plus three or more months of waiting before the intermediate stage, nighttime driving restriction, and either supervised driving of at least thirty hours or a passenger restriction.

PHYSICAL ACTIVITY AND OBESITY

Physical activity, nutrition, and obesity have received considerable interest among funders, policy makers, and researchers. Over time, children and adolescents have been engaging in less planned (or purposive) and incidental physical activity (Maibach, 2007). Childhood obesity has more than doubled for children and adolescents over the past three decades (Institute of Medicine, 2004), in part because they engage in less physical activity as compared to previous generations (Alderman, Smith, Fried, & Daynard, 2007).

Emblematic of the growing interest in childhood and adolescent obesity, the Robert Wood Johnson Foundation announced an unprecedented $500 million, five-year commitment to address the problem in 2006—in addition to the foundation's considerable investment in physical activity interventions (Kraft, Sallis, Vernez Moudon, & Linton, 2006). The latter work is focused on building a knowledge base about how the environment affects physical activity (through their Active Living Research program), engaging policy makers to promote active communities (through their Active Living Leadership program), and supporting demonstrations of community efforts to promote activity (through their Active Living by Design, Active Living Network, Active for Life, and Wheeling Walks programs). In the nutrition area, one sees a similar focus. A variety of policy interventions have been developed, including food labeling, improved nutrition and accessibility of school breakfast and lunch programs, and improvements in the federal dietary guidelines, to name a few (Alderman et al., 2007; Mello, Studdert, & Brennan, 2006).

Thus, while researchers and practitioners continue to devote resources and attention to the biomedical bases underlying obesity, there is considerable attention to studying and intervening in the environments that encourage or discourage related health behaviors (Huang & Horlick, 2007; Sallis & Glanz, 2006; Sallis et al., 2006; Schwartz & Brownell, 2007). In the words of Alderman and colleagues, "the law must shift focus away from individual risk factors and seek instead to shape the situational and environmental influences that create an environment conducive to health" (Alderman et al., 2007, p. 102). Similarly, Schwartz and Brownell (2007) write about the toxic or obesity-generating environment in which we live and how influences in the environment affect obesity. A variety of policy interventions to promote physical activity and reduce obesity have been initiated. While the evidence base is still developing and the efficacy of some intervention approaches remains uncertain, there is growing evidence of impact (Heath et al., 2006; Sallis & Glanz, 2006). For example, public health researchers have combined forces with urban planners and transportation experts to examine how zoning

"The law must shift focus away from individual risk factors and seek instead to shape the situational and environmental influences that create an environment conducive to health."

laws and the design of communities can facilitate physical activity (Pollard, 2003; Schilling & Linton, 2005). These efforts focus on interventions such as promoting mixed land use or street scale design (combining retail, housing, and public use space in a geographically dense area), higher residential density, pedestrian-friendly development (walking and bicycle trails and proximity between housing and schools), availability of public use space (such as parks, trails, and swimming pools) and greater street connectivity, which all make walking and cycling an attractive and realistic alternative to driving (Heath et al., 2006; Pollard, 2003; Schilling & Linton, 2005).

As in other areas of adolescent health, disparities exist with respect to physical activity. In a large national study that assessed the availability of physical activity facilities for over 20,000 adolescents and nearly 43,000 census block groups, researchers found that adolescents from neighborhoods with lower socioeconomic status and higher minority populations were less likely than other groups to have access to physical activity facilities. This lack of access was associated in turn with less physical activity and being more overweight among these groups (Gordon-Larsen, Nelson, Page, & Popkin, 2006).

VIOLENCE

Violence is a pervasive problem among adolescents and takes many forms including homicide, physical assault and other violent crimes, sexual assault, battering in intimate relationships, and suicide. Adolescents' exposure to violence can come in many forms as well: as a victim, perpetrator, witness, or viewer (as with media violence). Although there has been a significant decline since the mid-1990s in the incidence of fatal youth violence, more recent mortality data reveal that among children older than one year, homicide and suicide still cause more deaths than all natural causes combined (Champion & Sege, 2007).

Media Violence

The amount of violence on television is disproportionately high relative to real life. Although most children are not witnesses to severe violence in their own lives, by the time a child is eighteen, he or she will have seen more than 40,000 murders and over 200,000 other acts of physical violence on television (Huston et al., 1992). Violence on television is portrayed in ways that make it appealing to teens. Acts of violence are glamorized, trivialized, and rewarded, but the consequences of violent acts are rarely shown (Bushman & Huesmann, 2001). Decades of experimental and observational research led six prominent medical and psychological organizations to issue a Joint Statement on the Impact of Entertainment Violence on Children. The document reported a causal connection between viewing media violence and children's aggressive attitudes and behaviors (AMA et al., 2000).

To avoid criticisms about First Amendment rights and censorship, the policies surrounding children's exposure to media violence have focused largely on providing parents with information about the content of the media and allowing them the opportunity to make decisions about their children's exposure to violent media. One such policy was passed as part of the Telecommunications Act of 1996. This policy required all new television sets to include V-chip technology. The act also mandated that television program ratings be sent to the V-chip, allowing parents to block out content that had unacceptable ratings. Though designed to provide parents with information about television exposure, an inherent problem with the V-chip technology is that it relies on (1) the accuracy of the ratings and (2) the use of technology by parents. Per the Telecommunications Act of 1996, Congress gave the broadcast industry the opportunity to develop and implement a voluntary rating system. The rating system, also known as TV Parental Guidelines, was established by the National Association of Broadcasters, the National Cable Television Association, and the Motion Picture Association of America. Almost immediately, the system developed by broadcasters came under fire for their decision to use age-based ratings, which signify an appropriate viewer age, rather than content-based ratings (Kunkel & Wilcox, 2001). Research has supported the use of a content-based system, and in 1997 broadcasters agreed to amend their age-based ratings to include information on content as well. The ratings have also been criticized for their lack of accuracy, specifically as related to violent material (Kunkel et al., 1998). In addition, parents' low awareness and use of the ratings and the V-chip have come into question. In a 2007 survey, 50 percent of parents reported using the rating system; however, only one in six parents reported ever using the V-chip (Kaiser Family Foundation, 2007).

A Joint Statement on the Impact of Entertainment Violence on Children document reported a causal connection between viewing media violence and children's aggressive attitudes and behaviors.

Giving parents the tools and knowledge necessary to limit their children's exposure to violent media is one important and viable method for reducing aggression and violence among children and adolescents. The same is true of the rating system used for video games. Although these ratings have also been criticized for being confusing and lacking specificity, at the very least they provide parents with some information that they would not otherwise have. Many researchers in the field have called for the establishment of a universal media rating system that would include television, movies, video games, and even music.

Access to Firearms

Violence linked to firearms is a serious problem among adolescents (Duke, Resnick, & Borrowsky, 2005). In 2002, over 2,700 youth aged ten to nineteen were killed by firearms. Among adolescents aged fifteen to nineteen, firearm deaths rank number two after motor vehicle deaths and far outweigh deaths from disease. Approximately 43 percent of homes have one or more handguns; at least 30 percent of gun owners with children keep one or more loaded guns in the home. Thus, approximately nine million adolescents have access to handguns in their own homes (Champion & Sege, 2007). Considerable evidence exists linking access to firearms to increases in the risk of homicide, suicide, and unintentional injury (Duke, Resnick, & Borrowsky, 2005). When access to a handgun at home is available, a household member or friend is roughly forty-three times more likely to be the victim of the firearm than an intruder. (Kellerman & Rea, 1986) A gun stored in the home is associated with a fivefold increased risk of completed suicide (Kellermann et al., 1992). Policies related to gun violence have centered on access to firearms among youth. A review by the Task Force on Community Preventive Services was conducted to assess the impact of federal and state firearm laws on violent outcomes (Hahn et al., 2005). Laws included bans on specified firearms or ammunition, restrictions on firearm acquisition, waiting periods, registration and licensing, child access prevention laws, and zero tolerance laws for firearms in schools. For each of the laws reviewed, the task force found insufficient evidence of effectiveness. As is the case with any intervention, however, implementation and enforcement likely affect effectiveness.

Clinic-Based Violence Prevention

Given the public health issues surrounding violence among adolescents, bodies such as the American Medical Association (AMA) and American Academy of Pediatrics (AAP) have established policies for incorporating violence prevention into routine primary care (AMA, 1996; AAP, 1999). Pediatricians are encouraged to identify risk factors associated with violence (such as access to firearms) through routine screening and provide counseling and referrals if necessary. Research on the effectiveness of such interventions is limited. In terms of counseling about access to firearms, no effects on ownership were found (Duke et al., 2005). However, parents and youth report receptivity to counseling on firearms. In addition, research has shown that many pediatricians are not engaging in violence prevention, although some clinicians are beginning to incorporate violence prevention into well-child visits (Barkin, Ryan, & Gelberg, 1999; Barkin, Duan, Fink, Brook, & Gelberg, 1998). Although the research on clinic-based violence prevention is limited, these interventions are recommended by many governing health bodies, including AMA and AAP.

SEXUAL HEALTH

Key sexual health policy issues among adolescents include unintended teen pregnancy and sexually transmitted infections (STIs), including HIV/AIDS, and human papilloma virus (HPV). Teen pregnancy and birth rates in the United States have declined since the early 1990s. Even so, the United States continues to have the highest teen birth rate among all industrialized nations and a higher rate than over fifty developing nations. Declining rates have been attributed to a decrease in sexual activity and to a substantial increase in contraceptive use. Yet 63.1 percent of high schools seniors have had sexual intercourse (CDC, 2006), and millions of American youth are still engaging in high-risk behaviors. Annually, approximately 900,000 female adolescents in the United States become pregnant, nearly four million new STIs occur among fifteen- to nineteen-year-olds, and about 20,000 adolescents are newly infected with HIV (Feijoo & Grayton, 2004). In June 2006, the U.S. Food and Drug Administration (FDA) approved an HPV vaccine that protects against two types of HPV that cause 70 percent of all cervical cancers and two types of HPV that cause 90 percent of all genital warts. A key policy implication unique to HPV is supporting efforts to distribute the HPV vaccine and recommending or requiring the HPV vaccine for school. Policy-related strategies aimed at reducing unintended pregnancies and STIs focus primarily on decreasing sexual activity and increasing the accessibility and use of contraceptives, especially condoms, through sexual education programs and, to a lesser extent, youth development programs (Brindis, 2006).

In 1996, Congress signed into law the Personal Responsibility and Work Opportunities Reconciliation Act (PRWORA). It included a provision appropriating $250 million over five years for state initiatives promoting sexual abstinence outside of marriage as the only acceptable standard of behavior for young people. To examine changes in sexual behavior in relationship to Title V, Section 510, of the PRWORA, the prevalence of sexual behaviors from 1991 to 1997 was compared to 1999 to 2003. The former period corresponded to the widespread implementation of comprehensive sex education, whereas the latter covered the first five-year cycle of PRWORA Title V abstinence-only programs. Improvements in adolescent sexual risk taking were significantly greater from 1991 to 1997 than from 1999 to 2003 (Feijoo & Grayton, 2004). From 1991 to 1997, significant effects were reported on (1) the proportion of ninth to twelfth graders reporting ever having had sexual intercourse (decreased by 11 percent), (2) prevalence of multiple sexual partners (four or more in lifetime decreased by 9 percent), (3) current sexual activity among black males, and (4) condom use (increased by 23 percent). Likewise, a rigorous examination of four abstinence-only education programs found that youth in the four programs were no more likely than youth not in the programs to have abstained from sex in the four to six years after participation in the study (Trenholm et al., 2007). Youth in both groups who reported having had sex also had similar numbers of sexual partners and had initiated sex at the same average age. Youth in the abstinence education programs were no more likely to have engaged in unprotected sex than youth who did not participate in the programs.

Out of sixteen U.S.-based sex education programs and three youth development programs studied, a delay in the initiation of sex was demonstrated in twelve programs (Feijoo & Grayton, 2004). Seventeen programs had a positive impact on sexual behaviors among sexually experienced youth. Eight programs had a positive impact on incidence of STIs or on the number or rate of teen pregnancies. There is little support for abstinence-only sexual education programs. Although these programs do not appear to have a negative impact on risky sexual behaviors, there is no evidence for their effectiveness.

Although abstinence-only programs do not appear to have a negative impact on risky sexual behaviors, there is no evidence for their effectiveness.

Increasing access to contraceptives is another debated strategy for reducing teen pregnancies and STIs. Barriers to access include being unfamiliar with the health care system, inability to pay for services, fear that confidential information would be disclosed to family or friends, and concern about needing the consent of a parent of guardian (Brindis, 2006). Policies aimed at minimizing barriers to access contraceptives and health care services, including public funding for services, are needed and are more cost-effective than covering the costs associated with unintended pregnancies among teenagers.

Policies that support youth development are a relatively new approach to addressing teen sexual behavior. The premise of youth development programs is that the context in which young people make health-related decisions needs to be considered (Brindis, 2006). Providing youth with a supportive environment and a positive sense of the future promotes healthy adolescent development and is key in reducing adolescent pregnancy. Policies that support youth development include funding for programs and facilities that support youth development, youth employment, job readiness, youth-led business ventures, peer teaching and counseling, academic tutoring, recreation, mentoring, community service work, and life skills training.

SUMMARY

"Health policies will need to address both the collective lifestyles of modern societies and the social environments of modern life as they affect the health and quality of life of populations."

There have been calls for adolescent researchers to be more involved in the knowledge-to-practice-to-policy continuum. Some have called for researchers to pay more attention to building policy questions into their research, working with practitioners and community groups to use high-quality research in the field, and connecting directly to policy makers (Bleakley & Ellis, 2003). In this chapter, we have briefly reviewed some of the evidence linking policy-level variables to adolescent health, using the ecological model as a general organizing structure. From an ecological perspective, adolescent behavior and points of intervention leverage must be considered at multiple levels of analysis over time. We recognize that biological, cognitive, and interpersonal factors loom large for adolescents (Lerner & Galambos, 1998), and thus we do not want to minimize the important effect of behavioral choices made by adolescents. Rather, we suggest that it is equally important to consider the larger environment in which individual health decisions are made and actions are taken. Clearly, individual health is influenced by a confluence of individual and higher-order contextual factors. Kickbusch (2003) observed that the first public health revolution focused on sanitary conditions and infectious diseases (context). The second revolution focused on the relationship between health behaviors and premature death due to chronic diseases (individual behavior). The third revolution, which she contended we are in now, connects health to the higher-order concept of quality of life (context and individual behavior). In Kickbusch's words, "health policies will need to address both the collective lifestyles of modern societies and the social environments of modern life as they affect the health and quality of life of populations" (pp. 386–387).

KEY TERMS

Alcohol marketing

Cessation policies

Ecological model

Graduated drivers licensing (GDL)

Harm minimization

Master Settlement Agreement (MSA)

Secondhand smoke (SHS)

DISCUSSION QUESTIONS

1. Discuss ways in which health policy helps create the conditions in which adolescents will thrive (or not thrive). Provide examples.

2. What similarities or commonalities typically exist across policy approaches? Think of two policies not covered in this chapter: How are they similar? How are they different?

3. Choose an adolescent health risk behavior (such as drug use or smoking) and explain how policy can be strengthened in this area. Provide recommendations and suggestions for both policy makers and health care providers.

REFERENCES

Alderman, J., Smith, J. A., Fried, E. J., & Daynard, R. A. (2007). Application of law to the childhood obesity epidemic. *Journal of Law, Medicine and Ethics, 35*(1), 90–112.

American Academy of Pediatrics. (1999). The role of the pediatrician in youth violence prevention in clinical practice and at the community level. *Pediatrics, 103*(1), 173–181.

American Medical Association. (1996). Policy 145.99. In *AMA Policy Compendium.* Chicago, IL: American Medical Association.

American Medical Association, American Academy of Pediatrics, American Psychological Association, American Psychiatric Association, American Academy of Family Physicians, & the American Academy of Child & Adolescent Psychiatry. (2000). *Joint Statement on the Impact of Entertainment Violence on Children: Congressional Public Health Summit.* Retrieved August 16, 2007, from www.aap.org/advocacy/releases/jstmtEVC.htm.

Baker, S. P., Chen, L., & Li, G. (2006). National evaluation of graduated driver licensing programs (DOT HS 810 614). Washington, DC: National Highway Traffic Safety Administration.

Barkin, S., Duan, N., Fink, A., Brook, R. H., & Gerlberg, L. (1998). The smoking gun: Do clinicians follow guidelines on firearm safety counseling? *Archives of Pediatric and Adolescent Medicine, 152,* 749–756.

Barkin, S., Ryan, G., & Gelberg, L. (1999). What pediatricians can do to further youth violence prevention: A qualitative study. *Injury Prevention, 5,* 53–58.

Bleakley, A., & Ellis, J. A. (2003). A role for public health research in shaping adolescent health policy. *American Journal of Public Health, 93*(11), 1801–1802.

Braveman, P. (2006). Health disparities and health equity: Concepts and measurement. *Annual Review of Public Health, 27,* 167–194.

Brindis, C. D. (2006). A public health success: Understanding policy changes related to teen sexual activity and pregnancy. *Annual Review of Public Health, 27,* 277–295.

Brownson, R. C., Haire-Joshu, D., & Luke, D. A. (2006). Shaping the context of health: A review of environmental and policy approaches in the prevention of chronic diseases. *Annual Review of Public Health, 27,* 341–370.

Brownson, R. C., Newschaffer, C. J., & Ali-Abarghoui, F. (1997). Policy research for disease prevention: Challenges and practical recommendations. *American Journal of Public Health, 87*(5), 735–739.

Bushman, B. J., & Huesmann, L. R. (2001). Effects of television violence on aggression. In D. G. Singer & J. L. Singer (Eds.), *Handbook of children and the media* (pp. 223–254). Thousand Oaks, CA: Sage.

Campaign for Tobacco-Free Kids. (2003). *Summary of the Multistate Agreement (MSA).* Retrieved July 20, 2007, from www.tobaccofreekids.org/research/factsheets/index.php?CategoryID=8.

Centers for Disease Control and Prevention. (2002). Annual smoking-attributable mortality, years or potential life lost, and economic costs: United States, 1995–1999. *Morbidity and Mortality Weekly Reports, 51*(14), 300–320.

Centers for Disease Control and Prevention. (2006). Youth Risk Behavior Surveillance: United States, 2005. *Morbidity and Mortality Weekly Reports, 55*(SS-5).

Chaloupka, F. J., Grossman, M., & Saffer, H. (2002). The effects of price on alcohol consumption and alcohol-related problems. *Alcohol Research and Health, 26,* 22–34.

Champion, H., & Sege, R. (2007). Youth violence. In L. S. Neinstein & E. Woods (Eds.), *Adolescent health care: A practical guide* (5th ed; pp. 984–993.). Philadelphia, PA: Lippincott Williams & Wilkins.

Duke, N., Resnick, M. D., & Borowsky, I. W. (2005). Adolescent firearm violence: Position paper of the Society for Adolescent Medicine. *Journal of Adolescent Health, 37,* 171–174.

Etter, J. F. (2006). Laws prohibiting the sale of tobacco to minors: Impact and adverse consequences. *American Journal of Preventive Medicine, 31,* 47–51.

Farkas, A. J., Gilpin, E. A., White, M. M., & Pierce, J. P. (2000). Association between household and workplace smoking restrictions and adolescent smoking. *Journal of the American Medical Association, 284*(6), 717–722.

Feijoo, A. N., & Grayton, C. (2004). *Trends in sexual risk behaviors among high school students: United States, 1991 to 1997 and 1999 to 2003.* Washington, DC: Advocates for Youth. Retrieved August 3, 2007, from www.advocatesforyouth.org/publications/factsheet/fstrends.htm.

Gordon-Larsen, P., Nelson, M. C., Page, P., & Popkin, B. M. (2006). Inequality in the built environment underlies key health disparities in physical activity and obesity. *Pediatrics, 117,* 417–424.

Grant, B. F., & Dawson, D. A. (1998). Age at onset of drug use and its association with DSM-IV drug abuse and dependence: Results from the National Longitudinal Alcohol Epidemiologic Survey. *Journal of Substance Abuse, 10,* 163–173.

Green, L. W., & Kreuter, M. W. (1999). *Health promotion planning: An educational and ecological approach* (3rd ed.). Mountain View, CA: Mayfield.

Hahn, R. A., Bilukha, O., Crosby, A., Fullilove, M. T., Liberman, A., Moscicki, E., Snyder, S., Tuma, F., & Briss, P. A. (2005). Firearm laws and the reduction of violence: A systematic review. *American Journal of Preventive Medicine, 28*(2 Suppl. 1), 40–71.

Harrison, P. A., Fulkerson, J. A., & Park, E. (2000). The relative importance of social versus commercial sources in youth access to tobacco, alcohol, and other drugs. *Preventive Medicine, 31,* 39–48.

Hearst, M. O., Fulkerson, J. A., Maldonado-Molina, M. M., Perry, C. L., & Komro, K. A. (2007). Who needs liquor stores when parents will do? The importance of social sources of alcohol among young urban teens. *Preventive Medicine, 44,* 471–476.

Heath, G. W., Brownson, R. C., Kruger, J., Miles, R., Powell, K. E., Ramsey, L. T., & the Task Force on Community Preventive Services. (2006). The effectiveness of urban design and land use and transport policies and practices to increase physical activity: A systematic review. *Journal of Physical Activity and Health, 3*(Suppl. 1), S55–S76.

Hingson, R., & Kenkel, D. (2004). Social, health, and economic consequences of underage drinking. In R. J. Bonnie & M. E. O'Connell (Eds.), *Reducing underage drinking: A collective responsibility* (pp. 351–382). Washington, DC: National Academies Press.

Hopkins, D. P., Briss, P. A., Ricard, C. J., Husten, C. G., Carande-Kulis, V. G., Fielding, J. E., Alao, M. O., McKenna, J. W., Sharp, D. J., Harris, J. R., Woollery, T. A., & Harris, K. W. (2001). Reviews of evidence regarding interventions to reduce tobacco use and exposure to environmental tobacco smoke. *American Journal of Preventive Medicine, 20*(2S), 16–66.

Huang, T., & Horlick, M. N. (2007). Trends in childhood obesity research: A brief analysis of NIH-supported efforts. *Journal of Law, Medicine and Ethics, 35*(1), 148–153.

Huston, A. C., Donnerstein, E., Fairchild, H., Feshbach, N. D., Katz, P. A., Murray, J. P., Rubinstein, E. A., Wilcox, B. L., & Zuckerman, D. (1992). *Big world, small screen: The role of television in American Society.* Lincoln: University of Nebraska Press.

Institute of Medicine. (1988). *The future of public health.* Washington, DC: National Academies Press.

Institute of Medicine. (2004). *Preventing childhood obesity: Health in the balance.* Washington, DC: National Academies Press.

Johnston, L. D., O'Malley, P. M., Bachman, J. G., & Schulenberg, J. E. (2007). *Monitoring the Future national results on adolescent drug use: Overview of key findings, 2006* (NIH Publication No. 07–6202). Bethesda, MD: National Institute on Drug Abuse.

Jones-Webb, R., Toomey, T., Miner, K., Wagenaar, A. C., Wolfson, M., & Poon, R. (1997). Why and in what context adolescents obtain alcohol from adults: A pilot study. *Substance Use and Misuse, 32,* 219–228.

Kaiser Family Foundation. (2007). *Parents, children, and the media.* Retrieved on August 2, 2007, from www .kff.org/entmedia/upload/7638.pdf.

Kellermann, A, L., Rea, D. T. (1986). Protection or peril? An analysis of firearm-related deaths in the home. *New England Journal of Medicine*, 314, 1557-1560.

Kellermann, A. L., Rivara, F. P., Somes, G., Reay, D. T., Francisco, J., Banton, J. G., Prodzinski, J., Fligner, C., & Hackman, B. B. (1992). Suicide in the home in relation to gun ownership. *New England Journal of Medicine, 327,* 467–472.

Kickbusch, I. (2003). The contribution of the World Health Organization to a new public health and health promotion. *American Journal of Public Health, 93*(3), 383–388.

King, C., & Siegel, M. (2001). The Master Settlement Agreement with the tobacco industry and cigarette advertising in magazines. *New England Journal of Medicine, 345*(7), 504–511.

Kraft, M. K., Sallis, J. F., Vernez Moudon, A., & Linton, L. S. (2006). The second active living research conference: Signs of maturity. *Journal of Physical Activity and Health, 3*(Suppl. 1), S1–S5.

Kunkel, D., Farinola, W., Cope, K., Donnerstein, E., Biely, E., & Zwarun, L. (1998). *Rating the TV ratings: An assessment of the television industry's use of the C-chip ratings.* Menlo Park, CA: Kaiser Family Foundation.

Kunkel, D., & Wilcox, B. (2001). Children and media policy. *Handbook of children and the media* (pp. 589–604). Thousand Oaks, CA: Sage.

Lerner, R. M., & Galambos, N. L. (1998). Adolescent development: Challenges and opportunities for research, programs and policies. *Annual Review of Psychology, 49,* 413–446.

Maibach, E. (2007). The influence of the media environment on physical activity: Looking for the big picture. *Health Promotion, 21*(Suppl. 4), 353–362.

Mello, M. M., Studdert, D. M., & Brennan, T. A. (2006). Obesity: The new frontier of public health law. *New England Journal of Medicine, 354*(24), 2601–2610.

Mermelstein, R. (2003). Teen smoking cessation. *Tobacco Control, 12*(Suppl. 1), i25–i34.

Miniño, A. M., Heron, M. P., & Smith, B. L. (2006). Deaths: Preliminary data for 2004. *National Vital Statistics Report, 54* (19).

Mosher, J. (1995). The merchants, not the customers: Resisting the alcohol and tobacco industries' strategy to blame young people for illegal alcohol and tobacco sales. *Journal of Public Health Policy, 16*(4), 412–432.

National Cancer Institute. (2001). *Changing adolescent smoking prevalence.* Smoking and Tobacco Control Monograph No.14 (NIH Publication No. 02–5086). Retrieved July 18, 2007, from http://cancercontrol .cancer.gov/tcrb/monographs/14/index.html.

National Cancer Institute (1999). *Health Effects of Exposure to Environmental Tobacco Smoke: The Report of the California Environmental Protection Agency*, Smoking and Tobacco Control Monograph no. 10, NIH Pub. No. 99-4645.

National Highway Traffic Safety Administration. (1994, May 31). Research agenda for an improved novice driver education program: Report to Congress (Publication No. DOT-HS-808–161). Washington, DC: Author.

National Highway Traffic Safety Administration. (2003). Traffic safety facts 2002 (Publication No. DOT-HS-809-60). Washington, DC: NHTSA, National Center for Statistics and Analysis.

National Highway Traffic Safety Administration. (2007). Traffic safety facts 2007: Graduated driver licensing system (Publication No. DOT-HS-810-727W). Retrieved July 18, 2007, from www.nhtsa.dot.gov/people/injury/TSFLaws/PDFs/810727W.pdf.

National Research Council, Institute of Medicine. (2003). *Reducing underage drinking: A collective responsibility.* Washington, DC: National Academies Press.

National Toxicology Program. (2000). *Ninth report on carcinogens 2000.* Research Triangle Park, NC: U.S. Department of Health and Human Services, National Institute of Environmental Health Sciences.

Perry, C. L., Williams, C. L., Komro, K. A., Veblen-Mortenson, S., Stigler, M. H., Munson, K. A., Farbakhsh, K., Jones, R. M., & Forster, J. L. (2002). Project Northland: Long-term outcomes of community action to reduce adolescent alcohol use. *Health Education Research, 17,* 117–132.

Pollard, T. (2003). Policy prescriptions for healthier communities. *American Journal of Health Promotion, 18*(1), 109–113.

Robinson, T. N., & Sirard, J. R. (2005). Preventing childhood obesity: A solution-oriented research paradigm. *American Journal of Preventive Medicine, 28*(2S2), 194–201.

Sallis, J. F., Bauman, A., & Pratt, M. (1998). Environmental and policy interventions to promote physical activity. *American Journal of Preventive Medicine, 15*(4), 379–397.

Sallis, J. F., Cervero, R. B., Ascher, W., Henderson, K. A., Kraft, M. K., & Kerr, J. (2006). An ecological approach to creating active living communities. *Annual Review of Public Health, 27,* 297–322.

Sallis, J. F., & Glanz, K. (2006). The role of built environments in physical activity, eating, and obesity in childhood. *The Future of Children, 16*(1), 89–108.

Schilling, J., & Linton, L. S. (2005). The public health roots of zoning: In search of active living's legal genealogy. *American Journal of Preventive Medicine, 28*(2S2), 96–104.

Schmid, T. L., Pratt, M., & Witmer, L. (2006). A framework for physical activity policy research. *Journal of Physical Activity and Health, 3*(Suppl. 1), S20–1S29.

Schwartz, M. B., & Brownell, K. D. (2007). Actions necessary to prevent childhood obesity: Creating the climate for change. *Journal of Law, Medicine and Ethics, 35*(1), 78–89.

Shinn, M., & Toohey, S. M. (2003). Community contexts of human welfare. *Annual Review of Psychology, 54,* 427–459.

Slater, S. J., Chaloupka, F. J., Wakefield, M., Johnston, L. D., & O'Malley, P. M. (2007). The impact of retail cigarette marketing practices on youth smoking uptake. *Archives of Pediatrics and Adolescent Medicine, 161,* 440–445.

Smetana, J. G., Campione-Barr, N., & Metzger, A. (2006). Adolescent development in interpersonal and societal contexts. *Annual Review of Psychology, 57,* 255–284.

Stokols, D. (2006). Toward a science of transdisciplinary action research. *American Journal of Community Psychology, 38,* 63–77.

Substance Abuse and Mental Health Services Administration. (2004). *Results from the 2003 National Survey on Drug Use and Health: National findings* (DHHS Publication No. SMA 04–3964). Rockville, MD: Office of Applied Studies.

Task Force on Community Prevention Services. (2005). *The guide to community preventive services: What works to promote health?* New York: Oxford University Press.

Thompson, C. C., Hamilton, W. L., Siegel, M. B., Biener, L., & Rigotti, N. A. (2007). Effects of local youth-access regulations on progression to established smoking among youth in Massachusetts. *Tobacco Control, 16,* 119–126.

Trenholm, C., Devaney, B., Fortson, K., Quay, L., Wheeler, J., & Clark, M. (2007). *Impacts of four Title V, Section 510, abstinence educational programs.* Retrieved August 1, 2007, from www.mathematica-mpr.com.

Treno, A. J., Grube, J. W., & Martin, S. E. (2003). Alcohol availability as a predictor of youth drinking and driving: A hierarchical analysis of survey and archival data. *Alcoholism: Clinical and Experimental Research, 27,* 835–840.

U.S. Department of Health and Human Services. (1994). *Preventing tobacco use among young people: A report of the Surgeon General.* Atlanta: Author.

U.S. Department of Health and Human Services, Food and Drug Administration. (1996). Regulations restricting the sale and distribution of cigarettes and smokeless tobacco to protect children and adolescents: Final rule. 21 C.F.R. Part 801, *Federal Register, 61,* 44, 396–45,318.

U.S. Department of Health and Human Services. (2006). *The health consequences of involuntary exposure to tobacco smoke: A report of the Surgeon General.* Atlanta: Author.

U.S. Federal Trade Commission. (2001). Cigarette report for 1999. Retrieved August 8, 2007, from www.ftc.gov/reports/cigarettes/1999cigarettereport.pdf.

Voas, R. B., Tippetts, A. S., & Fell, J. C. (2003). Assessing the effectiveness of minimum legal drinking age and zero tolerance laws in the United States. *Accident Analysis and Prevention, 35*(4), 579–587.

Wagenaar, A. C., Murray, D. M., Gehan, J. P., Wolfson, M., Forster, J. L., Toomey, T. L., Perry, C. L., & Jones-Webb, R. (2000). Communities Mobilizing for Change on Alcohol: Outcomes from a randomized community trial. *Journal of Studies on Alcohol, 61,* 85–94.

Wagenaar, A. C, Murray, D. M., & Toomey, T. L. (2000). Communities Mobilizing for Change on Alcohol (CMCA): Effects of a randomized trial on arrests and traffic crashes. *Addiction, 95,* 209–217.

Wagenaar, A. C., & Toomey, T. L. (2002). Effects of minimum drinking age laws: Review and analyses of the literature from 1960 to 2000. *Journal of Studies on Alcohol,* (Suppl. 14), 206–225.

Wagenaar, A. C., Toomey, T. L., & Lenk, K. M. (2004/2005). Environmental influences on young adult drinking. *Alcohol Research and Health, 28*(4), 230–235.

Wakefield, M. A., Terry-McElrath, Y. M., Chaloupka, F. J., Barker, D. C., Slater, S. J., Clark, P. I., & Giovino, G. A. (2002). Tobacco industry marketing at point of purchase after the 1998 MSA billboard advertising ban. *American Journal of Public Health, 92*(6), 937–940.

Warner, K. E., Citrin, T., Pickett, G., Rabe, B. G., Wagenaar, A., & Stryker, J. (1990). Licit and illicit drug policies: A typology. *British Journal of Addiction, 85,* 255–262.

Wellman, R. J., Sugarman, D. B., DiFranza, J. R., & Winickoff, J. O. (2006). The extent to which tobacco marketing and tobacco use in films contribute to children's use of tobacco: A meta-analysis. *Archives of Pediatrics and Adolescent Medicine, 160*(12), 1285–1296.

World Health Organization. (2007). *Framework convention on tobacco control.* Retrieved July 18, 2007, from www.who.int/tobacco/framework/download/en/index.html.

Yancey, A. K., Fielding, J. E., Flores, G. R., Sallis, J. F., McCarthy, W. J., & Breslow, L. (2007). Creating a robust public health infrastructure for physical activity promotion. *American Journal of Preventive Medicine, 32*(1), 68–78.

CHAPTER

LEGAL AND ETHICAL ISSUES IN ADOLESCENT HEALTH CARE AND RESEARCH

ABIGAIL ENGLISH ▪ JOHN S. SANTELLI ▪ AUDREY SMITH ROGERS

LEARNING OBJECTIVES

After studying this chapter, you will be able to

- Evaluate legal and ethical contexts fundamental to the promotion of adolescent health.

- Explain the specific human rights of adolescents related to health.

- Differentiate between state and federal regulations that are associated with the health and medical privacy of minors.

Adolescents face diverse risks to their health and well-being, often as a result of behaviors that begin during the teen years. The health consequences of these behavioral risks may be aggravated or ameliorated by laws and ethical principles that inhibit or facilitate access to health care and participation in research. An understanding by health care professionals and by teenagers themselves of adolescents' legal rights may improve access to health care and health promotion. Moreover, recognition of key principles of ethics and human rights can also support health care access and health promotion for adolescents. This chapter explains the legal, ethical, and human rights contexts that are important for reducing the adverse effects of risk behaviors and promoting adolescent health.

HEALTH, HUMAN RIGHTS, AND ETHICAL PRINCIPLES

Both the principles of human rights embodied in international agreements and the principles of ethics articulated by official entities within the United States provide useful standards to guide policy development, clinical care, and advocacy on behalf of adolescents and their health. Documents of particular significance include the U.N. Convention on the Rights of the Child (United Nations, 1989) and the Belmont Report, issued by the National Commission for the Protection of Human Subjects of Biomedical and Behavioral Research (1979).

International Human Rights

Although important American leaders such as Eleanor Roosevelt and Jimmy Carter have been major champions of human rights, the United States has not fully accepted some of the most important embodiments of human rights principles that could be used to promote and protect the health of adolescents. Nevertheless, international human rights agreements and treaties provide a legal and ethical framework for health education and health services that may prevent or mitigate the negative impact of adolescent risk behaviors on health. The right to health is recognized in numerous international agreements (Freedman, 1995), including Article 25.1 of the Universal Declaration of Human Rights (United Nations, 1948), the United Nations Convention on the Rights of the Child (1989), and the Programme of Action of the International Conference on Population and Development, Cairo, 1994 (United Nations, 1994). Under these agreements, governments have an obligation to provide accurate health education information and access to health care services (Freedman, 1995).

Under Article 24 of the Convention on the Rights of the Child, signatories must "recognize the right of the child to the enjoyment of the highest attainable standard of health and to facilities for the treatment of illness and rehabilitation of health . . . [and] strive to ensure that no child is deprived of his or her right of access to such health care services." Although the United States is not a formal signatory to the convention, it sets forth an important international standard that should be consulted for guidance, even if it is not legally binding in the United States.

Moreover, under the Convention on the Rights of the Child, which is interpreted and updated by the Committee on the Rights of the Child, the special status of adolescents is recognized (United Nations, 2003). Adolescents are "active rights holders"—persons with their own human rights. Adolescents demonstrate emerging capacity for independent decisions about health, but also deserve continuing special protections in light of their unique vulnerabilities. The convention also recognizes the responsibilities, legal rights, and duties of parents to provide direction and guidance to children and adolescents. These rights and responsibilities should take account of the child's age and maturity while providing a safe and supportive environment.

The specific rights of adolescents related to health include the right to nondiscrimination, the right to express views freely, the right to legal protections about health care, the right to information, the right to privacy and confidentiality, and right to protection from abuse, neglect, violence, and exploitation (United Nations, 2003). The right to nondiscrimination is inclusive with regard to race, color, sex, language, religion, political opinion, disability, sexual orientation, and health status (including infection with HIV), and national, ethnic, or social origin. Governments have obligations to ensure these rights, including the provision of health and sexuality education and health services and the involvement of adolescents in their provision. Governments also have an obligation to create safe and supportive environments and to protect adolescents from labor exploitation and harmful traditional practices such as female genital mutilation. According to the committee's interpretation of the convention, primary health care services should be sensitive to the health needs and human rights of adolescents and should be available, accessible, acceptable to adolescents, and of good quality.

Under the Convention on the Rights of the Child, the special status of adolescents is recognized.

The Belmont Report

The Belmont Report, published in 1979, is an excellent primer on research ethics (National Commission, 1979). It provides an important ethical foundation for the conduct of research. These same principles are also highly applicable to the clinical practice of health care. Professional groups have used these ethical principles in creating standards for proper conduct for researchers and clinicians (Frankel, 1993; Rogers, Kinsman, Santelli, & Silber, 1999; Santelli et al., 2003). The Belmont Report describes three fundamental ethical principles: respect for persons, beneficence, and justice.

Respect for persons means treating people as autonomous beings and not as a means to an end. Within this principle are two basic obligations: honoring the autonomous choices of persons with the capacity to make their own decisions and protecting the welfare of those for whom this capacity is diminished.

The first tenet imposes obligations for fully informed and autonomous decision making in the provision of health care and in research participation. Individuals in both clinical and research settings are to be afforded their right to self-determination. The full exercise of this right demands that persons be provided with understandable information about a proposed intervention's intended benefits and potential risks, that they comprehend the information, and that they choose to participate freely and without undue influence, coercion, or intimidation.

Respect for persons also demands that special protections be extended to groups with diminished autonomy. These include persons with diminished capacity for informed decision making, such as children, and those with limited ability to exercise free choice, such as prisoners. The Belmont Report (National Commission, 1979) noted that individuals may "lose this capacity wholly or in part because of illness, mental disability, or circumstances that severely restrict liberty." The report further noted that self-determination is a capacity that "matures over an individual's life." When this capacity is limited or restricted, there exists an ethical obligation to protect the welfare of these individuals.

Adolescents who have not reached the age of majority in their respective jurisdictions represent individuals for whom both autonomy and protection might seem to apply. However, their near-complete cognitive development, their demonstrated capacity for life decisions, and their imminent legal status as adults combine to indicate that their situation is essentially different from that of younger children (Dubler & Nimmons, 1992, pp. 285–302). During early adolescence (circa age twelve to fourteen), most teens attain cognitive capacity similar to young adults (Weithorn & Scherer, 1994). Yet adolescents may lack the full set of experiences that inform good judgment and may therefore require some degree of protection. Moreover, no developmental theory supports a magical transformation on a specified birthday; the cognitive capacity of adolescents can vary considerably across individuals. Adolescents have a basic right to be supported in achieving full autonomy and realizing self-determination.

Beneficence is the ethical obligation to do good and to avoid harm. In clinical care and research, this means maximizing benefits and minimizing risks. Efforts to increase access to health care are prompted by this desire to do good.

Traditionally, this professional obligation to act for the benefit of others often has become confused with *paternalism* and unilateral decisions being made in behalf of the patient for his or her own good. This past century brought balance and clarity with new respect to the research subject's right to self-determination. Consequently, a newer understanding developed in health care as well. Thereafter, the obligation for beneficence expanded to include providing the individual patient with the information and support required for shared decision making.

Providing health care consistent with this principle of beneficence to adolescents as they transition into adulthood requires careful attention to the balance between possible "goods" and possible harms. In respecting the growing capacity of the adolescent to make decisions independently of his or her parent, the provider should not succumb to paternalism, becoming an alternate parent. Rather, the provider should seek to facilitate the development of a more mature relationship within the family unit, thus optimizing good.

Beneficence provides the ethical basis for conducting research that seeks to improve the health and well-being of participants. Such benefit may accrue to individuals or groups or both. It provides a general guideline that helps determine the acceptability of a research study by requiring consideration of a balance of the predicted benefits against the predicted risks. Researchers may not deliberately cause harm to a research participant to benefit others. To the extent that study design permits, study subjects can be provided opportunities for health education, social support, and linkage to needed or desired services (Santelli et al., 2003). The research experience can be an opportunity for the adolescent to develop empathy and compassion (Weithorn & Scherer, 1994, p. 147). Federal policies to extend the benefits of research to women, minorities, children, and adolescents by promoting their inclusion in research studies are motivated by this principle of beneficence.

Justice in the clinical realm demands fairness in access to health care and the distribution of benefits according to health needs. This principle of justice thus requires attention to disparities in access to care and disparities in health outcomes. Many public programs such as Medicaid and the State Children's Health Insurance Program are designed to redress disparities in health care access. Health and health care are increasingly seen as a human right to which all persons are entitled, consistent with the ethical principle of justice.

Justice in the realm of research entails a fair sharing of the benefits and burdens of research and is important in the selection of research participants. Research should not be conducted with groups or communities who are unlikely to benefit from the findings. Specific communities or specific groups should not be exploited for the benefits of others. For example, the conduct of pharmaceutical trials overseas by U.S. companies has been questioned, when citizens of those countries are unlikely to benefit directly from these new treatments.

Promoting participation by groups that historically have been excluded from research is also founded on the principle of justice. If certain groups of persons are systematically excluded from participation in research, these groups may not share in the beneficial results of that research. For example, women in the 1980s were excluded from certain cardiovascular prevention trials; thus, clinicians could not be sure that interventions tested with men would be effective with women. Similarly, adolescents have often been omitted or excluded from research studies due to uncertainties about their legal status and other factors, thus contributing to a paucity of knowledge about critical issues regarding clinical treatment and behavioral interventions.

Research should not be conducted with groups or communities who are unlikely to benefit from the findings.

The Belmont Report (National Commission, 1979) notes two important components of the principle of justice. First, research subjects cannot be "systematically selected . . . because of their easy availability, their compromised position, or their manipulability." Second, when research is publicly funded, the individuals who bear the risks of research must be "among the (likely) beneficiaries of subsequent applications of the research."

There are several common ways in which justice can be violated in the area of adolescent health research. There is a continuing need to design constructive preventive health programs for adolescents and to evaluate effective health care management for specific morbidities. When institutional review boards (IRBs) are overly focused on the protection of research subjects and are faced with the complexity of adolescent issues, they may choose to exclude adolescent study participants entirely. Alternatively, IRBs may be so concerned with potential parental reactions or may become so risk-averse that research efforts with adolescents are effectively stopped (Rogers, Schwarz, et al., 1999). IRBs and investigators need to work together to insure appropriate inclusion of adolescents in studies that may improve their health.

Professional Codes of Conduct

One hallmark of a profession is its capacity to delineate and impose obligations of competency and trustworthiness on its members (Beauchamp & Childress, 1994, p. 7). These obligations are promulgated in codes of conduct. Medical and allied health professions have established codes of conduct governing their corresponding professional practices; many have corresponding codes for the conduct of research. Codes of conduct fulfill multiple functions. The Society of Adolescent Medicine's Code of Research Ethics (Rogers, Kinsman, et al., 1999) notes that a *code* "reflects a collective professional conscience . . . based on collective experiences and distinct traditions" and "constitutes a basis for evaluating behavior and holding individual professionals accountable . . . and (responsible) for the collective integrity of the society." A code also serves to socialize new members into the ethical life of the profession and provides standards that can be used in judging allegations of misconduct (Frankel, 1993). These standards are based on ethical principles.

As noted earlier, the landmark Belmont Report (National Commission, 1979) stipulated three principles essential to the conduct of ethical research: respect for persons, beneficence, and justice. Beauchamp and Childress (1994) identified the principles underlying ethical medical practice as respecting the patient's autonomy, non-maleficence, beneficence, and justice. They noted that respect for the individual's autonomy and justice are relatively new additions to medical ethics.

Ethical codes are based on these fundamental principles, but cannot consist of principles alone. Their functionality derives from their applicability to guiding and judging the experience of professional practice. *Principles* are the skeleton of the code whose body is composed of critical information from professional traditions, collective experiences, relevant disciplines, and procedural and policy considerations (Beauchamp & Childress, 1994). Thus, the body of the professional code continues to be informed by these and other factors, while the skeleton endures as the code's fundamental base.

In the realm of health care, the practice codes of the major medical and allied health professions uniformly acknowledge the need to provide confidential services as a part of ethical and effective practice (Morreale, Stinnett, & Dowling, 2005). Physicians have duties to the patient specific to confidentiality, communication, and the disclosure of information. Here again, for adolescents as patients, there is a crucial balance between the protection of individuals with limited capacity and the empowerment of that developing capacity. In practice, achieving this balance requires a careful and sensitive delineation of the role of parents or guardians in the services provided to their adolescents. Adolescent patients certainly deserve privacy, but adolescents often engage in behaviors that can be unacceptable to their parents or guardians or actually harmful to themselves or others. Honoring the adolescent's person means clarifying the limits of confidentiality a priori; clearly the teen must be informed that potential harm to self or others will require disclosure in accordance with the provider's legal and ethical obligations, including in certain circumstances a duty to warn. At the same time, parents and adolescents need to appreciate the limits of disclosure specific to behaviors that are unacceptable to the parent, that may carry manageable risk, and whose unilateral disclosure may force the teen away from health care and guidance altogether. In these cases, providers should continue to work with the teen to facilitate the involvement and care of parents or guardians when sustained adult guidance is indicated.

LEGAL STATUS OF ADOLESCENTS AND ACCESS TO HEALTH CARE

During the second half of the twentieth century, the legal status of children evolved in ways that have major significance for both their health care and their participation in biomedical and behavioral research (English & Morreale, 2001). Under traditional English common law, children were considered the property (or "chattel") of their parents. The "personhood" of children received increasing legal recognition as states enacted child abuse reporting laws and medical consent laws affecting adolescents and as the United States Supreme Court began to extend constitutional protection to minors beginning in the 1960s. The United States Supreme Court explicitly extended the due process protection of the Fourteenth Amendment to children as well as adults in its 1967 decision *In re Gault* and extended the protection of the constitutional right of privacy to minors in a series of decisions beginning in 1976 with *Planned Parenthood of Central Missouri* v. *Danforth* (English & Morreale, 2001; Gardner & Wilcox, 1993). These legal developments acknowledged that although parents usually act in the best interest of their children, there is not always a congruence of interests among children, their parents, and the state. The state may need to intervene to protect the welfare of children and adolescents (Holder, 1992). Likewise, legal developments in the late twentieth century recognized adolescents' increasing capacity to make independent, rational decisions about their own health.

During the adolescent period, persons move from childhood to adulthood—from dependence and protection by parents to legal and functional autonomy. Their evolving legal status is expressed in several key concepts, such as age of majority, minor consent, emancipated minors, and mature minors. Although these concepts are applicable in different jurisdictions, the specific laws that embody them vary considerably among the states. Good sources of information on state laws regarding adolescents and consent for their health care are the Center for Adolescent Health and the Law (www.cahl.org) and the Guttmacher Institute (www.guttmacher.org/sections/adolescents.php). In addition, many organizations of health care professionals, such as the Society for Adolescent Medicine, the American Academy of Pediatrics, and the American Medical Association, have developed policies and ethical codes that provide guidance on the delivery of health care appropriate for adolescents, including confidential care when that best serves their health needs (Morreale, Stinnett, & Dowling, 2005).

All states recognize an *age of majority,* the age at which children become adults and are allowed to make independent decisions in many realms, including decisions about their own health. In most, but not all, states this is age eighteen (English, Matthews, Extavour, Palamountain, & Yang, 1995). Generally the consent of a parent is required for health care that is provided to a minor child, including an adolescent, under age eighteen. However, all states have also adopted a set of laws, known as *minor consent laws,* which allow adolescents to give their own consent for health care, depending either on their status or on the specific services they are seeking. Many of these laws were enacted in the 1960s and 1970s (English & Morreale, 2001; Melton, 1989).

Every state has laws that allow one or more of the following groups of minors to consent for their own health care: emancipated minors, minors living apart from their parents, married minors, minors in the armed services, pregnant minors, minor parents, high school graduates, or minors over a certain age. Minors who meet the legal criteria for emancipation would almost always be recognized as having the right to consent for their own health care, whether or not they have a legal declaration of emancipation issued pursuant to a formal state procedure. In addition, every state has laws that allow minors of varying ages to give their own consent for one or more of the following types of health care: general medical care, emergency care, family planning or contraceptive services, pregnancy-related care, diagnosis and treatment for sexually transmitted disease, HIV/AIDS care, diagnosis and treatment for reportable infectious or communicable disease, care for sexual assault, drug or alcohol care, and outpatient mental health services.

From an ethical perspective, autonomy in health care for adolescents includes both the right to consent to medical care and the right to privacy during the course of that treatment. A broad array of state and federal laws provide protection for the delivery of confidential health care to adolescents. For example, the minor consent laws themselves often contain confidentiality protections (English & Ford, 2003). Moreover, adolescents' interest in privacy has been protected in a long line of constitutional decisions by federal and state courts. The United States Supreme Court has recognized that the constitutional right of privacy protects minors as well as adults, particularly for reproductive health care, including contraceptives and abortion, albeit with some limitations related to abortion that do not apply in the case of adults (*Planned Parenthood of Missouri* v. *Danforth, 1976; Carey* v. *Population Services International, 1977: and Belloti* v. *Baird, 1979;* Gans, 1993;). Federal law has also provided confidentiality protection for family planning and drug and alcohol treatment services to minors (Gans, 1993; Department of Health and Human Services, 2002).The federal government has also promulgated broad medical privacy regulations, the *HIPAA Privacy*

Rule, which provides protection for the confidentiality of health care information of persons of all ages, including adolescents (English & Ford, 2004; Department of Health and Human Services, 2003.) The HIPAA Privacy Rule contains important provisions that affect the conduct of both clinical care and research (Department of Health and Human Services, 2002).The HIPAA Privacy Rule treats minors who consent for their own care as "individuals" who are afforded many of the same rights as adults. However, with respect to the specific issue of disclosure of information to parents and parents' access to protected records, the HIPAA Privacy Rule defers to the provisions of "state and other applicable law." If state or other law is silent, the rule defers to the discretion of health care professionals exercising medical judgment to determine whether information should be accessible to parents (English & Ford, 2004).

Laws that allow adolescents to consent for their own heath care and that provide confidentiality protections for that care acknowledge the importance of timely diagnosis and treatment, the deleterious public health impact of untreated conditions, the frequent failure of adolescents and parents to discuss health and behavior issues, and the emerging capacity of adolescents to make autonomous decisions. These laws are an essential component of any effort to address the health effects of adolescent risk behaviors.

RESEARCH REGULATION AND ETHICS

Research is essential to understanding adolescent health risk behavior and to promote the creation of programs that prevent risky behavior or interventions that ameliorate its consequences (Santelli et al., 2003). Prevention research can improve the practice of health promotion, and research on health services and clinical care can improve the care of adolescents. For adolescents to receive the full benefits of health research, they must be included as participants in that research. At the same time, the history of abuses in health research suggests that strong protections are needed to prevent harm to adolescents and other groups (Beecher, 1966; Lederer & Grodin, 1994). Research such as the Tuskegee study (in which prisoners were intentionally exposed to syphilis without being informed or treated) have created profound distrust, particularly within the African American community, about research and researchers, and such distrust has had serious repercussions in the environment for AIDS research in these communities (Thomas & Quinn, 1991). Tuskegee poignantly demonstrated the potential for initially well-intentioned researchers to fail profoundly in their ethical obligations to research subjects.

Protection from Harm

Current ethical thinking about research is shaped by twin and potentially conflicting imperatives to insure inclusion in research and to protect persons from the potential harmful consequences of research. These twin imperatives are reflected in federal regulations that promote inclusion in and protection from research. Adolescents are protected by the general federal regulations (45 CFR Part 46, DHHS 2001), as well as the regulations that address research with children (45 CFR Part 46, Subpart D, DHHS 2001). Although a separate set of regulations for adolescents does not exist, the regulations for children recognize the developmental changes of adolescence and the legal protections afforded adolescent minors in state laws that provide for minor consent for health care.

U.S. regulations on research (Department of Health and Human Services [DHHS], 2001) provide for a nationwide system of IRBs located within institutions conducting research (such as universities), which are regulated by the Office for Human Research Protections within the Department of Health and Human Services (Levine, 2001). For research involving living persons, IRBs must assess the risks and benefits to participants, ensure proper informed consent procedures, and provide special protections for vulnerable populations.

Honoring the principle of respecting persons requires the investigator to submit to independent review and oversight to ensure that a full informed consent process is in place and that the rights and welfare of research subjects are protected. The federal regulations spell out required elements of informed consent and special situations where the IRB may waive informed consent or modify informed consent procedures.

Specific subparts of the regulations (DHHS, 2001) include protections for vulnerable populations and provide special safeguards for pregnant women, fetuses, and neonates (Subpart B); prisoners (Subpart C); and children (Subpart D). Some issues of particular relevance for adolescents are addressed in Subpart D. Other populations such as persons who are cognitively impaired or socially disenfranchised do not have special sections in the regulations per se, but are nonetheless recognized as deserving special consideration.

Subpart D includes a definition of children, requirements for parental permission and the assent of the child, conditions under which parental permission may be waived, limitations on the kinds of research that is permitted, and protections for children who are wards of the state. Under Subpart D, research is categorized by its potential benefits and risks—requirements, balanced by the prospect of benefit, become more stringent as risk increases.

Parents or guardians are asked for permission for their children to participate in the research (only individuals can personally consent), and assent must be sought from children themselves, who are not yet capable of true informed consent. Children's assent is required, unless the research participation represents "the prospect of direct benefit that is important to the health or well-being of the children and is available only in the context of the research" (45 CFR 46.408; DHHS, 2001). The assent of older adolescents should carry more weight than that of younger children (Weithorn & Scherer, 1994, p. 154), and any move to waive their assent, particularly in the face of their active refusal, merits consideration by a properly constituted ethics board.

In Subpart D, *children* are defined as "persons who have not attained the *legal age for consent to treatments or procedures involved in the research,* under the applicable law of the jurisdiction in which the research will be conducted" (45 CFR 46.402; DHHS, 2005; emphasis added). This definition is important for determining whose permission or informed consent is required for an adolescent to participate in a research study—that of the parent or the adolescent. If the adolescent is classified as a child, parental permission and the assent of the adolescent is required, although the IRB may waive parental permission under specified circumstances. If the adolescent is not classified as a child, parental permission is not required and the informed consent of the adolescent is required.

The definition of children changed three times between 1973 and final publication in 1983 of the regulations for children in Subpart D (Santelli et al., 2003). This record is helpful in interpreting the definition of children in the current regulations. The original 1973 version defined children as "individuals who have not attained the *legal age of consent to participate in research* as determined under the applicable law of the jurisdiction in which the proposed research is to be conducted" (emphasis added). Because most states do not define an age of consent for research, a second definition was proposed in 1978. It referred to "persons who have not attained the *legal age of consent to general medical care.*" During the comment period, DHHS realized that many states allowed minors to consent to specific services such as STD treatment without parental permission under so-called "minor consent" statutes. The final definition in 1983 was changed to "persons who have not attained *the legal age for consent to treatments or procedures involved in the research.*" Thus, this final definition of children in the research regulations specifically references state laws on consent for medical treatment. These include laws defining the age of majority, emancipation, consent for general medical care, and consent by minors for their own health care in the treatment of specific conditions such as STDs, mental health disorders, and substance use.

If the adolescent is not classified as a child, parental permission is not required and the informed consent of the adolescent is required.

Based on a hierarchy of risk and benefit, Subpart D allows only four categories of research involving children: (1) research that involves no more than minimal risk; (2) research that involves more than minimal risk, but where there is a potential for direct benefit to individual research subjects; (3) research that involves a minor increase over minimal risk without direct benefit, but is likely to yield generalizable knowledge about the participant's disorder or condition; and (4) research that is not otherwise approvable but presents an opportunity to understand, prevent, or alleviate a serious problem affecting the health or welfare of children. Minimal risk is defined as "the probability and magnitude of harm or discomfort anticipated . . . are not greater . . . than those ordinarily encountered in daily life or during the performance of routine physical or psychological examinations or tests" (DHHS, 2001).

Specific requirements exist for each category of risk and benefit. All four categories require the assent of the child and the permission of one or both parents. *Assent* is the child's affirmative agreement to participate in research, whereas *permission* is the agreement of parent(s) or guardian(s) to their child's or ward's participation in research. The federal regulations use the terms *permission* and *assent* to distinguish these processes from the informed consent process with adults. Parents are not the research subjects and generally do not experience risks or benefits from the research. Younger children may lack the intellectual capacity or judgment to make decisions about research, although the concept of assent recognizes their emerging developmental capacity to provide informed consent as they mature. In accordance with the recommendations of the National Commission (1979), assent is commonly obtained from children aged seven and older. Beginning at twelve to fourteen years of age, assent forms for adolescents should closely resemble the consent forms used with adults.

Beginning at twelve to fourteen years of age, assent forms for adolescents should closely resemble the consent forms used with adults.

Subpart D also permits the waiver of parental or guardian permission, allowing the "older child" or adolescent to be the decision maker and consent independently to research participation. The U.S. regulations provide no guidance on how this determination of capacity should be made. Research by Weithorn and Scherer (1994, p. 152) suggests that "the cognitive functioning of fourteen-year-olds clearly appears sophisticated enough and sufficiently grounded in reason to meet legal criteria of competency to consent to most types of treatment and research." Teens older than age fourteen can be assumed to have adequate capacity. However, despite adult-level understanding and capacity, older adolescents can remain susceptible to pressures that compromise the voluntariness of their consent, such as institutional coercion. But unlike adults, these pressures may come from the very parents or guardians whose involvement has been required to "protect" them from such pressures.

The federal regulations governing research allow the IRB to waive parental permission in specific circumstances. Section 46.408 addresses the waiver of parental permission: "In addition to the provisions for waiver contained in 46.116 of Subpart A, if an IRB determines that a research protocol is designed for conditions or a subject population for which parental permission *is not a reasonable requirement* to protect subjects (e.g., neglected or abused children), it may waive consent requirements provided an appropriate mechanism for protecting the children who will participate as research subjects is substituted and provided the waiver is not inconsistent with federal, state, or local law" (DHHS, 2001; emphasis added).

In its report *Research Involving Children,* the National Commission listed other examples of appropriate situations for waiving parental permission: "research designed to identify factors related to the incidence or treatment of certain conditions in adolescents for which they may legally receive treatment without parental consent; research in which the subjects are 'mature minors' and the procedures involved entail essentially no more than minimal risk that such individuals might reasonably assume on their own; research designed to meet the needs of children designated by their parents as in 'need of supervision,' and research involving children whose parents are legally or functionally incompetent" (National Commission, 1977).

Similar to the protections provided to prisoners, special protections are also provided to children who are wards of the state, such as those in foster care (National

Commission, 1977). Research is limited to issues related to their status as wards or research conducted in schools, camps, hospitals, institutions, or similar settings in which the majority of children involved are not wards. IRBs are required to appoint an advocate for each child who is a ward, in addition to a legal guardian or other person in loco parentis. The advocate shall be an individual who must agree to act in the best interests of the child and cannot be associated in any way with the research, the investigators, or the guardian organization—except in the role as advocate or member of the IRB.

Research in Schools

Research studies conducted in schools are covered by two additional federal laws: the Family Educational Rights and Privacy Act (FERPA) and the Protection of Pupil Rights Amendment (PPRA). FERPA addresses the privacy of student educational records and the circumstances under which educational records may be accessed, amended, or disclosed. PPRA specifically addresses surveys administered in schools. PPRA requires that written parental permission be obtained for students who are not emancipated prior to participation in certain surveys or evaluations funded by the U.S. Department of Education (DOE) that collect information about the following eight specific topics:

1. Mental health and psychological problems

2. Sexual behaviors or attitudes

3. Illegal, antisocial, self-incriminating, or demeaning behaviors

4. Critical appraisals of individuals with whom respondents have close family relationships

5. Religious practices, affiliations, or beliefs

6. Political affiliations or beliefs

7. Income

8. Legally recognized privileged relationships such as those with physicians, lawyers, or ministers

Surveys not funded by the DOE that address any of these eight topics may be conducted after parental notification and after allowing parents the chance to opt out. In addition, parents have a right to inspect questionnaires and instructional materials used in conjunction with surveys, analyses, or evaluations. Local education agencies must notify parents at least annually about school policies regarding these rights and any upcoming surveys. These rights to privacy and informed consent transfer to students when they become adults or are emancipated. Additional information on these issues can be found at www.ed.gov/policy/gen/guid/fpco/index.html.

Ensuring Inclusion

During the 1990s, children and adolescents, women, and minority groups won increased rights to participation in research. Women's groups pointed out the frequent exclusion of women from many cardiovascular prevention trials, and AIDS activists demanded increased access to treatment, often available only through clinical trials. These groups successfully demanded increased access to research, leading the Congress to enact the National Institutes of Health (NIH) Revitalization Act of 1993 (NIH, 1994). This act is designed to ensure that women and members of minority groups are included in all NIH-funded clinical research. In 1998, given similar concerns about exclusion of children from research, the NIH issued the NIH Policy and Guidelines on the Inclusion of Children as Participants in Research Involving Human Subjects (NIH, 1998). The goal of this policy, which covers persons under the age of twenty-one, was "to increase the participation of children in research so that adequate data will be developed to support the treatment modalities for disorders and conditions that affect adults and may also affect children" (NIH, 1998). This policy states that children "must be included in all human subjects' research, conducted or supported by the NIH, unless there are scientific and ethical reasons not to include them" (NIH, 1998). Although much of the impetus for inclusion policies was fair access to clinical trials, notions of inclusion also apply broadly to health risk behavior research.

Federal inclusion policies are motivated by the ethical principles articulated in the Belmont Report. Given the prior history of research abuse, this report focused on protecting individuals from harmful research. Although research may entail risk, it also holds the potential to bring great benefit. The principles from Belmont, particularly justice, can be used to weigh both potential benefits and risks. Policies promoting inclusion in research are rooted in the principle of justice and the concept of nondiscrimination. Considering the ethics of access to research represents a fundamental shift in ethical and regulatory thinking (Levine, 1995). Protection remains essential, but these policies add an additional emphasis on inclusion. Research has been "transformed" from a fundamentally dangerous activity from which persons must be protected to one seen as entailing much promise of benefit (Levine, 1995). Thus, participation in research is essential if individuals and groups are to accrue the full benefits of research. The IRB takes on an expanded role—from thinking about risk and benefit for the individual to considering the balancing of protection and inclusion for groups as well.

SUMMARY

Current laws in the United States provide a strong set of legal protections for adolescents who need health care. They also establish a strong framework for protection and inclusion in biomedical and behavioral research. Inclusion in research on health behaviors is essential if we are to help adolescents prevent unhealthy risk taking and the outcomes of these behaviors. This body of law recognizes new health needs of adolescents and their developing capacity for autonomous decision making. Moreover, these laws reflect the thinking in most nations expressed in international human rights treatises and other agreements. Adolescent rights to health, health care, and health education are human rights. Human rights language is an appropriate and useful way to frame the legal protections for adolescents in clinical care and health research. The behavior of clinicians and researchers should be guided by the ethical codes created by their professional organizations and by a comprehensive understanding of adolescents' human and legal rights.

KEY TERMS

Age of majority	Justice
Assent	Minor consent laws
Beneficence	Permission
Children (final definition)	Principles
Code	Respect for persons
HIPAA Privacy Rule	The Belmont Report

DISCUSSION QUESTIONS

1. Compare and contrast the Belmont Report with the HIPAA Privacy Rule. What key features are most important to the protection of adolescents?

2. If you wanted to conduct a school-based health promotion study targeting children aged ten to fourteen years, what ethical considerations must be addressed in the institutional review board application? Why?

3. In most states, the age of majority is eighteen years. Would you argue for or against a lower age of majority in the United States? Defend your response.

REFERENCES

Beauchamp, T. L., & Childress, J. F. (1994). *Principles of biomedical ethics* (4th ed.). New York: Oxford University Press.

Beecher, H. K. (1966). Ethics and clinical research. *New England Journal of Medicine, 274,* 1364–1369.

Department of Health and Human Services. (2002). Standards for Privacy of Individually Identifiable Information: Final Rule. 67 Federal Register 53267; to be codified at 45 CFR 164.502(g)(3).

Department of Health and Human Services. (2003). Protecting personal health information in research: Understanding the HIPAA Privacy Rule. Washington, DC: Author.

Department of Health and Human Services, National Institutes of Health, Office for Protection from Research Risks. (2001, November 13). Code of Federal Regulations: Title 45; Public Welfare; Part 46: Protection of Human Subjects.

Dubler, N., & Nimmons, D. (1992). *Ethics on call.* New York: Harmony Books.

English, A., & Ford, A. (2004). The HIPAA Privacy Rule and adolescents: Legal questions and clinical challenges. *Perspectives on Sexual and Reproductive Health, 36,* 80–86.

English, A., Matthews, M., Extavour, K., Palamountain, C., & Yang, J. (1995). *State minor consent statutes: A summary.* San Francisco: National Center for Youth Law.

English, A., & Morreale, M. (2001). A legal and policy framework for adolescent health care: Past, present, and future. *Houston Journal of Health Law and Policy, 1,* 63–108.

Frankel, M. S. (1993). Professional societies and responsible research conduct. In *Responsible science: Ensuring the integrity of the research process—Vol. II* (pp. 26–49). Washington, DC: National Academy of Sciences, National Academy of Engineering, & Institute of Medicine.

Freedman, L. P. (1995). Censorship and manipulation of reproductive health information. In S. Coliver (Ed.), *The right to know: Human rights and access to reproductive health information.* Philadelphia: University of Pennsylvania Press.

Gans, J. (Ed.). (1993). *Policy compendium on confidential health services for adolescents.* Chicago: American Medical Association, National Coalition on Adolescent Health.

Gardner, W., & Wilcox, B. L. (1993). Political intervention in scientific peer review: Research on adolescent sexual behavior. *American Psychologist, 48,* 972–983.

Holder, A. R. (1992). Legal issues in adolescent sexual health. *Adolescent Medicine: State of the Art Reviews, 3,* 257–268.

Lederer, S. E., & Grodin, M. A. (1994). Historical overview: Pediatric experimentation. In M. A. Grodin & L. H. Glanz (Eds.), *Children as research subjects: Science, ethics, and law* (pp. 3–25). New York: Oxford University Press.

Levine, R. J. (1995). Adolescents as research subjects without permission of their parents or guardians: Ethical considerations. *Journal of Adolescent Health, 17*(5), 286–296.

Levine, R. J. (2001). Institutional review boards: A crisis in confidence. *Annals of Internal Medicine, 134,* 161–163.

Melton, G. B. (1989). Ethical and legal issues in research and intervention. *Journal of Adolescent Health Care, 10*(3 Suppl.), 36S–44S.

Morreale, M., Stinnett, A., & Dowling, E. (2005, September). *Policy compendium on confidential health services for adolescents* (2nd ed.). Chapel Hill, NC: Center for Adolescent Health & the Law.

National Commission for the Protection of Human Subjects of Biomedical and Behavioral Research. (1977). *Report and recommendations: Research involving children* (DHEW Publication No. OS 77–0004). Washington, DC: U.S. Government Printing Office.

National Commission for the Protection of Human Subjects of Biomedical and Behavioral Research. (1979). *The Belmont Report: Ethical principles and guidelines for the protection of human subjects of research.* Washington, DC: U.S. Government Printing Office. Retrieved June 5, 2008, http://ohsr.od.nih.gov/guidelines/belmont.html.

National Institutes of Health. (1994). Revitalization Act of 1993. Retrieved June 5, 2008, from http://grants.nih.gov/grants/OLAW/pl103–43.pdf.

National Institutes of Health. (1998). NIH policy and guidelines on the inclusion of children as participants in research involving human subjects. Retrieved June 5, 2008, from http://grants.nih.gov/grants/guide/notice-files/not98–024.html.

Rogers, A. S., Kinsman, S., Santelli, J. S., & Silber, T. J. (1999). Code of research ethics: A position paper of the Society for Adolescent Medicine. *Journal of Adolescent Health, 24,* 277–282.

Rogers, A. S, Schwarz, D. F., Weissman, G., & English, A. (1999). A case study in adolescent participation in clinical research: Eleven clinical sites, one common protocol, and eleven IRBs. *IRB: A Review of Human Subjects Research, 21,* 6–10.

Santelli, J. S., Smith Rogers, A., Rosenfeld, W. D., DuRant, R. H., Dubler, N., Morreale, M., English, A., Lyss, S., Wimberly, Y., & Schissel, A. (2003). Guidelines for adolescent health research: A position paper of the Society for Adolescent Medicine. *Journal of Adolescent Health, 32,* 443–451.

Thomas, S. B., & Quinn, S. C. (1991). The Tuskegee Syphilis study, 1932 to 1972: Implications for HIV education and AIDS risk education programs in the black community. *American Journal of Public Health, 81,* 1498–1504.

United Nations. (1948, December 10). Universal Declaration of Human Rights: Resolution 217 A (III). Geneva, Switzerland: Office of the United Nations High Commissioner for Human Rights.

United Nations. (1994). Report of the International Conference on Population and Development. New York: Author.

United Nations. (1989). Convention on the Rights of the Child. New York: Author.

United Nations. (2003). Adolescent health and development in the context of the Convention on the Rights of the Child: General Comment No. 4. Geneva, Switzerland: Office of the United Nations High Commissioner for Human Rights.

Weithorn, L. A., & Scherer, D. G. (1994). Children's involvement in research participation decisions: Psychological considerations. In M. A. Grodin & L. H. Glantz (Eds.), *Children as research subjects: Science, ethics, and law* (pp. 132–179). New York: Oxford University Press.

CHAPTER

27

ADOLESCENT RISK BEHAVIORS AND ADVERSE HEALTH OUTCOMES: FUTURE DIRECTIONS FOR RESEARCH, PRACTICE, AND POLICY

RALPH J. DICLEMENTE ▪ JOHN S. SANTELLI ▪ RICHARD A. CROSBY

LEARNING OBJECTIVES

After studying this chapter, you will be able to

- Recall the major foci of programs designed to decrease health risk behaviors among adolescents.

■ Summarize cross-cutting themes in research, practice, and policy for future adolescent health promotion efforts.

■ Recognize the importance of using an interdisciplinary approach in the development of adolescent prevention interventions.

Although adolescence can sometimes be a turbulent developmental period fraught with potential threats to mental and physical health, many adolescents traverse this period unscathed. Others, unfortunately, adopt health risk behaviors that significantly compromise their mental and physical well-being, thus limiting achievement of their full potential. Risk behaviors are not, however, random, inevitable, or uncontrollable. Indeed, there is ample empirical evidence indicating that they are preventable and amenable to change.

Recent advances in intervention technology such as innovative risk reduction programs have made important contributions to reducing adolescents' risk behaviors. In addition, advances in health promotion technology such as self-deploying airbags, better shock-absorbing bicycle helmets, and a broader and more effective range of contraception options can lead to marked reductions in adverse health outcomes. And, finally, policy changes represent an emerging and valuable strategy to protect the health of adolescents. Although intervening with adolescents in small groups or individually has demonstrated effectiveness in preventing and modifying risk behaviors, policy changes can be instrumental in enhancing adolescents' health at the population level. Policy changes include new and stricter laws to discourage driving under the influence of alcohol, the mandatory requirement for using seat belts, lower speed limits, better lit roadways, lower blood alcohol concentration levels for DUI status, an increase in the age limit to purchase alcohol and cigarettes, better nutritional diets at schools, and school-based health promotion education. Many of the policy and legal statute changes have helped prevent or reduce the adverse impact of risk behaviors and enhanced the prospects for reduced morbidity and survival for adolescents experiencing an adverse health outcome (such as an auto accident). Each of these advances, policy changes, legal changes, and other changes in adolescent health promotion rely at least in part on behavior to succeed.

Adolescent health promotion programs that directly encourage individuals to adopt and maintain health-protective behaviors remain an important and practical strategy. Laws and technology designed to enhance prevention are limited by people's willingness to use technology properly and adhere to laws. Thus, it may be useful to explore models in health promotion that typically implement a variety of strategies simultaneously to maximize the likelihood adolescents will adopt and sustain risk-reducing behaviors.

Programs designed to decrease health risk behaviors among adolescents can focus on several key behavioral determinants. They may (1) enhance adolescents' awareness of the threat posed by risk behaviors, (2) increase their perception of personal vulnerability, (3) modify their beliefs, norms, attitudes, motivations, and intentions, (4) enhance behavioral skills, and (5) increase their accessibility to and the affordability of products that are health-protective. Although modifying adolescents' risk behaviors is admittedly a formidable challenge, such changes are achievable.

Multifaceted, interdisciplinary approaches have succeeded in contributing to substantial changes in risk behaviors in the last two decades. An increasing number of well-designed controlled intervention trials are yielding effective strategies indicating that theory-based, carefully crafted, and well-implemented programs can succeed in preventing the initiation of risk behaviors or reducing existing risk behaviors before they result in adverse health outcomes.

In this volume, we document exciting advances in adolescent health promotion—from theory to intervention, policy, and advocacy. Nonetheless, we cannot stop to take solace in these advances, for there remains much that needs to be accomplished. Far too many adolescents suffer from the consequences of their health risk behaviors. As Robert Frost might have advised us, "we have miles to go. . . . " The aim of this concluding chapter is to highlight key cross-cutting themes in research, practice and policy, suggesting important directions for future research, practice, and policy approaches in the field of adolescent health promotion.

PREVENTION RESEARCH AND PRACTICE ARE INTERDISCIPLINARY

The success of prevention efforts is to a large extent attributable to the heterogeneity of disciplines actively involved in the science of adolescent health promotion. Advances in prevention are being made by transcending disciplinary boundaries in theory, methodology, implementation, and evaluation strategies. The most important advances have involved not just social and behavioral science researchers and health promotion practitioners, but clinicians, policy makers, and youth advocates.

Perhaps the best opportunity to develop a coherent, effective, and interdisciplinary approach to adolescent health promotion research is through the continued integration and collaboration among researchers in the behavioral and social sciences, public health practitioners, health educators, clinicians, law and policy experts, epidemiologists, and biostatisticians. Although the development of new and more effective health promotion programs is important, equally important is the efficiency with which programs can be disseminated and integrated into sustainable components of schools, community agencies, clinics, and other adolescent-serving venues. A key aspect of this translational research-to-practice agenda is the rapid diffusion of effective strategies and technologies and the widespread adoption of evidence-based strategies, whether these strategies are innovative behavior change programs, development of vaccines (for HPV, for example), or changes in public health policy.

There is also growing recognition and support for integrative biopsychosocial models of adolescent health behavior. Theoretical models of risk taking and psychosocial models of behavior, articulated in earlier chapters of this volume, have been at the core of behavior change strategies. In fact, the biopsychosocial model, while not recent, has become even more valuable given our enhanced understanding of the role of genetic and biological processes and health behavior. Likewise, existing frameworks for understanding adolescent mental processing and decision making, and emergent frameworks such as positive youth development theory may lead to rapid advances in primary and secondary prevention strategies, as well as the development of effective maintenance strategies designed to promote long-term adoption of health-protective behaviors.

ADOLESCENT HEALTH PROMOTION NEEDS TO ADDRESS MULTIPLE LEVELS OF CAUSALITY

Historically, adolescent health was largely viewed as an individual-level health phenomenon. This perspective dominated the early days of prevention efforts. Subsequently, we have witnessed a subtle, but continuing shift from the adolescent in isolation to an emphasis on the adolescent within his or her social and environmental context. It has become increasingly clear that myriad influences—those emanating from the adolescent, as well as from relationships with family, peer networks, friends, the community, and broader societal forces such as the media—all make an impact on adolescents' health risk behavior.

As researchers and practitioners alike increasingly acknowledge the importance of social context, the need to understand adolescents' behavior within their social environment and intervene on these broader social structural levels becomes critical. Although individual-level interventions can be effective at motivating behavior change, they may not be sufficient to sustain behavior changes over protracted periods of time, particularly in the face of pervasive countervailing social pressures that promote or reinforce risk behavior. Further, addressing behavior change within individual-level interventions often lacks sufficient breadth to reach large segments of an at-risk population.

One growing area of research is designing interventions targeted at the community level. These programs are designed to promote health-protective behavior adoption and maintenance by providing adolescents with information and skills to change behavior through naturally occurring channels of influence in the community and simultaneously to provide a supportive environment that encourages health-protective behaviors. Changing community norms also reinforces and maintains health-promoting behaviors. This approach provides one avenue for ensuring a social context in which adolescents will be reminded that the healthier alternative (safer behavior) is preferred and in accordance with community standards and norms.

Community-level interventions may have four interrelated outcomes. First, they may promote the adoption of health-protective behaviors among adolescents engaged in risky behaviors. Second, they may help sustain newly acquired health-protective behaviors and, we hope, solidify these changes so that they are maintained over protracted periods of time. Third, they may serve to amplify individual-level program effects over extended time periods, thereby reducing the potential for relapse to high-risk behaviors. And finally, community-level interventions may foster an atmosphere that discourages the initial adoption of high-risk behaviors. By changing the broader influences on adolescents' risk behavior, community-level interventions greatly contribute to improvements in population-level health.

More recently, and as a direct result of this shifting emphasis from the adolescent to the adolescent within a social context, there has been growing recognition of the need for complementary approaches to adolescent health promotion. These approaches integrate strategies designed to modify adolescents' behavior and their physical environment as part of a multifaceted, coordinated prevention program.

Theory development and application form an important cornerstone in this effort to better understand and harness the factors most influential in motivating adolescents' health behavior. Derived from theory, innovative complementary intervention strategies, coordinated and systematically implemented, are far more effective than programs implemented in a fragmentary manner. As an example, though group-based interventions designed to enhance the adoption of HIV-preventive behaviors have demonstrated effectiveness, newer approaches are evaluating *hybrid intervention models* (multisystemic interventions) that complement individual-level health promotion programs with programs implemented at other levels of causality. The objective is to develop multisystemic interventions designed to reinforce health-protective messages through diverse channels of influence. Of course, these programs need to be carefully calibrated, coordinated, and precisely implemented to maximize their influence. Misaligned programs may not be optimally effective. As these multistrategy programs continue to emerge and evolve, they will increase in sophistication, complexity, and scope. However, a caveat should be noted; we cannot substitute logic for empirical evidence. These programs will need to be rigorously evaluated to demonstrate their relative efficacy vis-à-vis traditional intervention strategies.

STRATEGIES ARE NEEDED TO IMPROVE THE SUSTAINABILITY OF HEALTH PROMOTION PROGRAMS

Another key area in adolescent health promotion research is in the development of strategies to sustain intervention program effects over time. There is ample evidence from health promotion research across diverse fields that both individual-level and community-level interventions can modify health risk behaviors. However, there are also data suggesting that intervention effects decay over time. In individual-level prevention interventions, one strategy that is frequently utilized to minimize decay (or attenuation of treatment effects) is to use booster sessions subsequent to delivering the primary "dose" of the intervention. Though this has shown efficacy in reconstituting treatment effects in long-term follow-up, it is clearly labor- and time-intensive and thus costly. Given our current cost-constrained environment, alternative approaches are needed and should be explored for specific application in adolescent health promotion.

One strategy that holds promise is the use of media interventions to enhance health risk communication, motivate adoption of health-protective behaviors, reinforce prevention messages, and sustain behavior change. Media are often thought to encompass only radio or television; however, other media strategies that may be equally, if not more, appropriate for adolescents are computer-based interventions or Internet-implemented interventions. These newer technologies provide exciting opportunities to develop tailored media-based interventions. As stand-alone interventions or in complementary models in conjunction with other intervention strategies, these health risk communication media-based interventions may create a social climate that encourages continued adherence to health-protective behaviors.

New media modalities—particularly the Internet—can help increase awareness of adolescent health risks, raise awareness of the benefits of prevention, and create a climate that encourages public or private funding for adolescent health promotion. The Internet can circumvent the reticence of other media such as television and of the public schools to address socially sensitive issues such as adolescent sexuality. Thus, the many types of media can be instrumental in creating a social climate that makes a wide spectrum of prevention strategies more acceptable at both the individual and community level. For example, it is widely recognized that media attention and education around motor vehicle safety issues such as seat belt use, bicycle helmet use, and the hazards of drinking and driving prepared the public for the mandatory legislation that followed, thereby facilitating an understanding and acceptance of new laws.

Although media-based interventions may be effective in preparing the public or stimulating adolescents to consider adopting health-promoting behaviors, media interventions can also be informative, entertaining, and personally relevant. In addition, messages about adolescent health risks disseminated through diverse media channels may facilitate more open discussion of risk behavior and its adverse health consequences. Generating such discussion and framing media messages to focus on needed policy changes are the basis for media advocacy, which has received much attention as a promising approach in public health and may be equally relevant in adolescent health promotion research and practice.

Media interventions are not a panacea. It is clear that media-based interventions remain an understudied intervention modality in the United States. Indeed, media may be particularly suitable as part of a complementary health promotion strategy in which media messages are coordinated to accompany an existing individual- or community-level intervention. Whether media campaigns—in isolation or in conjunction with existing health promotion—would enjoy widespread support and success in the United States is arguable. However, media programs, even less innovative ones, may still serve to create a social climate conducive to open discussion about the magnitude and extent of adverse health consequences posed by adolescents' risk behaviors. Finally, as previously noted, media messages may reinforce prevention messages for adolescents exposed to other more intensive interventions. In this way, media campaigns may directly affect adolescents' health behavior and influence behavior indirectly by affecting social norms to help sustain newly adopted health-protective behaviors or reinforce maintenance of low-risk behaviors in the face of countervailing social pressures.

NEW AND PROMISING THEORETICAL ORIENTATIONS

Theories are developed to predict and explain phenomena. In adolescent health promotion research and practice, theories are useful in predicting and explaining why adolescents do or do not engage in behaviors that increase their risk for adverse health outcomes. Many theories have been utilized to guide exploratory research designed to identify the antecedents and determinants of health risk behaviors. Likewise, theory has played an integral role in guiding the development of programs designed to eliminate or reduce risk behaviors associated with the likelihood of experiencing an adverse health outcome.

The range of theoretical approaches possible in adolescent health promotion is diverse. Theoretical approaches from a broad spectrum of disciplines have been utilized to guide observational research regarding the determinants of health risk behaviors as well as experimental research concerning behavior change intervention. Considerable evidence suggests that theory-based interventions can be effective in promoting the adoption of health-protective behaviors. However, many theories related to behavior, econometrics, environmental psychology, communications, anthropology, and other aspects of social science remain to be tested. Part of testing and refining theory involves change. As theories become less useful or fail to guide the design and implementation of prevention interventions, they should be modified or even discarded in favor of more useful explanatory models. This process of development, elimination, and replacement is incremental and cyclical, allowing new theories to emerge, be synthesized, and embraced. The current theoretical armamentarium has been very useful in furthering our understanding of the interplay of factors that can affect both risk and protective behaviors and for guiding program design and implementation.

Adolescent health promotion could also benefit from continued theory development. New models that ask broader questions and marshal different data can be instrumental in accelerating scientific progress and innovative applications or revisions of current models. These new theories and applications should be empirically tested. Likewise, as the focus of intervention research shifts from individual-level to broader contextual interventions, a different array of theories may be required to help guide these interventions. As with any science, the field of adolescent health promotion needs to be receptive to innovation and maintain rigorous evaluation standards in the development of new methods and models.

THE NEED TO IMPROVE PREVENTION PROGRAM TRANSFER

No health promotion intervention is perfect. It should be axiomatic that not every adolescent exposed to an intervention will adopt the appropriate preventive behaviors. Such a goal is unrealistic and unnecessary to alter risk trajectory on a population level. Striving for this goal may even be counterproductive, creating inertia among policy experts, practitioners, and other consumers of adolescent health promotion research while they search for the "magic bullet" intervention that will protect everyone automatically.

This does not mean that we lower the standard for determining effective health promotion interventions. Quite the contrary, failure to adopt and maintain rigorous standards for identifying effective interventions comes with the cost of wasting scarce resources on ineffective programs. It does mean, however, that while the continued efforts of scientists and practitioners need to be directed at developing more effective interventions, existing interventions that have demonstrated programmatic efficacy need to be widely disseminated, adopted, and scaled up to have optimal impact at a population level.

Ultimately, enhancing adolescents' health does not only depend on the development and evaluation of innovative behavior change approaches, but on how effectively these interventions can be translated and integrated (into clinic practice, school curricula, or community programs). Thus, future research should also focus on identifying mechanisms for the timely translation of effective interventions into sustainable community-, clinic- or school-based programs. Successful translation in adolescent health promotion can benefit from guidelines, theoretical constructs, and approaches already developed in other areas of public health.

Without a competent and fully operational infrastructure for dissemination, it is doubtful that intervention research will be translated thoroughly enough to fulfill the promise of promoting adolescents' health.

While the research "output" for behavioral approaches to promote adolescent health has been remarkable—particularly research in the past few years using models or theory-based interventions—the "uptake" and the integration of this information into ongoing sustainable, programmatic activities has been far less plentiful. Understanding the barriers that impede the rapid adoption of new health promotion programs by governmental and community-based organizations is a critical need in the field. As described in this volume, we have many interventions known to modify adolescents' risk behavior, but we have not paid sufficient attention to their dissemination and adoption. Further study is needed in advancing our understanding of how organizations, including the individual providers within organizations, are influenced to adopt innovations in prevention and risk reduction.

The development of sustainable systems and processes for the efficient transfer of health promotion programs is contingent on many factors. Foremost is the need for an infrastructure responsible for collecting and collating new information, as well as organizing, managing, and coordinating the active transfer of information to practitioners and other consumers (policy analysts, elected officials, health department officials, clinical and social service providers, and program managers in community-based organizations). For efficient program transfer, investing in the development of an infrastructure to design and continually monitor systems and processes needed to promote rapid and widespread use of evidence-based interventions is critical. Resources will need to be identified, mobilized, and committed to the ongoing maintenance and support of the infrastructure that promotes the rapid dissemination of adolescent health promotion programs.

There is a clear distinction between the passive transfer of intervention programs and the actions required to encourage and enable the implementation of these programs. The transfer of effective strategies for individual and community use is not automatic. Rather, it must be an active and purposive application of skills, systems, and resources dedicated to supporting both the transfer and the uptake of new prevention programs. Thus, gaps and inadequacies in the infrastructure responsible for supporting the transfer and uptake of new health promotion programs will clearly limit how efficiently systems and processes can be designed, implemented, maintained, and evaluated. Without a competent and fully operational infrastructure for dissemination, it is doubtful that intervention research will be translated thoroughly enough to fulfill the promise of promoting adolescents' health. To support the adoption of these programs, it will be necessary to invest in training, the provision of relevant materials, and an ongoing program of technical assistance.

THE NEED TO MEASURE COST-EFFECTIVENESS IN HEALTH PROMOTION RESEARCH

The increasing emphasis on cost containment, the emergence of the managed care environment and the disproportionate increase in the cost of health care versus other expenditures over the past decade, has prompted examining cost-effectiveness as one criterion for evaluating adolescent health promotion programs. In a constrained fiscal environment, it becomes imperative that we not only evaluate program efficacy in terms of impact (e.g., changes in behavior, attitudes, norms, knowledge) and outcomes (e.g., changes in morbidity, mortality, and quality of life) but also assess cost-effectiveness. Such information is vitally important to program planners, policy makers, practitioners and other persons involved in the design and implementation of health promotion and disease prevention programs.

Arguably, one might question whether adolescent health promotion programs should be held accountable to the standard that a program's economic benefits to society must outweigh its financial costs. However, whether or not one accepts that standard, the application of economic evaluation techniques is as appropriate to adolescent health promotion as they are to other health programs. For example, if two programs (i.e., smoking cessation among adolescents), using rigorous evaluation methodology, yielded similar impact and outcome evaluations, but one program cost $2 per participant to achieve cessation while the other program cost $10 per participant, the cost effectiveness differential would favor the former program. Indeed, the former program could be markedly expanded to reach many more people and still cost less than the latter program; yielding a substantial population-level benefit.

Unable to sidestep the issue of cost effectiveness, adolescent health promotion researchers, scientists, health care providers, policy analysts and program planners need to become familiar with the theory and methods used to conduct cost-effectiveness studies. This methodology represents an entirely different perspective for many adolescent health researchers and practitioners. Most often, adolescent health researchers and practitioners have had their philosophical, theoretical and methodological roots in their own particular discipline rather than economic research.

INTERACTIONS BETWEEN SPHERES OF INFLUENCE: LESSONS FOR THE FUTURE

Increasing require-ments to provide documented cost-effectiveness data to support inter-vention programs will require that adolescent health promotion pro-gram planners and interventionists have adequate research training.

Several converging spheres of influence—such as law, technology, behavioral science, and economics—will likely result in increased focus on adolescent health promotion, but some important caveats must be noted if this influence extends to adolescent health research. First, adolescent health promotion is a sci-ence of diverse disciplines. Much will be gained by embracing the breadth of perspectives from these different disciplines and subse-quently engaging in transdisciplinary work. However, it is incumbent upon both researchers and practitioners to work toward convergence of theories and methodologies to improve health promotion practice. In many ways, adolescent health promotion might be considered an *applied science,* borrowing from basic methods in other fields (such as behav-ioral and social science, adolescent medicine, and public health) and applying these methods to adolescent health promotion. Second, not only will the goal of converging the science of adolescent health promo-tion be advanced by using rigorous, empirically based methodologies, but such methodological rigor will soon be required as managed care organizations and governmental agencies, key resources in health pro-motion practice, will increasingly require demonstrable evidence of cost-effectiveness of these programs. It is clear, for example, that the use of theory and methodological rigor is not uniform across different areas of adolescent health promotion research. Indeed, there is marked variability in the use of theory-based interventions and in the use of rig-orous randomized controlled trials to assess programmatic efficacy. Third, these increasing requirements to provide documented cost-effectiveness data to support intervention programs will require that adolescent health promotion program planners and interventionists have adequate research training. This will require the training of scientist-practitioners who are capable of both implementing and evaluating health promotion programs. In fact, aca-demic researchers who are also trained as scientist-practitioners may be best able to appreciate the barriers of service program implementation and best able to advance the field while developing empirically validated programs capable of more broad-scale dis-semination than at present.

SUMMARY

This volume has attempted to outline the promising developments occurring in the-ory, program design, and evaluation methods and to explore their application to ado-lescent health promotion research, practice, and policy. We have highlighted different health risk behaviors, with varying individual and population risk profiles, in varying settings, and with different populations. From this overview, it is apparent that the field of adolescent health promotion is heterogeneous, multidisciplinary, and rapidly growing. The depth and breadth of this research—which has applied broad-based public health, clinical, and social and behavioral sciences to adolescent health promotion—is impressive. As new theoretical models and innovative intervention strategies are identified and as societal, health care, and regulatory influences increase their focus on effective health promotion programs, adolescent health researchers, practitioners, and policy analysts will need to understand the complex interplay between these multiple and at times competing forces.

Given the human suffering, economic costs, lost productivity, and medical care resources associated with adolescent morbidity and mortality, interventions that demonstrate programmatic efficacy will be an important component in any public health strategy to promote adolescent health. Further, given the monetary expenditure involved in developing and evaluating adolescent health promotion interventions, it is critical that these studies be adequately designed, conducted, analyzed, and reported. Although adolescent health promotion programs, adequately funded and innovative in design, offer great potential to effectively reduce risk behaviors and subsequent adverse health outcomes, this progress will not be rapid. Behavior change on a scale large enough to affect population level health will require a comprehensive sustained effort. New opportunities and new challenges lie ahead for researchers and practitioners to apply their tools, skills, and perspectives to promoting adolescent health. Indeed, this is an exciting time to be engaged in adolescent health promotion research and practice.

KEY TERMS

Applied science
Hybrid intervention models
Preventing intervention decay

DISCUSSION QUESTIONS

1. The authors state: "One might argue whether adolescent health promotion programs should be held accountable to the standard that a program's economic benefits to society must outweigh its financial costs." Should adolescent health programs be held accountable? Explain.

2. How has the study of adolescent health shifted over the last few decades? Describe reasons for this shift and discuss the growing trends in present-day research.

3. In what ways can programmatic efficacy be maximized to have a greater impact at the population level? Is it possible to develop a perfect intervention, one that will yield positive intervention effects for all adolescents exposed? Justify your response.

NAME INDEX

SUBJECT INDEX